GLOBAL HEALTH CARE
ISSUES AND POLICIES

Carol Holtz, PhD, RN
Professor of Nursing
WellStar School of Nursing
Kennesaw State University
Kennesaw, Georgia

JONES AND BARTLETT PUBLISHERS
Sudbury, Massachusetts
BOSTON   TORONTO   LONDON   SINGAPORE

362.1
G562

World Headquarters

Jones and Bartlett Publishers
40 Tall Pine Drive
Sudbury, MA 01776
978-443-5000
info@jbpub.com
www.jbpub.com

Jones and Bartlett Publishers
Canada
6339 Ormindale Way
Mississauga, Ontario L5V 1J2
Canada

Jones and Bartlett Publishers
International
Barb House, Barb Mews
London W6 7PA
United Kingdom

Jones and Bartlett's books and products are available through most bookstores and online booksellers. To contact Jones and Bartlett Publishers directly, call 800-832-0034, fax 978-443-8000, or visit our website, www.jbpub.com.

Substantial discounts on bulk quantities of Jones and Bartlett's publications are available to corporations, professional associations, and other qualified organizations. For details and specific discount information, contact the special sales department at Jones and Bartlett via the above contact information, or send an email to specialsales@jbpub.com.

The authors, editor, and publisher have made every effort to provide accurate information. However, they are not responsible for errors, omissions, or for any outcomes related to the use of the contents of this book and take no responsibility for the use of the products and procedures described. Treatments and side effects described in this book may not be applicable to all people; likewise, some people may require a dose or experience a side effect that is not described herein. Drugs and medical devices are discussed that may have limited availability controlled by the Food and Drug Administration (FDA) for use only in a research study or clinical trial. Research, clinical practice, and government regulations often change the accepted standard in this field. When consideration is being given to use of any drug in the clinical setting, the healthcare provider or reader is responsible for determining FDA status of the drug, reading the package insert, and reviewing prescribing information for the most up-to-date recommendations on dose, precautions, and contraindications, and determining the appropriate usage for the product. This is especially important in the case of drugs that are new or seldom used.

Production Credits

Executive Editor: Kevin Sullivan
Acquisitions Editor: Emily Ekle
Associate Editor: Amy Sibley
Editorial Assistant: Patricia Donnelly
Production Director: Amy Rose
Production Editor: Carolyn F. Rogers
Senior Marketing Manager: Katrina Gosek
Associate Marketing Manager: Rebecca Wasley

Manufacturing and Inventory Coordinator:
  Amy Bacus
Composition: Shepherd, Inc.
Cover Design: Kate Ternullo
Cover Images: Nurse administering an oral polio
  vaccine to a child in India: © S. Nagendra/Photo
  Researchers, Inc.; map image © Photos.com.
Printing and Binding: Malloy, Inc.
Cover Printing: Malloy, Inc.

Library of Congress Cataloging-in-Publication Data

Global health care : issues and policies / [edited by] Carol Holtz.
    p. ; cm.
  Includes bibliographical references and index.
  ISBN-13: 978-0-7637-3852-5 (pbk.)
  ISBN-10: 0-7637-3852-2 (pbk.)
  1. World health. 2. Medical policy—Cross-cultural studies. 3. Public health—Cross-cultural studies. 4. Medical care—Cross-cultural studies. I. Holtz, Carol.
  [DNLM: 1. World Health. 2. Cross-Cultural Comparison. 3. Delivery of Health Care.
  4. Health Policy. WA 530.1 G5628 2008]
  RA441.G573 2008
  362.1—dc22

  6048   2007031435

Printed in the United States of America
11 10 09   10 9 8 7 6 5 4 3

4/10

CONTENTS

Section I	Global Healthcare Policy, Methods, and Delivery

iii

| Section II | Special Global Healthcare Issues |

Section III   Lifespan Health Issues

INTRODUCTION

This textbook was designed to give a basic level perspective of world health issues and policies as described in the literature at the time of authorship of the book chapters. While impossible to be timely and inclusive of all world health issues, geographical regions, or world events, it is meant to give a background and summary of representative issues at the time the chapters were written.

Global Health

Tarantola (2005) states that *global health*, as applied to human development, is a political variable that relates to the health of the whole planet, which moves beyond geographical and political boundaries. These include both governmental and nongovernmental (NGO) agencies. During the 1960s the World Bank first advocated global thinking in relation to health issues by the phrase, "think globally and act locally."

Beaglehole and Yach (2003) report that globalization is now frequently used to describe the increasing global "interconnectedness" or global interdependence of humanity, which includes the health of all on the earth. Economic globalization has been affected by the last two decades of international trade, financial investments, human migration, travel, and tourism. The marketing and sales strategies of international tobacco companies, pharmaceutical companies, and international travel have had a huge influence on global health issues.

Negative aspects of globalization include global warming, cross border pollution, financial crises, the spread of HIV/AIDS and international crime. The globalization of disease began with European explorers and conquerors that came to the Americas and gave smallpox, measles, and yellow fever to the various indigenous populations. They also brought typhus, influenza, and the plague. The poorest were most vulnerable with the small elite wealthier groups having better nutrition, access to better health care, and better sanitary (hygienic) conditions. More recently the spread of HIV/AIDS, TB, SARS, West Nile virus, Ebola, and other infectious diseases have emerged. Rapid movement of people and food products by travel results in new emerging health problems such as mad cow disease and avian influenza. Globalization has recently changed the lifestyles of developing countries resulting in new chronic diseases from the importation of high sodium, high fat fast foods, and with newer technologies (TV, appliances, etc.) causing more sedentary life changes. Moreover, in developing countries today, people are acquiring chronic diseases (such as heart disease, cancer, stroke, obesity leading to diabetes), which are adding a double burden to the still challenging acute infectious diseases (Beaglehole & Yach, 2003).

History

The World Health Organization (WHO) was established just after World War II as an intergovernmental agency for the purpose of leading and coordinating worldwide health activities. Its activities are initiated when consensus regarding world health priorities is reached. Today's world health is improved when economic development of nations is improved with the cooperation of governmental and nongovernmental agencies. In the last decade, numerous efforts have been initiated, such as the Global Alliance for Vaccines and Immunizations, the Global Tuberculosis Partnership, and the Global Fund on HIV/AIDS (Ruger, 2005).

The World Bank began in 1946, originally established to finance European reconstruction, but is today a major resource for the health, nutrition, and population (HNP) for developing countries. A few examples of the historical activities of the World Bank include the appointment in 1968 of Robert McNamara, who became president of the World Bank. This resulted in the initiation of a program in Population Control, giving funding for family planning. In 1971 McNamara emphasized the need to combat malnutrition. Additionally, in 1974, the Onchocerciasis Control Program was developed in cooperation with the United Nations Development Program, Food and Agriculture Organization, and the World Health Organization. This program was created to eliminate river blindness in West Africa. After 30 years the onchocerciasis program protected an estimated 34 million people and also cleared an estimated 25 million hectares of land for agricultural use (Ruger, 2005).

In 1985 WHO gave $3 million US dollars in grants for the World Food Program for emergency food supplies to sub-Saharan Africa, followed by the WHO and the United Nations co-sponsoring, in 1987, a Safe Motherhood Project, the first of global initiatives for this area. In 1998 WHO lent 300 million US dollars for India's Women and Child Development Program (Ruger, 2005).

At present the World Bank is the world's largest financial contributor to health projects throughout the world, having an annual budget of $1 billion US dollars for health, nutrition, and population (HNP). In addition, it currently is giving $1.3 billion US dollars for HIV/AIDS, 50% of which goes to sub-Saharan Africa. It allows repayment periods up to

35–40 years and a 10-year grace period. Although one of the main purposes of the World Bank is to generate and disseminate knowledge, its main advantage over other global healthcare agencies is to generate and mobilize healthcare resources. One of the criticisms of the World Bank includes the user fees, which are said to cause a disproportionate burden on the poor and sick people of the world (Ruger, 2005).

State of the World Population

The United Nations Family Planning Association (UNFPA, 2004) further validates, across nations, the inadequate resources, gender bias, and gaps in serving the world's poor. Many developing countries have begun population projects to reduce poverty, develop laws and policies to protect the rights of women and girls, initiate reproductive health services into primary health care, increase the skills of birth attendants, and provide more prevention and treatment of HIV/AIDS. There are currently approximately 2.8 billion people in the world, while 350 million couples lack birth control access. Birth complications still remained the leading cause of death of women, with 5 million new cases being reported in 2003. In addition, unsustainable consumption and rapid population growth have been serious problems related to the world environment, resulting in clean water becoming scarce. Land is being deforested, and fish stocks are being harvested beyond sustainable limits. The problems are further compounded by people moving from rural to urban environments resulting in overcrowded cities that burden the caring capacity. By 2050 the expected world population will be 8.9 billion people, and the 50 poorest nations will triple in size to 1.7 billion people (UNFPA, 2004).

WHO (2005) reveals that of the 136 million births per year, fewer than two thirds of women in *less* developed countries, and only one third in *least* developed countries, have skilled birth attendants during deliveries. As a result, each year approximately 530,000 women die in pregnancy or childbirth, 3–4 million babies die within their first 4 weeks of life, and 10.6 million children die before the age of 5.

Predictions of Global Health Patterns

WHO (2005) indicates the following world health issues of the future.

1. Tobacco will be causing chronic obstructive pulmonary diseases (e.g., emphysema and lung cancer) and will kill more people than the HIV epidemic.

2. Males living in the former USSR and socialist economies in Europe will have poor and deteriorating health status, including a 28% risk of death in the 15–60 age groups.

3. Mental health diseases (depression, alcoholism, and schizophrenia) will have been underestimated in significance and will be responsible for 1% of deaths and 11% of the total world disease burden.

4. Communicable diseases, maternal and perinatal problems, and nutritional diseases will still be large problems in developing countries, while the noncommunicable diseases such as depression and heart diseases will also cause premature death and disability.

5. Deaths from noncommunicable diseases will increase by 77%, due to the aging of the world population and the decrease in birth rate.

6. Accidents and violence mortality (death) rates may compete with mortality rates of infectious diseases.

Predictions of the Leading Causes of Diseases or Injury Worldwide

In rank order:

1. Ischemic heart disease
2. Unipolar major depression
3. Road traffic accidents
4. Cerebrovascular disease (stroke)
5. Chronic obstructive pulmonary disease (COPD)
6. Lower respiratory infections
7. Tuberculosis
8. War
9. Diarrhea diseases
10. HIV
11. Perinatal conditions
12. Violence
13. Congenital anomalies
14. Self-inflicted injuries
15. Trachea, bronchus, and lung cancer

Greater investments in scientific research and technology will be needed in developing countries in order to meet the greater demand for the challenges of treatment of illness and disease prevention. UNFPA (2004) indicates that many of the world population challenges will include:

1. **Migration from rural areas to urban cities**—By the year 2007 half the world's population will be urban, which will create a greater need for social services including reproductive health, especially in poor urban areas.

2. **Stress on the global environment**—Global warming, population growth, resource consumption, deforestation, and decreases in water and cropland will further impact negative health outcomes.

3. **Increased demand for family planning**—Greater than 350 million couples will still lack family planning services and by 2025 demand will increase by 40%.

4. **Pregnancy and childbirth complications**—This will cause illness and death in women in developing countries resulting in 8 million women having life-threatening complications with 529,000 deaths.

5. **Lack of prenatal care**—Thirty-three percent of all pregnant women in the world will receive no prenatal care and 60% of all deliveries will be outside a hospital.

6. **Skilled birth attendants**—Only 50% of all pregnant women will be delivered by a skilled birth attendant.

7. **HIV/AIDS**—Thirty-eight million people will have HIV/AIDS.

Population Growth Issues

As of 2005, the global population of 6.7 billion continues to grow rapidly at a rate of approximately 76 million a year. By 2050, 2.5 billion new people will be added to the world population. The average family size has declined from 6 children per woman in 1960 to 3 children per woman presently, mainly due to family planning. Predicted projections are that family size will level off by 2050. Countries which have significant decreases in fertility will have increases in the aging population. Ninety-six percent of the world population growth will be from developing countries. Europe and Japan will have declining populations and North America will increase by 1% due to immigration. Population estimates and growth patterns have been lower than those predicted 10 years ago mainly due to the impact of HIV/AIDS. The 38 African countries most affected by HIV/AIDS are projected to have 823 million people by 2015, which constitutes 91 million fewer people than if no AIDS deaths had occurred (UNFPA, 2004).

Equality in Health Care

The world collectively lacks an equal rights-based approach in the distribution of health care. Disparities in health care are now a major challenge for health care agencies around the world. Nelson Mandela stated, "The greatest single challenge facing our globalized world is to combat and eradicate its disparities" (Mandela, 1998). The burden of disease is growing disproportionately in regions of the world, which are also commonly effected by "brain drain." Doctors and nurses from Africa, Asia, and Latin America are leaving the rural areas for cities while others are leaving their countries altogether and relocating in developed nations. The irony is that more health care providers in developed countries are now working, at least part of their working lives, in developing countries, while a "brain drain" is pulling some of the most competent health care providers out of their home countries in which they are most needed. Regardless of the causes, many developing countries, with the least amount of human and economic resources are confronted with the largest burden in public health. In the developed world, 15% of the world's population consumes more than 60% of world energy than the developing world (Farmer, Furin, & Katz, 2004).

At the end of 2002 there was still major evidence that socioeconomic as well as health inequalities existed within and among nations. Although the health of the world population has improved considerably, there are still areas of the world that have inadequate and inequitable health care within its borders and among its citizens. For example, within almost the entire continent of Africa at the end of 2002, there were 42 million people living with HIV/AIDS. The disappearance of an entire generation of productive men and women ages 18–45 is evidence that health care services have been inadequate, resulting in children and grandparents left behind (Ruger, 2005).

Adequate health care promotes social stability and economic growth. Countries that do not have adequate health care often have inadequate funding, poor government organization, and inadequate access for health care services for all of its population (Go & Given, 2005). Go and Given (2005) report that although developing countries such as India, Mexico, and China would like to expand their health care systems and have more high technology, they first must re-structure their systems to give more expenditure and emphasis on education and preventive medicine rather than trying to first invest in high technology health care. The three main criteria for an adequate health care system include: 1) **equitable access** to quality care by accessing both prevention and treatment services for rural and urban populations; 2) **affordability**, which means that even if people have no income or health insurance they may receive services; and 3) **sustainability**, which means that it will have long-term political and financial support.

For example, Mexico, China, and India are emerging economies which are rapidly industrializing and changing into a global market economy, each with their own unique culture, geography, and history. All three countries are working to improve access to their health care systems for all, and are emphasizing preventive health care as a major priority. Ninety percent of Mexicans now have access to preventive care and basic public health services, although some indigenous Indians in isolated rural areas still have none. Sixty-seven percent of India's population is immunized although many rural areas have less basic health care than urban areas. Previously the Indian government paid the entire cost of health care for individuals, but now a shift in health care cost has placed greater burden on the individuals to cover their health care needs. The Indian government is now spending less and expects that individuals pay for part of the services that were once completely paid for by the government. At present new medical treatments and medications are becoming more expensive and many people must also pay out-of-pocket for health care because they lack health insurance. For example, the percentage of people in Mexico, China, and India with health care insurance is 53%, 60–70%, and 82–85% respectively (Go & Given, 2005). The World Health Report (WHO, 2003) states that a key responsibility of a government's healthcare system is to decrease the health disparities. Lack of political power and basic education are barriers to accessing the healthcare system for all. The majority of the population has equal access, yet a small elite group has access to state of the art health care.

Emerging Health Threats

The WHO Report of 2003 indicates that public health issues evolve over time and as a result of planned and unplanned activities or changing environments, humans are in contact with many organisms which have the capacity to cause disease. With the development of antibiotics people are able to survive bacterial infections, which previously would have been the cause of certain death. Today infectious diseases are the main cause of new epidemics such as HIV/AIDS or Ebola or reoccurring epidemics, such as with tuberculosis or cholera. These emerging health threats are caused by resistance to antibiotics, new strains of bacteria which are resistant, or poor adherence to medical regimens (WHO, 2003).

Preventable diseases and injuries are seen more as humans migrate from rural to urban areas. Also seen more often are unintentional injuries such as traffic accidents, poisonings, and intentional injuries, such as war and street violence. More than 40% of the total disease burden due to urban air pollution occurs in developing countries, and children are most vulnerable to these environmental hazards, because they do not have the ability to detoxify pollutants related to their bodies' immaturity. It has been reported that in 2000 more than 90% of all deaths due to injuries occurred in low- and middle-income countries. Although tobacco use is declining in developed countries there continues to be an increasing use in developing countries (WHO, 2003).

Mental health, neurological disorders, and substance abuse are causing a great amount of disability and human suffering. Many people do not receive any health care for these problems because of inadequate infrastructures, and widely prevalent stigma and discrimination which prevents them from seeking care. Many countries lack mental health care policies, facilities, or budgets within their healthcare systems. Cost effective services are available and research clearly demonstrates that depression, schizophrenia, alcohol and drug problems can be treated at primary care centers with inexpensive medications and basic training of health care personnel. Intentional (suicide, violence, and war) and unintentional (traffic accidents) injuries, which primarily affect young adults, accounted for over 14% of the adult disease burden of the world in 2002, yet in parts of Europe and the Eastern Middle East region, it accounts for greater than 30% of the disease burden. In males, violence, traffic injuries, and self-inflicted injuries are within the top 10 disease burdens in the 15–44 year old groups (WHO, 2003).

Measures of Population Health

The CDC (2003) Summary Measures of Population Health Report, indicates that in order to evaluate the health of a population, one needs to examine the population's:

1. **Life expectancy**—A measure of mortality rates across the developmental life span, which is expressed in years of life.

2. **Healthy life expectancy (HLE)**—Years of active life, reflecting a person's ability to perform tasks which reflect self-care, called the activities of daily living. This is a way of measuring not just years of life, but expected years of life divided into healthy and unhealthy life. It is a way to more accurately measure the current health of a population, measuring the extent of morbidity and mortality of a population.

3. **Mortality**—The number of deaths within a specific population, which has often been used as a basic indicator of health.

4. **Disability**—Refers to a situation in which a person's abilities or limitations are determined by physical, mental or cognitive status within society which is determined by how well the personal environment accommodates the loss of functioning.

Global Health Indicators

Global monitoring of health changes across world populations requires global health indicators. The indicators provide estimates of a country's state of health and may reflect direct measurements of health phenomena, such as diseases and deaths, or indirect measurements such as education and poverty. With population statistics on education, access to safe water and sanitation, and rates of diseases, it is possible to fairly accurately measure a population's low, medium, or high burden of disease. Unfortunately, few developing countries are able to measure their health statistics accurately; therefore, numbers of births, deaths, those with specific diseases etc. can often be only estimates and may not actually be truly representative of the population. Criteria for good health indicators are the following:

1. **Definition**—The indicator must be well defined and be able to be used internationally.

2. **Validity**—The indicator must accurately measure what it is supposed to measure and must be reliable so that it can be replicable and consistent in different settings, and easy to interpret.

3. **Feasibility**—Obtaining the information must be easily affordable and not overburden the system.

4. **Utility**—The indicator must provide useful information for various levels of health decision makers (Larson & Mercer, 2004).

Global Health and Moral Values

The creation of global initiatives requires a review of ethical and moral values. In 2003 the Director General of the WHO, Lee Jong-Wook, stated that global health must be guided by an ethical vision. He reported that technical excellence and political commitment have no value unless they have an ethically sound purpose. The following are different schools of thought used to justify global initiatives:

1. **Humanitarianism**—Acting virtuously toward those in need. It is often the response to social problems. Humanitarianism is incorporated within all religions, based on compassion, empathy or altruism. It is the ethical basis of philanthropy by nongovernmental organizations (NGOs). It is also the basic philosophy behind US governmental foreign aid policy.

2. **Utilitarianism**—Maximizing happiness for many people. Improving the health of individuals living within a society will be in the best interest for all the people of a society.

3. **Equity by achieving a fair distribution of health capabilities**—Ensuring that all people in a society have a fair and equal chance to achieve good health.

4. **Rights: fulfilling obligations so others are dignified**—Ensures that health care respects human rights and dignity for all people living in a society.

5. **Knowledge and institutions**—Supports the basis for research and development of new health technologies and medications. For example, the recent development of HIV/AIDS antiretroviral drugs has created a new moral dilemma by the variety of affordability among nations. Corporations have what is perceived as "huge" profits by producing and selling the drugs; however, the cost of development and use of resources will have to be recouped.

6. **Consensus and advocacy groups**—People who are usually in powerful political positions who wish to have health policies established for others in the society.

Theoretical Solution Plans

The United Nations Millennium Summit in 2000 met with representatives of 189 countries to develop a road map with goals to improve the areas of: peace, security and disarmament, poverty eradication, environmental protection, human rights, democracy and good governance protecting the vulnerable populations, assisting with the special needs of Africa, and strengthening the United Nations. These goals were established to be achieved by 2015. While governments made commitments to work towards these millennium goals, practical solutions are yet to be fully identified or implemented (WHO, 2003).

Conclusion

This introduction, which serves to introduce the reader to this textbook, attempts to examine the overall perspective of various global health issues. Definitions of key terms and a brief discussion of global health history, the state of the world population, predictions of global health patterns, population growth issues, equity in accessing health care, emerging health threats, global health indicators, and global health and its relationship to moral values are briefly addressed. Within the following chapters, a great number and more specific issues are addressed.

Definitions of Key Terms

Demographic/Socioeconomic Conditions

1. **Population**—Total number of people
2. **Education level**—Percentage of the population 20 years and above with no education
3. **Unemployment rate**—Percentage of the population age 15–64 who do not have jobs
4. **Energy source for cooking**—Percentage of households using electricity, wood, paraffin, and other sources for cooking
5. **Water and sanitation**—Percentage of households with refuse removal, access to piped water, no toilet

Burden of Disease

1. **Infant mortality rate**—The number of children less than one year old who die in a year, per 1,000 live births
2. **Under 5 mortality rate**—The probability of a child dying before age 5 years per 1,000 live births per year (percentage of children who die before the age of 5 years)
3. **Adult mortality**—The probability of dying between the ages of 15 and 60 (percentage of 15 year olds who die before their 60th birthday)

4. **Life expectancy**—The average number of years a person could expect to live if current mortality trends were to continue for the rest of that person's life

5. **Cause of death profile**—Percentage of death in the population caused by a specific disease from the Nation Burden of Disease List

6. **Years of life lost**—The number of years lost based on the standard life expectancy for the age of death, with future years discounted at 3% and age weighting

7. **Prevalence of a disability**—Percentage of people with moderate to severe disability, which is a physical or mental handicap which has lasted for at least six months, or is expected to last at least six months, which prevents the person from carrying out the activities of daily living independently, or participating fully in educational, economic, or social activities.

Source: CDC, 2003.

References

Beaglehole, R. & Yach, D. (2003). Globalisation and the prevention and control of non-communicable disease: The neglected chronic disease of adults. *The Lancet, 362,* 903–908.

Centers for Disease Control and Prevention (CDC). (2003). *Summary measures of population health. Report of findings on methodologic and data issues.* Retrieved August 13, 2007, from http://www.cdc.gov/nchs/data/misc/pophealth.pdf

Centers for Disease Control and Prevention (CDC). (2004). *Chronic disease prevention.* Retrieved June 13, 2005, from http://www.cdc.gov/programs/chronic.htm

Chui, D., Lau, J. S. K., & Yau, I. T. Y. (2004). An outcome evaluation study of the Rheumatoid Arthritis Self-Management Programme in Hong Kong. *Psychology, Health & Medicine, 9*(3), 286–291.

Farmer, P., Furin, J. J., & Katz, J. T. (2004). Global health equity. *Lancet, 363,* 1832.

Go, R., & Given, R. (2005). *Sustainable healthcare.* Deloitte Research. Tuck Executive Education of Dartmouth. Retrieved September 4, 2007, from http://www.publicservice.co.uk/pdf/em/issue_3/EM3Robert%20Go%20Ruth%20Given%20ATL.pdf.

Hafstrom, I., & Hallengren, M. (2003). Physiotherapy in subtropic climate improves functional capacity and health-related quality of life in Swedish patients with rheumatoid arthritis and spondylarthropathies still after 6 months. *Scandanavian Journal of Rheumatology, 32,* 108–113.

Katz, D. (2004). The burden of chronic disease: The future is prevention. *Public Health Research, Practice, and Policy, 1*(2), 1. Retrieved June 29, 2005, from www.cdc.obv/pcd/issues/2004/apr/04_0006htm

Larson, C., & Mercer, A. (2004). Global health indicators: An overview. *Canadian Medical Association, 171*(10), 1.

Mandela, N. (1998). Transcript of the speech at the special convocation of an honorary doctoral degree, Harvard University, Cambridge, Massachusetts, September 18, 1998. Retrieved August 8, 2007, from http://www.cambridgeforum.org/cfmandela/13_nelson_mandela.html

Michalsen, A., Klotz, S., Ludtke, R., Moebus, S., Spahn, G., & Dobos, G. (2003). Effectiveness of leech therapy in osteoarthritis of the knee. *Annals of Internal Medicine, 139,* 724–730.

Porter, D. (2004). *Chronic diseases need global health attention.* Retrieved June 18, 2005, from http://www.eurekalert.org/pub_releases/2004-06/jaaj-cdn052704.php

Reddy, K. Srinath. (1999). *Chronic disease epidemics in developing countries: Can we telescope transition?* Retrieved June 18, 2005, from http://www.medguide.org.zm/diseases/chrondis.htm

Ruger, J. P. (2005). The changing role of the World Bank in global health. *American Journal of Public Health, 95,* 60–90.

Tarantola, D. (2005). Global health and national goverenance. *American Journal of Public Health Association, 95*(1), 8.

United Nations Family Planning Association. (2004). *State of the World population 2004. The Cairo Consensus at Ten: Population, reproductive health, and global effort to end poverty.* New York: United Nations Population Fund. Retrieved September 4, 2007, from: http://www.unfpa.org/upload/lib_pub_file/327_filename_en_swp04.pdf.

Woolf, A., & Pfleger, B. (2003). Burden of major musculoskeletal conditions. *Bulletin of the World Health Organization, 81*(9), 646–656.

World Health Organization. (2003). *World health report 2003—shaping the future.* Retrieved August 7, 2007, from http://www.who.int/whr/2003/en

World Health Organization. (2005). *Integrated chronic disease prevention and control.* Retrieved June 18, 2005, from http://www.who.int/chp/about/integrated_cd/en

WHO and the Bone and Joint Decade. (2001). *The global economic and healthcare burden of musculoskeletal disease.* Retrieved June 11, 2005, from www.boneandjointdecade.org

Zan-bar, T., Aron, A., & Shoenfeld, Y. (2004). Acupuncture therapy for rheumatoid arthritis. *APLAR Journal of Rheumatology, 7,* 207–214.

Acknowledgments

This textbook represents the combined efforts of many well-educated, dedicated, experienced, and hard working chapter contributors. The administrators of Kennesaw State University, including Dr. Richard Sowell, Dean of the WellStar College of Health and Human Services, and the research dean, Dr. Timothy Akers, gave me tremendous support and encouragement to complete this task. In addition, the fine editorial staff of Jones and Bartlett Publishers believed in my ideas and was excited about the concept of this book. They stood by and encouraged me in a professional manner to take this book forward to publication.

I would like to thank my husband, Dr. Noel Holtz, who gave me the encouragement and support to follow my dream to create the idea for this book. For my children, Pam Gilmore, Aaron and Stacy Holtz, and Daniel and Maggie Holtz, and my grandchildren Andrew, Brandon, Caroline, Sarah, and Meryl, I give you this legacy of scholarship, hard work, and perseverance that I learned from my previous generation and hope that you will also do something for which you are proud that will contribute to your next generation and further enrich our society. I also want to thank my mother, Barbara Weinberg, and my late father, William Smith, who always believed in me and encouraged me to achieve scholarly pursuits.

A special loving tribute is given to the memory of one of the contributing book authors, Dr. Robert Lipson, a magnificent corporate executive and inspiring community leader of the WellStar Health System of Marietta, Georgia. He, along with his coauthors, Dr. Govind Hariharan of Kennesaw State University, Dr. Marsha Burke, and Dr. Caroline Aultman of the WellStar Health System, submitted their book chapter only two weeks before his untimely death. For you, Dr. Lipson, we will continue to use your illustrious and visionary ideas as your legacy to your family and community.

CONTRIBUTORS

Kathie Aduddell, EdD, MSN, BSN
Kennesaw State University
Kennesaw, GA

Mary Ann Alabanza Akers, PhD
School of Environmental Design
University of Georgia
Athens, GA

Timothy A. Akers, PhD, MS, BS
Kennesaw State University
Kennesaw, GA

Linda G. Alley, PhD, RN
Epidemiologist
Centers for Disease Control and Prevention
National Center for Chronic Disease Prevention
    and Health Promotion
Division of Cancer Prevention and Control
Cancer Surveillance Branch
Atlanta, GA

Caroline Aultman
Director of Strategic Planning
WellStar Health System
Marietta, GA

David Bennett, PhD, RN
Kennesaw State University
Kennesaw, GA

Barbara J. Blake, PhD, ACRN
Kennesaw State University
Kennesaw, GA

Marsha Burke
WellStar Health System
Marietta, GA

Mary Ann Camann, PhD, RN
Kennesaw State University
Kennesaw, GA

Cheryll Cardinez, MSPH
Centers for Disease Control and Prevention
National Center for Chronic Disease Prevention
    and Health Promotion
Division of Cancer Prevention and Control
Cancer Surveillance Branch
Atlanta, GA

Deborah S. Cummins, PhD
University of Illinois at Chicago
Chicago, IL

Bowman O. Davis, Jr., PhD
Kennesaw State University
Kennesaw, GA

Richard B. Davis, MSFS
Centers for Disease Control and Prevention
Atlanta, GA

Temeika L. Fairley, PhD
Centers for Disease Control and Prevention
National Center for Chronic Disease Prevention
    and Health Promotion
Division of Cancer Prevention and Control
Atlanta, GA

Marvin Friedman, PhD
Toxicologist Consultant
Oviedo, FL

Suzanne Grisdale, RN, BSN

Robert A. Hanson, DO, MS
Pontiac Osteopathic Medical Center
Pontiac, MI

Govind Hariharan, PhD
Kennesaw State University
Kennesaw, GA

Ping Hu Johnson, MD, PhD
Kennesaw State University
Kennesaw, GA

Robert Lipson, MD, MBA
WellStar Health System
Marietta, GA

Janice Long, MS, RN
Kennesaw State Uinversity
Kennesaw, GA

David B. Mitchell, PhD
Kennesaw State University
Kennesaw, GA

Natia Partskhladze, MD
Partners for Health
Tbilisi, GA

Enrique Paz, MD, MPH
Former Minister of Health for Bolivia
Bolivia

Kathy Plitnick, PhD, RN, CNS, CCRN
Georgia State University
Atlanta, GA

Paran Pordell, MPH, CHES
Centers for Disease Control and Prevention
Division of HIV/AIDS Prevention
Epidemiology Branch
Atlanta, GA

Larry Purnell, PhD, RN, FAAN
University of Delaware
Newark, DE

Betsy Rodriguez, RN, MSN, DE

Alexandra Toma, MFFS
Director of Peace and Security Initiatives

Jonathan B. VanGeest, PhD
Kennesaw State University
Kennesaw, GA

H. Kenneth Walker, MD
Emory University School of Medicine
Atlanta, GA

Judith L. Wold, PhD, RN
Georgia State University
Atlanta, GA

Michelle Zebich-Knos, PhD
Kennesaw State University
Kennesaw, GA

Chapter 1

Global Health in Developed Societies: Examples in the United States, United Kingdom, Sweden, and Israel

Carol Holtz

This chapter will give examples of developed countries and their major health issues and trends. Many of the health issues will be reviewed in greater detail within other chapters of this text. These countries were chosen because they vary in healthcare systems and geographic areas.

Many of the developed countries are currently working on controversial legal, religious, and ethical issues that directly relate to health care and healthcare systems of delivery. Specifically, the following topics address:

- Access to health care for all residents
- Issues of funding for nonlegal residents (illegal aliens) and healthcare services provided by government and nongovernment organizations
- Options for termination of an unwanted pregnancy
- A women's right to determine what happens to her body (birth control, abortion, contraception, genital mutilation, sexual assault and/or abuse, sterilization, child molestation, prostitution)
- Sex education in schools, clinics, and public health facilities

United States

Location

The United States is located in North America, bordering both the Atlantic and Pacific Oceans, between Canada in the north, and Mexico in the south. It includes 50 states, the District of Columbia, and several territories and possessions.

Population Statistics

The US population as of 2005 was 295,734,000. Tables 1-1 through 1-4 show age distribution, health statistics, ethnicity, and religion.

TABLE 1-1   Age Distribution

0–14 yrs	26%
15–64 yrs	67%
65 yrs +	12.4%

Source: CIA, 2005.

TABLE 1-2   Population Size and Health Statistics

Population growth rate	.93%
Birth rate	14.14 per 1000 population
Death rate	8.25 per 1000 population
Net migration rate	3.31 immigrants per 1000 population
Infant mortality rate	6.5 per 1000 live births
Male life expectancy	74.89 years
Female life expectancy	80.67
Fertility rate	2.08 children born per woman
HIV prevalence rate	.6%
	950,000 people with HIV/AIDS

Source: CIA, 2005.

TABLE 1-3   Ethnic Groups

White (Caucasian or European-Americans)	77.1%
Black (African-Americans)	12.9%
Asians	4.2%
Native Americans and Pacific Islanders	.3%
Other	4%
*Hispanic	*13%

* The US Census Bureau does not include Hispanic (Latino) as a separate category because a Hispanic (Latino) can be of any race or ethnic group, yet 13% identified themselves as Hispanic, making this the largest minority group in the United States.

Source: CIA, 2005.

TABLE 1-4 Religions	
Protestant	52%
Roman Catholic	24%
Mormon	2%
Jewish	1%
Muslim	1%
Other	10%
None	10%

Source: CIA, 2005.

Economy

The United States has the largest and most technologically powerful economy in the world with a per capita GDP of $40,000 annually. It is a market-oriented economy. Twelve percent of the population lives below the poverty line. The unemployment rate is approximately 5.5%, but rates vary among ethnic groups, gender, socioeconomic groups, and geographic locations. It is the leading industrial power of the world, highly diversified and technologically advanced. Its products include steel, petroleum, motor vehicles, aerospace, telecommunications, chemicals, electronics, food processing, consumer goods, lumber, and mining. Products include wheat, corn, other grains, fruits, vegetables, cotton, beef, pork, poultry, dairy products, forest products, and fish (CIA, 2005).

Health Trends and Issues

Monitoring the health of any country is essential for identifying and prioritizing public health and research needs. It is necessary for identifying important information such as diseases and conditions and for determining new health policy priority areas, funding, and programs. The overall health of the United States is improving because of funding devoted to health education, public health programs, health research, and health care. During the past 50 years many diseases have been eradicated or greatly controlled. Heart disease deaths have declined because of public health education emphasizing healthy lifestyles, such as decreasing cigarette smoking, lowering cholesterol through medications and diet, and new technology in heart procedures and surgery. In spite of the 1964 Surgeon General's report published over 40 years ago, 25% of men and 20% of women in the United States continue to smoke. With respect to infectious diseases, HIV/AIDS rates have declined because of new antiretroviral medications. Home, workplace, and motor vehicle safety have also helped to extend lives by lowering unintentional injuries for adults and children. Rates of acute infectious diseases of children such as measles, mumps, and rubella have decreased due to immunizations (CDC, 2004a).

Although the United States is the most developed nation with a state-of-the-art healthcare system of delivery, it is important to note that the United States does not have the longest male and female life expectancy rate. For example, in 1999, life expectancy in Japan was 3 years longer for men and 4 years longer for women than the US life expectancies. In 2002 the infant mortality rate actually increased for the first time since 1958. Overweight, obesity, and physical inactivity are currently significant risk problems for adults and children and lead to chronic diseases such as diabetes, hypertension, and heart disease. For the first time ever, children are developing significantly high rates of type 2 diabetes. Overall rates for cancers have declined since the 1990s for males and have remained stable for females. For people over 65, activities of daily living (ADLs) have not declined since 1992 (CDC, 2004).

The National Governor's Association reports that the US healthcare system is not cost-effective for the amount of money spent yearly. The United States spends more than any other developed country ($1.7 trillion annually) in the world, which is equal to $5267 per person on health care. Neither public nor private funding can be sustained indefinitely. As costs continue to go upward, fewer people will be able to afford private health insurance and will need to apply for Medicaid and the State Children's Insurance Program (SCHIP) or Medicare (National Governors' Association, 2005).

The United States clearly is the leader in healthcare spending, as a percentage of GDP, as compared to other developed countries (see Figure 1-1).

A growing number of Americans, often referred to as *the working poor*, are caught in the middle by earning too much money to be eligible for Medicaid, are not old enough for Medicare, and also can not earn enough to pay for a private healthcare policy. In addition

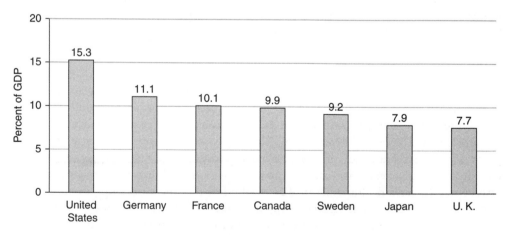

Note: Data for Sweden, Japan, and the United Kingdom are from 2002. All other data are for 2003.

Figure 1-1 The United States exceeds other industrialized nations in total health spending as a percentage of GDP.

Source: U.S. Government Accountability Office, 2005.

to cost, the problem is accessing health care. Many other industrialized countries, such as Iceland, Japan, and Sweden, spend less money and have even better health care than the United States. The National Governors' Association (2005) believes that the United States must increase the total efficiency of the healthcare system.

Tables 1-5 and 1-6 compare US male and female life expectancies with other selected developed countries.

US infant mortality in 2001 was the fifth highest of industrialized countries, with 6.8 deaths per 1000 live births, compared to Iceland, with the lowest rate of 2.7 deaths per 1000 live births. The United States also has one of the highest rates of all types of cancers also one of the highest obesity rates. In 2003 the United States reported deaths from medical errors ranging from 44,000 to 98,000. State governments are working towards developing an improved information technology system that will help make more efficient healthcare services to not only enhance patient healthcare delivery, but also to restructure medical data that could be better standardized, stored, and shared more easily. For more effective surveillance systems and research studies, healthcare providers could be rewarded for high quality and effective care. Consumers could make more informed decisions about choices of healthcare providers to compare prices with quality of services. Under certain circumstances the government has the potential to influence others to extend coverage to those who are currently uninsured (National Governors' Association, 2005).

TABLE 1-5   Male Life Expectancies in Selected Developed Countries for 2001

United States	74.4 yrs
Iceland	78.3 yrs
Japan	78.1 yrs
Sweden	77.6 years

Source: National Governors' Association, 2005.

TABLE 1-6   Female Life Expectancies in Selected Developed Countries for 2001

United States	79.8 yrs
Japan	84.9 yrs
Switzerland	83 yrs
Spain	82.9 yrs

Source: National Governors' Association, 2005.

Population Characteristics

The racial and ethnic composition of the United States has changed. The Hispanic (Latino) population and Asian and Pacific Islander ethnic groups have grown rapidly in the past 10–20 years. In 2002, the Hispanic population became the largest ethnic minority, representing 13% of the total population, and the Asian population made up 4% of the US population. During the past 50 years the US population of adults age 75 and older grew from 3% to 6%, and by 2050, the older adult population is projected to make up 12% of the US population. In 2002, greater than 50% of African-American and Hispanic children and those older than 65 years lived at or near poverty levels (CDC, 2004a).

Leading Health Indicators and Causes of Deaths

The following are the leading health indicators by rank order (CDC, 2002a):

- Physical activity
- Overweight and obesity
- Tobacco use
- Substance abuse (drugs and alcohol)
- Responsible sexual behavior
- Mental health
- Injury and violence
- Environmental quality
- Immunizations
- Access to health care

Table 1-7 gives the 10 leading causes of deaths in the United States in rank order.

Utilization of Health Care

The CDC (2004b) related that the US healthcare system has undergone a dramatic change over the last decade. New technology, drugs, procedures, and tests have changed the manner in which care is delivered. The growth of ambulatory surgery has been influenced by improvements in noninvasive and minimally invasive techniques. The growth of managed care and payment by insurers and other payers has been an attempt to control healthcare costs, which has also had a major impact on healthcare utilization.

The following are factors that decrease the utilization of health care (CDC, 2004a):

- Decreased supply of hospitals and healthcare providers
- Improvement in public health and sanitation, such as cleaner water
- Better public health education of risk factors and methods to make behavioral changes to reduce risks

TABLE 1-7   Ten Leading Causes of Deaths per 100,000 in 2001

Heart disease	29
Cancer	22.9
Stroke	6.8
Chronic lower respiratory diseases	5.1
Accidents	4.2
Diabetes mellitus types 1 and 2	3
Influenza and pneumonia	2.6
Alzheimer's disease	2.2
Kidney disease	1.6
Blood poisonings	1.3

Source: CDC, 2005a.

- New treatments or cures for diseases
- Public policy or guidelines that recommend decreased utilization
- Shifts of care sites, such as from inpatient to outpatient surgery
- Payer pressures to decrease costs
- Changes in practice patterns, such as those that emphasize more self-care, alternative sites, or alternative medicine

The following are factors that increase the utilization of health care (CDC, 2004a):

- Increased supply of healthcare facilities and providers
- Population growth
- Aging population
- New procedures and technologies
- Guidelines or policies that recommend increased utilization
- New threats, such as HIV or bioterrorism
- New drugs
- Increased healthcare coverage
- More aggressive treatments for patients
- Changes in consumer demand, such as cosmetic surgery and hip replacements

[handwritten margin note: things that can fix problem]

Many types of preventive care or treatment of illnesses are performed at an increasing rate in outpatient clinics or physicians' offices. For example, the use of prenatal care services, which begins in the first trimester of pregnancy, has been steadily rising. Children are receiving their childhood immunizations at a high level. The chickenpox vaccine (varicella) has been widely distributed as well. Women are getting Pap smears and mammograms at increasing rates, and older adults are increasingly getting vaccines for influenza and pneumonia (CDC, 2004a).

On the other hand, inpatient utilization health care has been declining. Admissions and length of hospitalization stays have decreased. Many procedures that used to be done within the hospital are now done in clinics, physicians' offices, outpatient surgery centers, and rehabilitation centers, leaving more complex procedures and illnesses to be treated within the hospital. Inpatients now have higher acuity levels whereas inpatient mental health treatment has significantly declined (CDC, 2004a).

Access to Health Care and Disparities in Access

The best health care in the world is meaningless for those who do not have access to health insurance coverage or who can not afford it. The continued increases in healthcare costs combined with economic changes have caused a number of US residents to be without any health insurance, giving them less access to health care.

With respect to healthcare cost, the highest expenditure is partly due to prescription drugs. In spite of the great expenditure, accessing health care is dependent on many variables. These include the supply of healthcare providers and the ability to pay for the services. Between 1994 and 2002, 16–17% of the US population younger than 65 years of age had *no* health insurance. In 2002 individuals with private insurance decreased, and those with Medicaid increased, with no significant changes for the rates of the uninsured. In 2002, 11% of children under 18 years lacked health insurance. Working males are less likely than working females to have health insurance (CDC, 2004a).

The United States has been growing more racially and ethnically diverse. Residents also are living longer. The National Center for Health Statistics (CDC, 2004a) describes major areas where disparities exist between race and ethnicity and socioeconomic status. Those residents who live in poverty are more likely to be in poor health and less likely to receive adequate health care. Poor people were four times more likely to have psychological stress. There are large disparities in infant mortality rates and life expectancy rates between those in poverty and others in the remainder of the population. In addition, adults under 64 years who are Latino or Native American (American Indian) are more likely to be uninsured than those in other racial or ethnic groups. Diseases or medical conditions such as diabetes or obesity increase with age and are more likely to be found in non-Hispanic blacks and Latinos than non-Hispanic whites (European-Americans). Some of these disparities may be the result of socioeconomic status, culture and health practices, stress, environmental exposures, discrimination, and access to health care (CDC, 2004a).

TABLE 1-8   Healthcare Utilization by Ethnic Groups Using Managed Care Insurance

	African-Americans (%)	European-Americans (%)
Mammograms	62.9	70.9
Diabetic retinal exams	43.6	50.4
Serious mental illness (posthospitalization follow-up exam)	33.2	54
Post heart attack (MI) (use of beta-blocker medications)	64.1	73.8

Source: Schneider, Zaslavsky, and Epstein, 2002.

Health and health care are unevenly distributed in the United States. Underrepresented minorities are less likely than the majority population to have good health care and health (see Table 1-8) and have fewer opportunities to access diagnostic procedures and tests, surgical procedures, and therapeutic medications.

Petersen, Wright, and Peterson (2002) studied African-American and Caucasian patients and interventional cardiac procedures and found that African-Americans had far fewer cardiac interventions and procedures.

Dr. David Satcher (former US Surgeon General) and colleagues (2005) reported that from 1960 to 2000, the United States made progress in decreasing the black–white gap in civil rights, housing, education, and income, but inequality still exits in health care and general health status. A study conducted by Callahan and Cooper (2005) reveals that young adults who were 19–24 years old are the most likely to be uninsured in the United States. The researchers collected data from 11,866 subjects. Results indicate that 27% of women and 33% of men had no health insurance. Almost one third of the young adults are uninsured. Only half of the employers of this group pay any health insurance for their employees. The consequences for this group of noninsured people are that these young adults are at the highest risk period for unintended pregnancy, sexually transmitted diseases, substance abuse, injuries, and other chronic medical diseases. Uninsurance in adults is related to less frequent healthcare screenings, delayed diagnosis of illnesses such as cancer, poor care for chronic diseases, and higher rates of mortality when hospitalized. This study also found that Latino young adults were more likely to be uninsured than any other ethnic group.

There are significant disparities in accessing health care in the United States depending on race, ethnicity, and socioeconomic status. Those living in poverty are significantly less likely to access health care and are generally in poorer health than others. In addition, those in poverty are four times more likely to have serious mental health problems. Infant mortality rates and life expectancy rates also differ among racial and ethnic groups (CDC, 2004a). The United States *does* ration health care by not providing universal coverage to its entire population, but rather relies on a market economy to adjust supply and demand. The United States provides less access to health care to more people than any other developed country. Those who get charity treatment are most likely to get less than adequate health care (Lamm & Blank, 2005).

Reschovsky and Staiti (2005) conducted a study that addressed both physicians' and patients' perspectives on quality of health care for rural America as compared to urban America. Data were collected from 12,406 physicians and 59,725 patients, representing 48 US states. Results of the study indicate that rural areas had far fewer physicians than urban areas, but the overall perception was that health care was adequate for this area. A decreased rural supply of healthcare providers did not necessarily mean lower quality of care. Because of a lower population density and fewer physicians, patients in rural areas often had to travel longer distances for care, wait longer for appointments, and wait longer in doctors' offices, yet there were no perceived differences of unmet medical needs within the two groups. Nevertheless, physicians in rural areas reported greater difficulty in helping patients (by referral) receive specialty medical care, when needed. This was because of a lack of qualified medical specialists in rural areas. Rural residents were poorer and more likely to lack adequate insurance or be able to pay out of pocket expenses for health care (CDC, 2004a).

Medication Usage

Utilization of medications differs according to third-party coverage (insurance) and availability. Noninstitutionalized Americans increased their drug usage from 39 to 44% from 1988–1994 to 1999–2000. Not only was drug usage higher, but the numbers of drugs used per person also increased. Nearly half of the US population takes at least one prescription medication, and almost 1 in 6 take three or more medications. These medications are predominately for lowering cholesterol to reduce the risk of heart disease, controlling depression, and/or controlling diabetes. Numbers of people taking medications and numbers of medications taken increase with age, with 5 out of 6 people 65 years or older taking at least one medication and nearly half taking three or more (CDC, 2004d).

Fertility

In 2002 birth rates for teenagers continued to decline with 43 births per 1000 women (2002), while birth rates for women aged 35–44 increased. More women are postponing birth for education and careers, and infertility interventions make it more possible for women to give birth at later ages (CDC, 2004a).

Other trends differ by racial and ethnic groups. In 2002, the birth rates for Hispanic (Latina) women ages 15–44 years was 64% higher than for non-Hispanic white women, with 94.4 births per 1000 Hispanic women as compared to 57.4 per 1000 white women (CDC, 2004a).

Health Behaviors

Cigarette smoking in the United States has decreased to 25% for men and 20% for women. It is strongly associated with low education and low socioeconomic levels. Between 1997 and 2003 teenage smoking had also decreased from 36% to 22%. Smoking during pregnancy, which causes a higher incidence of preterm and low-birth weight babies, declined from 20% in 1989 to 11% in 2002, yet teenage smoking during pregnancy for 2002 was higher at 18%. Low birthrate babies, who have higher risks for deaths or disabilities, have increased in numbers from 7% of all births in 1990 to 7.8% in 2002 (CDC, 2004a).

Cigarette smoking rates are decreasing in the United States and are expected to continue decreasing in the future (see Figure 1-2).

Overweight and obesity has become a nationwide problem among children and adults in all age groups. Obesity causes about 300,000 deaths per year in the United States and is perhaps second only to smoking as a preventable cause of death. Estimates of deaths from obesity are based on body mass index (BMI), which is defined as weight in kilograms divided by height in meters squared. BMI is correlated with body fat and is the measure recommended by the National Heart, Lung, and Blood Institute for use in clinical

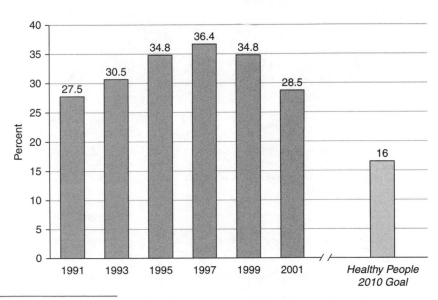

Figure 1-2   Smoking rates in the United States, 1991–2001.

Source: US Department of Health and Human Services, 2005.

practice. Much of this problem relates to inactivity and overeating, especially of the high-fat "junk" foods. In 2003, 33.3% of high school students had no moderate or vigorous physical activity, females having less activity than males. Within the adult population 20–74 years of age, obesity increased from 47% in 1976–1980 to 65% in 1999–2002. Obesity across the lifespan also varies by race and ethnicity. In 2002, 50% of non-Hispanic African-Americans, 39% of Mexican-Americans, and 31% of non-Hispanic white adults were obese. From the time period of 1976–1980 to the time period of 1999–2002, the rates of overweight and obesity in children 6–11 years of age went from 7% to 16%, and for adolescents 12–19 years, the obesity rate more than tripled from 5% to 16%, respectively (Flegal, Williamson, Pamuk, & Rosenberg, 2004; CDC, 2004a).

According to the CDC statistics, overweight and obesity are clearly rising for all age groups (see Figure 1-3).

Alcohol use for those 18 years and older was reported by 41% of males and 20% of females, with the most common usage by 18–24 year olds. Illegal drug use among 12–17 year olds was 12% in 2002. Males 26–34 years had a rate of 222 per 100,000 for cocaine-related visits to emergency rooms (CDC, 2004a).

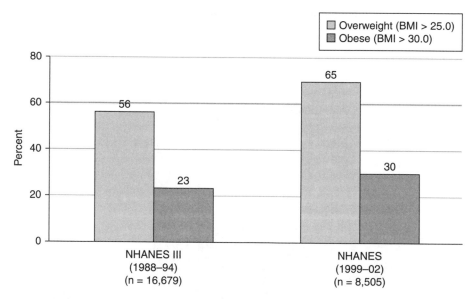

*Age-adjusted by the direct method to the year 2000 by U.S. Bureau of the Census estimates using the age groups 20–39, 40–59, and 60 years and over.

Figure 1-3 Age-adjusted* prevalence of overweight and obesity among US adults, age 20 years and over.

Source: CDC, 2004.

Morbidity

Morbidity (disease rate) includes the limitation of activities due to chronic illness. The rate was 6–7% for children under 18 years during 1997–2002. As adults age morbidity caused by chronic illness increases. In 2002, 14% of those 65 years and older were limited in at least one ADL (CDC, 2004a).

Mortality (death rate) reflects the statistics of life expectancy and infant mortality. They are the key measures to evaluate the overall health standard of a population. For the United States there is an upward trend in life expectancy. The total population life expectancy increased from 74.5 years in 1990, to 77.4 years in 2002. Yet, also in 2002, the infant mortality increased from 6.8 per 1000 live births to 7 per 1000 live births. Racial and ethnic disparities are evident in mortality statistics. A national health objective for 2000 was to reduce the infant mortality rate (IMR) in the United States to 7 per 1000 live births, and for 2010 further reduce the rate to 4.5 infant deaths per 1000 live births. In addition, a goal was to erase the racial and ethnic disparities of infant mortality. When examining the subregions of the United States (see Tables 1-9 and 1-10), the infant mortality disparity rates are evident (CDC, 2004a).

Despite the fact that Americans smoke less and have lowered their cholesterol and that deaths from heart disease and stroke are declining in the general population, deaths are not declining within specific racial and ethnic groups in the United States. Those who have no change in health statistics are African-Americans, Hispanics (Latinos), those who are poor, and those with less than a high school education. African-American men and women have the highest rates of hypertension, diabetes, and hospitalizations for stroke. African-American women also have higher rates of obesity. Hispanics (Latinos) were most likely to lack health insurance, have influenza or pneumonia vaccines, and had the poorest rates of good health. Native Americans (American Indians) had the highest rates of cigarette smoking and alcohol use. Reasons for the disparities include access to health

TABLE 1-9 US Regions with High Infant Mortality Rates (2002)	
US State/Region	**Per 1000 live births**
District of Columbia	13.5
Mississippi	10.4
Alabama	9.7
Louisiana	9.5
South Carolina	9.3
National infant mortality rate = 7 per 1000 live births	

Source: CDC, 2004a.

TABLE 1-10 US Infant Mortality Rates within Racial and Ethnic Groups (2002)

Race/Ethnic Group	Per 1000 live births
European-Americans (whites) (non-Hispanic)	7
African-Americans (blacks)	13.9
Hispanics	5.9
Asian/Pacific Islanders	5
American Indian/Alaskan Natives	9.1

Source: CDC, 2004a.

care, trust of the healthcare providers, cultural and language barriers, and genetic predisposition to heart diseases and stroke (Young, 2005).

Child Health

Wise (2004) revealed the following about the determinants of child health in the United States. In 2002 about 17% of all children and 18.5% of those under 6 years lived in poverty with incomes below 100% of the federal poverty level ($14,348 in 2002). Half of those living in poverty live at 50% of the federal poverty level, placing them within the "severely poor" group. Children who are poor disproportionately suffer more problems with low birth weight and overall higher infant and child mortality and morbidity rates. Medicaid eligibility expansion for poor children and the State Children's Health Insurance Program (SCHIP) for poor children eligible for Medicaid have made a significant difference in facilitating access to health care for poor children.

Almost 60% of all deaths in childhood occur during the first year of life, and 40% of all deaths in childhood occur during the first month of life. Death in newborns is usually from prematurity, low birth weight, congenital anomalies, or other genetic disorders. The United States has increased the survival rates of premature babies mainly through advances in technology and the neonatal intensive care units. In spite of this advanced technology the United States still does not rank among the best in infant mortality rates among developed countries. This is mainly because of the high rate of premature births in the United States. With the ever-increasing rates of survival of premature babies also comes long-term health problems. African-American babies continue to have twice the infant mortality rates as Caucasian babies. The difference is attributed to the higher rates of low birth weights and premature babies of African-American women who live in poverty (Wise, 2004).

The US mortality rates for children have fallen sharply during the past few decades. The greatest reduction has been from prevention and treatment of acute infectious diseases. Deaths from unintentional injury remain the leading cause of childhood death at present in the United States. Children having complex chronic conditions have the second highest death rates. Hospitalization costs for children ages 1–18 (from highest to lowest in cost) are from the following causes: asthma, mental disorders, trauma, respiratory infections, ear infections, other infections, epilepsy, diabetes, and congenital anomalies. Mortality rates for African-American male adolescents (15–19) rose dramatically, mainly because of homicide and suicide. In addition African-American children also had significant death rates from sickle cell disease (Wise, 2004).

Child health outcome trends (according to a study by the National Health Interview Survey of 40,000 households) revealed that little has changed in the rates from the years 1962 to 2000 of children with acute illnesses (any disease that requires restriction of activity for less than 3 months). For young children the rate remained stable and declined slightly for school-aged children. For chronic illnesses such as asthma, type 2 diabetes, and behavioral disorders, there was an increase in rates during the past several decades. Obesity is now considered a chronic problem with children, also causing other problems, such as type 2 diabetes (Wise, 2004).

The CDC reported that more children than ever had health insurance in 2003, but their parents often had less coverage (CDC, 2004c). More than 70% of indigent children under 18 years are covered by some form of public insurance, either federal or state. Still about 3.9 million children in 2003 did not have any form of health care. More specifically, 12% of Hispanic (Latino) children, 5% of non-Hispanic African-American children, and 3% of Caucasian children had no health care. Also, more than 4 million children aged 2 to 17 years lacked dental care.

Blumberg, Halfon, and Olson (2004) report that the first 3 years of a child's life are critical for development. Early exposure to malnutrition, viral infections, drugs, and environmental toxins can result in harmful consequences to the neurological development, resulting in alterations in cognitive and emotional development. These effects are not always recognized immediately and may not be discovered until the child is older. Other consequences of exposure to a compromised environment may result in cardiovascular disease or diabetes later in adulthood. Ideally, a child who has a positive caring relationship with parents and other caregivers will have opportunities for learning skills needed throughout the child's life. Today there are great obstacles that impede the growth of a child towards a safe and healthy life. Children need regular health checkups that include immunizations and treatment for illnesses, intellectual stimulation, as well as good nutrition and a safe and caring home environment.

Health Care for the Older Adult

Lamm and Blank (2005, p. 23) state, "One of the challenges in America's future is to retire the baby boomer without bankrupting the country or unduly burdening future generations." Ways to provide health care and services to the elderly include society (the government) funding of health care or social insurance. The US healthcare retirement system is now unsustainable and healthcare expenditures have grown in the past 40 years to 2.5 times the rate of inflation, which is now greater than 15% of the GDP. About 3 times more is spent on the elderly than on children in the United States.

The most rapidly growing segment of the US population during the past decade is the group of people 65 and older. With the increases in life expectancy, more health care is needed for maintaining and improving quality of life. The United States has made progress in vaccinating 90% of children by the time they are 2 years old, but immunization rates for adults 65 years and older range from 23% to 49% with great racial and ethnic disparities. The US Public Health Service has established a national health goal of 90% immunization rate for older adults by 2010 for influenza and pneumonia vaccines. These can be given in the traditional sites of physician offices or health clinics, but they can also be given in nontraditional sites, such as grocery stores and senior centers. Recommendations from the CDC for immunizations for older adults include (Weber, 2004):

- Tetanus-diphtheria vaccine—All adults, every 10 years
- Influenza vaccine—Adults 50 and older, annually
- Hepatitis A vaccine—Adults at risk
- Hepatitis B vaccine—Adults at risk
- Measles, mumps, and rubella vaccine—Susceptible adults
- Varicella (chicken pox) vaccine—Susceptible adults
- Meningococcal polysaccharide vaccine—Susceptible adults

For older adults, oral health care is not covered by Medicare, and many have difficulty in accessing this care. The well elderly as well as the chronically ill elderly will need good oral care for routine cleaning, problems with tooth loss, dental caries, and periodontal diseases. Periodontal diseases are chronic and can carry organisms and spread endotoxins causing other problems, such as systemic infections. At present there are not enough dentists trained to meet the needs of the elderly nor are there funds for many residents to pay for these services (Lamster, 2004; CDC, 2004e).

In addition to medical care benefits, the federal government also has a federal food and nutrition program for older adults who qualify. The US government appropriates about $1 billion annually for all food and nutrition assistance programs for older adults, funded through the Older Americans Act (OAA). OAA nutrition programs only reach 6–7% of the people who need them. This program is run by the US Department of Health and Human Services of the US Department of Agriculture. The federal government's special Supplemental Nutrition Program for Women, Infants and Children (WIC) is funded at $5 billion and reaches about 50% of eligible women, infants, and children. This program began in the 1970s (Friedland, 2005a; Wellman, 2004).

Occupational Health

Safety in the workplace continues to be a challenge. In 2002 workplace injury and illness affected 2.5 million people. This includes manufacturing, service industries, and mining, including gas and oil. Mining had the highest death rates with 24 deaths per 1000 employed workers. Pneumoconiosis deaths, which are related to occupational exposures to dust, remain a challenging problem. Fortunately, between 1992 and 2002 the overall occupational injury death rates have decreased 23% to 4 deaths per 1000 employed US workers (CDC, 2004a).

Medical research suffered recently when the medications Vioxx and Bextra were removed from the store shelves when the federal government revealed that the drug companies had overlooked potentially harmful side effects. In addition there were ethics investigations about medical research conducted for drug companies (Guterman, 2006). Seminario (2003) states that the scope of US workplace injury and illness is enormous. In 2002, there were more than 5000 work-related deaths from traumatic injuries and an estimated 50,000 to 60,000 died from occupational diseases. The number of reported workplace injuries was over 6 million. The Occupational Safety and Health Administration (OSHA) estimated that reported injuries are underestimated by as much as 50%. Much progress has been made in decreasing work-related diseases and deaths. Muscular and skeletal disorders are the biggest sources of problems reported. These come from repetitive motion injuries, which create medical problems such as carpel tunnel syndrome and back injuries.

Occupations with the most repetitive motion injuries are as follows (Seminario, 2003):

- Truck driver
- Nursing aids, orderlies, attendants
- Laborers, nonconstruction
- Assemblers
- Janitors
- Registered nurses
- Stock handlers and baggers
- Construction workers
- Supervisors, sales jobs
- Carpenters
- Cashiers
- Maids and housemen
- Sales workers
- Clerks
- Welders
- Cooks

Villarejo (2003) reported that of US hired farm workers, who are mostly Mexican immigrants, two-thirds of them are living in poverty. Very little data has been collected related to their health issues. At least half are undocumented; only 20% have any health insurance either from the government or their employer. The Federal Migrant Health Program serves about 13% of all workers plus their dependent families. Only 10% receive food stamps or WIC, and 13% receive Medicaid (federal health benefits for those eligible by low income and number of family members, under 65 years, and not able to receive Medicare). Half are under age 29, and 80% are male. Less than half earn below $10,000 per year. Most have only 6 years of education and the majority has access to health care only when absolutely necessary, visiting hospital emergency rooms or clinics. Less than half of the workers have ever been to a dentist. Infectious diseases most often reported were parasites from poor drinking water in work camps, and tuberculosis at a rate six times greater than the general US population. In addition, HIV/AIDS and sexually transmitted diseases were at much higher rates than the general US population.

Complementary and Alternative Medicine

The CDC (2004f) reports that 158 million people in the United States used complementary and alternative medicine (CAM) medical interventions for health, at a cost of $230 million. One study of 31,000 adults conducted by the CDC (2004f) revealed that 36% of the US adult population uses CAM. If prayer for health is also considered, the percent rises to 62%. CAM is defined as a group of diverse medical and healthcare systems, practices, and products that are not at present considered to be part of conventional medicine. When used with conventional medicine, it is considered complementary, and when used alone or in place of conventional medicine, it is considered alternative. Types of CAM include those offered by providers, such as acupuncture and chiropractic, plus others which do not need a provider, such as yoga, message, special diets, vitamins, herbs, or botanical products. Prayer for health was also included as a type of CAM. The CAM interventions were most often used to treat back pain, colds, neck pain, joint pain or stiffness, depression, or anxiety. Fifty-five percent of US residents use CAM with conventional methods, 26% use CAM at the suggestion of their conventional medical care providers, and 13% use CAM because they believe it is less expensive than conventional medicine. In addition, 28% use CAM because they believed that their conventional medicine was not helping them.

The CDC (2004f) reported that there is some strong scientific evidence from randomized clinical trials for the use of acupuncture and some herbal medicines and manual therapies. More research is necessary to prove the safety and efficacy for other practices and medicinal plants. Unregulated or inappropriate use of some CAM (traditional) medicines or practices can sometimes have harmful effects. For example, the herb ephedra (*ma huang* in Chinese) is traditionally used to treat respiratory congestion in China, but in the United States it was marketed as a diet additive, which has caused some deaths from heart attacks or strokes. Twenty-five percent of modern medicines are made from plants that were first used in traditional medicine. Many other traditional medicines from plants or herbs are currently being tested for prospective modern use for malaria, HIV, and sickle cell anemia.

The National Center for Complimentary and Alternative Medicine (NCCAM) of the National Institutes of Health recommends that people who are considering the use of CAM should review the following key points:

- As an informed consumer, review the scientific studies (published in refereed journals) done of the products that are being considered for use.
- Consult a conventional healthcare provider before starting any use.
- Learn more about the background and competency of a healthcare provider who is practicing a therapy such as acupuncture.
- Check for health insurance coverage before starting treatments or care.
- Check about the components or ingredients that make the products and where they come from.
- Check about the safety of the manufacturing process. How do they avoid contamination? The US Food and Drug Administration does not require testing of dietary supplements. If dietary supplements claim to diagnose, treat, cure, or prevent disease, they are considered an "unapproved new drug" which is being sold illegally.

Payment for Health Care

The United States spends $1.7 trillion or almost 15% of the gross domestic product (GDP) on health care. The United States spends $5267 per person on health care, which is 53% more than any other country, as shown in Table 1-11 (Anderson, Hussey, Frogner, & Waters, 2005).

Residents of the United States often must pay higher prices than other developed countries for pharmaceuticals, hospital stays, and physician visits. For example, the cost of an average hospital stay in the United States in 2002 was $2434 compared with $870 in Canada. Some of the possible reasons that the US costs are so high are that: (1) the United States is paying higher prices for health care; (2) the population is aging; (3) other countries have constrained the supply of healthcare resources, especially for elective healthcare procedures, creating long waiting lists and lower costs; (4) the threat of malpractice litigation creates a more costly defensive medicine practice in the United States; and (5) excessive costs of administering of US health care. From 1970 to 2002, the United States had a healthcare policy based on demand of the consumers, better access to new and expensive technologies, and shorter or nonexistent waiting lists. As compared to other Western European countries, the lengths of hospital stays are generally shorter with a greater use of high-technology equipment, such as CTs and MRI scanners. Administrative costs for health care in 2002 include 3% of the total budget for the federal

TABLE 1-11   Per Capita Expenditures on Health Care by Selected
Nations (2005)

Country	Per Capita Expenditure in US Dollars
United States	5267
United Kingdom	2160
Canada	2931
Japan	2077
Norway	3083
Switzerland	3446
Sweden	2517
Mexico	553
Turkey	446

Source: Anderson, Hussey, Frogner, & Waters, 2005.

Medicare program, 6.7% of the federal and state Medicaid program, compared with 12.8% for private insurance programs (Bodenheimer, 2005). During the 1990s the costs of health care were decreased because of decreased payments to physicians and hospitals, but more recently, hospitals increased their market power by consolidation and were able to demand higher prices (Bodenheimer, (2005).

The US healthcare system does not necessarily result in better health care nor patient satisfaction, as compared to other Western European countries that spend much less on health care (Anderson, Hussey, Frogner, & Waters, 2005). The federal government has predicted that with an average growth rate of 7.2% through 2013, costs will be rising from $1.6 trillion (14.9% of the gross domestic product) to $3.6 trillion (18.4% of the gross domestic product) (Bodenheimer, 2005).

The four major factors that make up the healthcare system include: (1) healthcare purchasers, which includes employers, governments, and individuals; (2) medical insurance groups, who receive money from the purchasers and reimburse the providers; (3) governments, who are insurers and purchasers in Medicare and Medicaid programs; and (4) payers, who are both purchasers and insurers. Healthcare providers include physicians, nurses, and other healthcare professionals. Also included are hospitals, nursing homes, home care agencies, and pharmacies. The suppliers include the pharmaceutical, medical suppliers, and computer industries. Each dollar spent on healthcare services is an expense to payers and income to providers and suppliers. Payers would like to reduce healthcare costs, and providers and suppliers generally resist cost containment (Bodenheimer, 2005).

Seventy-five percent of people in the United States who are under 65 have private health insurance, which is mainly obtained through the place of work. Health insurance is usually provided through a managed care organization such as a health maintenance organization (HMO), preferred provider organization (PPO), and point of service plans (POSs). For those over 65 years, and for those who are disabled, Medicare, a federally funded program, provides health care. Medicaid, a federal and state governmentally funded program, provides health care for low-income individuals and families (CDC, 2004a). There were 15.2% or 43.6 million within the US population in 2003 without any form of health insurance. Working age adults were more likely than children or older adults to lack coverage for health care. The minority population of the United States disproportionately lacks health insurance coverage. In 2003 about 33% of Latino/Hispanics lacked any type of healthcare insurance, while 17.4% of non-Hispanic African-Americans, and 11% of Caucasians lacked health insurance (Bodenheimer, 2005).

Medicaid was passed in 1965 under Title 19 of the Social Security Act to assist states to pay for health care for the very poor. It was designed to give states flexibility so that services would be provided for specific groups of people. To be eligible, a person must be aged, blind, disabled, or a member of a single-parent family with dependent children. Some are eligible who make a higher income, but have exceptionally high medical costs. Pregnant woman can be eligible for care with 133% of poverty level income. Also those who participate in adoption or foster care may be eligible. Each state, the District of Columbia, and the US territories have different eligibility programs. In 2004, 42.4 million people were enrolled in this program (Friedland, 2005b).

Sweden

The kingdom of Sweden is a Nordic country in Scandinavia, in Northern Europe. The present king is Carl XVI Gustaf and the prime minister is Goran Persson. It has a subarctic climate and has light all summer and very little light during the winter. It is divided into 21 different counties, each with a county administration board and a county council. Each council is divided into many municipalities. In 2004 there were 290 municipalities in Sweden. Sweden has a very high standard of living because of its high-tech capitalism and an extensive social welfare system (Government Offices of Sweden, Ministry of Health and Social Affairs, 2004).

Sweden has one of the highest levels of health care in the world, a very low infant mortality rate, and a high average life expectancy. Those in the population who have chronic illnesses have a good quality of life due to excellent health care. Death rates from diseases such as diabetes and heart disease are declining. The older adult population is growing, and more people are able to live a higher quality of life than in previous years (Government Offices of Sweden, Ministry of Health and Social Affairs, 2004).

Healthcare System

The goal of the Swedish healthcare system is for the entire population to have equal access to good health care, which is provided by need, and funded by the Swedish government, representing all of its citizens. The government health welfare system includes health and medical care, care of the elderly, pharmaceutical care, psychiatric care, and dental care. The healthcare system is directed by the Medical Responsibility Board, the Pharmaceutical Benefits Board, the Medical Products Agency, the National Board of Health and Welfare, the Swedish Council on Technology Assessment in Health Care, and the state-owned National Corporation of Swedish Pharmacies (Government Offices of Sweden, Ministry of Health and Social Affairs, 2004).

Health care is administered by 21 different county councils throughout the country. Eighty-nine percent of the councils' budgets are used for health and dental care. Municipalities are responsible for care of the elderly and psychiatric care. For those needing psychiatric care the municipalities also take care of their housing, employment, and financial support. Healthcare agencies within Sweden consist of 9 regional hospitals, 70 county and provincial hospitals, and 1000 health centers. The costs consist of 9.1% of the GDP, which is equal to $196.8 billion dollars. The out-of-pocket costs paid by patients are about 15% of the total healthcare expenditures (Government Offices of Sweden, Ministry of Health and Social Affairs, 2004).

There are different categories of charges for health care within the Swedish healthcare system:

- Outpatient healthcare charges—Charges are for visits to a district nurse, doctor, or specialist. Costs vary among the different councils and depend upon the type of healthcare provider used. The maximum that any one person pays for health visits per year is 900 SEK ($115 US). This maximum cost also includes children under 18 within the same family.

- Pharmaceutical charges—The maximum cost per year for medications is 1800 SEK ($230 US). After this cost is reached, a free pass is given, which is good for 12 months from the date of the first purchase.

- Charges for a portion of dental treatments—These charges vary depending on the type of treatment and materials used. It also covers orthodontia work.

- Costs for inpatient care—When a patient is admitted to a hospital the local council can charge the patient a maximum of 80 SEK ($10.24 US) per day (Government Offices of Sweden, Ministry of Health and Social Affairs, 2004).

Swedes have an extensive social welfare system in which the government pays for child care, maternity and paternity leave, healthcare costs above a ceiling amount, retirement pensions, and sick leave. Parents get 480 days paid leave of absence from their jobs from the time of the birth of a child to his or her eight year. Child care is free and guaranteed for all children 1–5 years old. For the aging adult, the Swedish Social Security Insurance

Agency provides an old age pension. It also provides for loss of income if a person is unable to work because of illness or is caring for a child (Government Offices of Sweden, Ministry of Health and Social Affairs, 2004). The government is concerned about environmental health and has recently passed a law concerning smoking in public restaurants. As of May 1, 2005, all pubs, restaurants, and cafes are smoke free (2004).

During the 1990s Sweden's welfare state was in crisis due to economic challenges and lack of political support. Some spending cuts and reforms were made, but the healthcare system was left mostly intact. For the first time, the private healthcare sector competed with the public healthcare providers. The new private healthcare services (5–15% of all health care) began to somewhat undermine the egalitarian system of equal quality health care for all the citizens. At present there are choices of health services, and the more wealthy citizens are using private healthcare services while the others use the traditional public health services (Government Offices of Sweden, Ministry of Health and Social Affairs, 2004).

Statistics

The country of Sweden has a population of 9 million people (Wikipedia, 2004). Its gross national product per capita is $27,271 USD, which is ranked as the 26th highest in the world. Life expectancy at birth is 78 years for males and 83 years for females. Healthy life expectancy is 71.9 years for men and 74.8 years for females. The infant mortality rate (under 12 months) is 3 per 100,000 live births, which is among the lowest in the world. The child mortality rate (under 5 years) is 5 per 100,000 males and 3 per 100,000 females. Total health expenditure per capita is $2512. The total fertility rate is 1.6. Because Sweden has socialized medicine, the government pays 85.3% of the total health expenditure. The remaining 14.7% of healthcare expenditure is paid privately by out-of-pocket payments. About 23% of the population is 60 years old or older (WHO, 2005).

Patient's Rights

The Swedish healthcare system is responsible for ensuring and maintaining patients' rights. Information is given to patients about their healthcare problems, treatments, options, and costs. Questions are answered about any other concerns about their health issues. The purpose is to prevent injuries and minimize risks resulting from injury or serious illness. Each council and municipality has a patients' committee. Patients may report problems to the Medical Responsibility Board (Government Offices of Sweden, Ministry of Health and Social Affairs, 2004).

Dental Care

The dental health of the nation has improved considerably for all age groups during the last few decades. The numbers of children who need tooth fillings has declined as well as the number of older adults who need total tooth extractions. There are still many differences in level of dental care among county councils. The criteria for good dental care consist of the following:

- Having high standards with a particular emphasis on preventive care
- Satisfying safety concerns
- Being easily accessible
- Respecting patients' rights
- Having good communication between patients and dental healthcare personnel

Mental Health

The Swedish government takes the responsibility of providing mental health care as a part of basic health and medical care. Patients with slight or moderate mental health needs can get care by primary care healthcare providers. Compulsory mental health care is regulated by the Compulsory Mental Care Act. Patients with serious mental health problems are treated in a special psychiatric care setting, even if they refuse care. This is especially true if he or she threatens the personal safety, physical, or mental health of others. Forensic mental health care provides for care for people who have committed serious crimes and also for those who suffer from mental illness (Government Offices of Sweden, Ministry of Health and Social Affairs, 2004).

Sex Education

Sweden is a pioneer country for family planning for the world. In Sweden attitudes toward teenage sex education are considered liberal. Sex education is a high priority and has been taught in schools since the 1950s. Since 1975, abortion has been free and given on demand. Contraceptive counseling is free, and Planned Parenthood is available in youth clinics. Screening for sexually transmitted diseases is included. Contraception and emergency contraception is low in cost and sold over the counter. Teenage pregnancy is rare. Since the 1990s the economy has been stagnant and rates for teen abortions, sexually transmitted diseases, smoking, and drug use have increased (Edgargth, 2002).

United Kingdom

The United Kingdom of Great Britain and Northern Ireland is a country located in Western Europe. As a member of the European Union, it is usually known as the United Kingdom or UK, or inaccurately known as Great Britain, Britain, or England. The United Kingdom has four parts consisting of England, Wales, and Scotland located on the Island of Great Britain; and Northern Ireland, located on the island of Ireland. The capital and largest city is London. The United Kingdom has a population of 59,553,800 people. As of August 2007, England's government is headed by Gordon Brown, who is prime minister, and Queen Elizabeth II. The queen's role is mainly ceremonial. The government is a constitutional monarchy with executive power given to the prime minister (Wikipedia, 2005).

The United Kingdom is a leading world financial power and trading center, with a capitalist economy. The economy is ranked fourth largest in the world, and the United Kingdom has a per capita income of $30,309 (2005 estimate), making it the 16th highest in the world. During the past 20 years the government has decreased private ownership and has continued the growth in the direction of a welfare state. This country produces 60% of its food and needs with only 1% of its labor force. It has coal, natural gas, and oil. Insurance, banking, and other business services contribute to the high per capita income. It is Europe's largest manufacturer of cars, armaments, computers, petroleum products, televisions, and mobile phones. It is ranked sixth in the world for tourism. Languages spoken are mainly English, but other indigenous languages include Welsh, Scottish Gaelic, Irish Gaelic, Cornish, Lowland Scots, Romany, and British Sign Language (Wikipedia, 2005).

Healthcare System

The National Healthcare System (NHS) was established in 1948 to provide free health care for all residents of the United Kingdom, designed to be free at the point of need, meaning that every time a resident needs to go to the doctor or receive inpatient hospital treatment, it is provided free of charge. This system is funded by federal taxation and run by the Department of Health. In addition there are also private healthcare providers, in which people pay either by insurance or out of pocket at the time of use (BBC, 2005).

The basic concepts are the following (Light, 2003):

- Health care should be "free at the point of service." No copayments are needed for services.
- Health care is funded through income taxes. The UK people believe that income taxes are more equitable and cost effective than insurance-based health care as in the United States.
- A strong primary healthcare base should be established for the NHS. Every UK resident should be able to choose a physician or healthcare service. The system also provides general practitioners (physicians) incentives to practice in underserved areas.
- Reduction in the inequalities of health care is made. Areas that have greater health problems and are poorer are now getting more funding.
- Bonuses are given to general practitioners who reach population-based targets for health prevention.
- All subspecialists are paid on the same salary scale.
- Basic prescription drugs are price controlled while research for new drugs is rewarded. The government works out an agreement with the private pharmaceutical companies to create price controls for drugs.

During the last few years the private sector has funded some of the buildings and structures within the National Healthcare System, and in addition some local communities are currently making some of their own healthcare decisions. Since 1997 a change in philosophy toward healthcare management has moved toward more partnerships and comprehensive planning. The New Labor government has emphasized cooperation with the competition of the private healthcare systems, better management, and improved organization (Muller, 2002). There are differences in the healthcare system within each country in the United Kingdom. There is a secretary of state for health, who must answer to the UK parliament. The Department of Health is responsible for local planning, regulation, inspection, and policy development. There are also 28 strategic health authorities who manage the health care of their region and are considered the link between the Department of Health and the National Healthcare System (BBC, 2005).

Healthcare services are divided into primary and secondary and are managed by the local NHS organizations called trusts. Primary care is delivered by local general practitioners, surgeons, dentists, and opticians, who are generally called *primary trusts*. The primary trusts decide the amount and quality of services provided by hospitals. They receive about 75% of the overall NHS budget. In addition they also control hospital funding. The hospitals and specialized services, such as mental health, are managed by organizations called *acute trusts*. The primary trusts are often outsourced to private companies. Usually the outpatient services such as surgery and ophthalmology generally have long waiting lists. Private health care has similar services, and patients who use this system of care generally pay by private health insurance. Insurance premiums are either paid by employers or individuals who pay out of pocket by themselves. There are over 300 private hospitals in the United Kingdom (BBC, 2005).

The UK healthcare system is currently far from ideal. Light (2003) comments about the current situation of the UK's NHS, reporting that the current system is no longer sustainable and no longer affordable. If services were limited to only emergency and welfare service it would have been economically feasible. Specialty care services will be united with primary care services. Muller (2002) states that the system is failing to meet expectations because of underfunding and the fact that it is centrally controlled.

Stevens (2004) reports that the National Health Service of England has a healthcare system with outdated old buildings and inadequate equipment. Health professionals consist of 2 physicians per 1000 people as compared to 2.8 in the United States and 3.3 in France and Germany. Long waits exist for routine surgery. In 2003, the UK taxes increased and policy makers began to pay more attention to improving the healthcare system. Recently some issues were identified, and the following changes were made as a result (Stevens, 2004):

- Increase the supply of physicians and nurses. The supply of physicians and nurses was increased by 55%.

- Modernize the infrastructure. Hospitals were rebuilt and record keeping, prescriptions, and scheduling went to an electronic system.

- Increased in-service learning help for doctors, nurses, and other health professionals to make great improvements in the new knowledge and technology of healthcare delivery.

- National standards were made in types of care given to patients. Goals were set to improve health statistics for specific illnesses such as reductions in rates of heart and cancer disease, access to care for all residents, and reductions in infant mortality rates.

- For the first time doctors were subject to mandatory relicensing every five years. Quality assurance is used to upgrade standards of care.

- Healthcare providers are individually rated by performance and the results are published as public information.

- Financial bonuses are given to healthcare providers who are doing an excellent job.

- Healthcare funding now goes to primary care trusts directly, which purchases some managed care for patient care.

- Patients are given a choice of any provider, which may be public, private, or not for profit.

- The NHS will be using the diagnosis related group (DRGs) system for keeping pricing for services more regulated.

- The NHS will be accountable to local citizens for its budget, spending, and services.

Health Issues

Within the United Kingdom the major health issues are cancer, coronary heart disease, stroke, accidents, and mental illness. New health problems are HIV/AIDs and Creutzfeldt-Jacob disease (Sproston and Primatesta, 2003).

Cardiovascular disease (CVD) and stroke are some of the biggest causes of death or disability per year. Life expectancy is 80 years for women and 75 years for men. A goal was set to reduce CVD and stroke death rates for people under 75 by two fifths by the year 2010. In a study conducted by the UK government, 13.6% of males and 13% of females reported a CVD or stroke diagnosis. Incidence increased as household income decreased (poorer people had greater incidence). Stroke is the single largest cause of severe disability and the third most common cause of death in the United Kingdom. Each year 11,000 die of stroke in England and Wales. Most people diagnosed with CVD or stroke took aspirin and lipid-reducing medications (Sproston & Primatesta, 2003; Youman, Wilson, Harraf, & Kalra, 2003).

Diabetes (types 1 and 2) was reported by people over 35 years at the rate of 4.3% for men and 3.4% for women. Incidence also increased as household income decreased (poorer people had greater incidence) (Sproston & Primatesta, 2003).

Hypertension (high blood pressure) was diagnosed in those people with a systolic blood pressure of 140 mm Hg or greater and a diastolic blood pressure of 90 mm Hg or more. The prevalence was 31.7% of men and 29.5% of women. Less than half the informants of the study were on treatment medications. Treatment rates were 46.3% for women and 36.8% for men. Uncontrolled hypertension is the greatest cause of stroke (Sproston & Primatesta, 2003). Lloyd, Schmieder, and Marchant (2003) report that in the United Kingdom about 5.7 million adults, which is 12% of the population over 16 years, have a blood pressure above 160 mm Hg/95 mm Hg. In addition, 10.3 million (21%) have a blood pressure of 140 mm Hg/90 mm Hg. An estimated 58,000 cardiovascular problems occur in these patients because of hypertension, which would not exist if their blood pressure were within normal limits. They concluded that failure to control blood pressure contributes to huge monetary costs to the NHS for treating cardiovascular problems.

Cancer causes problems for one in four people, with the most common form (one third) being lung cancer. Eighty to ninety percent of all lung cancers are from smoking. For women, 20% of cancer is due to breast cancer. England has one of the worst rates of breast cancer in all of Western Europe. Cancer in the United Kingdom is one of the three leading causes of death for all ages, except for preschool children. Cancer causes about 62,000 deaths per year (Sproston & Primatesta, 2003).

Smoking was identified as the single greatest preventable cause of illness and premature death in the United Kingdom. In the United Kingdom the overall smoking rates for all ages are 27% of men and 24% of women. These rates are higher for younger adults and lower for those 75 years or more. In 2004 the Public Service Agreement (PSA) set an objective of reducing adult smoking rates to 21% or less by 2010. Cigarette smoking increases as household income decreases (Sproston & Primatesta, 2003).

Alcohol consumption was reported by 42% of men and 26% of women, who stated that they consumed alcohol at least three days a week. The statistics on alcohol (2004) revealed that in 2002, 47% of men drank more than four units of alcohol at least one day in the previous week, and 22% of women drank at least three units of alcohol one day in the past week. Total expenditure on alcohol was 5.7% of family income in 2003 (Sproston & Primatesta, 2003).

Overweight and obesity were diagnosed for 65.4% of men and 55.5% of women in the United Kingdom. Overweight is defined as 25 kg/mm2 and obese as over 30 kg/mm^2. Obesity rates were higher in lower-income households (Sproston & Primatesta, 2003).

Accidents account for 10,000 deaths per year in England. England has lower death rates from car accidents than anywhere else in Europe, but rates of death of children from pedestrian accidents are one of the highest in Europe. Road accidents are higher in rural areas than larger cities. Older adults are at risk for death and disability from falls.

Osteoporosis affects more women and contributes to the number of broken bones, especially wrists and hips (Sproston & Primatesta, 2003).

Infant and Child Health

The infant mortality rate for the United Kingdom is 6 per 100,000 live births (Youman et al., 2003). Child poverty in the United Kingdom is about 19.4%, as measured by children who are living in households with less than 50% of median income. This compares with 22.4% in the United States, but other developed European countries, such as Sweden, Norway, or Belgium have rates less than 5%. The United Kingdom has experienced high levels of unemployment in the past 20 years. Socioeconomic status (SES) is among the most important health determinants during a person's lifetime. Poverty and low SES are associated with higher infant and childhood mortality rates, chronic childhood illnesses, and many acute illnesses. In addition there is a close relationship with birth weight and mental health problems (Spencer, 2003). National statistics (2004) reports that children's dental health is much improved. The 2003 Children's Dental Health Survey found that among 15-year-olds, cavity rates have fallen from 42% in 1983, to 30% in 1993, and to 13% in 2003 (National Statistics, 2004).

Herbal Supplements by Adults

The use of herbal extracts in the United Kingdom especially by older adults has been increasing. A recent survey found that 15% of those older than 65 years used over-the-counter herbal medicine during the last 12 months. The herbs are used to treat existing health problems, prevent illness, and promote general health. Older adults should report the use of herbs to their doctors. Doctors should have good information about potential herb and drug interactions (Canter & Ernst, 2004).

Israel

Israel was created as a nation in May 1948, in the area known as Palestine, which had been ruled by the British from 1920 to 1948 through a charter from the League of Nations. The creation of the nation of Israel resulted as the culmination of the Zionist Movement that began in the 1800s in Europe. Immigrants came mostly from Eastern Europe. After World War II and the Holocaust, larger numbers migrated to Israel. In addition, others came from Arab countries in Asia and Africa.

The country of Israel has a population of 6,433,000 people. Its 2003 GDP per capita was $20,780, and life expectancy was 78 years for males and 82 years for females. The population consists of 80% Jews, who speak Hebrew; 15% Muslims, who speak Arabic (Sunni); and the remainder are Christians and Druze. In the early 1990s a large number of immigrants came from the former USSR, increasing the population by 14%. This immigration doubled the number of physicians as well as the total healthcare needs of the country. The Arab population has a large number of children (40% under the age of 15) and a small portion of elderly (5.1% are older than 65 years). The Jewish population has 27% of its children younger than 15, and 11.1% of its adults older than 65. The country's older adult population is 9.5% of the total population, which is larger than any country in the European community or the United States. (Infoplease, 2005; Israel Ministry of Foreign Affairs, 2003).

Israel's system of government is a parliamentary democracy, with the highest authority of law run by the Parliament, called the Knesset. The Knesset has 120 members elected by the citizens every 4 years. The executive power is in the cabinet, headed by the prime minister. The head of state is the president, who is elected for a 5-year term. This person has mostly ceremonial duties and minimal authority. Unemployment is 8% for all residents, with a higher rate for the Arab minority population (Israel Ministry of Foreign Affairs, 2002).

Israel has a high rate of literacy (95%). There is free education for all children ages 5–15 years, and postprimary education is also free, lasting another 6 years (Infoplease, 2005; Israel Ministry of Foreign Affairs, 2003). Israel is one of the most highly educated countries in the world with the highest numbers of engineers, scientists, and PhDs per capita (135 per 10,000) (Israel Ministry of Foreign Affairs, 2003).

The agricultural economy is citrus fruits, vegetables, cotton, beef, poultry, and dairy products. Industry consists of high-tech products such as aviation, communications, and electronics, as well as wood and paper products, foods, beverages, tobacco, and diamond cutting. The cell phone and voice mail was originally developed in Israel by the Motorola Company (Infoplease, 2005; Israel Ministry of Foreign Affairs, 2003).

There are international disputes about the Israeli land. The West Bank and Gaza Strip are Israeli occupied, subject to the Israeli-Palestinian Interim agreement. Permanent status is to be determined by further negotiation. The Golan Heights is Israeli occupied, and Lebanon claims the Shab'a Farms of the Golan Heights. The capital is Jerusalem, but the United States and most other countries have embassies in Tel Aviv (Infoplease, 2005).

Culture

Although Israel has residents who differ greatly in racial and ethnic backgrounds, it is still possible to describe the Israeli culture. Israeli cultural values reflect that the family is central to Israeli life with great emphasis on children. Married children often live near their parents and care for their elderly parents. The father is considered the head of the household, but women also have input into family decision making (Israel Ministry of Foreign Affairs, 2002).

The predominant religion is Jewish. Jewish people believe that when death occurs, the body must be buried within 24 hours. Traditionally the body is in a white shroud and the casket is made of wood. Traditional Jewish diets consist of kosher food. The rules of kosher food dictate that only animals with cloven hooves who chew their cud may be eaten. Slaughtering and preparation of meat must be done in a certain way. Only fish with scales may be eaten, and no shellfish are allowed. Milk and meat may not be eaten in the same meal (Israel Ministry of Foreign Affairs, 2002).

Arab culture is the second most common culture of Israel. An Arab is defined as anyone who was born in an Arab-speaking country and speaks the Arabic language, and shares the beliefs and values of the Arabic culture. Arabs are either Muslim or Christian. Most Arabs value Western medicine and also have other strong beliefs, such as in the evil eye. Arab women are less likely to work outside their homes, due to the cultural practice of staying at home to care for the house and raise the children. When an Arab girl has her first menstrual period (menarche) she is considered a woman. She is not expected to socialize with boys and the family may put greater restrictions as to when she may leave the house and with whom. For the Muslim girl, she may start wearing the head scarf or hijab (Israel Ministry of Foreign Affairs, 2002).

Health Statistics

Israel has been a pioneer in modern public health and is one of the world's healthiest countries. Israel has absorbed numerous Holocaust survivors who had severe health problems and many immigrants diagnosed with TB, malnutrition, cancer, and heart disease. Many immigrants from the Ukraine and Belorussia were exposed to radiation from the Chernobyl nuclear plant meltdown in 1987 (Israel Ministry of Foreign Affairs, 2002).

Healthy life expectancy at birth is 70.5 years for males and 72.3 years for females for the year 2002. The infant mortality is 5.4 per 1000 live births, higher for Arabs, and lower for Jews and Christians (Looking at Israel-Health, 2003).The difference in infant mortality rates among Jews and Arabs is caused by consanguineous marriages among Arabs that produce more congenital abnormalities and also by the lower Arab use of prenatal care services. Arab child mortality is 7 per 1000 children. The fertility rate is 2.9, with a rate of 2.6 for Jews, and 4.6 for Moslems. Total fertility rate is higher in Israel than in all countries in Europe. Total expenditure for health care is $1890 per person, or 9.1% of the GDP (WHO, 2003).

Israel has a highly developed healthcare system with a comprehensive scope of services and high technology, which make it one of the most progressive in the world. The Israeli government has an active role in financing and setting up the network of services. Israel has a high level of immunizations (90%), compared to the European community; it ranks second in immunization rates for polio, sixth for diphtheria, and seventh for measles. Israel's life expectancy is higher for Jews and women than for Arabs and men. In comparison to European nations it has a very low rate of diseases and deaths due to alcoholism (Israel Ministry of Foreign Affairs, 2002). In 2002 Israel began giving smallpox vaccines to its healthcare workers, police officers, and others who may be in contact with people with smallpox. The HIV/AIDS prevalence rate is .1% for adults ages 15–49 years. About 1.5 to 4.9 per 1000 residents are living with HIV/AIDS (UNICEF, 2003).

Healthcare System

The ministry of health is responsible for licensing, supervising, and planning all health services in Israel. The government has a network of hospitals that represent about 50% of the total hospital beds in the country. These hospitals were developed by the government's general sick fund, which are presently called General Health Services (GHS). In 1994 the National Health Insurance (NHI) Law was passed to provide health care (health insurance and access) to all residents of Israel. Almost all services are available on a basis of need, rather than the ability to pay. There are four different sick funds available to residents who may choose one they wish. One problem is that the ministry of health does not provide incentives for quality assurance for the sick funds (Israel Ministry of Foreign Affairs, 2002).

Emergency care is available through Magen David Adom (Red Shield of David), a mobile ambulance service, similar to the Red Cross or Red Crescent in other countries. There are 354 general and specialized hospitals as well as a network of outpatient clinics, mother–child health centers, convalescent homes, rehabilitation centers, and school health programs, which include dental care (Israel Ministry of Foreign Affairs, 2003).

Israeli health researchers have made significant contributions in cancer, immunology, cardiology, brain, orthopedic, plastic surgery, and the treatment of burns. Israeli medical technological developments include computerized tomography, pacemakers, and lasers (Israel Ministry of Foreign Affairs, 2003).

Not all of Israel's residents and neighbors are happy with the system of accessing health care. The Palestinians believe that the new Israeli wall blocks some access to health care. The 10,000 chronically ill Palestinians and 100,000 pregnant women could face great hardships and be put at some risk. Yunis al Khatib, who heads the Palestinian Red Crescent Society, said that Palestinians living in 22 enclaves have been denied access to health care (Aljazeera.net, 2005).

Health Issues

The leading causes of death in Israel are heart disease, cancer, stroke, and injury. One quarter of the population is overweight, and this increases with age. Smoking levels are high, with 33% of males and 25% of females smoking (Israel Ministry of Foreign Affairs, 2002). HIV/AIDS in Israel dropped from a rate of .96 per 1000 in 1990 to .47 per 100,000 in 1996, due mainly to education. Human organ transplants have been performed in Israel since 1964, including kidney, liver, and heart. A national organ transplant center was established in 1993 (Israel Ministry of Foreign Affairs, 2002).

Financing Health Care

National healthcare spending has been steadily increasing. The National Health Insurance (NHI) Law was passed in 1995. Every employer must pay a health tax to finance a portion of his or her employees' health insurance. This health insurance has a capitation formula that puts limits on healthcare spending per person, depending on age, rather than ability to pay. Because care for the older adult is much more costly than younger residents, the sick funds receive 3.5 times more money per person for those 75 years and older than for younger residents. In addition, more money is funded for each person with a diagnosis of thalassemia, Gauche's disease, end-stage renal disease, multiple sclerosis, and HIV/AIDS. The national funds come from several resources, such as the taxable income from wages, the national budget, and some from out of pocket funds from consumers, which are from copayments. Dental services are not covered by national health insurance. Private physician fees and medications are not covered. The rate of out-of-pocket fees for medical care is among the highest in the European community. Health care covered by the National Health Insurance for all Israeli residents include the following (Israel Ministry of Foreign Affairs, 2002):

- Medical diagnosis and treatment
- Preventive medicine and health education
- Hospitalization (general, maternity, psychiatric, and chronic)
- Surgery and transplants (if medical treatment is not available, treatment abroad will be covered)
- Preventive dental care for children
- First aid and transportation to a hospital or clinic
- Medical services at the workplace
- Medical treatment for drug and alcohol abuse
- Medical equipment and appliances
- Obstetrics and fertility treatment
- Treatment of injuries caused by violence
- Medication, ordered by a health provider from the ministry of health
- Treatment for chronic illnesses
- Physical therapy, occupational therapy, and other therapies

Healthcare Resources

There are 26,000 physicians in Israel, most of whom are salaried employees of hospitals and sick funds. The ratio of physicians to residents is 4.6 to 1000 residents, which is among the highest in the world. One reason is the immigration of many physicians from the former Soviet Union. Primary and secondary health care is provided by sick funds. Mental health, chronic, and long-term care are covered by government funds, but no dental care is provided free of charge. Sick funds resemble the health maintenance organization (HMO) delivery system in the United States. Every permanent resident of Israel is eligible for membership in one of four types of sick funds, and may change from one type to another once a year. Sick funds must accept anyone regardless of gender, age, or health status (Israel Ministry of Foreign Affairs, 2002).

Reproductive Health

Modern contraception is available and legal. Most who use contraception, use the IUD. Sterilization is seldom used. Abortion is legal under certain circumstances. The Israeli Family Planning Association is run from Tel Aviv. It provides counseling for adults and teens and provides HIV/AIDS educational programs. It has specific training for working with Russian-speaking and Ethiopian immigrants (International Planned Parenthood Federation, n.d.). An estimated 68% of reproductive age adults use contraception of some type (UNICEF, 2003).

Violence and Health Care

A consequence of the daily terror situation in Israel is that residents must address the daily anxiety, stress, and fear directly relating to safety and security. Others must deal with post-traumatic stress syndrome, and for healthcare providers, compassion fatigue. Compassion fatigue relates to the trauma of those who provide care for the victims of trauma (Wiener, 2005). Wiener (2005) also states that since the beginning of the Intifada and until 2003, trauma and deaths have resulted from the Israeli–Palestinian conflict. More than 275 security persons and greater than 650 civilians have been killed by terrorism. In addition, 1700 security persons and over 4400 civilians have been injured by terrorism. These incidences take their toll in psychiatric disorders such as anxiety, stress, depression, and post-traumatic stress disorders.

A study by Aharonson-Daniel, Waisman, Dannon, and Peleg (2003) indicated that a relatively high number of children have been affected by terror-related injuries. They reported that besides the physical damage, the incidents have often dramatically upset the sense of safety, security, and well-being of surviving children. In Israel millions of children use a bus to get to and from school, and many terrorist explosions have occurred on buses or at bus stations. Often whole families are injured at one time. Powell (2004) also describes an organization called Physicians for Human Rights (PHR) representing Israeli and Palestinian physicians who work to promote peace through dialogue. They work with mobile medical clinics to bring health care to Palestinians who can not access care, which includes prisoners in Israeli jails. Under the Geneva Convention the Israeli government is still responsible for the health of Palestinian territories.

References

Aharonson-Daniel, L., Waisman, Y., Dannon, Y., & Peleg, K. (2003). Epidemiology of terror-related versus non-terror-related traumatic injury in children. *Pediatrics, 112*(4), e280–e284.

Anderson, G., Hussey, P., Frogner, B., & Waters, H. (2005). Health spending in the United States and the rest of the industrialized world. *Health Affairs, 24*(4), 903–914.

Aljazeera.net. (2005, February). *Israel wall prevents healthcare.* Retrieved June 27, 2005, from http://english.aljazeera.net/NR/exeres/B534582B-6D77-4781-9E8A0074C20F.htm

BBC. (2005). *Guide: How the healthcare system works in England.* Retrieved June 11, 2005, from http://www.bbx.co.uk/dna/ocam/A2454978

Blumberg, S., Halfon, N., & Olson, L. (2004). National survey of early childhood health. *Pediatrics, 113*(6), 1899–1906.

Bodenheimer, T. (2005). High and rising health care costs. Part 1: Seeking an explanation. *Annals of Internal Medicine, 142*(10), 847–854.

Callahan, S. T., & Cooper, W. (2005). Uninsurance and health care access among young adults in the United States. *Pediatrics, 116*(1), 88–95.

Canter, P., & Ernst, E. (2004). Herbal supplement use by persons over 50 years in Britain. *Drugs and Aging, 21*(9), 597–605.

CDC (Centers for Disease Control and Prevention). (2002a). Office of Disease Prevention and Health Promotion. *Healthy People 2010.* Leading health indicators. Retrieved June 1. 2005, from http://:www.healthypeople.gov/lhi

CDC. (2002b). National Center for Health Statistics. *Healthy People 2010.* Summary measures of population and health. Report of findings on methodologic and data issues. Retrieved July 9, 2005, from http://www.healthypeople.gov/About.whatis.htm

CDC. (2003). National Center for Health Statistics. *Health Care in America.* Trends in utilization. Retrieved June 1, 2005, from http://www.cdc.gov/nchs/data/misc/healthcare.pdf

CDC. (2004a). National Center for Health Statistics. Retrieved July 9, 2005, from http://www.cdc.gov/nchs/pubs/pubd/other/atlas/atlas.htm

CDC. (2004b). National Center for Health Statistics. *New chartbook examines health care utilization in America.* Retrieved June 1, 2005, from www.cdc.gov/nchs/pressroom/04facts/healthcare.htm.

CDC. (2004c). National Center for Health Statistics. *More children than ever had health insurance in 2003, but coverage for working-age adults declined.* Retrieved June 1, 2005, from http:///www.cdc/nchs/pressroom/04news/insur2003.htm

CDC. (2004d). National Center for Health Statistics. *Almost half of Americans use at least one prescription drug, annual report on nation's health shows.* Retrieved June 1, 2005, from http:www.cdc.gov/nchs/pressroom/04news/hus04.htm

CDC. (2004e). National Center for Health Statistics. *The state of aging and health in America 2004.* Retrieved June 1, 2005, from http://www.cdc.gov/aging/pdf/State_of_Aging_and_Health_in_America_2004.pdf

CDC. (2004f). *More than one third of U.S. adults use complementary and alternative medicine, according to new government survey.* Retrieved June 1, 2005, from http://www.cedc.gov/nchs/pressroom/04news/asultmedicine.htm

CDC. (2004g). National Center for Health Statistics. *Americans slightly taller, much heavier than four decades ago.* Retrieved June 1, 2005, from http://www.cdc.gov/nchs/pressroom/04news/americans.htm

CDC. (2005a). The 10 leading causes of death in the U.S., 2001. In *World almanac & book of facts.* Hyattsville, MD: National Center for Health Statistics.

CDC. (2005b). National Center for Health Statistics. *Annual update of the HHS poverty guidelines.* Retrieved July 9, 2005, from http://as0e.hhs.gov/poverty/05fedreg.htm

CDC. (2005c). Recent trends in vital statistics. In *World almanac & book of facts* (p. 73). Hyattsville, MD: National Center for Health Statistics.

CIA (US Central Intelligence Agency). (2005). *The World Factbook—United States.* Retrieved June 3, 2005, from http:www.cia.gov/cia/publications/factbook/index.html

Edgargth, K. (2002). Adolescent sexual health in Sweden. *Sexually Transmitted Infections, 78*(5), 352.

Flegel, K., Williamson, D., Pamuk, E., & Rosenberg, H. (2004). Estimating deaths attributable to obesity in the United States. *American Journal of Public Health, 94*(9), 1486–1489.

Friedland, R. (2005a). How Medicare works. *Generations, Spring*, 30–34.

Friedland, R. (2005b). How Medicaid works. *Generations, Spring*, 35–38.

Good Medicine—II. (2005). *Medical innovations in Israel.* Retrieved June 27, 2005, from http://www.jewishvirtuallibrary.org/jsource/med/four.html

Government Offices of Sweden. Ministry of Health and Social Affairs. (2004). *Homepage.* Retrieved June 1, 2005, from http://www.sweden.gov.se/sb/d/2061

Guterman, S. (Nov. 30, 2006). *Daily health policy report.* Accessed at www.kaisernetwork.org

Infoplease. (2005). *Israel.* Retrieved June 12, 2005, from www.infoplease.com/ipa/A0107652.html

International Planned Parenthood Association. (n.d.). *Israel.* Retrieved June 27, 2006, from http://ippfnet.org/pub/IPPF_Regions/IPPF_CountryProfile.asp?ISOCode=IL

Israel Ministry of Foreign Affairs. (2003). *Looking at Israel—Health.* Retrieved June 12, 2005, from http://www.mfa.gov.il/MFA/Facts%20About20Israel/Looking%20at%Israel/Looking

Israel Ministry of Foreign Affairs. (2002). *The health care system in Israel—An historical perspective.* Retrieved June 12, 2005, from http://mfa.gov.il/MFA/History/Mordern%20History/Israel%20at%2050/THE%20Heal.

Lamm, R. and Blank. (2005). The challenge of an aging society. *The Futurist, July–August*, 23–27.

Lamster, I. (2004). Oral health care services for older adults: A looming crisis. *American Journal of Public Health, 94*(5), 699–701.

Light, D. (2003). Universal health care: Lessons from the British experience. *American Journal of Public Health, 93*(1), 25–30.

Lloyd, A., Schmieder, C., & Marchant, N. (2003). Financing and health costs of uncontrolled blood pressure in the United Kingdom. *Pharmacoeconomics, 21*, 33–34.

Muller, R. (2002). *Enabling prospective health care: Great Britain's efforts to provide comprehensive health care.* Retrieved June 11, 2005, from http://conferences.mc.duke.edu/privatesector/dpsc2002/bj.html

National Governor's Association. (2005). *A national healthcare innovations program* (pp. 1–12). Washington, DC: National Governor's Association.

Peterson, L., Wright, S., & Peterson, E. (2002). Impact of race on cardiac care and outcomes in veterans with acute myocardial infarction. *Medical Care, 40*(Suppl. 1), 186–196.

Powell, S. (2004). Trauma in Palestine and Israel. *Washington Report on Middle East Affairs, 23*(3), 76.

Reschovsky, J., & Staiti, A. (2005). Access and quality: Does rural America lag behind? *Health Affairs, 24*(4), 1128–1139.

Satcher, D., Fryer, G., McCann, J., Troutman, A., Woolf, S. & Rust, G. (2005). What if we were equal? A comparison of the black-white mortality gap in 1960 and 2000. *Health Affairs, 24*(2), 459–463.

Saving lives: Our healthier nation. (1999). Retrieved June 6, 2005, from http:///www.archive.official-documents.co.uk/document/cm43/4386/4386-07.htm

Schneider, E., Zaslavsky, A., & Epstein, A. (2002). Racial disparities in the quality of health care for enrollees in Medicare managed care. *Journal of American Medical Association, 287*, 1288–1294.

Seminario, M. (2003). Workers at risk. The dangers on the job when the regulators don't try very hard. *Multinational Monitor, June*, 21–26.

Sproston, K., & Primatesta, P. (Eds.). (2003). *Health survey for England.* London: The Stationery Office.

Stevens, S. (2004). Reform strategies for the English NHS. *Health Affairs, 23*(3), 37–44.

The White House. (n.d.). *Leading causes of death in America.* Retrieved June 15, 2005, from http://www.whitehouse.gov/government/handbook/health.html

UNICEF. (2003). *At a glance: Israel—statistics*. Retrieved June 27, 2005, from www.unicef.org/infobycountry/israel_statistics.html

Vallarejo, D. (2003). The health of the U.S. farm workers. *Annual Review of Public Health, 24*, 175-193.

Weber, C. (2004). Update on immunizations for older adults. *Urologic Nursing, 24*(4), 352-353.

Wellman, N. (2004). Federal food and nutrition assistance programs for older people. *Generations, Fall*, 78-85.

Wiener, Z. (2005). Individual and societal reactions to ongoing terror in Israel. *Journal of Ambulatory Care Management, 28*(1), 80-85.

Wikipedia. (2004). *Sweden*. Retrieved June 11, 2005, from http://en.wikipedia.org/wiki/Sweden

Wikipedia. (2005). *United Kingdom*. Retrieved June 11, 2005, from http://en.wikipedia.org/wiki/United_Kingdom

Wise, P. (2004). The transformation of child health in the United States. *Health Affairs, 21*(3), 9-25.

World Almanac & Book Facts. (2004). *Israel*. Retrieved June 12, 2005, from http://epnet.com/DeliveryPrintSavwe.asp?tb=1&_ugsid+0D98B26F-D9E7-48E4-89

World Health Organization. (2003). *Israel*. Retrieved June 5, 2005, from www.who.int/countries/isr/en

World Health Organization. (2003). Sweden. Retrieved June 5, 2005, from www.who.int/countries/swe/en

Youman, P., Wilson, K., Harraf, F. & Kalra, L. (2003). The economic burden of stroke in the United Kingdom. *Pharmacoeconomics, 21*(Suppl. 1), 43-50.

Chapter 2

Developing Countries: Mexico, China, and South Africa

Carol Holtz

This chapter will address the health conditions of three developing countries: Mexico, China, and South Africa. These countries were selected because they differ in culture, economics, politics, geographic regions, and types of health issues. The following sections will discuss such things as:

- Family planning, infertility care, abortion, sterilization, and adoption practices in Mexico, China, and South Africa
- How communism affects health care in China
- The "one child per family" policy in China
- Women rights issues in South Africa

Mexico

Mexico is located in the southern region of North America; its northern neighbor is the United States, and its southern neighbors are Guatemala and Belize. Mexico's eastern coast is the Gulf of Mexico and the western coast is the Pacific Ocean. The capital and largest city is Mexico City. The government is a federal republic with 31 states and one federal district (World Almanac Education Group, 2004; WHO, 2004).

People

There are approximately 102 million people in Mexico, with about 10 million people living in Mexico City. Mexico City is one of the most populated cities in the world and has very diversified ethnic groups consisting of Mestizo (indigenous Indian and European mixture, about 60%), American Indian (30%), Caucasian (9%), and other (1%). The main religions are Roman Catholic (89%) and Protestant (6%) (World Almanac Education Group, 2004). Ninety-one percent of the people over 15 years of age are literate, but in selective areas, the literacy rate drops to approximately 20% (Pan American Health Organization, 2002). The principal language is Spanish, but 6 million indigenous Indians primarily use one of a variety of 92 other distinct languages (World Almanac Education Group, 2004; WHO, 2004).

Economy

The Mexican economy has industries of steel, food and beverages, chemicals, textiles, mining, and tourism. Approximately 12% of Mexico's land is used for farming, and 45% of the land is arid and difficult or impossible to farm. The per capita income is US$8500, reflecting the growth resulting from the 1994 North American Free Trade Agreement (NAFTA) with the United States and Canada (World Almanac Education Group, 2004).

Health

The health and healthcare system in Mexico has experienced numerous challenges in both primary and secondary healthcare delivery and statistical surveillance of healthcare issues. Tables 2-1 and 2-2 show selected epidemiologic data across Mexico. However, it is imperative to know that surveillance data collected in Mexico, just as collected in the United States by the Centers for Disease Control and Prevention (CDC), may vary, depending on regional systems of reporting.

Clean water has always been a challenge for preventing illness and maintaining health of the population. In a study conducted in Mexico City by Cifuentes, Mazari-Hiriart, Carneiro, Bianchi, and Gonzalez (2002), the risk of enteric diseases in children under 5, was linked with environmental indicators in the living area, such as water quality, sanitation, and socioeconomic status. The Mexico City area has 18 million people and has some of the poorest sanitation. The study results indicated that bacteria was found in 32% to 40% of well water, and rates for diarrhea in young children ranged up to 11.5%.

Healthcare System

Mexico has a variety of programs that cover healthcare costs for its residents. The Social Security Administration (SSA) provides leadership for the health system. In addition there are private health organizations that vary in quality and costs. Public health is provided

TABLE 2-1   Health and Vital Statistics for Mexico

Life expectancy	Males: 68.7 years
	Females: 74.9 years
Birth rate	22.77 births per 1000 people
Death rate	5.02 per 1000 people
Fertility rate	2.4 per 1000 people
Infant mortality	15 per 1000 live births

Source: Adapted from World Almanac Education Group, 2004.

TABLE 2-2   Leading Causes of Death in Mexico

1. Heart disease	71 per 100,000
2. Malignant neoplasms (cancer tumors)	55 per 100,000
3. Diabetes mellitus	47 per 100,000
4. Accidents	36 per 100,000
5. Liver diseases	28 per 100,000
6. CVA (strokes)	26 per 100,000
7. Birth defects	20 per 100,000
8. Infectious diseases	5.7 per 100,000
9. HIV/AIDS	4.3 per 100,000
10. Tuberculosis	3.3 per 100,000

Source: Adapted from Pan American Health Organization, 2002.

by the leadership of the secretariat of health, with support from the social security institutions, especially the IMSS (Instituto Mexicano del Seguro Social or Mexican Institute of Social Security). The IMSS gives complete coverage for all medical care including prescription medications except for preexisting medical conditions. The social security system covers workers in the economy and is made up of several agencies and funded by contributions from employers, employees, and the federal government. The IMSS is the largest institution in the system and serves 80% of the population, and includes the following (Pan American Health Organization, 2002):

- State Workers Social Security and Services Institute (ISSSTE)
- Petroleos Mexicanos (PEMEX)
- Armed forces (SEDENA)

Healthcare costs represent about 5.6% of the gross domestic product (GDP) of Mexico. The average per capita yearly healthcare spending is the equivalent of US$240. Only 13% of the 4000 hospitals in Mexico have been nationally certified as being quality healthcare delivery systems (Barraza-Llorens, Bertozzi, Gonzalez-Pier, & Gutierrez, 2002) (Figure 2-1).

Inequality in Health and Health Care

Barraza-Llorens et al. (2002) report that half of Mexico's 100 million people have some type of health insurance, and half of all its residents pay for health care out of pocket. Disparities in infant mortality rates exist in the poorest areas of Mexico and its more

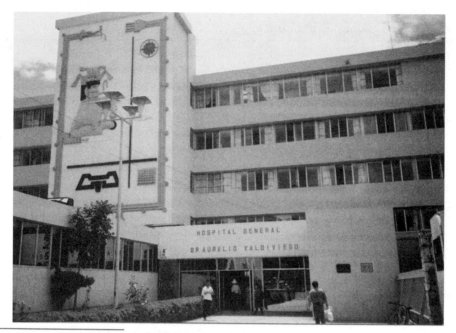

Figure 2-1 A municipal city hospital in Oaxaca, Mexico.

affluent areas. The range of infant mortality rates is from 103 per 1000 live births to 9 per 1000 live births, respectively. In some of the poorest indigenous rural communities (as in Oaxaca or Chiapas), the infant mortality rate is 58% higher and life expectancy is 5 years lower than the national average. Their life expectancy rate is 10 years lower than for those living in Mexico City or Monterrey (the more affluent areas).

For the more educated and wealthier Mexicans, excellent care can be easily obtained, but for the poorest, many get only vaccinations as part of their routine health care. The poor are also very much in need of health education in such areas as water quality, sanitation, nutrition, and safe sex. From a health education perspective, the minimum treatment for illnesses should include oral rehydration therapy (ORT, or the replacement of fluids and electrolytes) for the many intestinal infections causing diarrhea and dehydration, especially in small children. Forty percent of the indigenous Indians have been found to be anemic, compared with the national average of 26%. Much of the inequality of health and health care is also due to the rates of access to health care. The range of women delivering in a hospital setting varies from 10% to 80%, (Barraza-Llorens et al., 2002).

Nutrition

Mexico has experienced significant nutritional changes that have a tremendous effect on types of diseases challenging the population. There is a rise in the aging population caused by a shifting from high fertility to low fertility and mortality. More people are having fewer children, less acute illness, and living longer with more chronic diseases. Recently more people in Mexico are having problems related to having low-birth-weight babies, obesity and malnutrition, diabetes, and heart disease. Diets have shifted to higher fats and refined carbohydrates. Between the years 1988 to 1999 fat intake increased from 23.5% to 30.3%. Because of these changes there is a rise in overweight and obesity. Between two national nutritional health surveys, one in 1988 and one in 1999, the overweight and obesity rates of women ages 18–49 years increased significantly; in 1988 the rate was 33.4%, but in 1999 the rate increased to 59.6%. The obesity rates of children under 5 years also increased 26% from 1988 to 1999. Obesity is a known risk factor for morbidity and mortality, causing increased rates of diabetes, hypertension, cancer, stroke, and heart disease (Rivera, Barquera, Gonzalez-Cossio, Olaiz, & Sepulveda, 2004).

In a study of children in Mexico, by Gonzalez-Barranco and Rios-Tores (2004), the findings linked early malnutrition of children during their first year of life with latent chronic diseases, such as diabetes and cardiovascular disease. Statistics confirmed that in Mexico there has been a progressive increase in the rate of low-birth-weight babies who later develop type 2 diabetes and cardiovascular disease. The authors of this study report that diabetes mellitus is now the leading cause of mortality in Mexico.

Wyatt and Tejas (2000) conducted a study of nutrient intake and growth of preschool children of various socioeconomic groups in the city of Oaxaca, Mexico. The state of Oaxaca is known for its extreme poverty, especially among the indigenous Indian population. The primary protein and energy sources for children in the low income group, which is the majority of the population, are corn tortillas and beans, which constitute only about 63% of the recommended intake. Most children had very little milk products, fresh fruits, or vegetables, and consequently they had higher rates of malnutrition and infectious diseases. These diets are also associated with impaired growth.

Mexican Folk Medicine Practices

Because of the high cost of modern medicine and the barriers to accessing medical care, many Mexicans still use traditional or folk medical practices, especially in poorer rural areas. Traditional medical practitioners usually practice a more holistic approach to health maintenance, prevention, and treatment of illness. Table 2-3 lists some of the very common examples of plants or herbs used for illness prevention and treatment.

Some people who use traditional medical remedies believe that these treatments are not only cheaper, but are also safer, even though they may be slower to work. Folk medicine used in Mexico is a common practice of maintaining health and preventing and treating illnesses. Traditional Mexican folk medicine can be traced to 16th-century Spain, and also to the practices of indigenous Indians living in Mexico for many generations before the Spaniards arrived. Folk medicine involves a relationship of a person with their environment, emotions, and their social, spiritual, and physical world.

TABLE 2-3 Examples of Plants or Herbs Used for Illness Prevention and Treatment

Manzanilla	Chamomile, which can be purchased in tea bags or fresh and dried. It is used for stomach ailments, stimulating the appetite, for sore throats, and mouth infections.
Arnica	Sold in the form of a powder or as an infusion mixed with rubbing alcohol, used for wounds or bruises. Tea made from the flower of this plant is used for colds, clearing the lungs, and for fatigue.
Cilantro (coriander)	Used to strengthen the heart and as a stomach tonic, and to prevent parasites. It is often used in salads, soups, or in main dishes for flavoring
Nopales	Leaf of the prickly pear cactus believed to help with blood glucose and cholesterol. It can be served as a vegetable or salad, and even as a flavor for ice cream.
Berro (watercress)	Applied to the temples, it is used to relieve headaches
Romero (rosemary)	Massaged over joints to relieve aches
Albahaca (basil oil)	Inhaled to clear the sinuses
Tomillo (thyme)	Used as an antiseptic and also to aid digestion
Toronjil	Is similar to mint, and used for tea, to relieve an upset stomach, and to sleep well
Jamaica (hibiscus)	Used to make a tea, is very high in vitamin C, and is used also as a diuretic

Source: Adapted from Marsh & Hentges, 1988.

Within each unique area of Mexico are spiritual and physical healers. Healers often seek to balance the imbalances causing illness. Causes of illness may be a failure to relate properly to God, interpersonal relationship failures, or imbalances with food, water, air, or temperature. The following is a list of types of traditional healthcare providers (Hunt, Glantz, and Halperin, 2002; Vista Community Clinic, 2004):

- *Curanderos,* who are often called healers, are believed to be chosen and empowered by God.

- *Yerberos* are herbalists who specialize in using herbs and spices to treat or prevent illness.

- *Sobadors* are masseuses, who try to correct musculoskeletal imbalances by massage therapy.

- *Parteras* are lay midwives who have had training as a birth attendant from other family members or friends. They (females only) may be well experienced, but may not have a formal education, although some may have attended a special training program. Most use clean techniques, and others may not be as careful. Women with low-risk pregnancies will often use parteras for a home delivery. The cost is less and access may be easier than going to a physician, especially if the woman lives in a remote area. Twenty-five percent of women in Mexico use a traditional birth attendant. In rural areas of the indigenous Indians, such as in Chiapas, pregnant women have a 60% rate of using a partera. The partera will often promote a squatting position for delivery, rather than the supine (flat lying) position that physicians practice. Other women may prefer to use family members or friends rather than a partera for a home delivery.

- *Promotores* are women or men who have received basic training in first aid, taking vital signs (temperature, blood pressure, and pulse), are able to give medications including injections, do basic assessments, and make referrals when needed.

There are many common folk illnesses that are *not similar* to conventional medical terminology and beliefs. The following are examples of these diseases with explanations for why some diseases occur (Marsh & Hentges, 1988):

- *Empacho* (blocked intestine) is believed to be caused by a bolus of food that sticks to the wall of the intestine, by eating improperly cooked food (e.g., cold tortillas, not fully cooked meat), or eating food at the wrong time of the day (bananas eaten late at night). Symptoms include major bloating or stuffiness of the stomach, constipation, indigestion, diarrhea, vomiting, nausea, or anorexia.

- *Susto* (fright sickness) occurs when a victim experiences a startling event and becomes *asustado*. For example a person could be frightened by a dog or a car accident, or a bad dream. Symptoms include daytime drowsiness, nighttime insomnia, irritability, depression, or anxiety.

- *Mal de ojo* (evil eye) is caused by a person "with a strong or powerful eye," who looks at a person without touching the person. Symptoms include fever, vomiting, crying, or listlessness.

- *Caida de mollera* (fallen fontanelle) is believed to be caused by the baby pulling away from the breast too quickly, carrying the baby incorrectly, or letting the baby fall to the floor. Symptoms include diarrhea, vomiting, inability to suck, restlessness, sunken eyes, irritability, and reduced tears.

- *Aire de oido* (air in the ear) is when it is believed that air is trapped in the ear canal. Symptoms include fullness or popping of the ears, pulling on the ears, and earaches.

A Unique Case Study: An Example of Health Beliefs, Customs, Practices, and Health Problems and Issues for the State of Oaxaca and Nearby State of Chiapas, Mexico

Understanding the specific cultures within Mexico enables one to comprehend actual and potential health problems and enhances the cultural competence for healthcare providers to be proactive in understanding health issues and teaching preventive measures. To restate, Oaxaca has the highest infant and maternal mortality rates of any state in Mexico. The reason for these poor health indicators is extreme poverty, which results in the nutrition and health outcomes of the population (Figure 2-2).

The Oaxacan Zapotec Indian pueblo (village) of El Campanario has a malnutrition rate of 50% for both adults and children, and another pueblo of San Miguel Mixtepec has a rate of 15.8%, which is much higher compared to the national average of Mexico with a rate of 8%. In these impoverished communities the diet consists of mainly beans and tortillas, with some vegetables, which is usually chili or squash. Depending on the season, some fruits are eaten as well. Meat is seldom eaten, and when eaten, is from wild animals such as deer, rabbit, squirrel, or skunk. During pregnancy women try to add more fruits and vegetables to their diets if they can afford them. The culture includes beliefs in the "hot and cold" theory of balance. After delivery of their babies, the women believe that

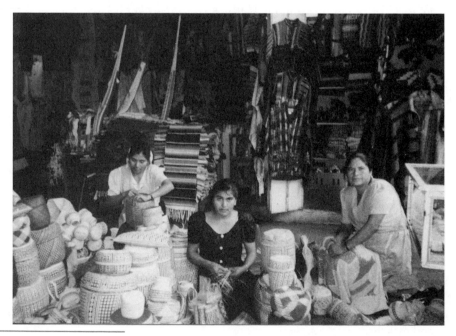

Figure 2-2   Zapotec women weaving baskets in the market in Oaxaca, Mexico.

they must consume foods considered "hot," because delivery is considered a "cold" experience. They eat hot (in temperature as well as spice) foods to give back the heat lost in labor. They consume fried eggs, fresh milk, and atole, a drink made from corn (maize) and herbs. These foods are believed to help in breast milk production. Babies are given breast milk and later, eggs, soup, rice, and vegetables. Malnutrition begins in the 8th month of life if the children are not given the necessary complementary foods. Often they are also given foods cooked in unsanitary water, which causes diarrhea and dehydration, which in turn, contributes to higher rates of infant morbidity and mortality (Marsh & Hentges, 1988).

In the state of Oaxaca, *chapulines* (grasshoppers) are considered a delicacy and are eaten frequently. The state director of health announced a warning to the population, particularly pregnant women and children, to beware of *chapulines* that are prepared with a red chili powder coating, lime juice, garlic, and salt. These chapulines contain high levels of lead and can cause lead poisoning, which is a threat, especially to children. Lead poisoning can cause neurological damage and mental retardation (San Joaquin County Health Department, 2002).

Another similar problem with lead poisoning comes from the lead-glazed ceramic pottery made in Oaxaca, which could be used to contain food for consumption. The lead in the glaze or lead paint to decorate the pottery can also cause lead toxicity in children as well as adults (Azcona-Cruz, Rothenberg, Schnaas, Zamora-Munoz, & Romero-Placeres, 2000).

A problem from corn fungi affecting birth defect rates is found in Oaxaca. In a research article entitled "Folic acid could ease threat from corn toxin (**fumonisin**)," the authors report that people in Mexico and Southwest United States who eat corn tortillas from corn contaminated with a toxic fungus could have fatal birth defects or babies born with neural tube defects such as anencephaly (underdeveloped brain) or spina bifida (an improperly closed spine). Pregnant women could reduce the harmful effects of this toxin if they consumed folic acid in their diets by eating such foods as leafy green vegetables, legumes, citrus fruits, cereals and grains fortified with folic acid, and tablets of folic acid (Wahlberg, 2004).

In Oaxaca HIV/AIDS is an increasing health issue for the community. According to d'Adesky, (2002), Mexico has two different worlds that experience the epidemic of HIV/AIDS differently. Within the isolated rural areas there is a lack of infrastructure and medical attention and lack of training of doctors to treat this disease. Often patients are dying without any medical attention at all. Patients suspected of having HIV are automatically referred to larger cities such as Oaxaca City for care. For residents of poor and isolated communities, the transportation for accessing health care, if affordable, can be 8–12 hours by bus or car. Many migrant workers from Oaxaca come to the United States and encounter the HIV virus, later bringing it back to their wives, newborns, and others in their local community. As of 2002 the Mexican government estimates the official cases at 46,000, while other unofficial estimates report about 150,000, including undocumented cases. Other sources estimate the number to be much higher, at 450,000 cases. The government reports that 60% of those with HIV/AIDS are eligible for medical treatment through the Social Security system. Most people who are receiving treatment live in the larger urban areas.

In the state of Oaxaca, with 2 million people, many live in small rural communities, composed of poor indigenous Indians who raise coffee. About 50% of this population is illiterate, and 15% speak no Spanish, only their indigenous dialects. Few are aware of HIV/AIDS, and within their cultures discussion about sex is taboo. This makes it difficult to educate the people about health prevention and treatment options. The public organization, Coesida, provides a range of preventive and treatment services. Nutrition is a difficult challenge in HIV patients because many are poor and have no funds. Also, limited access to clean water adds to the problem of susceptibility to infections (d'Adesky, 2002).

Another unique health problem is occurring in Chiapas, also an area of extreme poverty and high infant mortality. Since 1994, Chiapas, located in southern Mexico, has been the site of a low-intensity armed conflict between the Mexican government and the insurgents known as the Zapatistas. This conflict involves the local disputes about land, religion, access to health care and other issues. Mexican health statistics have revealed that this area constantly has very high infant and maternal mortality rates as compared to other parts of the country. The Zapatistas have refused to use all government health programs and choose to rely on nongovernmental organizations (NGOs) and to establish their own village primary healthcare workers. During the 1990s there have been reports of pertussis outbreaks in indigenous Indian villages that refused immunizations for political reasons. Strains of antibiotic-resistant tuberculosis and childhood malnutrition were the result of lack of adequate health care (Brentlinger, Sanchez-Perez, Cedeno, Morales, Hernan, Micek, & Ford, 2005).

Based on 1999 data the following information provides a background of the serious health issues facing the people of Oaxaca.

Infants and Children

- Infant mortality rate was 15 per 1000 live births.
- Mortality in children under 5 was 25 per 100,000.
- Leading causes of deaths were congenital malformations (birth defects) and infections due to influenza and pneumonia.
- Death rates for infant males was 30% higher than infant females.
- Intestinal tract diseases had a rate of 28,000 per 100,000.
- Anemia rate was 27%.
- Maternal mortality rate was 12 per 10,000 live births.
- Half or more of the state's population has *no* access to health care.
- Mortality rate for children 5–9 years was 34 per 100,000.

- The undersupply of primary care health providers in the state of Oaxaca has led to a death rate of 3% for children ages 5–14 years and 5.7% for those 15–24 years.

- Main causes for the mortality of children 5–14 years are: infectious intestinal diseases (20% of deaths); malnutrition (caloric and protein deficits are 20% and 24% respectively); and some specific areas that have extreme poverty.

- Respiratory infections and heart disease frequently cause many other deaths.

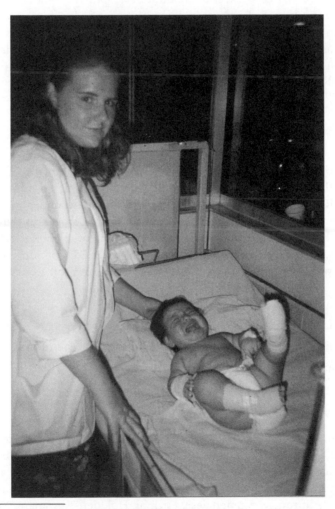

Figure 2-3 An American student nurse from Kennesaw State University, caring for a baby in the pediatric unit of a hospital in Oaxaca, Mexico.

Adolescents

- Accidents were the leading cause of death in the 15–24 age group with a rate of 31 deaths per 100,000.

- Homicide was the second cause of death with 14 deaths per 100,000.

- Malignant tumors (cancer) were the third cause of death with 6 per 100,000.

- The suicide rate was 6 per 100,000.

- Polysubstance use (alcohol, drugs, and tobacco) is also high for this group.

In the country of Mexico social and economic development, demographic changes, and improvement in health care have resulted in an increase in life expectancy and a rapidly expanding aging population. The improvement in the economy and a more stable political system has also helped change the healthcare status of the people of Mexico. As people are living longer they are also experiencing long-term noncommunicable diseases rather than only acute illness (Reyes-Beaman et al., 2005).

China

Description

China is the world's fourth largest country in area (after the countries of Russia, Canada, and the United States), and is located in east Asia, bordering on numerous countries, including the Russian Federal Republic, India, Pakistan, Vietnam, and Mongolia. China, slightly smaller than the United States, has climates varying from tropical in the south to subarctic in the north. At present it has a great amount of air pollution, mostly greenhouse gases and sulfur dioxide particles from use of coal and other carbon-based fuels. It also has water pollution, hazardous waste, deforestation, and soil erosion problems (CIA, 2005a).

Population

A graph of China's aging population and the forecast for the increased percentage of people 65 and older can be seen in Figure 2-4. A breakdown of China's health and vital statistics can be seen in Table 2-4.

Ethnic Groups in China

The Han ethnic group makes up 91.9% of the population, with the remainder being Zhaung, Uygur, Hui, Yi, Tibetan, Miao, Manchu, Mongol, Buyi, Korean, and other nationalities. The official religion of China is atheist; there are 1–2% who are Daoist, Buddhist, or Muslim; and 3–4% are Christian. The standard language is Mandarin with other dialects such as Cantonese, Shanghaiese, Fuzhou, Hokkien-Taiwanese, Xiang, Gan, and Hakka dialects. China has a 90.9% literacy rate (CIA, 2005a).

Figure 2-4 China's aging population.

Source: Quoted form the Web site of the National Bureau of Statistics of the People's Republic of China, www.stats.gov.cn.

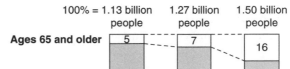
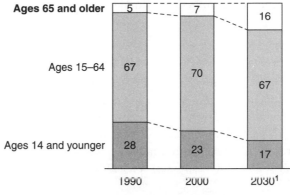

Percent

100% = 1.13 billion people   1.27 billion people   1.50 billion people

	1990	2000	2030¹
Ages 65 and older	5	7	16
Ages 15–64	67	70	67
Ages 14 and younger	28	23	17

¹Forecast

TABLE 2-4   China's Population (2005 Data)

Total population	1.3 billion people
Birth to 14 years	21.4%
15–64 years	71%
65+ years	7.6%
Population growth rate	.58%
Birth rate	13.14 per 1000 people
Death rate	6.9 per 1000 people
Gender ratio	1.06 males per 1 female
Infant mortality rate	24.18 deaths per 1000 live births
	Males: 21.21 per 1000 live births
	Females: 27.5 per 1000 live births
Life expectancy at birth	Males: 70.65 years
	Females: 74.09 years
Fertility rate	1.72 children per woman
HIV rate	.1%
	840,000 already have the disease

Source: CIA, 2005a.

Government

The government of China (also called the People's Republic of China or PRC) is communist, with the capital in Beijing. China has 23 provinces and 5 autonomous regions (CIA, 2005a).

Economy

Since 1978 the economy has moved from a centrally run and planned soviet-style of government to a market economy. Business and agriculture are more locally run, rather than by the central communist government. The economic system still continues to function within strict communist political control. The change in management style of business has increased the GDP four times. The GDP is US$7.262 trillion, and the per capita income is $5600 (2004 estimate) (CIA, 2005a).

Healthcare System

History

China has one of the longest historical records of medicine of any existing civilization in the world. Traditional medicine as well as new technology are both present in the Chinese healthcare system. In 1949 Chairman Mao Zedong established a rural preventive healthcare program, emphasizing disease prevention. The ministry of public health was responsible for all health care. Large numbers of more sophisticated urban physicians were sent to the countryside to practice. In addition, less trained "barefoot doctors" were sent to small rural communities to help supply the needs for local rural health care. They worked out of village medical centers, providing preventive and primary medical care. There were township health centers that had 10–30 bed hospitals. This was called the rural collective health system. Only seriously ill patients went to county hospitals, which served a much larger population base. In large urban areas, health care was provided by paramedical personnel, who were assigned to factories and neighborhood health stations. Patients with serious illness went to the district or municipal hospitals. In the 1950s China was isolated by the Western powers, and the Soviet Union was its only ally. Medical schools and hospitals were built with the help of Russians. There was an emphasis on public health and prevention of illness. The government mobilized the people to begin massive patriot health campaigns aimed at environmental sanitation and preventing disease. An example was the assault on the "four pests" (rats, sparrows, flies, and mosquitoes), as well as the efforts towards eradicating snails that carried schistosomia disease. Other health campaigns were devoted to water quality and waste management (Wikipedia, 2005; CIA, 2005a). Unfortunately much of the agriculture was ignored or handled poorly by overplanting and not harvesting all the crops, leaving them to rot. Thus many of the agricultural programs failed. As many as 20 to 30 million people starved to death, and infant mortality rose to 300 per 1000 (Hesketh & Zhu, 2002).

In the 1960s, campaigns to prevent sexually transmitted diseases, such as syphilis, were successful. By the 1970s China was able to set up affordable primary health care in the rural areas. During the 1980s China's health policy was restructured based on market-driven reforms. The barefoot doctors were then less needed. A more sophisticated system of health care was established. With a 1% growth rate of the 1.3 billion people, China became very concerned about population growth and began restricting family size by implementing the "one child per family" policy. Diseases such as tuberculosis, hepatitis, hookworm, and schistosomiasis still remained a problem. Later other more chronic diseases such as HIV/AIDS, cancer, cardiovascular disease, and heart diseases became frequent causes of mortality, similar to other industrialized societies (Wikipedia, 2005; CIA, 2005a).

According to the Freedom House, which is an organization that judges how much freedom citizens of various countries have, China is near the bottom of the list along with other countries limiting freedom. It is possible that these restrictions actually helped the health care in China. From the 1950s to the 1970s health care in China improved greatly under a very strict authoritarian rule. The brothels and opium dens were officially closed, the four pests (flies, mosquitoes, rats, and sparrows) were greatly reduced, and the training of a million "barefoot" lay doctors by urban doctors was accomplished. Healthcare through prevention was promoted. Claims by the communist government stated that sexually transmitted diseases, schistosomiasis, and leprosy were decreased, access to health care for all was promoted, and infant mortality decreased. It is almost impossible to verify all claims because China was a closed system allowing few outsiders to document facts. The irony today is that as China becomes freer and having a more market economy, some advances in health care have actually decreased. For example, universal access to health care for all is gone, and poor rural Chinese have great difficulty today getting prevention and treatment with the current partial out-of-pocket payment system (Hesketh & Zhu, 2002).

China, with its market reforms, has had tremendous economic growth. One of the results is a fee-for-service private medical practice with few governmental restrictions. Private medical practice was not allowed during the Cultural Revolution, but it reemerged in the 1980s after the dissolving of the Cooperative Medical System (CMS) during the Maoist times, when many lived in communes. At present rural families must pay out-of-pocket fees for medical services, which is often prohibitive in cost making it inaccessible for many (Lim, Yang, Feng, & Zhou, 2004).

The barefoot doctors today in the small remote villages of the far west are often supported by a very small government salary each month and often work out of their homes rather than a clinic so that they are also able to maintain their farms when there are no patients. The doctors charge a small fee to the patients for their services, and the remainder of their salaries comes from drug sales. Often doctors overprescribe medicines in order to increase their incomes. Village doctors have inadequate training and often do not take patient histories nor keep medical records as part of its economic reforms. The

Chinese government has increasingly cut the percentage of funds for health care, so that by 2000, 60% of the healthcare costs were paid for by the individual. The typical city doctor earns US$600–$1200 per month and sees 60–80 patients per day. The government has recently budgeted US$350 million dollars to establish disease control and prevention centers in poor areas. Many poor areas had difficulty treating SARS because of the inadequate resources ("Life as a Village Doctor," 1997).

Access to Health Care and Costs

Since the 1980s the Chinese government has had a laissez-faire policy for health care in rural areas and reverted to a self-pay system for clinic visits and hospitalization, which are now both very expensive relative to income. One average hospitalization costs 50% more than the average annual income. Access to health care in many areas is now on a sliding scale based on the ability to pay, yet many are still unable to afford health care. In urban areas medical care includes high technology. The government health insurance has given more equal access to health care, but cost inflation is now a major governmental concern. Copayments were first started to make the users more aware of health costs when accessing medical care. Medications and high-tech tests are now charged to patients and not covered by the government insurance.

A majority of China's population lives in rural areas. Those who live in urban areas are in many ways advantaged. The rural versus urban system is more intensified by a system of population registration that limits migration from rural to urban areas (Zimmer & Kwong, 2004). At present China has made great efforts to improve its public health system. Funds have been given to modify and enlarge the disease prevention and control centers and for the establishment of emergency centers and hospitals for the country. The major infrastructure has been improved. The ministry of health set up 10 national medical teams for disaster relief and disease prevention in some of the major cities. The SARS epidemic was controlled rapidly with the new infrastructure (Zheng, 2005)

The average cost of a hospital stay in Beijing is ¥11,500 or US$1400, which is the equivalent of 6 months pay for the typical Beijing resident. The largest cities in China are using 80% of the country's medical resources. China's total healthcare spending is 5.3% of the GDP (as of 2000), but 60% comes from out-of-pocket spending by individuals. In rural areas where 700 million of the population lives, most have no health insurance, and costs are much higher than most farmers can afford. The United Nations predicts that 10 million will die of HIV by 2010 (World Bank, 2002).

Serious health disparities exist in China according to Hsiao (2004). Greater than 500 million Chinese patients have inadequate basic health care and are not able to pay for care when they become seriously ill. A Chinese national health survey conducted in 1998 showed that 71% of the poor rural population was unable to pay for care when admitted to the hospital. Many refused care and left the hospitals because of financial reasons. Based on 2000 data, a comparison of rural and urban health conditions revealed that urban residents in 2000 had an infant mortality rate of 11.8 per 1000 live births as compared to 37 per 1000 in rural areas. Residents in western rural areas had an infant mortality rate of 52.3 per 1000 live births (Hsiao, 2004).

Health Priorities

China has had a rapid growth in social and economic development that has created a demand for high-quality health care. The life expectancy of the average person has increased, and this will create an aging population with chronic health problems. The leading cause of death in those 1–44 years is injuries. About 750,000 deaths and 3.5 million hospitalizations occur each year. More people are using motorcycles and cars, and fewer people are walking or using bicycles. As a result of changes in diet and activity, cardiovascular disease is increasing rapidly. About 2.6 million deaths occur annually from this problem. By 2020 it is projected that 13 million will die annually from this disease. Mental health problems account for about 20% of total diseases (George Institute for International Health, 2003).

Respiratory Problems

China's movement towards a market economy has increased incomes and improved health indicators; yet, there still remains a problem with pollution from coal combustion, which is damaging the air, water, and ultimately the agriculture, which in turn affects the residents' health. Of the 10 most polluted cities of the world, China has seven of them. China remains the world's second highest emitter (the United States is first) of carbon dioxide emissions, mainly from industry. With the help of the United Nations and the United States, China hopes to have a multimillion dollar energy strategy to combat pollution (Zhang & Cai, 2003).

Respiratory diseases are now a widespread and serious issue. With China's tremendous growth it is also taking a heavy toll on the environment and public health. Currently there are high rates of smog from industrial and traffic pollution that is causing very high rates of respiratory infections and chronic illnesses. China relies heavily on coal that contains high levels of sulfur; it is used for 70% of its domestic energy needs. A new environmental law was passed in 2003 by the Chinese government to encourage the country to burn less coal for fuel and use cleaner coal-burning technologies as used in Japan and the West (Zhang & Cai, 2003).

Tobacco smoking, especially among adult males, has been an increasingly growing problem in China and has caused many respiratory diseases and deaths. China makes and sells more cigarettes than any other country in the world and has more than 320 million smokers, which represents about 25% of the population. Rates are highest among adult men who have a 67% smoking rate. Four percent of all females smoke. This number is very significant because cigarette smoking has become the leading cause of preventable deaths in China and the rest of the world. It seems inevitable that China will have a tremendous increase in mortality from smoking-related diseases such as chronic obstructive pulmonary disease (COPD), lung cancer, and pulmonary tuberculosis (Watts, 2004a; Zhang & Cai, 2003).

Mental Health

Mental health is a major issue in China today because of the rapid social and economic changes. Changes today include financial losses from bad business deals and gambling; higher rates of extramarital affairs, family violence, and divorce; rising rates of substance use and abuse; weakening of the traditional family values and relationships; large numbers of rural migrants seeking employment in larger urban environments; a widening gap between the rich and poor; work-related stress; and a faster pace of life. Eighty percent of the country's healthcare budget goes to the urban residents; yet, the urban people represent only 30% of the total population. Funds for mental health are very limited for the rural population who cannot afford the out-of-pocket costs for mental health care. Shanghai, the largest population in China, boasts having the most comprehensive mental healthcare system in the country (Chang & Kleinman, 2002).

According to the World Health Organization's 2003 data, 13% of the population has psychological problems, and 16 million people in China suffer from serious mental illness. Every year in China there are 280,000 people who commit suicide, accounting for 25% of the entire world's suicide statistics. Another 20–50 million people per year attempt suicide. Suicide accounts for the fifth leading cause of death of people 15–35 years of age. The suicide rate in China is three times higher in rural areas as compared to urban areas. This rate is 25% higher among women than men, which is contrary to many other nations of the world. Reasons for the higher rates for female suicides in rural areas are due primarily to poverty, low status of rural women, forced marriages, family violence and conflict, chronic stress, and no hope for the future. Men in rural areas are often absent from the homes for long periods of time, leaving the women to work in the fields, take care of children, cook, and care for the house (Pochagina, n.d.).

Nutrition

Throughout China there has been a change in diet and physical activity and overall body composition patterns. During the past 10 years, the number of people living in China in absolute poverty has significantly been reduced. The proportion of those extremely poor decreased from 20% to 6% during the same period. As a result of this change in economics, the prevalence of obesity and diet-related noncommunicable diseases has increased more rapidly than in industrialized societies. Diets have shifted from high carbohydrates to high fat and high-density energy foods leading to diseases from overweight and obesity such as diabetes, stroke, cancer, and cardiovascular diseases (Du, Mroz, Zhai, & Popkin, 2004).

Cardiovascular disease is the leading cause of mortality in the world, and that includes China and other developing countries. China and other developing nations have been experiencing an epidemic in cardiovascular disease during the last few decades mainly because of lifestyle and diet changes. Currently there is a prevalence of metabolic syndrome and overweight individuals among adults in China. Metabolic syndrome is characterized by a cluster of problems that consists of abdominal obesity, increased blood pressure and glucose concentration, and elevated cholesterol levels. Obesity is a risk factor not only for cardiovascular disease but also type 2 diabetes, hypertension, and cancer. Excess weight is also a cause for osteoarthritis and gall bladder disease (Gu et al., 2005; Dang, Yan, Yamamoto, Wang, & Zeng, 2004).

HIV/AIDS

HIV/AIDS entered China in 1985, and 20 years later the epidemic has continued to spread at an alarming rate (see Figure 2-5). The government estimates that there are about 3 million paid blood donors in China, and 12.5% are HIV positive. The number of yearly reported AIDS cases has increased at an average rate of 30% per year from 1995 to 2000. In 2001 the increase was 58%, and in 2003 the rate increased to 122%. The WHO and the U.S. CDC estimate that 840,000 people are living in China with HIV, and 80,000 have AIDS. Inadequate surveillance systems make it difficult to assess the full magnitude of the epidemic. About 80% of China's HIV/AIDS population lives in rural areas of the country. Most of those with this disease are IV drug users and blood donators, who gave the disease

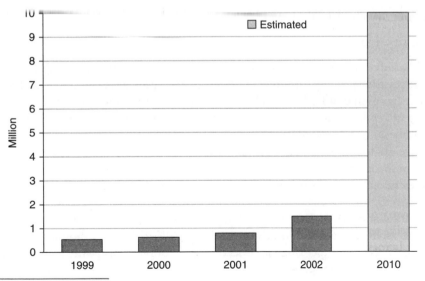

Figure 2-5 Current and future estimates of people with AIDS in China.

Source: Data from UNAIDS.

to their wives and then to their babies. Homosexuality is forbidden in this communist country, yet 17.7% received this disease from homosexual transmission. The central government is now considering the possibility of supplying free antiretroviral drugs to AIDS patients not covered by health insurance. Few people (6%) in China who have HIV/AIDS have been tested, and they continue to spread the disease to their partners and babies. Unless effective prevention strategies are quickly begun, 10 million are estimated to become infected by the end of 2010 (Wu, Rou, & Cui, 2004).

The general population of China knows little about the sexual practices that increase the risk of contracting HIV infection. HIV/AIDS prevention in the general population has been rare. Those now living in China with HIV/AIDS face severe discrimination and have limited access to healthcare services, especially in the rural areas (Chen, Han, & Holzemer, 2004). Recently the government promised to provide free HIV tests to anyone who wanted one, and fully cover treatment costs for poorer patients (Watts, 2004b; Kanabus, 2005).

Tuberculosis

Dye (2004) reported that China has an estimated 1.4 million tuberculosis cases per year, which is greater than any other country in the world except India. The World Bank funded the first TB survey and a new project followed, which aimed to treat the cases and prevent new ones. The prevalence of the disease fell by 30% in seven years. Hu, (2004) reported in a recent study that the prevalence of TB is down 30% after the World Health project was initiated to prevent and reduce TB in China. Only 30–40% of people with TB are diagnosed and treated each year.

Population Control

China has only 7% arable land and has 22% of the world's population. To feed, house, and promote good health care the "one child per family" policy was established. The advantages are that each child will have a healthier life, family costs will be lower, and the child will get a better education. Women will be able to focus on their careers as well as care for their families. The government claims that this policy has prevented mass starvation. One problem is that Chinese parents usually rely on their children, especially their sons, for support in their old age. The result is that most couples want a male child if they can have only one child. As a result many female babies have been killed, and female fetuses have been aborted. Some women have stated that they have had forced abortions of their second child, and others have stated that they have had forced sterilization. At present there is a surplus of men and some men are having difficulty in finding wives. Also as the population is getting older there is concern about couples not having a child to care for them in old age (Population–China, 2004).

Traditional Medicine

The practice of traditional Chinese medicine was strongly promoted by Chinese leaders, and it has remained a major part of health care. Western medicine gained acceptance in the 1970s and 1980s. The goal of China's medical personnel is to synthesize the use of both Western and traditional Chinese medicine; yet, this practice has not always worked out so easily. Physicians trained in traditional medicine and those trained in Western medicine are very separate groups with different basic ideas. Traditional Chinese medicine uses herbal treatments, acupuncture, acupressure, moxibustion, and cupping of skin with heated bamboo. These approaches are very effective in treating minor ailments and chronic diseases, and produce far fewer side effects. Some more serious and acute problems are also treated by traditional medicine (Wikipedia, 2007b).

South Africa

Geography

South Africa is located at the southern tip of the continent of Africa. It borders on Botswana, Lesotho, Mozambique, Namibia, Swaziland, and Zimbabwe, as well as the Atlantic and Indian Oceans. Its climate is mostly arid, with a subtropical region along the east coast. Natural resources include gold, chromium, antimony, coal, iron ore, manganese, nickel, phosphates, tin, uranium, gem diamonds, platinum, copper, vanadium, salt, and natural gas (CIA, 2005b).

Population

South Africa's population as of 2005 is approximately 44 million. The country is currently experiencing the world's highest rate of people with HIV/AIDS, as well as the world's highest mortality rate from this disease (see Table 2-5).

Ethnic groups include the following (CIA, 2005b):

- Black African (79%)
- White (9.6%)
- Colored (8.9%)
- Indian/Asian (2.5%)

Religions practiced include the following (CIA, 2005b):

- Zion Christian (11.1%)
- Pentecostal/Charismatic (8.2%)
- Catholic (7.1%)
- Methodist (6.8%)
- Dutch Reformed (6.7%)
- Anglican (3.8%)
- Other Christian (36%)
- Islam (1.5%)

TABLE 2-5   Rate of South Africans with HIV/AIDS

Population	44 million
Birth–14 years	30.3%
15–64 years	64.5%
65+ years	5.2%
Population growth rate	–.31%
Death rate	21.32 per 1000 people
Infant mortality	61.81 per 1000 live births
Life expectancy	43.27 years
HIV/AIDS adult prevalence rate	21.5 % (2003 estimate)
	5 million people (20% of 15–49-year-old population and 35% of all women of childbearing age)

Source: Adapted from US Department of State, Bureau of African Affairs, 2005.

- Other (2.3%)
- Unspecified (1.4%)
- None (15.1%)

Languages spoken in South Africa include the following (CIA, 2005b):

- IsiZulu (23.8%)
- IsiXhosa (17.6%)
- Afrikaans (13.3%)
- Sepedi (9.4%)
- English (8.2%)
- Setswana 8.2%
- Sesotho 7.9%
- Xitsonga 4.4%
- Other 7.2%

The literacy rate of the total population is 86.4%.

South Africa has the largest population of people of European descent in Africa, the largest Indian population in Africa, as well as the largest colored (mixed European and African) group in Africa. It is one of the most ethnically diverse countries in Africa. The country has had a history of racial problems between the black majority and the white minority. The Apartheid policy was introduced in 1948 and ended in 1990. Crime remains a big problem in South Africa, ranking first in the world in murder by firearms, manslaughter, rape, and assault. It also ranks fourth in the world for robbery, according to a survey done by the United Nations during 1998–2000. Problems also persist with illegal drug transportation and sales (Wikipedia, 2007a).

The population is relatively young, with about one-third of the people under age 15. Fertility is declining, and there is an increase in persons over 60 years. The healthcare services accommodate not only services for obstetrics, pediatrics, and adolescents, but also for the aging population as well. A large number of the populations (18% in some areas) are illiterate. Half of all households use electricity for cooking (Bradshaw & Nannan, 2004).

Government

The government is a republic, formally named the Republic of South Africa (RSA), with a legal system based on Roman-Dutch law and English common law. The system of government is also called a parliamentary democracy, with its capital located in the city of Pretoria, and comprising nine provinces. (CIA, 2005b; US Department of State, Bureau of African Affairs, 2005).

Economy

South Africa has a two-tiered economy. One is similar to other economically strong developed countries, and the other is more like developing countries with only the basic infrastructure. South Africa has well-developed financial, legal, communication, energy and transportation systems. It has the world's 10th largest stock exchange and a modern infrastructure. It has the best telecommunications system in Africa. But it also has a very high unemployment rate of 26.2% (40% according to Wikipedia, 2005), much of which is a remainder of the Apartheid era (CIA, 2005b; US Department of State, Dept. of African Affairs, 2005).

The country's wealth is unevenly distributed, with the minority whites having a much larger portion of the wealth and the majority blacks having a very challenging existence with difficulty finding well-paying jobs. The country has an overall gross domestic product (GDP) per capita of US$11,100 (2004 estimate). Its industries include mining (the world's largest producer of platinum, gold, and chromium), auto assembly, metalworking, machinery, textile, iron and steel, chemicals, fertilizers, ship repair, and foods. The main agricultural products are corn, wheat, sugarcane, fruits, vegetables, beef, poultry, mutton, wool, and dairy products (CIA, 2005b; US Department of State, Dept. of African Affairs, 2005).

Healthcare System

South Africa's healthcare system consists of a large public sector and a smaller, yet fast-growing private sector. Basic primary health care is offered free to all residents of the country, but is highly specialized; high-tech care is limited to only those who can afford private care. The dilemma is that the government contributes about 40% of health care costs for the public health, yet 80% of the population uses the services. The public hospitals are continuously growing in numbers, and the mining industry has their own 60 hospitals and clinics in different locations within the country (US Department of State, Dept. of African Affairs, 2005).

Since 1978 the country has decentralized the basic primary healthcare system and has focused on a district healthcare system run by local governments. Disparities exist between municipalities, depending on the funding from the local area. Poor municipalities with little funding have little allocated for their healthcare budgets. Rural areas are poorly funded as compared to urban areas. Poor women, especially in rural areas, are often seen by a nurse or nurse midwife for prenatal care and delivery as compared to urban women who more often receive prenatal care and delivery from a physician (Harrison, 2005).

State of Health in South Africa

The general state of health in South Africa is dependent upon the quadruple burden of disease, including the tremendous impact of HIV/AIDS. Also included are the high rates of injury, the problem of underdevelopment of the country as a whole, and numerous residents with chronic diseases. The largest rise in death rates of adults is in the young adult group, who are dying in increasing numbers from AIDS. Deaths from tuberculosis, pneumonia, and diarrhea are also increasing rapidly. The greatest cause of death in South Africa is HIV/AIDS (infants and young adults), followed by homicide (young adult men), tuberculosis, road traffic accidents, and diarrhea. Noncommunicable disease deaths are found in high numbers in the 60 and older group of the population. Causes of death for children under 5 years are ranked as follows (Bradshaw & Nannan, 2004):

1. HIV/AIDS
2. Low birth weight
3. Diarrhea
4. Lower respiratory infections
5. Protein–energy malnutrition
6. Neonatal infections
7. Birth asphyxia and birth trauma
8. Congenital heart disease
9. Road traffic accidents
10. Bacterial meningitis

There is a significant increase in the use of tobacco, which in turn is causing more lung diseases, especially lung cancer. Campaigns to deter youth from smoking and encourage smokers to stop are being led by healthcare organizations in increasing numbers. Throughout South Africa there is a major change in diet in types and quantity, with movement away from traditional plant foods to high fat and high sugar foods, with low fiber. As a result of this change overweight and obesity are now chronic problems among South African people. Urban people are more likely to be obese than rural people, and those over 65 years are less likely to be obese. South Africans are now more sedentary than previously. Alcohol consumption is now also increasing especially among males. It not only is causing chronic diseases such as liver and esophageal cancer, but also contributing to homicides, violence and motor vehicle accidents (Bradshaw & Nannan, 2004).

Racial Inequalities

Numerous racial inequalities continue to exist in the wake of Apartheid. Unemployment is much higher within the black or African population compared to the other ethnic groups. Whites are the most employed group. Half of Africans live in formal housing (solid structures with indoor plumbing and electricity) compared with 95% of whites (Bradshaw & Nannan, 2004).

Healthcare Personnel

There is a shortage of nursing and other healthcare personnel in South Africa, as well as a maldistribution problem. The majority of trained nursing and allied health professionals work in the private sector that serves much less of the general population than the public sector. In addition more trained health personnel work in urban rather than rural areas. Doctors, especially those with more subspecialty training, are more likely to be working also in the private sector and in urban areas. Also there is a problem with skilled health personnel leaving South Africa for other countries, such as the United States, Canada, New Zealand, the United Kingdom, and Australia. South Africa is actively trying to recruit nurses and doctors especially to work in the underserved areas. In addition, to healthcare personnel trained in Western medicine, there are 200,000 traditional healers who practice in South Africa (Padarath, Ntuli, & Berthiaume, 2004).

Chronic Diseases

South Africa, a developing country, currently is experiencing a vast increase in the prevalence of chronic diseases, which historically were more associated with developed countries. Health problems such as hypertension, elevated cholesterol, alcohol and tobacco use, and obesity are now being observed in South Africa in greater frequencies. Risks for chronic diseases include: age, gender, tobacco and alcohol use, diet, and physical activity. Others include family history and genetic background. Most chronic diseases are preventable with modification of lifestyle behaviors. Changes in activity and diet can greatly influence the risk for numerous chronic diseases. The greatest causes of deaths in South Africa include:

- HIV/AIDS
- Heart disease
- Homicide and violence
- Stroke
- Tuberculosis
- Lower respiratory infections
- Road traffic accidents
- Diarrhea diseases
- Hypertension
- Diabetes

All of the above are chronic diseases, with the exception of homicide and violence and traffic accidents.

Communicable Diseases

Sexually transmitted infections (STIs) continue to be one of the most common problems in adolescents and young adults in South Africa. About 10% of adults who go to a health clinic have concerns about a STI. About 4 million people have these diseases per year. Healthcare workers are involved in treatments and prevention measures, such as counseling, condom promotion, and partner notification (Shabalala et al., 2002).

Tuberculosis is a chronic pulmonary and extrapulmonary disease characterized by positive acid-fast stains or cultures of *Mycobacterium tuberculosis*. A TB skin test provides evidence of the infection, if positive. A chest X-ray is taken to confirm shadowing, reflecting lung invasions. Cervical lymph node swelling may also be present. Tuberculosis is a huge problem in South Africa. South Africa ranks seventh in the world in highest number of cases, with 556 cases per 10,000 people. Part of the reason for the high prevalence is improved case detection brought on by the HIV/AIDS epidemic, especially among young adults. Poverty and overcrowding are also related to the high rate. Other factors include the increase and extent of drug resistance, particularly multidrug resistance (MDR) (Mwinga & Fourie, 2004). A recent study reported that 55% of the people with TB were also HIV positive. Those affected by HIV/AIDS are five times more likely to develop TB. One third of the 40 million in all of Africa with HIV/AIDS also have TB. In sub-Saharan Africa, the numbers are actually even much higher. The South African Medical Research Council forecasts that there will be 300,000 cases of TB this year and 30,000 deaths from it in the country—a fatality rate of 10% compared to having one of the lowest rates in Africa before the advent of HIV/AIDS (Bamford, Loveday, & Verkuijl, 2004; Nullis-Kapp, 2005).

At present approximately 54% of patients have documentation of being cured of TB as a result of treatment. The Eastern Cape, a very poor rural area with limited resources, has an extremely high incidence of TB with 675 per 100,000 (Bamford, Loveday, & Verkuijl, 2004).

Cholera is an intestinal malady caused by the *Vibrio cholerae* organism. Cholera results in loss of large volumes of watery stool (excrement), leading to rapid dehydration and shock, resulting in death without treatment. Fatality for untreated cholera is 50%. Those with cholera get rapid breathing, vomiting and painless diarrhea, and go into metabolic acidosis. Appropriate oral or intravenous rehydration therapy is needed to replace lost fluids and electrolytes. It is epidemic in Asia, Africa, India, and South America (Sack, Sack, Nair, & Siddique, 2005). Cholera has been a significant burden in South Africa. It is one of the diseases requiring notification of the World Health Organization. In 2000–2001 a cholera epidemic occurred, with 106,389 reported cases. Cholera deaths result from poor sanitation and poor water supply. An estimated 18 million South Africans have no basic sanitation. Of this group, 75.8% live in rural areas. Almost 50% of those children go to schools where there is only a pit for toilet use. By 2002, after initiatives were taken for those without water and sanitation, the rate of cholera infection was reduced to 7 million (Duse, da Silva, & Zeitsman, 2003; Mudzanani, Ratsaka-Mathokoa, Mahlasela, Netshidzivhani, & Mugero, 2004).

In the continent of Africa greater than 38% of the people have no access to safe water, which is higher than any other place in the world. In South Africa there were 12 million people without safe water and 20 million without sanitation facilities. By the year 2020 South Africa's population demands will exceed its water supply by 8%. Health maintenance is dependent on an adequate water supply and adequate sanitation facilities (toilets). It is vital in hospitals and healthcare clinics to have adequate clean water and sanitation for prevention and treatment of diseases and illnesses. A clean and adequate supply is necessary for simple handwashing in patient care. In short supply areas it is necessary for healthcare workers to disinfect water if unclean and teach techniques to patients. Several techniques include boiling, chorine tablets, filtration, and clean storage (Duse, da Silva, & Zeitsman, 2003).

Malaria is a serious disease transmitted to humans by the bite of the Anopheles mosquito. Symptoms include fever and a flulike illness including chills, headache, muscle aches, and fatigue. It can also cause anemia and jaundice. If not treated promptly it can cause kidney failure, coma, and death. Malaria can be prevented by antimalaria drugs, such as atovaquone/proguanil, doxycycline, and mefloquine. Chloroquine is *not* effective for malaria prevention in South Africa. Protection from mosquito bites is also very important (CDC, 2004).

Malaria is a major health problem in sub-Saharan Africa and affects great numbers of young children and pregnant women. It is the main cause of 20% of all deaths of young children in Africa. About 95% of the infections in South Africa are due to *Plasmodium falciparum*, the microbe that lives in the gut of the Anopheles mosquito. Transmission is seasonal, with October to February having the most cases. Use of drugs for treatment and vector control by spraying has been effective. South Africa along with five other countries was given permission by the United Nations Environmental Programme to use DDT for public health use only. The use of DDT in 2000 made a significant change in the mortality and morbidity of this disease. It should be noted however, that DDT is a banned pesticide in the United States and most developed and developing countries (Moonasar et al, 2004).

South Africa has an estimated 4–6 million people living with HIV/AIDS. The national prevalence of HIV in pregnant women is 26.2%. A study published on AIDS by the South African Medical Research Council concluded that for 2000–2001, the prevalence of HIV/AIDS was almost three times as high as listed in a government statistical report. Eighty percent of the causes of mortality due to AIDS in men, and 70% in women, was written on death certificates as TB or lower respiratory tract infections. In children, three times as many deaths due to AIDS was written as lower respiratory tract infections, diarrheal disease, and protein-energy malnutrition (South Africa needs to face the truth, 2005).

Greater than 280,000 babies were born exposed to HIV. The highest rates are among newborns and breast-fed children. Poverty increases the vulnerability to HIV infection somewhat, because those people usually have less education and less access to information about safe sex practices. High unemployment rates and lack of support may deny mothers access to receiving care in clinics. Access to antiretroviral therapy (ART) drugs for HIV/AIDS patients in South Africa is very limited. In 2002, of the 500,000 who could immediately benefit from the medications, 20,000 to 40,000 were receiving treatment, and of those who were receiving treatment, most were receiving care in the private sector. In 2003 the government made ART more available to the public sector. One problem in providing these drugs is the very high cost for the medications and tests (Doherty & Colvin, 2004).

In 2005 in South Africa, where less than 3% of people who need ART actually receive it, private companies are supplying drugs directly to employees who are HIV positive. The corporate sector is presently taking more responsibility than ever before (Venter, 2005). Some of the social factors that make South African women vulnerable to HIV/AIDS relate to the position of women in society and practice of safe sex. Women are often born into a low social status in South Africa. Physiologically men are able to pass the virus to women more easily than women to men, making a woman twice as likely to become infected. Women are exposed to the HIV virus and many other STIs because of the greater mucosal surface exposed to pathogens during sexual activity, particularly young girls, who are not fully mature. In addition violence against women is very high in South Africa. Incidents of rape in South Africa are considered one of the highest in the world, yet are seldom reported. Rapes of female children are exceptionally high. A myth that "having sex with a virgin will cure AIDS" remains part of the increase in child rape. In addition, a very high incidence of husband–boyfriend violence also occurs. Women can be beaten if they refuse to have sex with their partners. Women often remain in abusive relationships for financial dependency reasons. No matter what the reason, violence against women increases the risk of HIV and STI infections. In South Africa 30% of women are head of the households, are often poor, have no financial aid from men, and consequently have a very unfavorable economic position and little power. Selling sex can often be a survival strategy and can also make them even more vulnerable to HIV. Young girls may trade sex for money, clothes, or food (Ackermann & de Klerk, 2001).

Another problem in South Africans is the increasing number of orphans who are left because both of their parents have died of AIDS. Grandparents are trying to provide care for as many as 10 to 20 grandchildren after they have lost their children. Also many AIDS orphans are left alone to care for themselves. There is a lost generation of street children who have no education and have few economic resources. Some sell sex in order to keep themselves and siblings fed. Some are HIV infected and some are not, but many will die regardless of their situation (Sowell, 2000).

Aging

The South African population is aging because of declining fertility rates and decreases in life expectancy with those infected with HIV. The proportion of older people is 7.3% (2001). Those in their 70s represent 3.2% of the population, and those in their 80s represent 1%. Even with the AIDS epidemic the numbers of aging adults is expected to be 30 per 100 in 2015. There will be a large number of adults 65 and older, as compared to the number of children. AIDS affects the number of older adults the least. By 2015 there will be 4.25 million older adults, representing 9.5% of the total population (Joubert & Bradshaw, 2004).

The older black adults of South Africa are among the poorest people in the country and often lack credit or employment. Most have lived through Apartheid and have been poor all their lives. Fifty-eight percent of older adult Africans have no education; in Limpopa the rate is 74%, and in Mpurmalanga the rate is 66%. Many older adults, especially the Africans, who live in poverty and have little or no formal education, are now taking care of their children and/or grandchildren, which is a very difficult burden. The main source of income is Social Protection (Old Age Pension), which is provided for men 65 and older and for women 60 and older (Joubert & Bradshaw, 2004).

Traditional Medicine

The Alma Ata Declaration on primary health care, in conjunction with the World Health Organization (WHO), and the United Nations International Children's Emergency Fund (UNICEF) gave international recognition to the positive role of traditional indigenous healthcare providers. Traditional practitioners and birth attendants are recognized as important people in the primary healthcare team, but not as part of the public health service. Historically Western-style health practitioners, such as Dr. David Livingston, consulted with indigenous healers on drug treatment for fevers. Within South Africa many traditional healers believe that illness cannot be directly explained in physical terms, and some believe in supernatural entities, such as spirits, that bring about illness. Some also believe in direct causal connections comparable to Western medicine. Different health-care ideologies and systems have stood side by side together in South Africa for many years. Patients may want to use both types of medicine "just to play it safe." Up to 80% of the indigenous African people are accustomed to using traditional medicine as a first means for treatment of illness. Noristan Laboratories, a large pharmaceutical company, tested 350 herbs used by indigenous healers and found that 80% had some medicinal properties. Patients are faced with two healthcare system perspectives and will most likely continue to seek care from either as they see fit. At present there is limited cooperation between the two systems (Muller & Steyn, 1999).

The indigenous flora of South Africa contains 23,404 higher plant species, and the use of many of these species for medicinal use dates back to the San people in the region more than 20,000 years ago. Traditional medicine use in South Africa is often unacknowledged by the Western-style healthcare system yet pharmacists are often well equipped to bridge the gap between indigenous medicines and Western ones (Scott, Springfield, & Coldrey, 2004).

References

Ackerman, L., & de Klerk, G. (2002). Social factors that make South African women vulnerable to HIV infection. *Health Care for Women International, 23,* 163–172.

Azcona-Cruz, M., Rothenberg, S., Schnaas, L., Zamora-Munoz, J., & Romero-Placeres, M. (2000). Lead-glazed ceramic wear and blood levels of children. *Archives of Environment Health, 55*(31), 217–222.

Bamford, L., Loveday, M., & Verkuijl, S. (2004). Health Systems Trust. *South African Health Review.* Tuberculosis. 23. Chapter 15. 213–228.

Barraza-Llorens, M., Bertozzi, S., Gonzalez-Pier, E., & Gutierrez, J. (2002). Addressing inequality in health and health care in Mexico. *Health Affairs, May/June.* Retrieved June 27, 2005, from http://www.healthaffairs.org/freecontent.v21n3/s8.htm

Booysen, F. (2003). Urban-rural inequalities in health care delivery in South Africa. *Development of Southern Africa, 20*(5), 660–674.

Bradshaw, D., & Nannan, N. (2004). Health Systems Trust. *South African Health Review.* Health Status. 23. Chapter 4. 45–58.

Brentlinger, P., Sanchez-Perez, H. J., Cedeno, M. A., Morales, G. V., Hernan, M., Micek, A., et al. (2005). Pregnancy outcomes, site of delivery, and community schisms in regions affected by the armed conflict in Chiapas, Mexico. *Social Science and Medicine, 61*(5), 1001–1014.

Centers for Disease Control and Prevention. (2004). *Malaria information for travelers to South Africa.* Retrieved June 12, 2005, from http://www.cdc.gov/travel/regionalmalaria/safrica.htm

Chang, D., & Kleinman, A. (2002). Growing pains: Mental health care in a developing China. In A. Cohen, A. Kleinman, & B. Saraceno (Eds.), *The world mental health casebook* (pp. 85–97). New York: Kluwer.

Chen, W., Han, M., & Holzemer, W. (2004). Nurse's knowledge, attitudes, and practice related to HIV transmission in Northeastern China. *AIDS Patient Care and STDs, 18*(7), 417–422.

Central Intelligence Agency. (2005a). China. *The World Factbook*. Retrieved June 12, 2005, from http://cia/goov/cia/publications/factbook/goes/ch.html

Central Intelligence Agency. (2005b). South Africa. *The World Factbook*. Retrieved August 24, 2005, from http://www.cia.gov/cia/publications/factbook/geos/sf.html

Cifuentes, E., Mazari-Hiriart, M., Carneiro, F., Bianchi, F., and Gonzalez, D. (2002). The risk of enteric diseases in young children and environmental indicators in sentinel areas of Mexico City. *International Journal of Environmental Health Research, 12,* 53–62.

d'Adesky, A. (2002). *Mexico's other AIDS epidemic elicits scant response*. Retrieved June 18, 2005, from http://www.egis.com/pubs/amfar/2002/AM021001.html

Dang, S., Yan, H., Yamamoto, S., Wang, X., & Zeng, L. (2004). Poor nutritional status of younger Tibetan children living at high altitudes. *European Journal of Clinical Nutrition, 58,* 938–946.

Day, C. & Hedberg, C. (2004). Health Systems Trust. *South African Health Review*. 23. Human Resources. Chapter 23. 349–405.

Doherty, T., & Colvin, M. (2004). Health Systems Trust. *South African Health Review*. HIV/AIDS. 23. 191–212.

Du, S., Mroz, T., Zhai, F. & Popkin, B. (2004). Rapid income growth adversely affects diet quality in China—particularly the poor. *Social Science and Medicine, 59,* 1505–1515.

Duse, A., da Silva, M., & Zeitsman, I. (2003). Coping with hygiene in South Africa, a water scarce country. *International Journal of Environmental Research, 13,* S95–S105.

Dye, C. (2004). The effect of tuberculosis control in China. *Lancet, 363,* 417–422.

George Institute for International Health. (2003). China program. Factsheet.

Gu, D., Reynolds, K., Wu, X., Chen, J., Duan, X., Reynolds, R., et al. (2005). Prevalence of the metabolic syndrome and overweight among adults in China. *Lancet, 365,* 1398–1405.

Harrison, S. (2004). Health Systems Trust. *South African Health Review*. 23. Medical Schemes. Chapter 21. 291–293.

Hesketh, T., & Zhu, W. (2002). *Health in China: from Mao to market reform*. United Nations Development Programme, China.

Hsiao, W. (2004). Disparity in health: The underbelly of China's economic development. *Harvard China Review, Spring,* 64–70.

Hu, T. (2004). Financing and organization of China's health care. *Bulletin of the World Health Organization, 82*(7), 532–538.

Hunt, L., Glantz, N., & Halperin, D. (2002). Childbirth care-seeking behavior in Chiapas. *Health Care for Women International, 23,* 98–118.

International Youth Foundation. (n.d.). *The situation of children and youth in Oaxaca, Mexico*. Retrieved June 27, 2005, from http://www.ivfnet.org/document.cfm/41/section2/19

Joubert, J., & Bradshaw, D. (2004). Health Systems Trust. *South African Health Review*. 23. Health of Older Persons. Chapter 11. 147–162.

Kanabus, A. (2005). *HIV and AIDS in China*. Retrieved June 12, 2005, from http://www.avert.org/aidschina.htm

Life as a village doctor in southwest China. (1997). *Newsweek/Healthweek*. Retrieved June 12, 2005, from http://www.nurseweek.com/features/dispatches/China/971023.html

Lim, M., Yang, H., Zhang, T., Feng, W., & Zhou, Z. (2004). Public perceptions of private health care in socialist China. *Data Watch, Nov/Dec,* 222–234.

Markus, F. (2004). *China's ailing health care*. Retrieved June 12, 2005, from http://news.bbc.co.uk/2/hi/asia-pacific/4062523.stm

Marsh, W., & Hentges, K. (1988). Mexican folk remedies and conventional medical care. *Texas Medicine, 37*(3), 257–262.

Mexico: Basic health care for indigenous people. (2000). Retrieved June 27, 2005, from http://www.msf.org/content/page.cfm?articleid=6589CA90-DC2C-11D4-2010060084A6

Moonasar, D., Johnson, C., Maloba, B., Kruger, P., le Grange, K., Mthembu, J., et al. (2004). Health Systems Trust. *South African Health Review.* Malaria . Chapter 17. 23. 243–256.

Mudzanani, L., Ratsaka-Mathokoa, M., Mahlasela, L., Netshidzivhani, P., & Mugero, C. (2004). Health Systems Trust. *South African Health Review.* Cholera. 23. Chapter 18. 257–264.

Muller, A., & Steyn, M. (1999). Culture and the feasibility of a partnership between Westernized medical practitioners and traditional healers. *Society in Transition, 30*(2), 142–156.

Mwinga, A., & Fourie, B. (2004). Prospects for new tuberculosis treatment in Africa. *Tropical Medicine and International Health, 9*(7), 827–832.

Nullis-Kapp, C. (2005). Africa is worst hit by dual epidemic. *Bulletin of the World Health Organization, 83*(3), 165–166.

Padarath, A., Ntuli, A., & Berthiaume, L. (2004). Health Systems Trust. *South African Health Review.* 23. Human Resources. Chapter 22. 299–318.

Pan American Health Organization. (2002). *Mexico. Core health data selected indicators.* Retrieved July 22, 2002, from http://paho.org/English/DD?AIS/ep_484.htm

Pochagina, O. (n.d.). Suicide in present day China. *Far Eastern Affairs.*

Population–China. (2004). Putting on the breaks on reproduction. *Canada and the World, December,* 18–21.

Reyes-Beaman, S., Jagger, C., Garcia-Pena, C., Munoz, O., Beaman, P., Stafford, B., et al. (2005). Active life expectancy of older people in Mexico. *Disability and Rehabilitation, 27*(5), 213–219.

Rivera, J., Barquera, S., Gonzalez-Cossio, T., Olaiz, G., & Sepulveda, J. (2004). Nutritional transition in Mexico and other Latin American countries. *Nutrition Reviews, 62*(7), S149–S157.

Sack, D., Sack, R. B., Nair, G. B., & Siddique, A. K. (2005). Cholera. *Lancet, 363,* 223–33.

San Joaquin County Health Department. (2002). *State health department issues health warning on lead-contaminated chapulines (grasshoppers).* Retrieved June 18, 2005, from http://www.co.san-joaquin.ca.us/EHS/General_Info/News_and_Health_Warnings/Articles

Scott, G., Springfield, E. P., & Coldrey, N. (2004). A pharmacognostical study of 26 South African plant species used in traditional medicine. *Pharmaceutical Biology, 42*(3), 186–213.

Shabalala, N., Strebel, A., Shefer, T., Simbayi, L, Wilson, T., Ratele, K., et al. (2002). Evaluation of the quality of care for sexually transmitted infections in primary care centers in South Africa. *South African Journal of Psychology, 32*(4), 33–40.

Smith, N. (2003). *Nutrition among the Zapotec Indians of Oaxaca: Perceptions and practices during pregnancy and infancy.* New York: The Tinker Foundation.

South Africa needs to face the truth about HIV mortality. (2005). *Lancet, 365,* 546.

Sowell, R. (2000). AIDS orphans: The cost of doing nothing. *Journal of the Association of Nurses in AIDS Care, 11*(6), 15–16.

US Department of State, Bureau of African Affairs. (2005). *South Africa.* Retrieved June 12, 2005, from http://www.state.gov.r/pa/ei/bgn/2898.htm

Venter, L. (2005). Firms fill antiretroviral gap in South Africa. *Lancet, 365,* 1215–1216.

Vista Community Clinic. (2004). *Cultural awareness program. Cultural facts.* Retrieved July 22, 2005, from http://www.clas-sd.org/Cultural%20Facts%20-Past/culturalfacts%202004-04.htm

Wahlberg, D. (2004). *Folic acid could ease threat from corn toxin.* Retrieved June 1, 2005, from http://ajc.printthis.clickability.com/pt/cpt?action=cpt&title=folic+acid+could+easde+threat

Watts, J. (2004a). China promises to dash hopes of tobacco industry giants. *Lancet, 363.* 50.

Watts, J. (2004b). China's shift in HIV/AIDS policy marks turnaround on health. *Lancet, 363,* 1370–1371.

World Health Organization. (2004). Country: Mexico. Retrieved June 27, 2005, from http://www3.who.int/whosis/country/indicators.cfm?country=mex

Wikipedia. (2005). *China.* Retrieved June 11, 2005, from http://wikipedia.org/wiki/china

Wikipedia. (2007a). *South Africa.* Retrieved August 6, 2007, from http://en.wikipedia.org/wiki/South_Africa

Wikipedia. (2007b). *Traditional chinese medicine.* Retrieved August 6, 2007, from http://en.wikipedia.org/wiki/Traditional_Chinese_Medicine

World Almanac Education Group. (2004). Mexico. *World almanac and book of facts.* 817.

World Bank Group. (2002). *Beyond transition. Curing China's ailing health care system.* Retrieved June 12, 2005, from http://www.worldbank.org/transitionnewsletter/aprmayjun03/pg9.htm

Wu, Z., Rou, K., & Cui, H. (2004). The HIV/AIDS epidemic in China: History, current strategies and future challenges. *AIDS Education and Prevention, 16*(suppl A), 7–17.

Wyatt, C. J., & Tejas, M. A. (2000). Nutrient intake and growth of preschool children from different socioeconomic regions in the City of Oaxaca, Mexico. *Annals of Nutrition and Metabolism, 44,* 14–20.

Zhang, H., & Cai, B. (2003). The impact of tobacco on lung health in China. *Respirology, 8,* 17–21.

Zheng, C. (2005). China making big progress in public health care. *China Education and Research Network.* Retrieved June 12, 2005, from http://www.edu.cn/20050114/3126783.shtml

Zimmer, Z., & Kwong, J. (2004). Socioeconomic status and health among older adults in rural and urban China. *Journal of Aging and Health, 16*(1), 44–70.

Chapter 3

Global Perspectives on Economics and Health Care

Marsha Burke, Govind Hariharan, Robert A. Lipson, and Caroline Aultman

> A girl born in Chile in 1910 could expect to live only to age 33. Since then, her life expectancy has more than doubled to its current level of 78 years. . . . Her life is not only much longer, it is much healthier as well.
>
> —Jamison, 2006

Introduction

Across the world there is tremendous variation in the way health care is provided and funded and most importantly in healthcare outcomes. Yet concern about the financing of health care has become a matter of great concern in every economy. In developed countries, rapid growth in medical innovations and technology and the cost of caring for an aging population have combined to make soaring healthcare costs a primary concern. Developing countries plagued with a struggling economy find themselves hard-pressed to find sources of funding for providing even basic medical care for a growing population.

Economics is the study of how to allocate scarce resources across unlimited wants and needs. It is no wonder then that in a world faced with the problem of ever-growing demands on its healthcare resources amid tightening budgets, the field of health economics has grown exponentially more important in academic and policy settings. Health economists are often interested in analyzing whether healthcare resources are utilized efficiently and whether the proper incentives and healthcare systems exist or can be created to ensure efficiency. The current system for the provision of health care in countries such as the United States is rather complex, often with the patient receiving care from providers who are paid by a third party such as a private or public health insurance organization. However, there are currently more than 45 million people in the United States without insurance coverage. Providing unpaid medical care for these uninsured segments of the population results in cost shifting that makes health insurance more expensive. Since the early 1970s, the emergence of managed care organizations in the United States (often centered around health insurance companies) with its emphasis on cost effectiveness, return

73

on investments, and aligning incentives properly, highlighted the importance of utilizing economic principles in health care.

In this chapter, we compare and contrast five countries, Canada, India, Japan, Ukraine, and the United States. The choice of these particular countries for analysis was driven by the stark differences in their systems for providing health care and in their economic strength. Of these five countries, Canada, Japan, and the United States are highly industrialized countries with high per capita gross domestic product (GDP) and high levels of expenditure on health care. Yet there are significant differences between them in the levels of public and private expenditures on health care, the type of health systems they use, and, by some measures, the levels of health of their population. India has a rapidly growing economy with the second largest population in the world faced with problems of inequality. Ukraine is a newly independent former Soviet republic recovering from an economic recession and has an archaic healthcare system.

In the first section, we briefly describe the history and structure of the healthcare systems in each country, pointing out some of the critical problems in each. In the second section, we conduct a comparative analysis. In the third section, we develop the economic concept of productivity, explain the various techniques for applying it in healthcare settings, and analyze the productivity of healthcare resources in each country. In the final section, we discuss some of the key issues in the development of an ideal healthcare system.

Profiles of Five Healthcare Systems

The five countries under analysis here show a wide range of structures from predominantly private systems in Japan to the central universal program in Canada, from a health insurance based system in the United States to a Ukrainian system with no health insurance. In this section, we begin with a profile of each country's healthcare system and then briefly conducting a comparatives study.

Profile of the Canadian Healthcare System

Canada is the second largest country in land area in the world and has a relatively small population of slightly over 30 million. Prior to 1971, the Canadian healthcare system was very similar to the United States. It was predominantly based on employer-provided health insurance with a smaller role played by various government programs. Both hospitals and physicians operated privately with physician's fees determined by the market and hospitals paid on a negotiated fee-for-service basis. During this period a little over 7% of the GDP was spent on health care.

In 1971, Canada adopted a system of universal health insurance (Canadian Medicare System) provided by the government and funded by value-added taxes and income tax. All basic services were covered and patient copayments were nominal. Physicians were paid on the basis of a fee schedule determined by the government, and hospitals were allocated a budget by the provincial government with the overall budget set nationally. Although health insurance was provided to all by the government, the provision of health care remained largely in private hands. However, the private health providers in Canada are heavily regulated with price controls on most activities, services, and products. Hospitals also are restricted from raising funds on their own for capital investments and instead have to obtain funds from the provincial government. Although there are significant differences in overall spending on health care between Canada and the United States, Canadian health expenditures have not grown as rapidly as those in the United States, mostly as a result of the government regulation of prices and the government setting the budget allocation for health care.

In the early 1990s, Canada went through an economic recession that resulted in significant cost-cutting measures. This significantly affected healthcare expenditures as such expenditures were the largest single item in the provincial government budgets. As a result, between 1992 and 1997, health expenditure as a percentage of GDP declined significantly. Since then it has continued to increase and was 9.3% in 1999. Over 70% of total health expenditure is public. Hospitals occupy an important role in the Canadian Health system and hospital costs represented 31.4% of total health expenditure in 1999. Payment to physicians accounts for about 14%, with over 80% of this payment being of the fee for service variety. Much of the increase in healthcare costs can be attributed to pharmaceutical costs; such costs account for 15% of total health expenditure and have almost tripled since the late 1970s. The average per capita expenditure on drugs was $353 in 1998. In 2003, there were 2.1 physicians per 1000 people and 9.95 nurses per 1000 people. Waiting times for medical care are often extremely high.

Canadians have enjoyed significant improvements in life expectancy over the last four decades. Canadian life expectancy is among the highest in the countries belonging to the Organization for Economic Cooperation and Development (OECD, 2001): 75.8 years for men and 81.4 years for women in 1997. The interesting aspect of Canadian life expectancy patterns recently has been the narrowing of the gap between men and women. According to Or (2000) per capita GDP and tobacco, alcohol, and fat consumption are all strongly correlated with premature mortality. Over the last three decades, there has been a 39% reduction in male smoking rates, and alcohol consumption has declined. However, obesity, especially among women, remains a problem with one out of seven Canadians classified as being obese. The reduction in male smoking and the higher rates of female obesity may be responsible for the narrowing gap in life expectancy across gender.

Canada has often been cited by some as an example of the type of system the United States should adopt to provide universal coverage, though it has at least as many non-supporters.

Profile of the Indian Healthcare System

With a population of over a billion, India is the second largest country in the world (second only to China). It is a country of haves and have-nots with significant proportions of the population living in poverty while some segments are extremely well off. The economy grew very rapidly during the 1990s. Growth rates during some years were in the double digits, and the economy has continued on the fast track in this century. Like China, India has benefited greatly from participating in the global economy and is fast approaching an economic superpower.

India obtained its independence in 1947 from Great Britain and has for much of its postindependent life adopted a socialist approach to the provision of most services. However, the provision of healthcare services has to a large extent been provided and funded by private entities. Over 50% of all inpatient services and 60% of outpatient services are provided by the private sector. Many of the newer private hospitals are staffed by Western-educated medical personnel with the latest medical technologies available to them. Health care for the poorer and disadvantaged segments of the population, on the other hand, are primarily provided for by government-owned and ill-equipped health facilities. Public ownership is divided between central (national), state, municipal, and *panchayat* (village) governments. Public facilities own and operate many teaching hospitals, secondary hospitals, rural referral hospitals, primary health centers, and clinics or dispensaries.

In 1951 life expectancy at birth was only 36.7 years. It increased steadily to 64.6 years by 2000. Similarly, infant mortality was 146 per 1000 live births in 1950 and declined to 70 by 2000. Although significant progress has been made since independence, communicable diseases such as tuberculosis continue to affect large segments of the population. In addition HIV/AIDS has assumed virulent proportions. The 1990s also saw increases in mortality from lifestyle factors. An increased trend in smoking among youth and a lack of physical activity have been cited as key factors.

Health care is financed mostly with out-of-pocket payments. India annually spends about $23 per capita on health of which only about $4 is public. Although total health expenditure is 5% of GDP, 4% is private, which can be further broken down to 3.6% being out of pocket. The high out-of-pocket payments often poses a problem since, according to a World Bank report by Peters et al. in 2002, almost a quarter of all hospitalizations push people into poverty because of the loss of jobs and the high cost of private medical facilities. Within public expenditure the central government allocation for health out of its total budget remained stagnant in the 1990s while state allocations actually declined.

Health insurance covers about 10% of the population, with government employees covered under government plans and some private-sector employees covered under employer-provided plans. Since 2000 various plans have been rolled out by the government to provide affordable health insurance for the needy, but coverage for those insured in such plans is often restricted to ill-equipped public health facilities.

India has about 0.6 physicians per 1000 population and about 1.2 nurses and midwives per 1000 population. Primary care physicians working in the public sector are paid a low and fixed salary set at the national level. As a result most physicians work in their own clinics where fees are determined in competitive factors. During the 1990s with liberalization of controls many private hospitals and hospital chains with large capital investments in advanced technology and with highly trained staff began to grow rapidly. These new facilities provide care for the many beneficiaries of the booming economy. In addition, these new facilities have made significant inroads into providing services for the *health tourists* from Western economies attracted by the lower cost of advanced care in these facilities.

The stark disparity in healthcare utilization between different socioeconomic classes and rural–urban regions in India has been a matter of great concern for the government of India for many decades now. The best indicator of this is the disparity in infant mortality rates. The under 5 mortality rates for the lowest wealth quintile is triple that of the highest quintile. It is also twice as high for rural regions compared to urban and for mothers with no education compared to mothers with higher education. Similar disparities also exist with immunizations. Such disparities in health care at young ages are undoubtedly likely to result in widening disparities at older ages.

In addition to the inequalities between rural and urban regions, there are also significant variations across states in India in every aspect of income and health. The state of Punjab has the highest per capita income and the lowest percent of it population below poverty. The best-performing state in health is the state of Kerala; it also has the highest literacy rates (especially for women) and density of physicians and healthcare facilities per capita. Excluding Kerala, a positive relationship between high incomes and better health appears to hold in India.

As one of the fastest growing economies in the world India has to take urgent steps to address the huge disparities in healthcare provision. Sustained growth in the economy requires a source of healthy manpower.

Profile of the Japanese Healthcare System

Since the end of WWII, Japan has evolved from being an economy devastated by war to the second largest economy in the world with a GDP of $33,727 per capita in 2003. It has a population of around 130 million of which 19.5% are 65 years or older. By 2020 this segment is expected to be over a quarter of the population. The rapid aging of the population is a matter of great concern especially for healthcare provision and funding. Japan has some of the best health outcomes in the world, and it continues to improve in the health status of the population. There is also very little disparity within the country in healthcare access.

Life expectancy in Japan was 50 years for men and 54 years for women at the end of WWII. It has since grown to the highest among developed countries at 78 years for men and 85 years for women. Infant mortality is very low at 3 per 1000 live births. The leading cause of death in Japan is malignant neoplasm followed by cardiovascular disease. High stress levels have been blamed for the very high levels of suicides (around 32,109 in 2003) especially among working men. Although the prevalence of smoking is decreasing, it is still high compared to other industrialized countries. Over 50% of men smoke, and it is becoming increasingly prevalent among women.

The Japanese enjoy universal coverage and free access to all health facilities. Enrollment in an insurance plan was made mandatory for all Japanese in 1961. Most people (around 75 million) obtain their insurance through employer-related groups. The rest are covered under a national health insurance plan. Employers contribute around 4.5%, and employees contribute 3.5% of their pay toward the insurance premium. Both the employer groups and the national plans have copayments and catastrophic caps on out-of-pocket payments. Balance billing, which is the practice of charging full fees and billing the patient for the amount unpaid by the insurer, is prohibited, and prices to providers are set by the government. The fees for physicians are lower than in the Medicare Relative Value Scale used in the United States and is an important reason for the lower health cost in Japan (Phelps, 2003). Hospitals are mostly private, but the large hospitals and teaching hospitals are public. Most doctors work in private clinics and earn much more than the specialists working in the hospitals. The Japanese public visits their physicians regularly at an average rate of 15 times per year (Phelps, 2003). However, the number of minutes spent with the doctor is lower than in the United States. The prevalence of a fee-for-service system makes usage levels high for physician visits as the patient does not bear much additional cost from frequent visits. Due to the same reason, pharmaceutical spending is very high in Japan at 20% of total spending on health.

Total health expenditure went up considerably during the 1990s at around 3% and was $260 billion in 2002 accounting for 8.6% of GDP (WHO, 2005). The rapid aging of the population has been a primary cause of high health expenditures in Japan as in many other countries. A sizeable portion of total health expenditure (around one third) was for the aged. Likewise per capita expenditure for the aged was three times the average of $2,046. In 2000 in response to the large increase in long-term nursing care, the government introduced long-term care insurance. Although hospital admissions are lower than the United States, the average length of stay is much higher in Japan at over 3 weeks. This explains why 40% of total health spending was for inpatient care with hospitals providing over 90% of it. Public funds were used for 81.35% of total health expenditure with 65.4% coming from the Social Security Fund. Private expenditure accounted for 18.7% with most of it being household copayment. The lack of incentives often results in patients going directly to specialists even for minor ailments. The fee-for-service system also results in overtreatment and has been blamed for the high average length of stay. In 2002 there were 262,687 doctors at a rate of 1.98 per 1,000 population and a million nurses at a rate of 8 per 1,000 people.

Profile of the Ukrainian Healthcare System

Ukraine is the second largest country in Europe. It is a newly independent state formed as a result of the break up of the Soviet Union in 1991. In the 2001 census it had a population of 48.4 million, with 67% living in urban areas. During the era of the Soviet republic,

Ukraine was severely affected by major disasters including civil wars, famines, German invasion, and the Second World War. The Chernobyl nuclear accident in 1986 was a major catastrophe with significant consequences to life. The Ukrainian economy similarly suffered through a major economic recession from which it has only recently begun to recover. Since obtaining independence, Ukraine has developed the foundations for a more democratic system, but its healthcare system continues to be shackled by Soviet-style incentive systems.

Since its independence the population of Ukraine has fallen by 3.6 million or around 7.5%. The country finds itself faced with the unfortunate situation of poor economic health and a shrinking and aging population. Its fertility rate is the lowest in Europe, and its birth rate fell by 40% during the 1990s. This has been attributed by some to the increased rates of abortion. For example, in 2002, there were 82.8 abortions for every 100 live births. As a result of the low birth rates the proportion of the population under age 15 has declined over the last 10 years.

Ukraine faced a severe health crisis in the early 1990s when life expectancy actually fell by 4.4 years for men and 2.4 years for women. Although it has recovered from that crisis, in 2002 life expectancy was still only 62.2 years for men and 73.3 years for women. Cardiovascular disease is the primary cause of death in Ukraine. Because smoking is very prevalent (67% among men), alcohol consumption is very high, and 1% of adults have HIV/AIDS, the potential for significant health improvements is bleak.

Between 1990 and 1999 gross domestic product in Ukraine fell by 62%. This was not only a period of declining incomes, but it was accompanied by hyperinflation. Economic recovery since that time has been very slow. In 2000, only around 66% of the adult population is actively employed, and more than one quarter of the population lives in poverty. Thus, the ability of the government to finance the growing demand for health care is very limited.

In the postwar Soviet state, healthcare services with universal access to care was provided in a multitier structure with much of the responsibility for care being at the district (*rayon*) level and regional (*oblasts*) level. The republic provided more of the guidelines and norms governing the lower tiers. Healthcare services were provide at hospitals, sanitary and epidemiological stations, polyclinics, and specialized healthcare facilities. Size and staffing of these facilities was determined by population size. Much of the provision of care was initiated at the clinics and by primary physicians. During the 1970s and 1980s, there was considerable growth in the network of specialized facilities and units. This shifted priority away from primary care and physicians to specialists (WHO, 1999). The goal of the planning authorities was to increase capacity as measured by beds and personnel, and as a result Ukraine had the highest number of beds and physicians per capita in the world. The incentive structure was such that 80% of healthcare expenditure went toward inpatient care, and long hospital stays were common even for minor disorders. During the waning years of the Soviet Republic a new economic mechanism (NEM) was introduced to transform the system to a performance-based system rather than a capacity-based system.

After independence in 1991, the economy experienced a painful restructuring stage with very little ability to fund the increasing need for health care. This phase of transition to a free market economy, as with many other former soviet economies saw dramatic increases in prices of pharmaceuticals as well as basic necessities such as energy. The Ukrainian Constitution in 1996 stated that the function of the state was to "create conditions for effective medical services accessible to all citizens." Although Ukraine has universal access to health care for its citizens, most medical expenses are not covered except for children and other socially vulnerable groups. Thus, out-of-pocket payments are quite high.

The structure of the present day system continues to be similar to the Soviet system. Most of the primary health clinics or PHCs (6456 of them in 2000) are funded and operated at the district (*rayon*) levels. The regions fund and operate both the multispecialty, and specialized hospitals. They also establish the number of beds and staffing levels. The area serviced by a PHC is broken up into catchment areas (*uchastok*) each with a certain number of residents and a primary care physician. Although patients have free choice of physicians on paper there are many obstacles to it. They can also go to a specialist directly, and more than 60% do so. The incentive system is such that this is even lucrative for primary care physicians who get paid for referrals. Over 80% of public healthcare expenditure is funded locally. This results in significant inequalities across regions in the level of healthcare provision, and in 2001 a system of inter budget transfers was set up to remove regional imbalances. The budget allocation is based on the number of beds for hospitals and visits for clinics. There is very little incentive to be efficient, and the system encourages use of consultants and admissions.

Since 1991, healthcare expenditure in Ukraine has declined by 60%. The vast majority of healthcare facilities are publicly owned (24,166 such facilities in 2000) (WHO, 2000). Since 2000, there has been an attempt to increase the role played by privately owned facilities, but such a development is still nascent. The share of inpatient expenditure has dropped since independence but continues to be high at over 60% of total healthcare expenditure, mostly as a result of reductions in the number of beds. Capital investments in health care, while it has increased during the 1990s, remains low at only 7% of total health expenditures. Replacement of outdated medical technology and equipment has been very low at about 2%.

Private health insurance remains very limited with only 2% of the population covered by such policies in 2000. This is primarily a result of the high cost of such insurance and the inability of much of the population to afford it. In 1998, Ukraine developed a plan to provide mandatory state social insurance. This was to cover the entire population with insurance premiums paid by employers and employees equally with employee premium levels set at a fixed proportion of income. However the high rates of unemployment and a poor state revenue base made this impractical and the plan was rejected by parliament in 2003.

Ukraine has a very large number of physicians per capita. In 2003, there were 2.95 physicians per 1000 people, according to WHO. Of this only 26.6% are primary care physicians with the remaining being specialists. The staffing model and low remuneration has resulted in about 1300 vacant positions for physicians in 2000. The number of medical graduates rose by 20% from 1996 to 2001. Supply of nurses has been falling steadily. In 1991 it was the highest at 11.9 nurses per 1000 and had fallen to 7.8 by 2002. This is primarily because of low pay and low social prestige. Healthcare professionals are paid fixed salaries based on a national pay scale. Since 2000, the government has been making efforts to provide performance-based salary increments.

Profile of the United States Healthcare System

The United States is the richest country in the world and is a leader in technological innovation. It is no wonder then that it has evolved into a leader in the provision of sophisticated health care. In 2004, total health spending as a share of GDP was 15.3%, and health expenditures per capita were $6,100. This was higher than any other country. The United States also has one of the fastest growth rates in real health expenditures per capita (over 5% for most of the last decade) and spent the most on pharmaceuticals among Organization for Economic Cooperation and Development (OECD) member countries at $752 per capita in 2004. Yet over the past four decades the increase in life expectancy at birth of 7.6 years is less than the 14 years gained in Japan and 8.6 years in Canada over the same time period. This has resulted in the claim by many that the United States has reached a level of production of health care at which further improvements in health care will require very large increases in expenditure, an issue that we will explore further in the next section.

The US healthcare system relies extensively on private insurance to provide financial coverage for its people. More than 70% of the population under age 65 are enrolled in private health insurance plans, mostly through their employers. The American health system is distinguished by the unique role of managed care organizations. Managed care organizations evolved in the early 1970s primarily as a response to the rapidly growing cost of care in the United States. In the previously common practice known as *fee for service* providers charged a fee per unit of service rendered. Such a fee for service method resulted in significant overprovision of services since providers would be paid a greater amount the more services they provided. In managed care organizations, payment for services rendered by providers of care is usually a negotiated capitation or per enrollee rate. In the early days of managed care, health maintenance organizations, in which the same organization that provided insurance itself provided care, were the norm. Since then numerous other variants with different degrees of contractual arrangements between the insurance company and healthcare providers have evolved.

Government provision of health insurance in the United States is undertaken through Medicare and Medicaid, which were initiated in 1966. Health insurance for the population aged 65 and older is provided through Medicare. Part A of Medicare covers hospitalization and some skilled nursing facility charges, and the supplemental Part B covers physician and laboratory charges and medical supplies. Most prescription drugs are not covered under Medicare, but the passage of the Prescription Drug Act in 2005 provides some relief from the soaring costs of pharmaceutical products. The working population pays a Medicare tax to pay for the benefits received by the elderly. The rapid growth in the elderly population caused by the aging of the baby boomer generation and their longer life spans, coupled with low birth rates and working populations, has made the financial viability of such a program a matter of immediate and great concern. The Medicare system has been unable to meet present obligations with current revenue since around 1995, and it is expected that it will deplete all of its accumulated funds within the next decade. Numerous attempts have been made to rein in the growth of Medicare expenditures including contracting with managed care organizations and stricter controls on charges by hospitals and physicians.

Medicaid is a safety net program for people with low income, mostly women, children, and the elderly and disabled, who receive federal or state financial assistance. The program typically covers charges for physician visits, inpatient and outpatient hospital stays, and nursing home stays. However each state has tremendous discretion in determining benefits covered. As a result, there are significant variations across states in the level of benefits provided by Medicaid. Although initially it was a federal-state program with matching federal funds, this program has increasingly become reliant on state tax revenue. As a result of escalating healthcare costs, Medicaid programs have become the largest single item in many states budgets. As with Medicare, attempts to control growing Medicaid expenditures have included contracting with managed care organizations.

In 2002, there were 5794 hospitals in the United States, and 3025 of them were non-government owned. Most of these hospitals are not for profit with only about 766 of them being investor owned. Hospital charges account for over one third of healthcare costs in the United States with a total bill of $650 billion. Medicare paid 43.5% of this bill, private insurance paid 31.2%, Medicaid paid 18.3%, and the uninsured accounted for 3.8%. Those aged 65 years and older make up about 13% of the total population but accounted for about 35% of all hospital stays. The top three principal diagnoses for this age group were hardening of the heart arteries, pneumonia, and congestive heart failure. The mean charge per stay was $17,300 with infant respiratory distress syndrome having the highest average charge at $91,400 (see Table 3-1).

In the United States, as opposed to most other OECD countries, private expenditure on health is larger than public expenditure, mostly financed through private insurance. The share of private insurance is therefore higher than in any other country in the OECD. However around 15% of the population does not have any form of insurance and ends up relying on emergency rooms for medical care. Emergency rooms are required by law to provide essential care regardless of insurance status. The cost of providing uncompensated care to them is recovered by hospitals when feasible by charging more for their insured patients. Faced with the strong forces of competition from other providers, healthcare facilities in locations where such uncompensated care is large often are faced with an inability to pass on much of the costs and hospital bankruptcies are quite preva-

TABLE 3-1   Mean Hospital Charges

Principal Diagnoses With the Highest Mean Charges	Mean Charges	Mean Length of Stay (in days)
1. Infant respiratory distress syndrome	$91,400	24.2
2. Premature birth and low birth weight	$79,300	24.2
3. Spinal cord injury	$76,800	12.8
4. Leukemia (cancer of blood)	$74,500	14.1
5. Intrauterine hypoxia and birth asphyxia (lack of oxygen to baby in uterus or during birth)	$72,800	15.6
6. Cardiac and circulatory birth defects	$71,400	8.9
7. Heart valve disorders	$70,900	8.8
8. Polio and other brain or spinal infections	$63,200	13.0
9. Aneurysm (ballooning or rupture of an artery)	$55,300	7.7
10. Adult respiratory failure or arrest	$48,500	10.0

Source: AHRQ, 2003.

lent. The high cost of inefficiency to the hospitals under the new reimbursement mechanisms has also resulted in significant reductions in the number of hospital beds. The United States now has the fewest number of hospital beds per capita among OECD countries.

The United States has fewer physicians and nurses per capita than the OECD average (OECD, 2006). In 2000, there were 730,801 physicians with a density of 2.50 per 1000 and 26,669,603 nurses with a density of 9.37 per 1000. Because of the increasing prevalence of managed care organizations and the adoption of the relative value fee schedule for physician reimbursement rates the number of general practitioners has been growing while the number of some specialists (anesthesiologists, for example) has been declining. Smoking prevalence among adults has decreased to 17% in 2004, which is lower than Japan but higher than Canada. Obesity rates among adults were 30.2% in 2002—the highest in the OECD.

The question of why the United States with the prevalence of managed care and other cost-control mechanisms finds its healthcare costs soaring has been a question that has puzzled many. Three reasons are often cited for the rapid increase in healthcare costs: pharmaceutical price increases, utilization of new technology, and healthcare costs associated with aging.

Retail prescription drugs accounted for about 11% of national health expenditures in 2003, according to Smith et al. (2003). According to a study done by the American

Association of Retired Persons (AARP, 2006), during the 2000–2005 period manufacturer's prices for the most widely used brand name prescription drugs grew at an average annual rate of around 6%. Without exception prescription drug prices grew faster than the overall inflation rate during the last two decades. The growth in utilization of expensive new technology has been another key driver of the rising cost of health care in the United States according to many studies (Price Waterhouse Cooper, 2002; Hay, 2003). According to Rothenberg (2003), "Changes in medical technology accounted for 20–40% of the yearly rise in healthcare spending in the late 1990s."

As pointed out in the earlier discussion of hospital costs, the elderly (65 and older) make up 13% of the population but consume 36% of health care. According to Stanton and Rutherford (2005), the elderly had an average healthcare expenditure of $11,089 compared to $3,352 for working age people in 2002. Figure 3-1 shows that 43% of the highest spenders are in the 65 and older age group. This age group is the fastest growing group in the US population. The number of centenarians in the United States grew by over 6% during the 1990s according to Krach and Welkoff (1999). There were 120 centenarians per 10,000 population aged 85 and older in 1990 while in Japan there were about 29. Manton and Waupal (1995) found that life expectancy at age 85 is significantly higher in the United States than in England, France, Japan, or Sweden. Although this can be seen as a feather in the cap for our healthcare system, it is also a cause for great concern due to the associated high healthcare costs.

Comparative Analysis of Healthcare Systems

The five countries under study here show tremendous variation in the size of expenditures, role of government, and health insurance (see Figure 3-2). For consistency we have

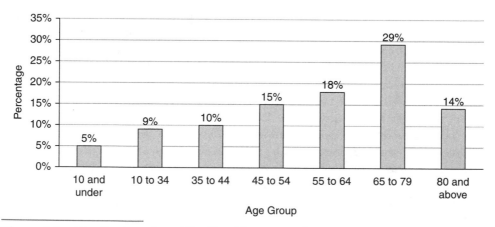

Figure 3-1 Distribution of top 5% of healthcare spenders.

Source: Adapted from Conwell & Cohen, 2005.

used the same data source extracted from the World Health Organization Statistical Information System (WHOSIS) for our analysis. WHOSIS is one of the few data sets that collects comparable data for these five countries. The OECD has much more detailed data on some variables, but it does not collect data on Ukraine and India and hence is of limited value here.

The United States leads in healthcare spending and spends about seven times as much on total health expenditures per capita as does India. The share of government expenditure in total health expenditure is similarly very different across countries. While the government in India spends only $20 per capita annually on health care, the United States government spends over a hundred times as much. Canada has a universal healthcare system, and private spending is only about 30% of total spending. In the United States the majority (55%) is private spending, and in India three quarters of all healthcare spending is private. Ukraine, which has universal coverage, still has a high share of private spending as benefits provided are so limited that patients are forced to make sizeable out-of-pocket payments. In India where private provision of health care is dominant but where private health insurance is at a nascent stage, out-of-pocket expenditures account for almost all of private spending on health care, but out-of-pocket expenditures account for only about 25% of all private spending on health care in the United States. Private health insurance pays for over 65% of private spending in the United States while it pays for less than 1% in India where health expenditures are mostly financed by out-of-pocket payments. Thus,

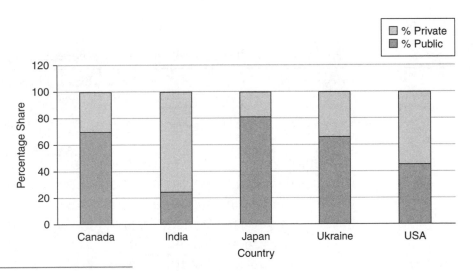

Figure 3-2 Per capita health expenditure shares.

Source: Adapted from WHOSIS, 2006.

India is the most private in healthcare financing, and the United States is the most privately insured economy.

The next question we can ask is does the type of system matter for the healthcare outcomes? Measures of health outcomes that are commonly used are life expectancy and infant mortality rates. The mostly public health financing system in Japan appears to do the best under either measure followed by Canada, which is also the second most in public financing of health care. In addition to the health system, lifestyle and other differences often play a big role as well here as we point out later.

Because measures of life expectancy do not always reflect the true health of the person, an alternate measure called healthy activity life expectancy (HALE) has recently been developed. HALE attempts to measure the number of healthy life years the person can expect to live.

The structure of the healthcare system and the reimbursement arrangements (capitation versus fee for service) can influence how much health care is provided per dollar spent. A crude illustration of this notion is displayed in Table 3-2. A more accurate investigation is undertaken in the next section. We compute the number of expected years of life at birth per dollar of per capita health expenditure by dividing life expectancy at birth and infant mortality rates by per capita health expenditure. Life expectancy per dollar spent (and HALE per dollar spent) is lowest in the United States across gender. Canada has the lowest outcome per dollar spent on infant mortality rate. The huge disparity in healthcare expenditures per capita across countries without an equally large disparity in outcomes is what drives this result, but the point still remains.

TABLE 3-2 Health Outcome per Dollar of per Capita Health Expenditure

Country	Life Expectancy per Capita Dollar		Infant Mortality Rate per Capita Dollar	Healthy Life Expectancy per Capita Dollar			
	Males	Females		Male	Female	Male	Female
	At Birth	At Birth		At Birth	At Birth	At Age 60	At Age 60
Canada	0.02281	0.02394	0.00167	0.022812	0.005122	0.02394	0.00599
India	0.62846	0.62557	0.75610	0.628459	0.118146	0.62557	0.12439
Japan	0.03181	0.03376	0.00134	0.031808	0.007615	0.03376	0.00922
Ukraine	0.17358	0.20276	0.00245	0.17358	0.028725	0.20276	0.04000
United States	0.01162	0.01205	0.01205	0.01162	0.002603	0.01205	0.00291

Source: Computations by authors.

There exists a good deal of evidence in the literature that shows that lifestyle factors play a major role in determining the level of health. The Japanese diet rich in fish has often been argued to be a principal reason for the healthier Japanese population. Smoking is highly prevalent among Japanese males and is second only to Ukrainian males. Obesity is most prevalent in the United States, and given the links between obesity, diabetes, and heart disease it is a cause for major concern. India has very low levels of obesity but high levels of smoking prevalence amongst males.

Thus, it is clear that there are wide variations in healthcare systems, expenditures, and outcomes across this selection of countries. In the following section, we describe and analyze production and productivity of health care in these countries.

Healthcare Productivity and Costs

In this section, we describe the concept of productivity and costs in health care and how they are used in making healthcare expenditure decisions. We then use cross-country data to estimate the production and cost of health improvements. We also compare the productivity and cost of health care across the sample of five countries.

Why does the United States have such high levels of medical expenditure per capita compared to the other countries but not much better outcomes? Phelps (2003), using data on perinatal mortality rates for five industrialized nations including Canada, Japan, and the United States points out that the "United States with higher medical spending than any other country is closer to the "flat of the curve" than other countries in the sense that additional spending on medical care is less likely to produce increases in health outcomes."

In Figure 3-3 we plot per capita healthcare spending on male life expectancy at birth for our sample of five countries. As per capita healthcare spending increases from a low of $82 in India to $2,244 in Japan, life expectancy increases rapidly from 61 years to 79 years. Further increases in spending such as for Canada at $2,989 and United States at $5,711

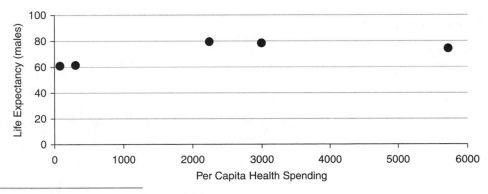

Figure 3-3 Health spending and life expectancy.

actually see lower life expectancy of 78 and 75 years respectively. This could be taken to suggest that healthcare spending in Canada and United States is beyond the stage of effectiveness in increasing medical outcomes, which is an issue that we explore further in this section. The association depicted here must be taken with great caution because of the very small number of observations and other factors such as lifestyle that play a role.

Economists often describe the production of health care using the concept of a production function. A production function describes the relationship between inputs and outcomes. It specifies for any given technology of production, the maximum amount of output that could be produced by a given combination of amounts of inputs. Outputs or outcomes could be cancer detection, mortality rates, length of hospital stay, or other measures of morbidity, and inputs could be tests, treatment procedures, and expenditures. With better technology, methods, and processes the same amount of inputs, such as physician time, can produce more output. The average product of an input (often referred to as productivity of an input) is the amount of output produced per unit of input whereas marginal product of an input refers to the amount of additional output produced using an additional unit of that input. At very low levels of health care, every additional test (unit of treatment) has a large and positive effect in improving health outcome. As the number of tests and procedures performed on the patient increases, each additional test has a smaller and smaller effect on outcomes. Such a tendency is what is referred to as diminishing marginal productivity. Across disease groups, across countries, and across patients this pattern often tends to occur and may explain why the United States does not do much better in some measures of health outcomes while spending significantly more than many other developed countries.

Neuhauser and Lewicki (1975) were one of the first to use economic analysis to advise medical decision making. They looked at the use of the sixth stool guaiac test for detecting colon cancer cases. The stool guaiac test can be repeated in order to detect more cases because of the existence of false positives or negatives in each round of testing. Table 3-3 below shows the number of tests conducted and the resulting number of cases

TABLE 3-3	Cancer Detection	
Number of Tests	Number of Cancer Cases Detected	Additional Cases Detected
1	65.9469	65.9469
2	71.4425	5.4956
3	71.9005	0.458
4	71.9387	0.0382
5	71.9419	0.0032
6	71.9422	0.0003

detected. As can be seen, while more cases are detected with more tests each additional test detects fewer and fewer additional cases of colon cancer. Moving from the fifth to the sixth test almost no additional cases are detected. Figure 3-4 plots the production function for cancer detection using the sixth stool guaiac test. The curve flattens out from the third test on indicating that very little additional cases are detected through additional testing. Figure 3-5 plots the marginal product of the sixth stool guaiac test showing the number of additional cases detected through additional tests.

Many studies such as Pritchett and Summer (1996) and Bhargava, Jamison, and Murray (2001) find evidence that higher incomes permit individuals to afford better nutrition, health care, and thereby health. Similarly studies (McGinnis & Foege, 1993) have shown that education and lifestyle factors play an important role in many

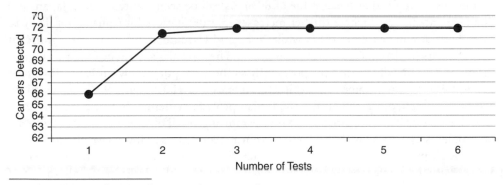

Figure 3-4 Production function for cancer detection.

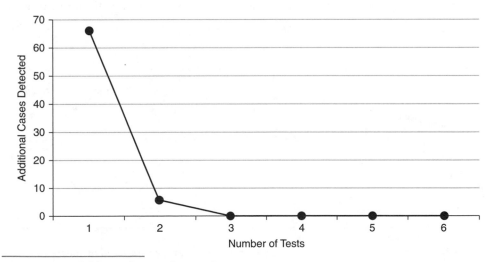

Figure 3-5 Additional cases detected.

dimensions of health. At a cross-country level, the production of health (as measured by HALE) should depend on the country's income (per capita gross national income [GNI]) and education (literacy rate) as well as lifestyle factors (smoking prevalence). We extracted data from the World Health Organization World Health Statistics data base for 58 countries (the reduction in sample size is due to the lack of data on smoking prevalence in many countries). Our regression result below suggests that not only does HALE increase with literacy rate and GNI, the effect of GNI on HALE gets smaller as GNI increases suggesting that it becomes less and less effective at generating higher HALE. Smoking prevalence was not significant probably because GNI already captures most of its effect.

$$\text{HALE} = 35.6 + 0.186 \text{ ALR} + 0.00141 \text{ GNI} - 0.0000003 \text{ GNI2}$$

Figure 3-6 shows the position of each of our sample of countries in this relationship (with literacy rate fixed at mean value of 80%). As can be seen, United States, Japan, and Canada are at the stage where further increases in gross national income is not likely to bring about any increase in HALE, while India and Ukraine are likely to see significant improvements in HALE as their economy grows. These results should be taken with great caution and are for illustrative purposes only as there are potentially multiple directions of causality between income and health (Chapman and Hariharan, 1994) for which we have not controlled. Bloom et al. (2004) also provide evidence that improvements in health have a significant positive effect on the rate of growth of GDP per capita. There are also problems associated with using cross-country regressions that we have not addressed.

Although productivity studies can characterize which tests or treatments or which countries are most effective in providing health care, to make decisions on allocation of scarce resources, the cost of treatments must play a central role. In a world faced with growing demands on its scarce healthcare budgets, the most pressing and controversial decisions are often associated with the questions of how much health care to provide?

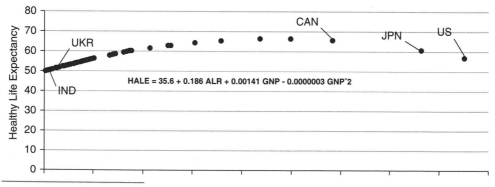

Figure 3-6 Health activity life expectancy vs. GNP (literacy rate fixed at mean value of 80%).

Whether it is governments, healthcare providers, or private individuals making such decisions, cost considerations invariably become critical in addressing them.

There are many methods developed by economists and others to include cost considerations in making better decisions. The most controversial of these is benefit-cost analysis (BCA). In BCA the monetized value of all the benefits (better or longer life for example) is compared against the cost of obtaining such a benefit. The controversy in the use of BCA to allocate healthcare resources is often centered on the methods for monetization of health benefits. For example, one commonly used dollar value for increases in life expectancy is the value of a statistical life (VSL) (Viscusi & Aldy, 2002). The VSL is often arrived at by using the amount individuals have been willing to accept as appropriate compensation for a reduction in life expectancy (for example accepting a wage premium for jobs with a higher risk of death). Table 3-4 lists some estimates of VSL for a sample of countries. For example, the value of a statistical life in India is $3.3 million compared to $9.7 million in Japan.

Critics of this approach point to the difficulty of inferring from a small increase in risk of death to a large increase, as well as the wide range of these estimates and measurement errors in these studies. In a recent report (Jamison, 2006) the authors calculate the value of investments in health by comparing changes in annual healthcare costs to changes in annual population health outcomes monetized using VSL. They calculate that in the United States, the cost per disability adjusted life year in US$ ranges from as low a cost as

TABLE 3-4   International Estimates of VSL

Country	Estimates of Value of Statistical Life (millions of US$)
UK	5.7–74.1
Canada	5.1–5.3
India	4.1
Taiwan	0.7
Japan	9.7
Hong Kong	1.7
Australia	11.3–19.1
South Korea	0.8
Austria	3.9– 6.5
United States	5–12
Ukraine	3.3

Source: Adapted from Viscusi & Aldy, 2001; Wallsten & Kosec, 2005.

$3 for taxing tobacco products over $25,000 for performing coronary artery bypass surgery. In a study on the effects of technological change on cost and care, Cutler and Mcclellan (2001) identified two channels through which improved medical technology affects health: substitution of newer technology for older less effective technology, and expansion, in which more people are treated with the new technology. Their results suggest that while improved technology comes at a higher cost the benefit from them outweighs the cost.

As a result of some of these criticisms and the difficulties in identifying all of the costs and benefits across generations, other approaches have become popular in healthcare decision making. Perhaps the most popular method for advising decision making in the allocation of scarce medical resources is cost-effectiveness analysis (CEA). CEA measures the cost per additional or incremental unit of health outcome and uses that to guide decisions on which procedure or test should be used and how much of it should be undertaken. The popularity of CEA over benefit-cost analysis (BCA) comes from the lack of a need to monetize health outcomes or benefits. CEA can be used for both the decision on which test or intervention to use as well as for how much of any given test or treatment. In the Neuhauser and Lewicki (1975) study, the cost per additional case detected increases rapidly with each additional test (Table 3-5). The first screening test is highly cost effective: it gains an additional cancer detected for only $1,175. Further tests detect fewer and fewer cases and thus entail progressively higher costs per case detected. The additional costs per cancer detected gained due to the sixth test are over $40 million, making it highly cost ineffective. However, in order to decide on the number of tests that is reasonable to conduct it becomes necessary to draw a subjective line. One attempt to do this can be found in Chapman and Hariharan (1994, 1996) in which the value of statistical life provides the cutoff.

TABLE 3-5   Stool Guaiac Test Cost-Effectiveness

Number of Tests	Total Cost of Diagnosis	Additional Cost of Detection	Cost per Cancer Detected	Marginal Cost per Cancer Detected
1	77,511	77,511	1,175.354717	1,175.354717
2	107,690	30,179	1,507.366064	5,491.484096
3	130,199	22,509	1,810.8219	49,146.28821
4	148,116	17,917	2,058.919608	469,031.4136
5	163,141	15,025	2,267.677112	4,695,312.5
6	176,331	13,190	2,451.009282	43,966,666.67

International Comparisons of Cost

Because of a lack of comparable data across countries, especially for developing countries, international comparisons of healthcare productivity has until recently been difficult. The World Health Organization in 1998 began an elaborate study to compute the costs of health care for a wide range of countries using a standardized metric. They computed the unit cost of care for primary, secondary, and tertiary care bed days and outpatient visits as well as for health centers at different levels of population coverage. Table 3-6 lists the unit cost of care for hospitalization (bed days), outpatient visits, and health center visits for our sample of five countries. As expected the differences are quite stark. While Canada and Japan have similar unit costs, the United States has inpatient and outpatient costs that are about seven times as high. India has the lowest unit costs across the board followed by Ukraine. Unlike inpatient and outpatient costs, health center care costs for the three wealthier countries are not significantly different from each other indicating that the major cost difference between the United States and other industrialized countries must be found in hospitals.

To make any reasonable statements, sample sizes much larger than our five countries are required. We therefore extracted a set of 58 countries from the WHO-Choice data with recent information on healthy activity life expectancy (HALE) and unit cost per primary bed day. If the higher unit costs in developed countries are from better quality of care it should be reflected in higher HALE in those countries. We used unit cost per bed day

TABLE 3-6   Unit Cost for Health Care

	Canada	India	Japan	Ukraine	USA
Cost per bed day					
Primary	140.09	14.71	138.85	30.11	906.64
Secondary	182.76	19.19	181.14	39.29	1,182.81
Tertiary	249.64	26.21	247.42	53.66	1,615.58
Cost per outpatient visit					
Primary	55.43	3.96	54.85	9.16	366.17
Secondary	78.62	5.62	77.80	12.99	519.38
Tertiary	116.30	8.31	115.09	19.22	768.31
Cost per health center visit					
50%	29.05	6.43	28.95	6.79	30.46
80%	29.05	6.43	28.95	6.79	30.46
95%	31.58	6.99	31.47	7.38	33.11

Source: Adapted from WHO-Choice, 2006.

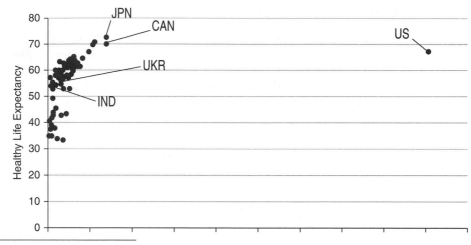

Figure 3-7   Healthy life expectancy vs. unit costs (health).

rather than per outpatient or health center visit because hospitalization is more often required for treating ailments with a high risk of death. As can be seen in the Figure 3-7, omitting the United States as an extreme outlier, the data does show that higher unit costs result in higher healthy life expectancy.

Figure 3-7 is a scatter plot of healthy life expectancy and unit costs of primary bed care for the 58 countries. The United States is an extreme outlier here because of its very high unit cost of inpatient care.

We also regressed healthy life expectancy on unit cost and unit cost squared to see if the increase in HALE gets progressively smaller as unit costs increase and find that to be true:

$$\text{HALE} = 41.4 + 0.454 \text{ UNIT COSTS} - 0.00194 \text{ UNITCOST2}$$

Figure 3-8 shows the positive relationship between unit costs and health outcomes (as measured by healthy life expectancy. Thus there is some evidence that higher unit costs do translate into better health outcomes.

To summarize, there appears to be some evidence suggesting that perhaps as Phelps and others have pointed out the United States may be at a stage where additional improvements in health are more difficult to achieve while countries such as India and Ukraine may find it easy and less expensive to achieve improvements in health.

Key Components of an Ideal Healthcare System

In the first three sections of this chapter, we explored the similarities and differences of healthcare systems across five countries and looked at key inputs (cost) and outputs (outcomes) of existing systems. Each country is grappling with ways to improve healthcare

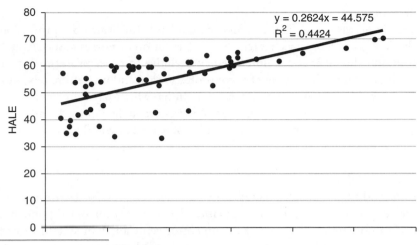

Figure 3-8 Unit costs and health outcomes.

delivery systems. While India and the Ukraine are focused on improving life expectancy and access to care, the United States is focused on improving the efficiency of the American system to lower cost while maintaining quality. Each system has evolved over time based on its unique circumstances around politics, culture, religion, and economic resources. A great deal can be learned by comparing and contrasting healthcare systems around the world. In this section, we discuss the key economic components that drive health care in any country.

Imagine that you are responsible for developing an ideal healthcare system in a newly established country. Economics deals with the best allocation of scarce resources and can provide guidance for the design of an ideal health system in order to determine "who gets what care when with the available resources." The challenges of developing an "ideal" model of care would be difficult to navigate. Here are a few key factors to be addressed in developing an ideal model of health care.

Access to Care

Access to care involves allocation of scarce resources based on the value assigned to human life. One of the foundational decisions to be made in any healthcare system is how much care will be provided. Based on the population to be served, a decision must be made about how many hospital beds are required, how much diagnostic equipment is provided and how many physicians and nurses are needed. These decisions will determine if and when individuals receive care. Capacity decisions are the biggest driver of cost, thus determining how much of the country's GDP will be spent on health care. Important considerations in determining the access to care include the following.

Healthcare Professionals

A key factor in access to care is the compensation levels for healthcare professionals. As seen in the first section of this chapter, the compensation of nurses and doctors both in the amount and the manner of reimbursement, relative to other professions within the country, will determine the supply of these professionals, and will ultimately impact the level of access to care. Some countries, such as India, which pay a low relative wage to nurses, have seen a reduction in the number of nurses available to provide care. In a global economy, healthcare providers can select other professions or travel to other countries to practice their profession.

Infrastructure and Technology

The amount and type of medical equipment and hospitals can be determined based on factors such as population, age of the population, health condition of the population, and willingness to wait for services. The government-driven Canadian system provides less high-tech diagnostic equipment than the entrepreneurial American system. As a result, wait times for Canadian citizens are often longer than they deem acceptable. Canadians routinely augment the care they receive by coming to the United States and paying out of pocket for diagnostic tests, surgeries, and even hospitalizations. If Canadians did not have the option of American care available to them, they might demand that the government invest in more technology and infrastructure.

Financing Systems

One of the biggest drivers of the overall healthcare system relates to the financing system. In most countries, financing systems have largely evolved over time based on the type of government in place. Public funding is described as funding provided by governments, such as Medicare and Medicaid in the United States. Private funding is paid either by individuals, employers, or insurance companies. Ultimately, the party financing health care will determine how much care they are willing to purchase.

Public Financing

When governments pay for care, they are entitled to establish payment rates and must determine what is purchased. Some governments have imposed strict guidelines on what they will pay for, while others allow more individual choice in care. In developing a healthcare model, it is necessary to determine what populations public funding will cover. Options for coverage range from universal coverage or may be limited to a certain age or economic level.

Private Funding

Private funding refers to the healthcare funding provided by individuals, or in some cases, by insurance companies. In the United States, the employer has historically purchased health insurance on behalf of the employee. The United States has the lowest out-of-pocket expenditure as a percentage of private expenditure on health. The result has been a disconnect between the amount of care obtained by the insured patient and the amount he or she pays for the care. Many would argue that the lack of personal financial responsibility has resulted in higher cost of healthcare services in the United States. This is known as the price-quantity relation. On the other extreme, in India individuals are required to pay for most care, but often lack the resources to do so, resulting in poor health status. Striking the proper balance of responsibility for funding is a key driver in developing an economically sound healthcare system.

Payment Methodology

Determining the payment methodology to providers is a key decision in the healthcare model. The goal is to encourage medical providers to provide the appropriate amount of care. If providers are reimbursed on a fee-for-service basis, the more tests they perform, the more money they receive. If however, providers are paid a fixed amount to care for a given population, known as capitation, there may be an incentive not to provide needed care. Another alternative is a cost-based approach, which pays the provider cost, plus a reasonable profit. Cost-based reimbursement does not encourage efficiency in delivering care. In the United States, the most recent trend is toward high-deductible insurance plans with health savings accounts. The design of these plans is to shift more financial responsibility to the consumer, and to encourage consumers to "shop" for the best price for the care they need. The goal is to force providers to offer competitive prices for their services.

Public Policy Decisions

There are a variety of public policy decisions that must be addressed regarding health care.

Public Health

A sound healthcare model must address how to provide incentives for healthy behaviors and lifestyles. Many countries have found that requiring certain immunizations can improve the health status of the entire country. Other countries, such as Canada, have seen large improvements in health status as lifestyle factors such as smoking have improved. For citizens covered by publicly funded programs, healthcare benefits could be linked to healthy behaviors. For example, government-funded programs could require vaccinations, routine exercise, or smoking cessation to receive government funding for their care.

Safety Net

Many healthcare models address providing care for those who can not afford to pay. Many studies show that the effective treatment of these patients reduces the overall cost of care in the long term. According to the HCUP fact book *Hospitalization in the United States 2002*, about 15% of the US population is uninsured, and the aggregate bill for them that year was $25 billion (AHRQ, 2003). Around 5 percent of infants born in the hospital are uninsured, and providing care at an early age will prevent later costly disease states. Diabetes is a disease that should not require costly hospitalization in many cases if appropriate outpatient care is received. More than 8% of all diabetes hospitalizations occur in patients who are uninsured. Similarly a report by the Families USA Foundation (2005) finds that the uninsured are three to four times more likely than insured to go without preventive care services, and uninsured children are one eighth less likely to have a regular source of care as insured children. Uninsured patients when hospitalized are in worse health and three times more likely to die in the hospital. As a result of cross-subsidization of uncompensated care, health insurance premiums were $922 higher in 2005 for the insured. Between $65 and $130 billion of productivity is lost in the United States annually because the uninsured population does not receive care, is sick more often, and loses productive hours.

End-of-Life Care

As mentioned, there is a correlation between dollar of per capita health expenditure and life expectancy. But at some point, there ceases to be a direct correlation between these two variables. In the Ukraine, it would be rare to see a 70-year-old receiving heart surgery. In the United States, however, it is quite common. According to HCUP fact book *Hospitalization in the United States 2002*, the most common reason for hospitalization for Medicare beneficiaries is congestive heart failure with 745,000 discharges in 2002 (AHRQ, 2003). Hogan and colleagues (2001) calculate that over a quarter of Medicare outlays went to medical care in the last year of life. Decisions about how much care to provide at the end of life have a significant impact on the total cost of health care for a given country.

Litigation Costs

Another important public policy decision is how to compensate a victim who is harmed by the healthcare system. The frequency and size of awards can impact the overall cost of health care by resulting in defensive medicine, higher insurance premiums, and significant legal costs.

Healthcare systems are extremely complex and involve thousands of decisions about how to provide care. The end result of all of these decisions can be measured in a variety of ways as described earlier. The most common global economic measure of healthcare systems is the percent of GDP spent on health. The United States GDP expenditure on health care of 15.2% is 92% higher than Japan's expenditure on health care of 7.9%. Healthcare expenditures have a major impact on the competitiveness of countries in the global economy. One notable example of how healthcare costs can impact global economics is the automobile industry. American automotive companies have had difficulty competing with Japanese carmakers because of higher production costs resulting from disproportionate healthcare costs. This competitive economic problem has been exacerbated by American automotive industry union contracts that require generous health benefits for current employees and continued insurance coverage for retirees. In 2002 for example, Toyota turned down hundreds of millions of dollars in subsidies from many US states and chose to build a 1,300-worker factory in Ontario. According to Canadian Industry Minister David Emmerson, "Canadian workers are also $4–5 cheaper to employ partly thanks to a taxpayer-funded healthcare system in Canada (CBC 2002). According to Ben Carliner at the Economic Strategy Institute, "Rising healthcare and pension costs are draining funds from Detroit's coffers and choking off research and design funding. Last year GM spent over $5.2 billion on medical benefits for over 1.1 million workers and retirees. That works out to over $1,400 per vehicle! There is more health care than steel in the cost of each GM vehicle sold. The other American automakers are in the same boat. In 2002, Ford spent $2.5 billion on healthcare benefits, and DaimlerChrysler spent $1.4 billion. In Japan and Europe, national healthcare plans mean that corporations pay little or nothing to maintain a healthy workforce. Healthcare costs are thus the source of a significant competitive disadvantage for the American auto industry and manufacturers generally" (Carliner, 2005).

When a disproportionate share of the cost of doing business is diverted to any sector of the GDP, it creates a competitive disadvantage in a global economy. In contrast, countries that do not provide adequate health care can be noncompetitive because of an unhealthy and unproductive workforce. A healthcare system that is significantly above or below the statistical norm for healthcare spending will result in consequences in the global economy. The globalization of trade forces all countries to consider how to provide appropriate levels of care through the most efficient delivery systems possible.

Acknowledgments

Marsha Burke, Dr. Robert Lipson (late), and Caroline Aultman are at WellStar Health Systems, and Dr. Govind Hariharan is at the Department of Economics, Finance, and Quantitative Analysis, Kennesaw State University. This chapter is dedicated to the memory of Dr. Lipson, a health care visionary, leader, and mentor. Our thanks to Jomon Paul for helpful comments.

References

AARP. (2006). Trends in manufacturer prices of brand name prescription drugs used by older Americans—2005 year end update. *AARP Public Policy Institute Data Digest, 134.*

AHRQ (Agency for Healthcare Research and Quality). (2003). Hospitalization in the United States. *HCUP Fact Book, 6.* Rockville, MD: Author.

Bhargava, A. D. T., Jamison Lau, L. J., & Murray, C. J. L. (2001). Modeling the effects of health on economic growth. *Journal of Health Economics, 20,* 423–440.

Carliner, B. (2005). Health care costs cripple US manufacturers. Economic Strategy Institute, blog post October 10, 2005. Retrieved June 27, 2006, from http://www.econstrat.org/blog/?p=26

CBC (Canadian Broadcast Corporation). (2002). 1,000,000 vehicles per year in Woodstock, Ont., starting 2008. Oct. 2002, CBC, Toronto, Ontario.

Chapman, K. S., & Hariharan, G. (1994). Controlling for causality in the link from income to mortality. *Journal of Risk and Uncertainty, 8*(1), 85–94.

Chapman, K. S., & Hariharan, G. (1996). Do poor people have a stronger relationship between income and mortality than the rich: Implications of panel data for health-health analysis. *Journal of Risk and Uncertainty, 12*, 51–63

Conwell, L., & Cohen, J. (2005). Characteristics of persons with high medical expenditures in the U.S. civilian noninstitutionalized population, 2002. *MEPS Statistical Brief* No. 73. Retrieved June 27, 2006, from http://www.meps.ahrq.gov/mepsweb/data_files/publications/st73/stat73.pdf

Cutler, D. M., & McClellan, M. (2001). Is technological change in medicine worth it?" *Health Affairs, 20*, 11–29.

Families USA Foundation. (2005). *Paying a premium: The added cost of uninsured.* Washington, D.C.: Author.

Government of India. (2005). Financing and delivery of health care services in India. (*Background Papers*, table 1, p. 7). National Commission on Macroeconomics and Health, New Delhi, India.

Hay, J. W. (2003). Hospital cost drivers: An evaluation of 1998–2001 state-level data. *American Journal of Managed Care, 9,* 13–24.

United BioSource. (2002). Estimating the value of investments in health care: Better care, better lives.6-14-2006 http://www.unitedbiosource.com/pdfs/HP_FullReport.pdf

Hogan, C., Lunney, J., Gabel, J., & Lynn, J. (2001). Medicare beneficiaries' cost of care in the last year of life. *Health Affairs, 20*(4), 188–194.

Pan American Health Organization. (1999). *United States of America.* Retrieved June 27, 2006, from http://www.paho.org/English/DD/AIS/unitedstates_graf_eng.pdf

Krach, C. A., & Velkoff, V. A. (1999). Centenarians in the United States. *Current population report, Special studies.* Washington, DC: US Census Bureau.

Jamison, D. T. (2006). *Economics and cost effectiveness, Disease Control Priorities Project.* International Bank for Reconstruction and Development/World Bank.

Lekhan, V., Rudiy, V., & Nolte, E. (2004). *Health care systems in transition: Ukraine.* WHO Regional Office for Europe, European Observatory on Health Systems and Policies.

Manton, K. J., & Vaupal, E. W. (1995). Survival after the age of 80 in the United States, England, France, Japan and Sweden. *New England Journal of Medicine, 333*(18), 1232–1235.

McGinnis, J.M. and Foege, W.H., (2004) "Actual Causes of Death in the United States, 2000" *JAMA* March 10; 291 (10): 1238-45

Neuhauser, D., & Lewicki, A. M. (1975). What do we gain from the sixth stool guaiac? *New England Journal of Medicine, 293*, 226–228.

OECD. (2001). OECD health a glance—How Canada compares. *OECD Policy Brief, Oct.*

OECD. (2006). How does the United States compare? *OECD health data 2006.* Retrieved June 27, 2006, from http://www.oecd.org/dataoecd/29/52/36960035.pdf

Or, Z. (2000). Determinants of health in industrialized countries: A pooled cross-country time series analysis. *OECD Economic Studies, 30*, 53–77.

Phelps, C. E. (2003). *Health economics* (3rd ed.). Boston: Addison-Wesley.

Price Waterhouse Cooper. (2002). The factors fueling rising healthcare costs (prepared for the American Association of Health Plans). Washington, DC: Author.

Pritchett, L., & Summers, L. H. (1996). Wealthier is healthier. *Journal of Human Resources, 31*, 841–868.

Rothenberg, B. M. (2003). *Medical technology as a driver of healthcare costs: Diagnostic imaging.* Retrieved June 27, 2006, from http://www.bcbs.com/betterknowledge/cost/diagnostic-imaging.html

Smith, C., Cowan, C., Sensenig, A., Catlin, A., Health Accounts Team. (2003). Health spending growth slows in 2003. *Health Affairs, 24*(1), 185–194.

Stanton, M. W., & Rutherford, M. K. (2005). The high concentration of US healthcare expenditures (Agency for Healthcare Quality and Research Pub. No. 06-0060). *Research in Action*, 19.

Viscusi, K. W., & Aldy, J. E. (2003). The value of a statistical life: A critical review of market estimates throughout the world. *Journal of Risk and Uncertainty*, *27*(1), 5–76.

Wallsten, S., & Kosec, K. (2005). The economic cost of the war in Iraq (Working Paper 05-19). Washington, D.C.: AEI-Brookings Joint Center for Regulatory Studies.

World Health Organization (WHO). (1999). *Ukraine country health report*. Kiev, Ukraine: WHO Liaison Office.

WHO. (2000). *Highlights on health in Ukraine*. Retrieved June 27, 2006, from http://www.euro.who.int/document/e72372.pdf

WHO. (2004). *Regional overview of social health insurance in South-East Asia*. Regional Office for South East Asia, India: Author.

WHO. (2005). *Country profile: Japan*. Retrieved June 27, 2006, from http://www.wpro.who.int/countries/05jpn/JPN.htm

WHO. 2006. *World health statistics 2006*. Geneva: Author.

WHOSIS. (2006). *Statistical information system*. Geneva: Author.

Peters, D. H., Yazbeck, A. S., Sharma, R. P., Ramana, G. N. V., Pritchett, L. H., & Wagstaff, A. (2002). *Better health systems for India's poor: findings, analysis, and options*. Washington, D. C.: World Bank.

World Bank. (1993). *Ukraine: The social sectors during transition—A World Bank country study*. Washington, D.C.: Author.

Chapter 4

Global Perspectives on Politics and Public Health Policy

Alexandra Toma, Michele Zebich-Knos, Richard B. Davis, and Enrique Paz

Introduction

The creation of public health policies, like other policies such as foreign policy or education policy, requires that ideas about problem identification and problem solving be transformed into measurable standards that require government involvement. Sometimes the need for creating a policy evolves from societal movements or nongovernment actors advocating for government to set policies or standards that affect the society in an equitable and efficient manner. This chapter introduces three avenues for discussing the role of government and politics in policy making—the United States, Bolivia, and a multilateral setting.

The first example is that of the United States, where the policy-making process will be outlined in a case study on US global AIDS policy. You will be able to understand the difference between several prime actors in the policy-making process—both official and unofficial. In the United States, the official policy-making actors are the three branches of government (the executive, legislative, and judicial branches). The unofficial actors constitute a diverse universe, including interest (or citizen) groups, sometimes called *lobbyists*, and the news media. Additionally, policy making can be significantly influenced by current events, which are often unpredictable and create a dynamic policy-making environment.

In the second example, we examine the South American country of Bolivia. The development of public health policy in Bolivia is much like that of the United States, since both share democratic principles; however, in Bolivia, additional actors, such as donor organizations and foreign governments, play a role to assist the government in undertaking expensive policies, such as vaccination campaigns or the eradication of certain types of diseases. This section will also explore the various challenges Bolivia faces in developing its public health policy.

Finally, in the last piece, we will explore examples of how policy is set in a multilateral organization. In this section, the United Nations World Health Organization (WHO) is seen as the primary driver to proactively develop and institute public health policies on a global scale. To understand how policy is created by a multilateral organization, we will describe how WHO operates and how WHO was successful in gaining enough worldwide support to have a treaty ratified on the control of tobacco products, all the while mitigating conflicting values among member countries.

The United States Perspective

Introduction

A famous policy maker once said: "No [foreign] policy—no matter how ingenious—has any chance of success if it is born in the minds of a few and carried out in the hearts of none." Although former Secretary of State Henry A. Kissinger was describing foreign policy making, his wise adage can certainly be applied to global health policy in the United States. *Policy* can be defined as a "definite course or method of action selected from among alternatives and in light of given conditions to guide and determine present and future decisions."[1]

The United States Constitution lays out the skeleton of policy making through its delineation of separation of powers—legislative, executive, and judicial—and the concept of checks and balances. Separation of powers was created so that no single branch of the US government would dominate the others and that all three would effectively work together in the best interests of the American people. The United States of America was established in part because the British monarchy was seen as a repressive force, not a representative one. The framers of the Constitution, therefore, wanted to ensure that when setting up a government, it would equitably represent the interests of the people it governed. This principle is clearly presented in the way that the legislative branch or Congress—which represents the citizenry of the United States—is favored as the main policy-making body of the US government. Section 8, Article I, of the Constitution states: "All Legislative Powers herein granted shall be vested in a Congress of the United States, which shall consist of a Senate and a House of Representatives."

Although some may argue that policy making occurs principally within the marble halls of Congress, and although it is true that the chief function of Congress is indeed the making of laws, overall policy making is a more complex process. This involves a multitude of actors throughout the process—from the idea phase to the legislative genesis, to formulating policy into law and, finally, to implementing or carrying out the intent of the legislation.

In this section, we will explore these steps as applied to global health policy. This process will be illustrated in a case study on US global AIDS policy. Throughout this section, it is important for the student to keep in mind several prime actors in the policy-making process—both official and unofficial. The official policy-making actors are the

---

[1]Merriam-Webster Dictionary.

three branches of the government; namely: (1) the executive, (2) the legislative, and (3) the judicial. The unofficial actors constitute a diverse universe, including interest or citizen groups, also called *lobbyists*, and the news media. As we said earlier, policy making can be significantly influenced by current events, which are often unpredictable yet help shape the policy-making environment.

Genesis of Global Health Policy in the United States

There are many actors that can influence how a policy is formulated. Policy ideas can come from members of Congress or from the president, from current events and the news media, or from an interest group, or individual US citizen.[2]

Executive Branch

The president of the United States has some degree of choice in setting the administration's agenda.[3] Presidents concentrate on issues that match their personal and political goals—not because of statutory requirements or abstract responsibilities. Although interest groups are a prominent force in policy making, the executive branch tends to make a conscious decision not to engage them.[4] Unless the interest group is a key member of the president's electoral coalition, there is only limited contact, partly because of the sheer number of interest groups in Washington, DC, and partly because there are numerically more opportunities on Capitol Hill to influence policy. Congress has 435 representatives and 100 senators while there is only one president.

As more people organize, as the political process expands to include more groups and classes than ever before, and as demands and needs of competing interests are weighed and mediated in the political process, the power of the president and Congress to insularly control policy is reduced.[5]

Interest Groups, Citizen Groups, and Lobbyists

In the classic formulation of representative government known as pluralism, of which the United States is an example, competing interests balance each other by bringing resources and arguments to bear on different sides of important public policy decisions.[6] Interest groups serve this function in American policy making.

---

[2]For more information on the genesis of policy, see the Library of Congress's THOMAS Web site, http://thomas.loc.gov.

[3]Paul C. Light, "The President's Agenda: Domestic Policy Choice from Kennedy to Clinton," Third Edition, p. 63.

[4]Ibidem, p. 94.

[5]James A. Thurber (editor), "Rivals for Power: Presidential-Congressional Relations," Second Edition, p. 15.

[6]Texas Politics Web site, http://texaspolitics.laits.utexas.edu/html/ig/print_ig.html

An interest group can be defined as a group of people or organizations with similar policy goals that enter the political process to try to achieve those goals.[7] It can be argued that interest groups are the most effective demanders of policies and exist because desired outcomes (i.e., policies) are enhanced through collective action within the political marketplace. By combining and concentrating the resources of their members, interest groups can have a greater impact in the political arena than either individuals or organizations.

In the face of a large and growing number of interest groups, some have noted that the pluralist approach of encouraging and facilitating the formation of interest groups is out of control.[8] In 2006, there were more than 22,000 associations of national scope, all actively pursuing a variety of public policy interest on behalf of their members. Beaufort B. Longest, Jr., (2006) does an excellent job at summarizing the competing arguments regarding interest groups' influence in policy making.

The importance of interest groups lies in the fact that they are able to present a unified position to policy makers on their preferences regarding a particular problem or its solution, by organizing and focusing the opinions of their members.[9] A unified position is much easier for policy makers to assess and respond to than the diverse opinions and preferences of many individuals acting alone. Interest groups or lobbyists are also a significant source of information for policy makers.[10] Lobbyists become experts in the specific policy issue they are representing. Third, interest groups can help policy makers develop and execute both legislation and a political strategy to implement it. Finally, interest groups can assist policy makers in their reelection bids, including through campaign contributions, votes, and volunteering for campaigns.

Obviously, interest groups will seek to elect to office those policy makers that are sympathetic to their cause. This unique aspect of American politics is very closely monitored by the Federal Election Commission (FEC), which was created in 1975 to administer and enforce the Federal Election Campaign Act (FECA). The FEC discloses campaign finance information, enforces the provisions of the law (i.e., the limits and prohibitions on contributions), and oversees the public funding of presidential elections.[11] In addition, only certain types of interest groups are allowed to engage in political activity.[12] The Center for Responsive Politics (www.opensecrets.org), a nonpartisan, nonprofit research organization, is an excellent source of information on campaign finance and policy making.

Another way in which an interest group can influence policy making is through litigation. This is successfully done by challenging existing policies, seeking to stimulate new

---

[7]Beaufort B. Longest, Jr., "Health Policymaking in the United States," Fourth Edition, pp. 82–83.
[8]Ibidem, p. 85.
[9]Ibidem, p. 177.
[10]Ibidem, p. 185.
[11]Ibidem, p. 186.
[12]For a more detailed explanation of these, see Longest, pp. 186–187.

policies, or trying to alter certain aspects of the implementation process through the legal system. Groups can file *amicus curiae* (friend-of-the-court) briefs, which are written depositions stating the group's position on certain issues and describing how the court's decision in the case will affect their membership.[13]

Finally, interest groups can influence policy making through shaping public opinion about a certain policy or issue. Policy makers, who are influenced by the opinions held by their constituents, will tend to listen more attentively to an interest group that has something to say regarding an issue that is of concern to their constituencies. Likewise, if constituents contact their representatives with specific policy issues in mind, that representative is more likely to consider the issue if it comes from those who directly elect them.[14]

Interest Groups in Policy Formulation

Individuals, health-related organizations and interest groups can participate directly in originating ideas for legislation, help with the actual drafting of legislative proposals, and participate in the committee hearings regarding the topics of specific interest to them.[15]

Well-funded and well-staffed interest groups can draw on the services of legislative draftspersons, from within their own organization or from an outside source in order to help draft preferred ideas and concepts into appropriate legislative language. Longest (2006) rightfully points out that an increasingly important source of ideas for legislation is "executive communication" from members of the executive branch to members of the legislative branch.[16] These types of ideas for legislation are typically in the form of a letter from a senior member of the executive branch, from the head of an independent agency, or even from the president himself. These letters are sent to the Speaker of the House of Representatives and, simultaneously, to the president of the Senate, who can then choose to insert them into the legislation development procedures. Another source of executive branch legislative ideas can be the president's annual State of the Union address, where he highlights his priorities and possible legislative initiatives.

A last important consideration regarding policy formulation is the role that the Office of Legislative Counsel plays in crafting legislation. "Leg counsel," as it is referred to on Capitol Hill, is composed of 30 or more attorneys that transform legislative ideas or proposals into actual legislative language appropriate for US laws and statutes. For more information on the Office of Legislative Counsel, visit http://legcoun.house.gov/public.htm (House) or http://slc.senate.gov/index.htm (Senate).

---

[13]Longest, p. 190.
[14]Another good Web site on interest group influence in policy making is the Library of Congress's THOMAS, "How Congress Makes Laws" (http://thomas.loc.gov).
[15]Longest, p. 206.
[16]Ibidem, p. 207.

Policy Development: How a Law is Made

Procedures for introducing legislation are similar in the House and Senate.[17] First, the legislation is crafted by a member of Congress (with input from the various actors discussed above) and introduced either solely, with a cosponsor, or with several original cosponsors. Then the legislation is sent to the "hopper" in the cloakroom on the House or Senate floor, or it is given to the clerk, who assigns the bill a number. Thirdly, the bill is referred to the appropriate committees or subcommittees for consideration. This step is accomplished through committee or subcommittee hearings and through "mark-up" of the bill. During mark-up, the committee either votes to approve the bill (supporting the legislative intent) or pass it along with an unfavorable recommendation. Then the bill is moved into the full House or Senate and debated. After this debate, the full House or Senate will take a vote on whether to pass or reject the legislation. For a bill to become a law, the House and the Senate must pass identical bills. If there are differences in the bills that are passed, the House and Senate will appoint members to a "conference committee," whose goal is to work out the differences between the two bills. Finally, the president must sign the bill for it to become law. For a more detailed explanation of the legislative process, visit the Library of Congress's THOMAS Web site (www.loc.gov) and read "How Our Laws Are Made" or visit the FirstGov Web site (www.firstgov.gov).

Legislation concerning global health policy will typically be assigned to the House Committee on Energy and Commerce's Subcommittee on Health or the House Committee on Ways and Means' Subcommittee on Health. In the Senate, global health policy legislation will be assigned to the Senate Committee on Health, Education, Labor, and Pensions or the Senate Special Committee on Aging. Once the bill is assigned to one of the aforementioned committees, the process of hearings, mark-up, and debate occurs, as described above.

Policy Implementation

A thoughtful, well-drafted law offers no guarantee that the policy intentions of the legislators will be carried out. Well-written laws always include clearly articulated goals and objectives; the "spirit" of the law should also be clear, making it easier for those implementing the legislation to carry out its intent.[18] Unfortunately, flaws can exist within several aspects of a piece of legislation, creating a disconnection between legislative intention and reality. As Longest (2006) writes, "Multiple goals and objectives embedded in a single policy can make its implementation extremely difficult, especially if [these goals] conflict or are not mutually supportive."[19] When this aspect is compounded with a flawed under-

---

[17]Walter J. Oleszek (2003) does a great job at summarizing the major differences between the two chambers.
[18]Longest, pp. 270–272.
[19]Ibidem, p. 270.

lying paradigm—a hypothesis of why the policy will fix an existing situation—the public law as drafted and passed in Congress will be difficult to implement in reality. Another factor to take into consideration when analyzing the implementation of any given law is the degree of flexibility in implementing the policy.[20]

Laws are sometimes left deliberately vague in order to give those institutions implementing them the flexibility to adapt a law to the daily realities involved in implementation. Another factor that directly impacts the implementation of a certain law is what is termed the "fit" between the policy and the implementing agency itself.[21] Two factors to consider here are the level of sympathy an implementing institution has towards the policy's goals and objectives and whether the institution has the necessary resources, in terms of authority, funds, personnel, prestige, information and expertise, technological know-how, equipment, and so on to properly implement the legislation. This degree of fit will oftentimes determine whether a policy will be successfully implemented and how fully the law will be carried out.

Policy Oversight

Even though during the implementation phase much of the responsibility for policy making shifts from the legislative to the executive branch, the former maintains control over the implementation process via congressional oversight. Legislative oversight is the continuing review by Congress of how effectively the executive branch is carrying out congressional mandates.[22] One way in which Congress can exercise its oversight responsibilities is through the "power of the purse," whereby Congress does not appropriate funds to adequately implement certain legislation if it deems the implementation as not consistent with legislative intent. Another way members of Congress are kept informed on whether legislation is properly being carried out is through holding committee hearings on the legislation and its impact (or lack thereof) on the problem or issue(s) it sought to address.

The Government Accountability Office (GAO) and the Congressional Budget Office (CBO) also exercise policy oversight roles.[23] These two independent agencies are specifically tasked by Congress to report back about the effects of policy making.

Finally, there is judicial oversight, in which administrative law judges in implementing agencies hear appeals of people or organizations that are dissatisfied with the way the implementation of a policy affects them.[24]

---

[20]Ibid., p. 272.
[21]Ibid., p. 277.
[22]This role was codified by the Legislative Reorganization Act of 1946 and is today carried out via congressional committees.
[23]More information on the GAO and CBO and how they provide legislative oversight can be found at www.gao.gov and www.cbo.gov, respectively.
[24]Longest, p. 251.

In sum, global health policies are formulated, implemented, and managed (through oversight) by all three branches of the United States government. These laws are also heavily influenced by outside actors, such as interest groups and the news media.

Case Study: HIV/AIDS and US Policy Making

Although the human immunodeficiency virus (HIV) and its consequences, acquired immunodeficiency syndrome (AIDS), were discovered in the early 1980s, the world lay silent on the topic for nearly 2 decades. The policy shift on the global AIDS pandemic came gradually in the United States, and there was no one actor nor was there a pivotal moment that alone shifted US AIDS policy toward a more proactive one. Instead, the January 2000 policy shift occurred as a result of a continuous process involving interest groups and executive–congressional turf battles.

In the late 1990s, an unexpected synergy between AIDS activists and critics of globalization started eating away at the political framework that supported the boom in the pharmaceutical industry. AIDS advocates, such as ACT-UP, tormented Vice President Al Gore's presidential campaign and chained themselves to desks in Trade Representative Charlene Barshefsky's office, pressing the Clinton administration to stop backing the pharmaceutical industry against generic competitors.[25]

Although drug pricing remained an issue of contention for the remainder of Clinton's term in office, the various interest groups pushing for change including gay groups, AIDS advocates, antiglobalization activists, and the media, finally managed to bring the global AIDS pandemic into the spotlight.

These actors would not have had access to the Clinton administration had it not been for two necessary political catalysts influencing the administration. The first was the creation on January 1, 1996, of UNAIDS. The establishment of a United Nations (UN) agency singly devoted to AIDS began to focus attention on the enormity of the problem and identified it as a global health priority among UN member states. Never before had the United Nations created a specialized agency solely for the purpose of dealing with one disease. UNAIDS's creation, therefore, was a strong signal that HIV/AIDS had reached crisis levels. Adding to this pressure, UNAIDS published a report in 1999 that pointed to HIV/AIDS as the lead cause of death in Africa.[26] The United States was thus forced to recognize HIV/AIDS as a global problem of gargantuan proportions.

The second catalyst that helped mold the convergence of events and actors upon changing the global health policy agenda was pressure from within the Clinton administration itself. The ever-present interest of several key members of Congress, the White

---

[25]Barton Gellman, "Death Watch: AIDS, Drugs and Africa: A Turning Point That Left Millions Behind," Washington Post, December 28, 2000.
[26]Previously, African governments had used these reports to cite malaria and tuberculosis as the main causes of death in Africa, thereby justifying their denial of HIV/AIDS as a problem.

House HIV/AIDS "czarina," Sandra Thurman, and, most importantly, Gore's National Security Adviser and member of the Principals Committee, Leon Fuerth, helped bring HIV/AIDS to the forefront. In Congress, longtime advocates of the battle against HIV/AIDS included Representative Nancy Pelosi (D-CA), and Senators Patrick Leahy (D-VT) and Bill Frist (R-TN). Their lobbying efforts helped to maintain constant pressure on the administration to acknowledge and combat the domestic and global AIDS pandemic. By far the most influential congressperson, and, it can be argued, the one who made the connection between global HIV/AIDS and domestic national security is Representative Barbara Lee (D-CA).

Rep. Lee pushed recognition of HIV/AIDS as a national security threat because of its detrimental effect in the areas of trade and social and democratic institutions. She joined Clinton on his 1998 trip to Ghana where she urged him to start addressing the AIDS pandemic.

On the congressional front, Rep. Lee's introduction of the *AIDS Marshall Plan for Africa (AMPA)* bill in July 1999, with full support of the Congressional Black Caucus, got the congressional ball rolling on multilateral funding for an AIDS trust fund in Africa. While Rep. Lee was gathering support for AMPA, Republican Congressmen Jim Leach (R-IA) introduced a similar bill. In February 2000, Reps. Lee and Leach teamed up and produced the bipartisan House Resolution 3519 (H.R. 3519), the *World Bank AIDS Trust Fund Act*, authorizing $100 million for AIDS programs in Africa. H.R. 3519 passed unanimously in the House (May 2000) and brought together disparate Senators (e.g., Helms, Boxer, Feingold, Kennedy, Hatch, Kerry, Durban) who passed it to President Clinton for signing in August 2000. By creating bipartisan support for the issue, Reps. Lee and Leach successfully detached AIDS from party lines; Democrats and Republicans were now working together to manage the global HIV/AIDS problem. There were two reasons, though, that AIDS was now more palatable to Congress: technological breakthroughs and demographics.

The numbers of AIDS patients dying were extraordinary, but the demographics of the infections were what pushed Congress to take notice. The patterns of the pandemic showed that HIV was no longer a gay men's disease. In Africa, more women than men were HIV positive. Additionally, girls were six times more likely than boys to contract the virus, and hundreds of thousands of children were being orphaned by the pandemic. These new victims were more palatable for conservative congressional Republicans to sell to their constituencies at home.

As demographics gave Congress a way to justify its support for global HIV/AIDS, technological breakthroughs pressured Congress into recognizing that there was indeed something that it could do to combat HIV/AIDS. In 1999, Nevaripine therapy to prevent mother-to-child transmission of HIV was released. Previously, there was no selling point with AIDS treatment and prevention: there was no cure, and there was no way to stop the spread. A series of success stories in Uganda, Senegal, and Thailand bolstered the belief that Congress could now begin to tackle the global AIDS problem.

With advocates such as Representative Lee and Senator Helms on the congressional side of the agenda-setting equation, Sandra Thurman and Leon Fuerth on the executive side acted to cement the link between the domestic AIDS battle and its global AIDS counterpart. Thurman organized a 1999 trip to Africa for an executive and legislative delegation. She was receptive to and worked with interest groups active on global AIDS (i.e., Global Health Crisis). She testified before Congress on the need to involve the United States globally, and she caught the attention of the Office of Management and Budget (OMB) in her lobbying for drastically increased spending on global AIDS programs. A 1999 White House report, written by Thurman's office, states:

> As goes Africa, so will go India, Southeast Asia, and the newly independent states of the former Soviet Union, and by 2005, more than 100 million people worldwide will have been infected with HIV. Leadership and resources are desperately needed to turn the tide.[27]

Leon Fuerth picked up on the connection at which Thurman only hinted that global HIV/AIDS is becoming a national security issue. At the time the White House report came out, Fuerth had already been briefed on the growing number of AIDS cases in Africa. In January 2000, US Ambassador to the United Nations, Richard Holbrooke, orchestrated a special session of the UN Security Council (UNSC) to discuss AIDS. Looking around the policy landscape, Holbrooke came to see AIDS as "the most important problem."[28] He found a ready ally in Leon Fuerth.

Holbrooke proposed a visit by Gore to the UNSC to dramatize American urgency for global HIV/AIDS. It did not hurt that Gore had been ceaselessly tormented by AIDS activists throughout his campaign for the Democratic nomination. On January 10, 2000, Gore spoke to the UNSC of the world's moral duty to "wage and win a great and peaceful war" against AIDS.[29]

Conclusion

As the AIDS case study illustrates, many actors including the various branches of the US government, the news media, interest groups, and, often, the unpredictable collusion of current events and public opinion serve to impact global health policy making. There are many routes to influencing, implementing, and overseeing the implementation of policies affecting global health, all of which make for a dynamic process in US policy making.

---

[27]Pooven Moodley, "Drugs Alone Will Not Stop AIDS in Africa," Milwaukee Journal Sentinel, July 23, 2000.
[28]Gellmann, July 5, 2000.
[29]Ibidem.

The Bolivian Perspective

Introduction

Bolivia is a small country with big problems. Situated in central South America, Bolivia covers 1,084,380 square kilometers (418,681 square miles) and, according to the latest estimation, there are 8,989,046 inhabitants.[30] Although 64% of Bolivia's population is urban, its 36% rural population is higher than the rural percentage for many of its neighbors. One measure of poverty linked to the urban–rural divide is the disparity in basic sanitation services. In 2004, 65% of the population had access to piped water services, but if we break down this statistic into its urban and rural components, we notice that 87% of those in urban areas had access, while only 27% of rural inhabitants had access to piped water.[31] Before we delve into Bolivian health policy, it is important to examine some basic socioeconomic indicators and trends that influence health issues. These indicators help shape the current political debate that is taking place under the current presidency of Evo Morales.[32]

From the latest available statistics in 2005, Bolivia's gross domestic product (GDP) per capita is US$1061, which places it much lower than its upper-middle income neighbor Argentina, whose GDP per capita is US$8,096. Not only is economic growth traditionally slow, but the World Bank calculates that Bolivian real per capita income has actually declined by 1% in the last 50 years, whereas Brazil's real per capita income increased by 350%, Chile's by 200%, and Argentina's by 75%. Not only has Bolivia experienced lower economic growth rates than its neighbors Chile, Argentina, and Brazil, it also suffers from significant income inequality. The World Bank and many Latin America experts attribute Bolivia's poverty to its rigid social structure that offers little opportunity for advancement out of the lower socioeconomic strata and helps perpetuate this income inequality.[33]

As evidenced by the aforementioned economic indicators, Bolivia is one of the poorest countries in Latin America; for example, a life expectancy at birth of only 64.5 years is just another statistic that mirrors the ill effects of poverty on the country's citizenry. This is considerably lower than Argentina's life expectancy of 74.6 years or Mexico's at 75 years. Bolivia's neighbor Peru is most similar in terms of ethnic composition, yet its life expectancy at birth is 5.5 years greater than that of Bolivia.[34]

---

[30]World Fact Book, Central Intelligence Agency, https://www.cia.gov/cia/publications/factbook/geos/bl.html.

[31]United Nations, Economic Commission for Latin America, *Statistical Yearbook for Latin American and the Caribbean, 2005*, p. 71.

[32]Morales was inaugurated as president of Bolivia in January 2006 and is leader of the Movement for Socialism (MAS).

[33]World Bank, *Bolivia Country Brief*, September 2006, http://www.worldbank.org.

[34]World Bank Development Indicators Database, April 2006. http://devdata.wordlbank.org. World Development Report, 2007, World Bank, September 23, 2006.

As we will discover in this section, Bolivia does have an extensive health policy that attempts to alleviate many poverty-related problems within its borders. As a result, some of the country's health indicators improved in the 1990s. Its mortality rate for children under the age of 5 years declined from 125 per 1,000 in 1990 to 69 per 1,000 in 2004, while the number of Bolivians with access to potable water increased from 72% in 1990 to 85% in 2003.[35]

One important distinguishing factor that influences health policy is Bolivia's ethnic composition. Bolivia has a large indigenous population: 56% of the population identify themselves ethnically as either Aymara or Quechua. Indigenous peoples are especially concentrated in Bolivia's rural areas. It is in these areas that are lacking adequate roads, potable water, sanitation, and basic health facilities. Indigenous rural areas are also most likely to be economically depressed.

Bolivia's poverty is best described by the Ministry of Health and Sport (MOH) when it summarized the poor quality of life that is so widespread throughout the country. In its report *Health Situation, 2004*, the MOH noted the following:

- 58% of the population had inadequate access to water and sanitation.
- 48% of the population had inadequate caloric intake.
- 39% of the population live in substandard housing.
- 29% of the urban population lives in abject poverty while 59% of rural dwellers fall into this category.[36]

Clearly, Bolivia faces considerable challenges in the area of health policy, many of which are largely socioeconomic in nature.

Politics, Policy, and Cultural Influences in the Healthcare System

Bolivia is a country that adopted a representative democratic system in 1982. Similar to the United States, Bolivia's government is divided between the executive, legislative and judicial branches. Bolivia is not a stranger to political turmoil: from 2000 to 2006, Bolivia had five presidents. In 2006, though, Bolivians democratically elected their current president, Evo Morales, who won by a clear majority of the vote.

Morales is Bolivia's first indigenous president and a socialist who actively pursues policies to alleviate poverty and raise living standards for the country's large indigenous population. His emphasis on centralized government control, nationalization of natural gas resources, and friendly relations with Cuba's Fidel Castro and Venezuelan President Hugo Chavez make his term in office controversial to certain sectors of Bolivian society.

---

[35]World Bank, *Bolivia Country Brief*, September 2006.
[36]Ministerio de Salud y Deportes (MOH), *Situación de Salud, Bolivia 2004*, pp. 16, 34.

As a former union leader for coca growers, Morales' stance on coca production distances him from the US government. The United States is more concerned about illegal drug production than the commercialization of coca leaf as a traditional health product—something Morales hopes will contribute to Bolivia's economy. In a September 2006 speech to the United Nations, Morales explained that coca is "part of our national identity [and] represents the community and its collectivity for the indigenous people."[37] Citing a Harvard University study on the health benefits of the coca leaf, he distinguished coca's medicinal properties from cocaine and was quoted as saying that "coca is green, not white like cocaine."[38] This example reveals the importance of Bolivia's traditions among its indigenous peoples and should not be overlooked when dealing with its healthcare system.

Universal coverage and access to health services for all citizens has long been an accepted goal for most Latin American governments.[39] Bolivia is no exception and shares this political philosophy toward health care coverage. For this reason it created the Basic Health Insurance (BHI) social security program to offer access to a wide variety of health provisions from prevention to cure. Yet for a variety of socioeconomic reasons, particularly in rural areas, public-sector health care within the BHI only reaches 43–48% of the population.[40]

Political influence on public health policy in Bolivia has been driven by powerful unions in the public health and social security systems. These unions were created to fight dictatorships of the 1980s, but remain in place today. Unions use methods such as strikes to obtain salary increases, reduced labor hours, and extraordinary privileges. Although the debate on how to provide universal health care rages on in Bolivia, no government to date has been able to reform the healthcare social security system in order to achieve this goal.

Decentralization Versus Centralization in Bolivia's Health Sector

To maximize improvements and bring health care closer to the people, the Bolivian government implemented a decentralized healthcare policy that President Morales is trying to alter with a renewed shift toward centralization. We will first examine the origin of the decentralization policy that still operates at the time of this writing.

---

[37]Haider Rivzi, "Bolivia: Morales Takes Coca Campaign—and a Leaf—to U.N" Global Information Network, p. 1.

[38]"Bolivian Leader Defends His Drug Policy," *The Guardian*, September 20, 2006.

[39]Cristian C. Baeza and Truman G. Packard, "Beyond Survival: Protecting Households From Health Shocks in Latin America," p. 128.

[40]Pan American Health Organization, "Bolivia: Country Profile," *Epidemiological Bulletin/PAHO*, March 2003, vol. 24, no. 1, p. 8. The MOH estimates that 77 percent of the population has no access to health care. See: Ministry of Health and Sports, *Situación de Salud: Bolivia 2004*, La Paz, Bolivia: MOH, January 2006, p. 157.

In April 1994, the Bolivian government passed the Community Involvement Act that provided the country's 314 municipalities with autonomy over resource management. This law marked a shift toward decentralization of Bolivia's healthcare structures and greatly modified the organization of healthcare services and delivery. The decentralization policy shifted 20% of central government revenues to these 314 municipalities; part of this percentage was resources that the central government used to finance healthcare programs.

In the public health sector the 1994 law transferred ownership of health infrastructure, health investment, and infrastructure maintenance to the municipalities. Within this context, public health is coordinated with municipal authorities and community representatives, through the four main actors in the healthcare system: (1) the Ministry of Health and Sports (MOH); (2) the state governor's Office of Health (SEDES); (3) the municipal government (DILOS); and (4) civil society, meaning the private sector. These four entities are responsible for providing health services to Bolivia's population. The decentralization policy was intended to make services more accessible to healthcare users and to empower municipalities who are in contact with their constituents to better meet their needs. A World Bank study noted that "it also gave local governments the authority to decide autonomously whether or not to fund health care, including the option to use the central government transfers for other purposes."[41]

The debate over introducing centralization in healthcare policy corresponds to Morales' desire to consolidate power in the central government in order to achieve his stated goals of poverty reduction. The decentralization policy in effect since 1994 is now challenged.

The most basic challenge Bolivia faces surrounds the creation of a Constitutional Assembly in July 2006 to rewrite the Bolivian Constitution. The result is an ideological battle between Bolivia's indigenous and nonindigenous peoples. Some might say that the current debate about Bolivia's political future is an ideological one that pits the "haves," or white Bolivian conservatives on the political right, against the "have-nots," or indigenous socialists on the left. Although most Bolivians recognize the pressing socioeconomic problems in the country, some citizens believe that this ideological struggle overshadows the real economic and social problems impeding the country's development. These problems include economic growth, revenue generation, distribution of wealth, and widespread poverty especially among Bolivia's native peoples. A new constitution modeled after Morales' vision will likely have a trickle down effect and further reinforce centralization of health care.

Cultural and Indigenous Influences on Health Policy

Approximately 62% of the Bolivian population belongs to one of Bolivia's various indigenous peoples. This ethnic diversity translates into different concepts of health, disease,

---

[41]World Bank, *Health Sector Reform in Bolivia: A Decentralization Case Study*, pp. 1–2.

and the coexistence of multiple medical systems ranging from biomedical (Western) to indigenous (traditional) medicine. The 2004 per capita healthcare expenditure was $5,711 in the United States and a mere US$60 per person in Bolivia.[42] Although private medicine is an important avenue for upper- and middle-class sectors of society in the United States, health policy making in developing countries such as Bolivia is affected by populations with fewer resources who often avail themselves of traditional health options as their only viable alternative. Such options usually cost less than Western medicine and also have cultural bonds to local society. Vandebroek, Calewaert, De Jonckheere, Sanca, and others describe, for example, how antibiotics are sold one pill at a time because local villagers could not afford the full dosage at once.[43] It is in this overall context that we must view the Bolivian health system complete with its own unique constituents.

There is still a high level of inequality and exclusion—some of which results from personal and cultural reasons. Clinics may be too far from home and inaccessible to those without transportation. Andean cultural norms also influence how citizens react to health care. In their study on traditional medicine in Bolivia, Vandebroek and colleagues write of an "Andean medical cosmology . . . full of images of human vulnerability to a hostile and unpredictable environment as reflected by the *wayras* [airborne or windborne diseases]."[44] Some inequality and exclusion are inadvertently sanctioned by the government through administrative requirements that impede certain citizens' access to health programs. For example, a birth certificate is required for access to infant health care; this translates into 12% of children under the age of 10 being excluded from such care.[45]

Sixty percent of those excluded can be attributed to external, or administrative barriers, while 40% are caused by personal or cultural reasons. Even though a significant portion of Bolivia's population lacks health care, there has not been significant improvement in the cultural adaptation of health services to accommodate the variety of indigenous populations in Bolivia. The current Minister of Health, Nila Heredia, hopes this system will change because the hospital-based healthcare system does not adequately recognize traditional culture in healing and prevention. Heredia believes that imported healthcare models fail when they ignore local customs. She cites the example of childbirth:

> In many cultures the placenta has a profound symbolic value. Therefore, it must be kept, and must be buried in the right way, so as to guarantee the survival and life of the child. According to medical logic, the placenta is useless and is thrown away.

---

[42]World Bank, *World Bank Development Indicators/2005*. March 2005.
[43]Ina Vandebroek, Jan-Bart Calewaert, Stijn De Jonckheere, Sabino Sanca, et al. "Use of Medicinal Plants and Pharmaceuticals by Indigenous Communities in the Bolivian Andes and Amazon," *Bulletin of the World Health Organization*, April 2004, vol. 82, no. 4, p. 248.
[44]Ibid., p. 248.
[45]UNICEF, "Health Insurance for Children and Mothers Slows Child Mortality in Bolivia," http://www.unicef.org.

This creates a huge gulf. And then, the woman would not go back for medical attention, because a part of her child, a part of life, has been thrown away.[46]

Heredia's approach to health policy is pragmatic—that is, it does not make sense to ignore the culture of more than 60% of Bolivia's population.

The new Vice Ministry of Indigenous Health and Traditional Medicine created in 2006 within the MOH seeks to bridge this gap. This ministry will have the challenging task of creating an intercultural model that integrates various aspects of culture, language, and knowledge of Western practices with traditional medicine from indigenous and native populations. Giving traditional medicine a high level of formal recognition will help to generate a greater degree of social cohesion in the country.[47] In their survey of traditional Bolivian medicine, Vandebroek et al. confirm the important role that traditional medicine plays in primary health care in rural areas. They point to the use of traditional healers in the area of Apillapampa, who were trained in Western medicine and work weekends in the primary healthcare facility when the regular medical staff is absent.[48] What this vice-ministerial-level office does is give formal acceptance of already existing practices.

Another way to incorporate indigenous peoples into Bolivia's health policy is through a program called EXTENSA which expands health coverage in rural areas. EXTENSA focuses primarily on infant and maternal health and incorporates mobile health units and personnel into their healthcare delivery plan.[49] Although not exclusively devoted to indigenous health, Law 2426 (passed in November 2002 as part of Bolivia's Poverty Reduction Strategy and implemented in 2003) created the Universal Maternal and Child Insurance (SUMI) program, which also offers added healthcare benefits to mothers and children. In the Andean region of South America, which includes Bolivia, Chile, Colombia, Ecuador, Peru, and Venezuela, mortality during pregnancy, delivery, or postdelivery is 30 times greater than in Canada, making maternal care a crucial part of Bolivia's health policy.[50]

Refining National Health Care

The 1997–2000 and 2001–2002 strategic health plans were designed to develop the Bolivian health system as proposed by Senator Mario Paz Zamora in his Universal Access and Bolivian Health System legislation, which would ensure universal access through individual, family, and community primary health care. To this was added an "epidemio-

---

[46]Gustavo Capdevila, "Bolivia: Wanted—Health Care Adapted to Indigenous Cultures," *Global Information Network*, May 26, 2006, p. 1.
[47]Perspectiva Global de Salud Publica y el Rol del Gobierno de Bolivia, UMSA.
[48]Ina Vandebroek, Jan-Bart Calewaert, Stijn De Jonckheere, Sabino Sanca, et al., p. 248.
[49]See: Ministry of Health and Sports, *Programa EXTENSA, Manual de Procedimientos Administrativos : Brigadas Integrales de Salud.*
[50]Ministry of Health and Sports Bolivia.

logical shield." The epidemiological shield concept was part of the 1999 health sector reforms and tackles Bolivia's communicable and vector-borne diseases, namely Chagas disease, tuberculosis, dengue, and malaria. The "shield" also includes vaccination programs and the establishment of an epidemiological surveillance system.[51]

The main pillar supporting these health sector reforms is the Basic Health Insurance, followed by its expansion to the Indian and Native Basic Health Insurance (SBSIO), and the Maternal and Infant Universal Insurance System (SUMI). These programs are designed to guarantee that all inhabitants have permanent access to preventive and other health benefits essential to mitigating the causes and consequences of disease and death in the country. The reforms provide health care and nutrition for children less than 5 years of age; immunization and promotion of nutrition; and attention to high-priority problems including diagnosis and treatment of the country's principal epidemics—tuberculosis, malaria, cholera, and sexually transmitted diseases.

The Ministry of Health and Sports is responsible for health sector regulation and for issuing and applying policies and national standards. A recent cause for debate in 2006 was the arrival of 600 Cuban doctors to Bolivia. Invited by President Morales, the doctors provoked an outcry from the medical community concerned about the lack of credential verification as required by law.

More subtle concern surrounded the fear that Cuban doctors may take Bolivian medical jobs away from Bolivian physicians. This resulted in a national strike organized by the Bolivian Medical Board. According to Deputy Health Minister Juan Alberto Nogales, the Cuban physicians only work in underserved rural areas and provide their own medical equipment.[52] Although approximately 43–48% of the population uses the public services of the BHI, between 20–25% of the population lacks access to health services altogether. This healthcare gap coupled with low capacity to adequately fund health care makes it more understandable why the Cuban medical teams were welcomed by the Morales government. As long as there is an absence of policy and enforcement to keep health workers in rural areas from migrating to cities, the urban–rural divide will continue to exist in Bolivia's healthcare system.

Case Study: Executive Branch Policy Making

Determining policy at the ministerial level is both challenging and a long-term endeavor. Nothing can be changed in one day. Public health policy is a process subject to political, economic, and social cycles. As Minister of Health and Sports in 2001, coauthor of this chapter, Dr. Enrique Paz, realized that you have to set short-term goals for yourself and long-term goals for the ministry. Paz cites an example of how the president requested that he design a health plan based on the General Economic and Social Development Plan of

---

[51]*Bolivian National Epidemiology Report*, Ministry of Health and Social Prevision.
[52]Colin Leslie, "Bolivian MDs Protest Free Cuban Care," *Medical Post* (Toronto), p. 48.

1997–2002 (PGDES) that would incorporate Bolivia's international commitments with the 5-year National Health Strategic Plan 1997-2002 (PES) to fight poverty.

Paz called the plan a "Bolivian Health and Social Security 12-Month Plan, 2001–2002" (P-12M) and it had six important points:

1. Implement the National Dialogue Law that Congress approved in 2001 to help fight poverty in coordination with all social, economical, and community-based organizations.

2. Develop a plan to create a civil service career system within the social security system. Paz created a presidential decree that approved a board of nine persons— three from the private sector, three from the labor sector, and three from the government.

3. Strengthen Bolivian health reform, assuring loans and international cooperation. The mandate was to expand BHI and free health insurance ranging from the elderly to indigenous populations and schools.

4. Consolidate the "epidemiological shield," the information platform, the Chagas program for pesticide fumigation and treatment, and other programs.

5. Strengthen the public health system with the creation of the National Institute of Public Health (INSP), whose goal it was to regroup all the research and public laboratories as a technical entity within the Ministry of Health.

6. Create the National Direction of Environmental Health (DGSAyP) and Health Promotion, whose goal it was to implement cross-collaborations with other government entities to address risk factors and treatments within the public health domain.

Indian and Native Basic Health Insurance (SBSIO)

Paz notes that during his service as Minister of Health, the MOH formed the Indian and Native Basic Health Insurance (SBSIO). This created a new paradigm, or permanent bridge, between traditional and formal, or Western, medicine. The main objective was to have a common language for prevalent health conditions within both systems and a mutual acceptance of knowledge and therapies associated with each of the cultures in Bolivia.

The other important piece of the SBSIO is the *Manual of Native Pharmacopoeia*. Thirty-six medicines used by traditional and nontraditional doctors were examined. It was expected that conditions would be created for small business to devote more time and resources to find plants and transform them into medicines. While Costa Rica's National Biodiversity Institute (InBio) illustrates the importance of searching for medicinal plants, or bio-prospecting, classifying them, and negotiating royalty contracts with large pharmaceutical companies, the Bolivian example is more modest and calls for the transformation of medic-inal plants into commercially marketed medicines by small businesses whose area of opera-tion is more limited than the multinational corporations with whom InBio negotiates.

Conclusion

Although Bolivian healthcare practices have progressed over the past 34 years, it is also true that the results achieved are not adequate. Most resources are allocated to fight infectious diseases, leaving the system without resources, or vision to focus on long-term planning processes. Bolivia also needs a multi-sector and interdisciplinary approach to address determinants of public health that contribute to the management of disease. Other sectors can contribute meaningfully to this interdisciplinary endeavor. Bolivia has not been able to expand more health promotion programs because of political circumstances and limited resources.[53]

In many countries, both developing and developed, the healthcare debate revolves around how to achieve universal coverage in medical services, how to best combine private and institutional medicine, how to finance increased costs, and how to achieve healthcare equity. Health care is becoming more important because of biomedical advances and increasing societal expectations. Health care takes up more budget dollars in almost every country as needs grow over time. This is Bolivia's challenge in the future.

A Multilateral Perspective

In this era of expanding global trade and interdependence, travel, and international awareness of domestic events within countries, international health becomes an increasingly important policy issue. Disease is a transnational phenomenon that knows no borders and, for this reason, has become especially worrisome as busy executives fly, for example, from Europe to Asia and Africa, with the United States as final destination—all in a matter of days.

News of infectious disease outbreaks in the developing world (e.g., severe acute respiratory syndrome [SARS]) and avian influenza (pandemic flu), which heretofore went unnoticed, now attracts great attention in the European, Canadian, and US media. Such attention is as much about fear of spreading disease to the developed world, often called the "North," than it is about the well-being of persons in Africa, Asia, or Latin America who contract debilitating or even deadly diseases. As the global "South," or developing world, expands its connections within the global marketplace, health issues once relegated to populations of the developed North (e.g., cancer, diabetes, obesity) also emerge as real health concerns. With increased disposable income comes access to products such as cigarettes, which are linked to cancer in humans. This means that global policy makers must now confront communicable, or infectious, diseases, as well as noncommunicable, or chronic diseases.

The policy debate continues to revolve around whether to stress communicable diseases prevalent among the South's poor or noncommunicable diseases that are

---

[53]Enrique Paz, *Informe de Gestión 1997–2002*, Ministerio de Salud y Previsión Social, Republica de Bolivia, 2002.

responsible for most deaths in the developed world (Lancet, 2000). Many in the developing world argue, as Reddy (2005) does, that we should emphasize both communicable and noncommunicable diseases rather than emphasize only those infectious diseases that commonly afflict the poorest 20% of the developing world. Reddy et al. point out that India has the most oral cancers in the world attributed to the use of chewing tobacco as well as the highest number of diabetics.[54] Even in our previous case of Bolivia, communicable diseases only account for 12% of all deaths.[55]

Reddy urges us not to forget that noncommunicable, chronic diseases such as cancer or cardiovascular disease afflict the middle 60% of those who live in the global South.[56,57] Because of his status as a respected Indian cardiologist, and a proponent of dealing with chronic diseases, Reddy achieved the status of an innovator within the World Health Organization's (WHO) Network of Innovators intended to encourage the diffusion of new ideas for disease prevention. Scarce resources also influence this policy debate. Put simply, how should countries allocate their money toward communicable or noncommunicable diseases? This same question applies in the global arena when WHO makes decisions within its own United Nations (UN) budgetary constraints.

We know that health policy can be made within countries at the local, provincial or state, and national levels. However, policy can also be made in international organizations by member countries. One very important international organization responsible for health policy making that influences countries around the globe is the World Health Organization. In this section we examine how WHO member countries strive to create effective global health policies that meet the needs of many countries both in the developed North and developing South. This is not an easy task because member countries maintain sovereignty within their own borders and have a final say over whether or not to accept a WHO policy and implement it.

One recent example of a successful WHO creation is the international treaty called the Framework Convention on Tobacco Control (FCTC), which has the signatures of many developed and developing countries. The FCTC is the world's first public health treaty currently in force that globally addresses a major health issue. Expansion of such wellness-related treaties narrows the health gap worldwide and contributes to a rapidly evolving relationship between North and South that reflects a new health paradigm, or model. This paradigm's major objective is the improvement of health worldwide, but also reflects a two-way path between the developed and developing world in order to achieve that

---

[54]Srinath K. Reddy, Bela Shah, Cherian Varghese, and Anbumani Ramadoss. 2005. Responding to the Threat of Chronic Diseases in India. *Lancet* 366: 1746–51.

[55]Pan-American Health Organization, "Basic Country Health Profiles for the Americas, Bolivia," (September 2002) http://www.paho.org.

[56]Srinath K. Reddy, Bela Shah, Cherian Varghese, and Anbumani Ramadoss. 2005. Responding to the Threat of Chronic Diseases in India. *Lancet* 366: 1746–51.

[57]Srinath K. Reddy, Bela Shah, Cherian Varghese, and Anbumani Ramadoss. 2005. Responding to the Threat of Chronic Diseases in India. *Lancet* 366: 1746–51.

objective. One way to achieve this objective is through the expansion of global health policies by means of international treaties, agreements, and conventions. Such documents possess greater legal clout than the mere existence of a global health program or regulation. That is how the WHO functioned until the FCTC came into force.

This section treats the WHO as the primary catalyst for this paradigm shift to a proactive, multilateral treaty-based method of improving global health. To better understand how the WHO operates we should ask ourselves what factors contribute to make the FCTC an innovative global health initiative within the UN umbrella. By asking this question we will gain a deeper appreciation of how the WHO operates and what that organization values in the global health policy-making process. Arriving at an organization's values, however, is a complex task and involves not only agreement, but also struggles and conflict among member countries—some of whom do not share a similar approach to solving health problems.

World Health Organization: Objectives and Governance Structures

Before examining programs, treaties, and activities it behooves us to understand what the WHO is and how it operates. The World Health Organization was founded on April 7, 1948, as a specialized agency within the United Nations designed to deal with health issues. Its constitution recognizes the totality of health, ranging from physical and mental aspects to social well-being, and not simply disease eradication. In fact, its comprehensive approach aspires to the "attainment by all peoples of the highest possible level of health."[58]

The WHO constitution emphasizes cooperation by individuals and states in its promotion of health and wellness and also recognizes unequal development patterns among states. The WHO constitution asserts that "Governments have a responsibility for the health of their peoples which can be fulfilled only by the provision of adequate health and social measures."[59] From its inception, the WHO has operated on the premise that health is a public good requiring governmental action to achieve its objectives. To achieve its objectives the WHO engages in coordinating international health work and enabling governments to strengthen their own health systems. Its functions also include supplying technical assistance and emergency aid when requested by host governments. In addition, the WHO functions as a statistical clearinghouse for epidemiological information and assists in disease eradication. The WHO's *Weekly Epidemiological Record*,[60] for example, is an outcome of its information dissemination function and is a useful tool for health policy

---

[58]World Health Organization. 1948a. *Constitution of the World Health Organization*. Geneva, Switzerland. http://www.who.int/about/en.

[59]World Health Organization (WHO), 1948a. *Constitution of the World Health Organization*. http://www.who.int/about/en.

[60]WHO, 2006a. *Weekly Epidemiological Record*. www.who.inter/wer.

makers worldwide as is its annual publication, *World Health Statistics*.[61] The WHO also promotes international standards for food and biological and other products.

The World Health Organization is actively involved in data gathering, research, and policy applications that contribute to the goal of improved health for the world's peoples. Its first notable project, the creation of international sanitary regulations, was unveiled in 1951 and later renamed the International Health Regulations (IHR). The IHR are a binding legal instrument on all WHO members who have not specifically deposited a reservation or rejection of these regulations. The 1969 regulations are currently in force and aim to stop the international spread of disease. Revised IHR were adopted in May 2005 and will enter into force on June 15, 2007.[62,63] Toward establishment of uniform world standards, the new regulations create a "single code of procedures and practices for routine public health measures at international airports and ports and some ground crossings."[64]

So emotionally charged is the global spread of infectious disease that it becomes less controversial and acts as a unifying force among states. Regardless of their political beliefs or systems, afflicted states share one commonality—a fear of disease. This is not the case for product-induced illnesses such as the link between tobacco and chronic diseases—especially cancer. By the very fact that tobacco products such as cigarettes or cigars are commercially produced and sold globally, their health ramifications become mired in a trade-related debate. This is not the case for malaria, or dengue fever. In one current example, the avian flu does involve the poultry industry worldwide. However, the poultry industry does not willfully produce a product it knows will harm people's health.

To manage its numerous programs and achieve its objectives, the WHO relies on what some consider a vast bureaucracy. However, as the new IHR reveal, this organizational structure has shown itself capable of rapid response. The new regulations are a post-9/11 recognition of global health security and incorporate standards not only for natural occurrences but also for "accidental release or deliberate use of biological and chemical agents or radionuclear material that affect health."[65]

The WHO's administrative headquarters is in Geneva, Switzerland, and the World Health Assembly (WHA) is its main decision and policy-making body. Each May the WHA holds an annual meeting for delegates from all 192 member countries with the goal of policy and financial review. The WHA appoints the director-general and also approves the budget. The 32-member executive board meets in January each year to discuss current issues and concerns which the board formulates into a formal agenda for WHA's annual meeting in May. The executive board elects its members who serve 3-year terms.

[61]WHO, 2006b. *World Health Statistics*. www.who.inter/wer.

[62]WHO, 2005. Revision of the International Health Regulations. WHA58.3, May 23.

[63]WHO, 2006c. *International Health Regulations*, http://www.who.int/csr/ihr/en.

[64]WHO, 2006c. *International Health Regulations*, http://www.who.int/csr/ihr/en.

[65]WHO, 2005. Revision of the International Health Regulations. WHA58.3, May 23.

The WHO Secretariat includes a 3,500-employee team of health experts and support personnel who work at headquarters, in the WHO's six regional offices worldwide (Africa, Eastern Mediterranean, Europe, Latin America, Southeast Asia, and Western Pacific), or as needed throughout the world. Reflecting the unavoidably political nature of this specialized agency, the WHO also maintains offices at the African Union (AU) and Economic Commission for Africa (Addis Ababa, Ethiopia), the European Union (Brussels), United Nations (New York), and the World Bank and International Monetary Fund (Washington, DC).

Collaboration with Nongovernmental Organizations

Although the WHO's current Civil Society Initiative encourages working relations between itself and nongovernmental organizations (NGOs), it is the constitution that delineates this relationship. An appendix to the WHO's Basic (Constitutional) Text is called the "Principles Governing Relations Between the World Health Organization and Nongovernmental Organizations." This constitutional appendix states that NGOs play a vital role in support of international health needs especially as they harmonize various interests within countries and regions.[66] The WHO's desire to collaborate with NGOs stems from its constitutional beginnings and appears on its Web site: "The objectives of WHO's relations with NGOs are to promote the policies, strategies, and activities of WHO and, where appropriate, to collaborate with NGOs in jointly agreed activities to implement them." [67]

The World Health Organization recognizes that informal or ad hoc contacts with NGOs can develop into an official relationship sanctioned by the executive board. Privileges awarded to officially sanctioned NGOs are outlined in the "Principles" text and include the right to:

- Appoint a nonvoting representative to WHO meetings and conferences.
- Provide statements upon request by the meeting chairperson.
- Request that the director-general make documentation available.
- Access nonconfidential documents that the director-general makes available to NGOs.[68]

The relevance of these governance structures and collaborative relationship with NGOs becomes apparent when moving to the next step—that of examining how the WHO transitioned from relatively politically risk-free health policies to a bolder, more innovative

---

[66]WHO, 1948b. *Principles Governing Relations Between the World Health Organization and Nongovernmental Organizations.* http://www.who.int/about/en.
[67]WHO, 2000d. *Framework Convention on Tobacco Control.* WHA53.16.
[68]World Health Organization. 1948a. *Constitution of the World Health Organization.* http://www.who.int/about/en.

approach that tackles not only tobacco-related diseases, but also the tobacco companies themselves.

Politicization of Global Health

The WHO is not new to allegations of politicization of the global health agenda, which manifested itself primarily as Cold War or Arab-Israeli cleavages, and in the post-Cold War era as a North-South cleavage. Amid the Cold War-era impasse and in an effort to accomplish what it set out to do in its constitutional objectives—to deal with health issues—many of the WHO's policies shied away from aggressively tackling social or commerce-related health issues. Siddiqi (1995) reminds us that such allegations span the WHO's history and go as far back as 1949 when the Soviet Union walked out in protest over accusations of politicization.

As mentioned earlier, the constitution put WHO philosophically at odds with the United States from its inception in 1948 because of its view that health is a *public good* and that government has an inherent responsibility for the health of its citizens. While providing some of the world's best health care and demonstrating a strong commitment to public health issues such as creation of a sanitary infrastructure (e.g., clean drinking water, sewage control, disease control), the United States has long regarded personal health care as a private matter—not as a defined right over which government has responsibility. Only as medical costs rose dramatically and the pool of uninsured increased did the debate expand to include whether Americans have a right to universal health care.

The role of government as having a responsibility for every American's health then entered the national debate in the United States, but it remains just that—a debate. However, very real fears of socialized medicine tainted the WHO's constitutional preamble from the beginning as it clearly stated that "governments have a responsibility for the health of their peoples."[69]

Siddiqi (1995) notes that, as early as 1946 and prior to the actual creation of the WHO, there was a rift over the new organization's responsibilities. The US adversity to socialized medicine from an insurance standpoint put it at odds with the Soviet Union, the Scandinavian countries, and most European countries. Objections over health insurance issues in this new health body delayed US ratification by 2 years.[70] The notion of political blocs is not new to the UN in the General Assembly or the Security Council, and the WHO is not immune to such political maneuvering either. The WHA has occasionally split over North-South issues. The one state-one vote method in the WHA means that African states, for example, can "produce as many as 30 or 35 votes, compared to the 1 vote for the United States or even some 20 votes for the major, developed states that supply most of

---

[69]World Health Organization. 1948a. *Constitution of the World Health Organization.* http://www.who.int/about/en.
[70]Javed Siddiqi, *World Health and World Politics: The World Health Organization and the UN System.*

the funds of the WHO."[71] The voting structure within the main policy-making and legislative body of the WHO provides the South with an inherent advantage when formulating policies.

Since both European, socialist, and developing countries share a broader interpretation of what public health should encompass and how to solve related health problems, voting becomes yet another structural advantage for pushing the innovative envelope—and expanding the global health agenda to include the negative affects of commercially produced tobacco products. It is not surprising that, within this environment, a more comprehensive interpretation of health issues eventually made it to the forefront in the form of the FCTC.

The move of Eastern European countries into one European bloc strengthens the argument of government responsibility for health care because both eastern and western Europe share the belief of health as a public good. Both are prone to accept greater government regulation as means for achieving a health objective. This puts Europe in greater harmony with the global South, which also favors a regulatory approach to the tobacco industry.

By 1978 the WHO became bolder in its assertions that health is a totality of aspects, not only the absence of disease. The WHO-sponsored International Conference on Primary Health Care produced the Declaration of Alma Ata in September 1978, called health a "fundamental human right," and clarified the WHO's position that optimal health requires "the action of many other social and economic sectors in addition to the health sector."[72] Further emboldened by the global South to move beyond health into the economic realm, the declaration went on to state:

> Economic and social development, based on a New International Economic Order, is of basic importance to the fullest attainment of health for all and to the reduction of the gap between the health status of the developing and developed countries.[73]

The Alma Ata Declaration wrote of health as a human right, but the WHO's publication, *Health for All in the Twenty-first Century* (1998), went a step further to affirm a "global public health good" within the context of trade liberalization. The document urged "greater compatibility in policy objectives to be developed between international and intergovernmental agencies and multinationals involved in trade and health."[74] This is an

[71]Javed Siddiqi, *World Health and World Politics: The World Health Organization and the UN System.*

[72]WHO, 1978, *Declaration of Alma-Ata.* International Conference on Primary Health Care, Alma-Ata, USSR. September 6–12.

[73]WHO, 1978, *Declaration of Alma-Ata.* International Conference on Primary Health Care, Alma-Ata, USSR. September 6–12.

[74]WHO, 1998, *Health for All in the Twenty-first Century.* A51/5.

earlier first step toward linking multinational companies to health and would later prove useful in formulating a tobacco treaty.

In support of the 2000 UN Millennium Declaration, the WHO set about implementing the following goals by the year 2015. The millennium development goals (MDGs) are development oriented and seek to eradicate poverty and hunger, achieve universal primary education, promote gender equality, reduce child mortality, improve maternal health, combat disease, promote environmental sustainability, and develop a global partnership for development (UN Millennium Project, 2006). The WHO interprets the MDGs as a means for developed countries to contribute money and expertise to developing countries in order to improve global health. The link reflects an expanded approach to health "through trade, development assistance, debt relief, access to essential medicines, and technology transfer."[75] While *Health for All* set the stage for making multinationals a responsible health actor in WHO policies, the MDGs closed the loop around economic and global trade as a means to improving health ends. Debt relief and technology transfer were now linked to health policy. Naturally, the creation of a global tobacco treaty seeking to curb a major industry would not be unanimously received by all states, especially a major tobacco exporter such as the United States.

Global Environmental Policy: A Model for Health Policy Making?

Policy makers often examine other policies and policy mechanisms to help enhance their own specific policy needs. One place global health policy makers look is within the realm of environmental policy and its many treaties. The similarity between global environmental and health issues is striking because, as Sands and Peel (2005)[76] assert, states can not act single-handedly within their own borders and expect to adequately address the problem. This is evident in the example of air pollution where one country's carbon dioxide or sulfur dioxide emissions affects its neighbors. Although many environmental problems are "transboundary" by nature (i.e., they cross boundaries), so too are health problems—one nation's avian flu outbreak can quickly become a cross-border problem and move from one country to another.

International cooperation becomes the norm, and most states are apt to increase cooperation if spread of a feared disease is imminent. However, the same degree of cooperation is not always as rapidly forthcoming for noncommunicable, or chronic, diseases resulting from tobacco or alcohol use, for example, or from the adverse affects of poverty. States might be tempted to regard such health issues as largely domestic and nonthreatening to their own populations.

---

[75]WHO, 2006e, *Health and the MDGs: Background*, www.who.int/mdg/background/en/index.html.
[76]Phillipe Sands and Jacqueline Peel. "Environmental Protection in the Twenty-first Century: Sustainable Development and International Law," in Regina S. Axelrod, David L. Downie and Norman J. Vig, eds., *The Global Environment: Institutions, Law, and Policy.* pp. 43-63.

Although lung cancer or malnutrition are health problems, they do not evoke fear of cross-border contamination as does avian flu or SARS. Also, when a disease such as lung cancer implicates a globally sold product such as cigarettes, solutions become highly charged and more controversial as the discussion shifts from the health sector to free trade. Accomplishing meaningful change becomes all the more difficult, making the use of treaties with binding components increasingly more attractive. Binding components are those parts of a treaty that countries are obligated to obey, provided they ratify the treaty.

Since World War II, the world has seen the proliferation of many environmental treaties brokered by the UN, yet only one treaty exists for global health policy. Today there are approximately 200 multilateral environmental agreements (MEAs) of global importance.[77] However, as the FCTC illustrates, this is changing. Countries can ultimately use international law in the form of multilateral treaties as a mechanism with which to expand their impact on health issues in a legally binding manner. Developing countries stand to gain the most from treaties that are written in a manner that recognizes "common, but differentiated responsibilities"—to borrow a term from global environmental policy and law. This means that while both developed and developing countries agree upon the objectives of a given treaty, both groups recognize that each other's contributions will vary over time based on levels of development and economic viability.

Although sources of international law include treaties, binding acts of international organizations, rules of customary international law, and judgments from international courts or tribunals, the treaty is the most important mechanism available in the global arena.[78] A framework convention or treaty, such as the FCTC, does not contain binding obligations and is usually negotiated with the idea that a binding protocol will follow at a later date.[79] For example, the 1997 Kyoto Protocol creates binding obligations for the UN Framework Convention on Climate Change signatories much as the 1987 Montreal Protocol on Substances that Deplete the Ozone Layer did for the 1985 Vienna Convention for the Protection of the Ozone Layer. Presumably the Framework Convention on Tobacco Control (FCTC) will also have its own binding protocol at a later date.

In the meantime, several principles of international environmental law serve as applicable strategies to health issues. These environmental principles include the following:

- "Cause no harm" and be a good neighbor to other states.
- "Common but differentiated responsibility," or the recognition that all states share common responsibility for protecting the environment, but differences

---

[77]Regina S. Axelrod, David L. Downie, and Norman J. Vig. *The Global Environment: Institutions, Law, and Policy.*

[78]Philippe Sands and Jacqueline Peel. "Environmental Protection in the Twenty-first Century: Sustainable Development and International Law," in Regina S. Axelrod, David L. Downie, and Norman J. Vig, eds., *The Global Environment: Institutions, Law, and Policy.* pp. 43–63.

[79]Brent S. Steel, Richard L. Clinton, and Nicholas P. Lovrich. 2003. *Environmental Politics and Policy: A Comparative Approach.*

among states means that not all of them are required to simultaneously pursue identical solutions to the problem.

- The "precautionary principle," or lack of full information should not prevent preemptive cooperation before the problem gets worse.

- "Polluter pays," or the idea that pollution costs should be the responsibility of those who cause the pollution. A similar concept is that of "producer pays" and is often applied to the disposal of European waste packaging.

- "Sustainable development," in its strict sense implies that humans must preserve our natural resources for the benefit of present and future generations (World Commission on Environment and Development, 1987, p. 8). *Our Common Future* also expanded this definition to include the notion of equitable resource use while inferring that economic and general development planning must incorporate environmental concerns into the process.

As we will see upon closer examination in the tobacco treaty case study, both European and developing states saw the relevance of applying such principles to WHO policy. They also found an ally in Gro Harlem Brundtland who is both an environmentalist and global health advocate. A former Norwegian prime minister and physician, Brundtland chaired the 1987 World Commission on Environment and Development—commonly known as the Brundtland Commission—which produced the historic document *Our Common Future*. *Our Common Future* introduced the world to an environmentally conscious way of thinking and inspired the creation of two major international treaties on climate change and biodiversity as well as the *Agenda 21* action plan for sustainable development. Implementation for this sustainable development goal occurred at the famous UN Conference on Environment and Development (UNCED), commonly called the Earth Summit, and held in Rio de Janeiro, Brazil.[80] These efforts created the realization among policy makers that development and environmental issues can not be solved in a vacuum. Instead they must be viewed as goals into which economic and social aspects must be incorporated in a manner that harnesses the strengths of the North for the good of the entire planet with a special focus on the needs of the global South.

Brundtland served as the WHO's fifth director-general from 1998–2003 and set the tone for policy priorities that would include both communicable and noncommunicable diseases. This was a period in which the FCTC was being refined in working group sessions, ultimately to be signed in 2003. From the start as director-general, Brundtland made her support of the global South clear when she stated early in her term of office that, "I envisage a world where solidarity binds the fortunate with those less favoured. . . . Where our collective efforts will help roll back all diseases of the poor."[81]

---

[80]Regina S. Axelrod, David L. Downie, and Norman J. Vig. *The Global Environment: Institutions, Law, and Policy.*
[81]Gro Harlem Brundtland, 1998. Speech to the Fifty-first World Health Assembly. A51/DIV/6. Geneva, Switzerland, May 13.

Brundtland believes that the role of developed countries must be to help developing countries achieve their health objectives even if that means going beyond financial assistance to actually curbing the North's commercial interests in harmful products such as tobacco. Brundtland was not shy about attacking the behemoth tobacco industry and, in 2003, she viewed the Framework Convention as an avenue for developing "efforts to build legal and regulatory protection against marketing efforts of the large tobacco companies."[82]

"Change Agents"

In this chapter we see that members of both the global North and South are proponents of global health governance through treaties. Nation states from the North and South that propose new ways to conceptualize global health policy become what Rogers and Shoemaker (1971) call "change agents." A change agent is a person or group "who influences innovation decisions in a direction deemed desirable by a change agency" (Rogers and Shoemaker, 1971, p. 227).[83] In this case the change agency is the World Health Organization and the change agents are nation states.

Political learning gained from environmental treaty successes has spilled over into the global health arena and made the developing South, in particular, a driving force, a primary innovator for a paradigm shift toward the use of multilateral treaties in global health policy. Hinrichs (2002) reminds us that "the prospects of successfully 'learning from others' are better the more it is possible to construct a direct link between a unanimously defined problem and a concrete policy."[84] While existing WHO programs, such as the Malaria Program, attempt to overcome a unanimously defined problem of malaria's often-deadly effects through the creation of a concrete malaria policy, the global weight of a program is not the same as that of a treaty. Thus, expanded global cooperation to achieve health policy goals is more likely to occur if such policy problems, goals, and solutions were couched in a formal treaty having the status of hard international law.

Case Study: Tackling Big Tobacco: A Bold New Path Toward Implementing Global Health Standards?

The WHO-initiated tobacco treaty known as the Framework Convention on Tobacco Control (FCTC) is a response to the increasing use of tobacco products worldwide. The increased usage rate in the developing world was a particular cause for alarm among WHO member states that sought to reduce the incidence of smoking by opening negotiations

---

[82]Gro Harlem Brundtland, 2003. Burden of Disease and Best Practices. Speech given at the WHO High-level Roundtable on Tobacco Control and Development Policy. Brussels, Belgium, February 3.
[83]Everett M. Rogers and F. Floyd Shoemaker. 1971. *Communication of Innovations: A Cross-Cultural Approach.*
[84]Karl Hinrichs, 2002. What can be Learned from Whom? Germany's Employment Problem in Comparative Perspective. *Innovation* 15 (2): 89–97.

on a global treaty in October 1999. These negotiations culminated in the first-ever global health treaty adopted in June 2003 and which came into force on February 27, 2005.

The World Health Organization knew about the harmful effects of tobacco as early as 1970 when the 23rd WHA passed Resolution 23.32, "Health Consequences of Smoking." This quiet start recognized the serious health effects of smoking that can lead to pulmonary and cardiac disease, including cancer and chronic bronchitis. Yet, recommendations fell far short of an international treaty, were fairly benign, and lacked authority. Instead, the WHA resolution called for WHO members to refrain from smoking at assembly meetings and for the WHO to generally discourage smoking in all countries especially through education of young people. The WHO resolution also called on the Food and Agriculture Organization to study crop-substitution alternatives in tobacco-producing countries.[85]

By May 1992, the WHO began a serious tobacco campaign at the 45th World Health Assembly (WHA) and which took shape in Resolution 45.20. This resolution passed by the WHA encouraged collaboration among international organizations to deal with the issue that the WHO called: "tobacco or health." In 1992, the WHO sought to balance health concerns alongside economic implications raised by tobacco-growing countries of the global South. Although the WHO recognized the health effects of tobacco use, it was "concerned about the economic effects of reduced production in the tobacco-producing countries that are still unable to develop a viable economic alternative to tobacco."[86] In order of importance, economic and health issues were equally divided.

However, by May 1995, the 48th WHA officially shifted its views and weighed in favor of controlling tobacco's negative-health ramifications.[87] The Ninth World Conference on Tobacco and Health held in Paris in October 1994 resulted in the first international strategy for tobacco control. This strategy was later adopted by the WHA in May 1995. Resolution 48.11, "An International Strategy for Tobacco Control." It was a product of the 48th Assembly in May 1995 and called for the creation of an international instrument—guidelines, a declaration, or international convention—on tobacco control to be adopted by the United Nations.[88] The 49th WHA in May 1996 called for the fast-track creation of a tobacco treaty.

The 1995 Resolution and its subsequent 1996 fast-tracking marked the starting point for a tobacco control treaty, but it was not until 1999 that negotiations within the intergovernmental working group actually began formulation of the Framework Convention on Tobacco Control. Once the working group began its treaty-making task, a clear shift toward use of environmental techniques also became evident.

---

[85]WHO, 1970. *Health Consequences of Smoking.* WHA23.32.

[86]WHO, 1992. *Multisectoral Collaboration on WHO's Programme on Tobacco or Health.* WHA45.20.

[87]WHO, 1995. *An International Strategy for Tobacco Control.* WHA48.11.

[88]WHO, 1995. *An International Strategy for Tobacco Control.* WHA48.11.

Setting the Stage

The *Report of the First Meeting of the Working Group* recognized that not only was tobacco a cross-border issue, but it also transcended the "bounds of public health." [89] This recognition made it easier for WHO to create a treaty that emphasized trade and regulatory controls as well as financial sharing of the enforcement burden. This latter point was also linked to the recognition that tobacco-growing countries of the South may need financial support for crop substitution. However, the fear about adverse economic impact on developing countries was assuaged by World Bank findings in the book *Curbing the Epidemic: Governments and the Economics of Tobacco Control* (1999).

The World Bank findings pointed to tobacco control as more economically cost-effective in the long term due to the millions of lives saved. It recognized the disease burden of this addictive substance and estimated that by the year 2000 tobacco would kill nearly four million people around the globe. While one in ten deaths is currently attributed to tobacco's harmful effects, by 2030 the ratio is expected to be one in six—or 10 million deaths annually.[90] Moreover, the book emphasized the increasing use of tobacco in the developing world and especially in China, where 25% of the world's smokers reside. Chinese smoking rates in the 1990s were comparable to those of the United States in 1950.[91] The World Bank call for action reminded readers, including working group members, that only two causes of death are growing worldwide—HIV and tobacco. While fighting HIV is universally accepted, the global response to tobacco was limited at best and largely focused within developed countries.

Curbing the Epidemic suggests that the need for tobacco controls is most acute in developing countries. According to the World Bank, the impact of reduced tobacco production on the economy of developing countries would be negligible or have little impact on employment or revenue. Any impact would be gradual and nearly inconsequential. *Curbing the Epidemic* (1999) thus gave WHO the green light to proceed with a comprehensive treaty that incorporates an environmental approach to treaty making. In fact, the book explicitly recognizes the successes of the environmental approach and urges its application to tobacco: "The framework convention-protocol approach has been used to address other global problems, for example, the Vienna Convention for the Protection of the Ozone Layer and the Montreal Protocol." [92]

The one difference between environmental issues and tobacco use is that the World Bank urged actions to curb demand rather than restrict or ban supply. This is markedly different from the phase-out approach to harmful pollutants contained in many environmental treaties. Neither the World Bank nor the WHO working group called for the

---

[89]WHO, 1999. *WHO Framework Convention on Tobacco Control: Report of the First Meeting of the Working Group.* A/FCTC/WG1/7.

[90]World Bank. 1999. *Curbing the Epidemic: Governments and the Economics of Tobacco Control.*

[91]World Bank. 1999. *Curbing the Epidemic: Governments and the Economics of Tobacco Control.*

[92]World Bank. 1999. *Curbing the Epidemic: Governments and the Economics of Tobacco Control.*

phase-out of tobacco products—only a reduction in consumer use through various means. Perhaps a phase-out will become acceptable in the future, but it is not presently an option under discussion, nor was it in the working group meetings leading up to the FCTC.

The working group felt that "treaties make a difference" and can take the form of a framework convention and subsequent amendments and protocols. While a framework convention has as its objective garnering widespread global support, the protocol will elaborate upon the details and binding obligations at a later date. This is so similar an approach to the environmental arena that the working group report recognized that "this type of instrument had proved its worth in disarmament and environmental protection."[93] Merging even closer to environmental tactics, the working group went so far as to recognize the principle of polluter pays and urged that it be "explored as a means of holding the tobacco industry accountable for the harm it causes."[94]

While the working group met to formulate the treaty, concomitant tobacco-control projects were undertaken simultaneously by the WHO's Tobacco Free Initiative. These projects ranged from advice on the policy effects of scientific aspects of the tobacco problem to better understanding of regulation and media as tobacco-limiting tools. The Tobacco Free Initiative also explored antitobacco legislative capacity, youth activities, and improved data gathering and surveillance in collaboration with the US Centers for Disease Control and Prevention, which is a US government agency within the Department of Health and Human Services.[95] The utility of these parallel projects was complementary to the treaty process.

The Tobacco Free Initiative projects reinforced the notion that tobacco was a high priority for the WHO. In other words, the WHO prepared the world incrementally through these various projects and facilitated global acceptance of a controversial and groundbreaking health treaty that painted commercially marketed tobacco products as a grave health risk. The WHO thus prepared potentially reticent countries by creating a link from tobacco initiative projects to a treaty having the force of international law behind it.

Director-General Brundtland was also a strong treaty supporter and, at every opportunity, smoothed the transition to its eventual entry into force in February 2005. In her 2000 report on noncommunicable diseases, Brundtland reminded the 53rd WHA of the link between cancer, diabetes, and chronic pulmonary disease and lifestyle factors such as diet, physical inactivity, and tobacco use.[96] Brundtland did not shy from innovation and men-

---

[93]WHO, 1999. *WHO Framework Convention on Tobacco Control: Report of the First Meeting of the Working Group.* A/FCTC/WG1/7.

[94]WHO, 1999. *WHO Framework Convention on Tobacco Control: Report of the First Meeting of the Working Group.* A/FCTC/WG1/7.

[95]WHO, 2000a. *Tobacco Free Initiative: Report by the Director-General.* A53/13.

[96]WHO, 2000b. *Global Strategy for the Prevention and Control of Noncommunicable Diseases: Report by the Director-General.* A53/14.

tioned the need for "innovative organizational models" throughout her report.[97] Her report was essentially a call to action that spurred the development of the tobacco treaty.

By May 11, 2000, the framework convention was ready in draft form.[98] The idea was to create a treaty that would set standards while not discouraging countries with harsh rhetoric and obligations—that could come later in a protocol. The draft treaty received WHA approval for the negotiation phase to begin in October 2000 and an intergovernmental negotiating body was formed to begin the task of finalizing the document.[99]

Between 2000 and May 21, 2003, the WHO continually revisited the tobacco issue in its assembly. In May 2001, for example, the WHA addressed the issue of transparency in the tobacco control process and used stronger language to portray the role of big tobacco interests: "The tobacco industry has operated for years with the expressed intention of subverting the role of government and of WHO in implementing public health policies to combat the tobacco epidemic."[100] The tobacco industry was thus portrayed as a formidable public enemy. WHO member states were encouraged to be mindful should tobacco interests attempt to infiltrate their midst. Any member delegation affiliated with the tobacco industry was encouraged to be forthcoming with this relationship.[101]

Framework Convention on Tobacco Control
The final product was adopted on May 21, 2003, in Geneva and contained most of the important elements discussed in preliminary working group sessions. The treaty was a victory for developing countries, and its preamble reinforced the serious concern for the increase in global tobacco product consumption "particularly in developing countries."[102] This was a treaty aimed at empowering countries worldwide, but with special emphasis given to the global South. Part VII, Article 20, calls for parties to provide financial and technical resources for the purpose of helping developing countries as well as countries in transition (e.g., former communist countries).

Article 22 of the treaty is more explicit in its assertion that parties should take into account developing country needs and "promote the transfer of technical, scientific and legal expertise and technology, as mutually agreed, to establish and strengthen national tobacco control strategies."[103] The WHO made a groundbreaking contribution to the body of international law in the form of the world's first global health treaty and

---

[97]WHO, 2000b. *Global Strategy for the Prevention and Control of Noncommunicable Diseases: Report by the Director-General.* A53/14.

[98]WHO, 2000c. *WHO Framework Convention on Tobacco Control: Report of the Working Group, Corrigendum.* A53/12 Corr.1.

[99]2000d. *Framework Convention on Tobacco Control.* WHA53.16.

[100]WHO, 2001. *Transparency in Tobacco Control Process.* WHA54.18.

[101]WHO, 2001. *Transparency in Tobacco Control Process.* WHA54.18.

[102]WHO, 2003. *WHO Framework Convention on Tobacco Control.*

[103]WHO, 2003. *WHO Framework Convention on Tobacco Control.*

reinforced that tobacco consumption and exposure to tobacco smoke cause disease and death were "unequivocally established" by the scientific community.[104]

Harsh words were reserved for the industry's use of carcinogenic chemicals in cigarettes to foster human dependence on tobacco, and any attempt by the tobacco industry to undermine or subvert tobacco control efforts should be an ongoing concern for signatory states.[105] In short, the treaty demonstrated its acceptance of the premise that tobacco is harmful to health, and the tobacco industry was to blame. Unlike the Vienna Convention for the Protection of the Ozone Layer, the FCTC did not call for such drastic action on tobacco—only its control. The phase-out of the most harmful ozone-depleting chemicals was possible because more ozone-friendly substitutes were created. Perhaps industry will respond to the FCTC by creating a harmless cigarette that meets health standards; unfortunately, this appears unlikely as long as it contains tobacco.

Although CFC manufacturers were encouraged to create safer alternatives, the global community does not encourage creating safer cigarettes. The treaty's ultimate intent is to stamp out tobacco entirely, from a health perspective, yet the WHO is unable to say this explicitly at this time. The "polluter pays" concept indirectly appears in Part VI, Article 19, of the treaty where liability is seen as a tactic to achieve the goal of decreasing tobacco use:

> For the purpose of tobacco control, the Parties shall consider taking legislative action or promoting their existing laws, where necessary, to deal with criminal and civil liability, including compensation where appropriate.[106]

Reference to appropriate compensation is a generalized attempt to recognize the polluter pays concept without implying a cause and effect relationship between tobacco manufacturers and end users—or victims.

Article 19 encourages member states to pursue product liability as a means of bringing attention to the problem. The treaty focuses on the need to take measures to protect everyone from tobacco's harmful effects. To achieve this goal the treaty urges member states to take concrete steps such as reducing demand through price and tax measures, regulation of packaging and labeling, educational and public awareness campaigns, cessation of tobacco advertising where constitutionally feasible, and through reduction in illegal supply. The treaty encourages member states to take appropriate measures, but does not require them to do so. Creating specific and required benchmarks in tobacco control (i.e., binding obligations) will come at a later date in a protocol.

Conclusion

The momentum created by the first-ever global health treaty is an innovative start to tackling health problems—especially those caused by lifestyle choices. The treaty was a result

---

[104]WHO, 2003. *WHO Framework Convention on Tobacco Control.*
[105]WHO, 2003. *WHO Framework Convention on Tobacco Control.*
[106]WHO, 2003. *WHO Framework Convention on Tobacco Control.*

of cooperative efforts among actors from the North and South and benefited from strong guidance of the WHO's director-general Gro Brundtland, who vigorously lobbied for its creation. While the United States, the second top tobacco-producing state after China, signed the treaty, it has yet to ratify the document.[107] At first glance this may appear detrimental to global antitobacco goals, but is less troublesome than we may think because 84% of the world's smokers live in developing and transitional, or former communist, countries.[108] These countries overwhelmingly ratified the treaty and should thus reap benefits with or without US participation.

Unlike transboundary greenhouse gas pollution from a major emitter nation to which we may fall victim regardless of our country of residence, tobacco use is largely a self-contained lifestyle issue. It is more easily controlled through lifestyle changes resulting from education and personal decisions not to smoke. The FCTC thus provides tools and facilitates one's ability to say no to smoking.

However, future protocols could go farther by pressing for mandatory reductions in tobacco production or manufacture. The FCTC creates a future avenue for global health policy that leads the way toward more aggressive options to deal with tobacco—even to the extent of calling for a gradual phase-out of its manufacture into cigarettes, smokeless, or chewing products.

Health innovation continues to evolve toward international cooperative efforts that take a proactive approach to the disease burden. Pandemic spread of avian flu is one problem that the WHO and other regional health organizations take seriously and currently tackle at this writing. Yet, innovation in the global health arena will have a greater impact if it takes the form of a law that a treaty provides.

Conclusion

In this chapter, you have learned through three different examples—the United States, Bolivia, and a multilateral organization, WHO—how public health policy making can be accomplished. As illustrated in the AIDS case study, global health policy making is truly impacted by several actors, including the various branches of the US government, the news media, interest groups, and, oftentimes, the unpredictable collusion of current events and public opinion. There are many routes to influencing, implementing, and overseeing the implementation of policies affecting public health policy, all of which make for a dynamic process in US policy making.

During the last 34 democratic years, Bolivia has moved forward on many issues regarding the control of disease and the implementation of public health and healthcare policies that can improve the quality of life of Bolivians; however, there is a long road

---

[107]WHO, 1999. *WHO Framework Convention on Tobacco Control: Report of the First Meeting of the Working Group.* A/FCTC/WG1/7.
[108]WHO, 2006f. *The First Session of the Conference of the Parties to the WHO Framework Convention on Tobacco Control.* www.who.int/tobacco/fctc/cop/en.

ahead for all segments of Bolivian society to enjoy the level of health in developed countries. As in many parts of the developing world, most resources devoted to public health are targeted for fighting infectious diseases, which leaves the system without resources or vision to focus on long-term planning processes.

The WHO example seems to illustrate that health innovation continues to evolve toward international cooperative efforts that take a proactive approach to the burden of disease. A pandemic threat, such as the spread of avian flu, is one problem that the WHO and other regional health organizations take seriously and currently tackle along with controlling the reemergent threats of diseases thought long eradicated. Yet, innovation in the global health arena will have a greater impact if it takes the form of a "hard" law that a treaty provides, instead of guidelines that can be ignored or only partially instituted in member states that chose to implement them. The bold first step was taken thanks to a North–South coalition that recognized that a treaty would attract global attention like no other WHO documents or pronouncements have done previously. In short, this action goes "beyond a 'business as usual' approach" and can strengthen the WHO's ability to address global health inequalities.

References

USA

The Center for Responsive Politics. 2006. http://www.opensecrets.org.

Congressional Budget Office. 2006. http://www.cbo.gov.

FirstGov. 2006. http://www.firstgov.gov.

Gellman, Barton, "Death Watch: AIDS, Drugs and Africa: A Turning Point That Left Millions Behind," *The Washington Post,* December 28, 2000.

Government Accountability Office. 2006. http://www.gao.gov.

The Library of Congress. 2006. http://thomas.loc.gov.

Light, Paul C. *The President's Agenda: Domestic Policy Choice From Kennedy to Clinton.* Third Edition. Baltimore, MD: Johns Hopkins University Press, 1999.

Longest, Beaufort B. *Health Policymaking in the United States.* Fourth Edition. Chicago: Health Administration Press; Washington, DC: AUPHA Press, 2006.

Moodley, Pooven, "Drugs Alone Will Not Stop AIDS in Africa." *Milwaukee Journal Sentinel,* July 23, 2000.

Office of Legislative Counsel, U.S. House of Representatives. 2006. http://legcoun.house.gov/public.htm.

Office of Legislative Counsel, U.S. Senate. 2006. http://slc.senate.gov/index.htm.

Oleszek, Walter J. *Congressional Procedures and the Policy Process.* Sixth Edition. Washington, DC: CQ Press, 2004.

Texas Politics. 2006. http://texaspolitics.laits.utexas.edu/html/ig/print_ig.html.

Thurber, James A. (Ed). *Rivals for Power: Presidential-Congressional Relations.* Second Edition. Lanham, MD: Rowman & Littlefield Publishers, 2006.

Bolivia

Baeza, Cristian C. and Truman G. Packard. *Beyond Survival: Protecting Households From Health Shocks in Latin America*, Palo Alto, CA: Stanford University Press, 2006, p. 128.

Bolivian National Epidemiology Report, Ministry of Health and Social Prevision, 2002.

Capdevila, Gustavo. "Bolivia: Wanted—Health Care Adapted to Indigenous Cultures." Global Information Network, May 26, 2006, p. 1.

Kumate, Jesus, Gonzalo Gutierrez, and Juan Manuel Sotelo. *Sistemas Nacionales de Salud en Las Americas*, México: Secretaria de Salud, 1994, pp. 11–12.

Leslie, Colin. "Bolivian MDs Protest Free Cuban Care." *Medical Post* (Toronto), July 4, 2006, p. 48.

Ministerio de Salud y Deportes. *Situación de Salud, Bolivia 2004*. La Paz, Bolivia: January 2006, pp. 16, 34.

Ministerio de Salud y Deportes, *Programa EXTENSA, Manual de Procedimientos Administrativos: Brigadas Integrales de Salud*. La Paz, Bolivia: MOH June 2003.

Pan American Health Organization. "Bolivia: Country Profile," *Epidemiological Bulletin/PAHO*, March 2003, vol. 24, no. 1, p. 8.

Paz, Enrique. Informe de Gestión 1997–2002., Ministerio de Salud y Previsión Social, Republica de Bolivia, 2002.

Rivizi, Haider. "Bolivia: Morales Takes Coca Campaign—and a Leaf—to U.N." Global Information Network, September 22, 2006, p. 1

The Guardian. "Bolivian Leader Defends His Drug Policy." September 20, 2006, http://www.guardian.co.uk.

UNICEF. "Health Insurance for Children and Mothers Slows Child Mortality in Bolivia." http://www.unicef.org.

United Nations, Economic Commission for Latin America. *Statistical Yearbook for Latin American and the Caribbean, 2005*. New York: United Nations Publications, 2006, p. 71.

Vandebroek, Ina, Jan-Bart Calewaert, Stijn De Jonckheere, Sabino Sanca, et al. "Use of Medicinal Plants and Pharmaceuticals by Indigenous Communities in the Bolivian Andes and Amazon." *Bulletin of the World Health Organization.* April 2004, vol. 82, no. 4, p. 248.

World Bank. *Bolivia Country Brief*, September 2006, http://www.worldbank.org.

World Bank. *Health Sector Reform in Bolivia: A Decentralization Case Study*. Washington, DC: World Bank, 2004, pp. 1–2.

World Bank Development Indicators Database. April 2006, http://devdata.worldbank.org.

World Bank. World Development Report, 2007. Washington, DC: World Bank, September 23, 2006.

World Fact Book. *Bolivia Country Report*. Central Intelligence Agency, https://www.cia.gov/cia/publications/factbook/geos/bl.html.

Multilateral

Brundtland, Gro Harlem. "Burden of Disease and Best Practices." Speech given at the WHO High-level Roundtable on Tobacco Control and Development Policy. Brussels, Belgium, 2003.

———. 1998. Speech to the Fifty-first World Health Assembly. A51/DIV/6. Geneva, Switzerland, May 13.

Axelrod, Regina S., David L. Downie, and Norman J. Vig. *The Global Environment: Institutions, Law, and Policy*. Washington, DC: CQ Press, 2005.

Global Equity Gauge Alliance, Durban, South Africa and People's Health Movement, Bangalore, India. *Global Health Watch 2005-2006: An alternative world health report.* New York: Zed Books, 2005.

Hinrichs, Karl. 2002. What Can Be Learned from Whom? Germany's Employment Problem in Comparative Perspective. *Innovation* 15 (2): 89-97.

Lee, Jong-Wook. 2003. Global Health Improvement and WHO: Shaping the Future. *Lancet,* 362: 2083–88.

A Manipulated Dichotomy in Global Health Policy. 2000. *Lancet* 355 (9219): 1923.

McLendon, Michael K., Donald E. Heller, and Steven P. Young. 2005. State Postsecondary Policy Innovation: Politics, Competition, and the Interstate Migration of Policy Ideas. *Journal of Higher Education* 76 (4): 363–400.

Reddy, Srinath K., Bela Shah, Cherian Varghese, and Anbumani Ramadoss. 2005. Responding to the threat of chronic diseases in India. *Lancet* 366: 1746–51.

Rogers, Everett M. and F. Floyd Shoemaker. *Communication of Innovations: A Cross-Cultural Approach.* New York: Free Press, 1971.

Sands, Philippe and Jacqueline Peel. Environmental protection in the twenty-first century: sustainable development and international law, in Regina S. Axelrod, David L. Downie, and Norman J. Vig, Eds., *The Global Environment: Institutions, Law, and Policy.* Washington, DC: CQ Press, 2005, pp. 43–63.

Siddiqi, Javed. *World Health and World Politics: The World Health Organization and the UN System.* Columbus, SC: University of South Carolina Press, 1995.

Steel, Brent S., Richard L. Clinton, and Nicholas P. Lovrich. *Environmental Politics and Policy: A Comparative Approach.* Boston, MA: McGraw-Hill, 2003.

Walker, Jack L. 1969. The Diffusion of Innovations Among the American States. *American Political Science Review* 63 (3): 880–99.

World Bank. *Curbing the Epidemic: Governments and the Economics of Tobacco Control.* Washington, DC: World Bank, 1999.

World Commission on Environment and Development. *Our Common Future.* New York: Oxford University Press, 1987.

World Health Organization. 1948a. *Constitution of the World Health Organization.* Geneva, Switzerland. http://www.who.int/about/en/.

——. 1948b. *Principles Governing Relations Between the World Health Organization and Nongovernmental Organizations.* Geneva, Switzerland. http://www.who.int/about/en/.

——. 1970. *Health Consequences of Smoking.* WHA23.32. Geneva, Switzerland, May 19.

——. 1978. *Declaration of Alma-Ata.* International Conference on Primary Health Care, Alma-Ata, USSR. September 6–12.

——. 1992. *Multisectoral Collaboration on WHO's Programme on Tobacco or Health.* WHA45.20. Geneva, Switzerland, May 13.

——. 1995. *An International Strategy for Tobacco Control.* WHA48.11. Geneva, Switzerland, May 12.

——. 1998. *Health for all in the Twenty-first Century.* A51/5. Geneva, Switzerland, May 7–16.

——. 1999. *WHO Framework Convention on Tobacco Control: Report of the First Meeting of the Working Group.* A/FCTC/WG1/7. Geneva, Switzerland, October 28.

——. 2000a. *Tobacco Free Initiative: Report by the Director-General.* A53/13. Geneva, Switzerland, March 10.

——. 2000b. *Global Strategy for the Prevention and Control of Noncommunicable Diseases: Report by the Director-General.* A53/14. Geneva, Switzerland, March 22.

——. 2000c. *WHO Framework Convention on Tobacco Control: Report of the Working Group, Corrigendum.* A53/12 Corr. 1, Geneva, Switzerland, May 11.

———. 2000d. *Framework Convention on Tobacco Control*. WHA53.16, Geneva, Switzerland, May 20.

———. 2001. *Transparency in Tobacco Control Process*. WHA54.18, Geneva, Switzerland, May 22.

———. 2003. *WHO Framework Convention on Tobacco Control*. Geneva, Switzerland, May 21.

———. 2004. *Public Health problems Caused by Alcohol*. EB115/37, Geneva, Switzerland, December 23.

———. 2005. Revision of the International Health Regulations. WHA58.3, May 23.

———. 2006. WHO, *Executive Board Members* www.who.int/governance/eb/eb_members/en/print.html:.

———. 2006a. *Weekly Epidemiological Record*. www.who.inter/wer.

———. 2006b. *World Health Statistics*. www.who.inter/wer.

———. 2006c. *International Health Regulations*. http://www.who.int/csr/ihr/en/.

———. 2006d. The Civil Society Initiative. http://www.who.int/civilsociety/en/.

———. 2006e. *Health and the MDGs: Background*. www.who.int/mdg/background/en/index.html.

———. 2006f. *The First Session of the Conference of the Parties to the WHO Framework Convention on Tobacco Control*. Geneva, Switzerland, February 6-17. www.who.int/tobacco/fctc/cop/en.

Chapter 5

Global Health Research Methods

Timothy A. Akers

Mary Anne Alabanza Akers

Global health research (GHR) is an international enterprise that transcends national boundaries and political ideologies while embracing shared responsibilities and cooperative problem solving (Bloom, Michaud, La Montagne, & Simonsen, 2006; Research!America, 2005; Labonte & Spiegel, 2003). The global community of nations is increasingly relying on diverse bodies of research from other countries to help compare and contrast health indicators. As nations advance socially, economically, technologically, medically, educationally, and environmentally, their awareness of the importance of global health research becomes more sophisticated by examining health from an interdisciplinary perspective. The complexities surrounding the many diverse dimensions of health demand an awareness of the interdependency of people, systems, and nations (Bloom et al., 2006). Global health can range from a healthy economy to a healthy lifestyle to the immediate identification of a major superspread of an infectious disease or rapidly increasing levels of noncommunicable diseases, injuries, and disabilities, especially in developing countries.

As international travel increases, urban centers become denser, environmental and climate changes continue, and new and reemerging infectious diseases take center stage, there will continue to exist a need for a better understanding in how best to obtain, integrate, share, and use high-quality health data. These data, however conceptualized, may take into account, in part, health as measured by the economics and policies of a nation; the physical landscapes in which people live, work, and play; their quality of life; technological advances; and general health outcomes (Hanney, Gonzalez-Block, Buxton, & Kogan, 2003). Though whatever data are used and made available for global consumption and scrutiny, researchers interested in the many dimensions of global health are left to the mercy of the quality of the data and the citizenry and governments willing to participate in global health research.

How a nation is perceived by the global community generally and global research community specifically may depend, in part, on the quality of the data used in reporting their international health standing to the global community. A country's national standing may be looked upon with suspicion if its data are suspect and not viewed as credible by the global research or traveling community; or if the data are viewed as being too

143

controlled or contrived by the state, this may drastically affect the amount of international investment nations provide to countries seeking global health research funding or cooperation. Communist China, for example, has long been viewed as a nation that controls the release of its health data, which has inhibited progress and strained international cooperation (Uhlir & Esanu, 2006).

The inverse, however, is that within the context of democratic developed nations, they are also concerned in making sure that their developed status does not regress to a point where it will affect the well-being of its citizens, their health, environment, and economy. Making data access a top priority and having the data openly available for public scrutiny and scientific challenges has enabled developed nations (and developing nations with an open access policy to health data) to create Internet-based access points where data can be readily downloaded and analyzed by anyone throughout the world community and compared against other international benchmarks of health. The need for shifting the paradigm from "us against them," to more of a commonality of equals can strengthen the global health community's understanding around global health problems, such as data access, which lies at the core of global health research priority setting (Bloom et al., 2006).

However, the complexity or simplicity of the priority setting around data access may depend on whether it is in a raw, case-by-case format, or tabular, in which the data are based on aggregate analysis only. Whatever form, the important issue to consider is whether the data are open to public analysis. If data are made openly available, one thing is certain—the more the global community has access to it, the more valuable the data become.

Lastly, this chapter will summarize some salient issues that need to be considered before any new or seasoned global health researcher undertakes a global health research (GHR) project. The authors of this chapter maintain the position that global health research is more than drug and vaccine development. But rather, GHR is a tapestry of complexity that takes on many different dimensions, from vaccine and drug development to microenterprise development. Although GHR can take on many forms and perspectives, we will only address some of the contextual issue and, to a lesser degree, the methodological processes that should be considered from an interdisciplinary research perspective.

Planning for Global Health Research: The 10/90 Debate

Planning a global health research study may be stimulated by recognizing a health disparity that has been internationally disseminated through a diverse body of research publications and mass media communication, as in the case of HIV/AIDS, tuberculosis, SARS, bird flu, malaria, and other diseases. However, other areas of health disparities may not be as well known throughout the world or GHR community with respect to the relationship among health, environment, and the economy and their impact when brought together. For example, street vendors (e.g., microentrepreneurs) in the Philippines, Mexico, South America, Africa, India, the Middle East, and other nations and regions throughout the world contribute substantially to local and national economies. It is through this awareness of seemingly innocuous relationships where global health researchers begin their quest for searching out interdisciplinary reasons why health disparities or comorbidities exist.

The Global Forum for Health Research (2006) raised the specter of concern around the 10/90 debate that has stimulated a vast amount of GHR interest. What the 10/90 gap refers to is that 10% of the resources spent on research and development for health research is directed to diseases that account for 90% of the total global burden of disease. This disparity clearly exemplifies underfunding across the full spectrum of diseases. It is through this awareness that we can begin shifting our priorities to less known areas that still need research funding though not necessarily deemed as priority areas, such as environmental health and its impact on people, communities, economies, nations, regions, and the world health community (Labonte & Spiegel, 2003).

As of 2001, it is estimated that the world community has been increasing its spending on health research, with the latest estimates placing the figure at US$105.9 billion. Figure 5-1 shows the percentages of funding provided by each sector.

Clearly, the amount of funding by the public sector and private for-profit sector is approaching almost parity, with the private sector slightly in the lead. In spite of these positive increases, the "10/90 gap" persists with low- and middle-income nations continuing to experience underinvestment in health research (Global Forum for Health Research, 2006).

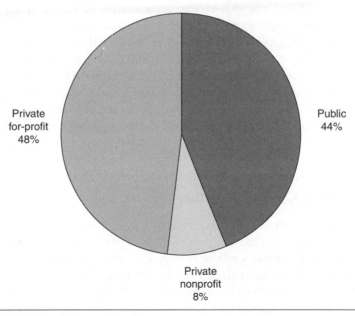

Figure 5-1 World health spending by sector.

Although funding clearly helps in directing greater resources to tackle a health disparity problem, notwithstanding underinvestment, part of the solution can also depend on whether access to or the development of interdisciplinary databases are made available that can be merged and integrated for more systematic analysis across nations and regions. The integrated and interdisciplinary overlap amongst and between surveillance systems and databases is sometimes referred to as the "informatics revolution" (Bloom et al., 2006).

Once a global health problem has been identified and verified, ideally through multiple interdisciplinary systems of analysis, the GHR community begins planning how to access data or target populations in the area or region of interest. Whatever the motive for conducting a GHR project, it should be based on a research question that may be beneficial to the basic or applied research community. A researcher interested in GHR may simply ask the question of "Why are so many people in a region disproportionately infected with the HIV/AIDS disease?" Or, "How does the physical environment in the central business district impact street vendor health?" Such questions begin the process of trying to find an answer.

Other questions may be raised based on a review of the most recent health data reported or through experiential knowledge gained while traveling in various regions throughout the world. Whatever the reason or rationale, GHR can take on many forms, ranging from the most basic and seemingly innocuous form of secondary data collection, to the more hands-on, total cultural immersion experience. The total immersion experience can range from the conducting of survey research; focus groups or key informant interviews; and the collecting of air, water, or other environmental samples; to more clinically based health screenings, as in the case of clinical trials. Whatever approach is undertaken, it is imperative that a GHR team plan their study well in advance of collecting the data, while recognizing at times that research in the field (e.g., local community) is an unpredictable process and may require immediate readjustment in the middle of the data collection phase. Although this can at times be viewed as inconsistent with rigid scientific protocols from a deductive reasoning point of view, the readjustments in protocols in the process of data collection can be quite appropriate when framing a research study from an interdisciplinary perspective, which may require reexamining a complex problem more inductively.

Accessing Data: Secondary Data

Some global health researchers invariably begin their quest for answers in the great citadels for intellectual exchange and learning—universities and libraries. These grand cathedrals of knowledge house some of the world's richest sources of literature on the research conducted throughout the world. However, because global health research affects the entire planet, access to such information, if not physically within the reaches of all, should be at their fingertips, such as through open access portals to the Internet and computers. And, with the advent of the Internet, volumes of data sources are being made readily available electronically, as compared to printed resources that can be costly, time consuming in printing, and not immediately available for international dissemination. The Canadian Coalition for Global Health Research reports that greater than 90% of the scientific publications in the health field are published by researchers from developed nations (Forti, 2005). By making global health data more easily accessible on the Internet, the diverse pool of global health researchers can begin to expand exponentially.

To varying degrees, secondary and tabulated data, or research reports, have been and continue to be made available to global health researchers in many different forms. For example, taxonomy of data sources may consist of, but not necessarily be limited to, the following:

- Abstracts and summaries on global health issues
- Nationally sponsored reports by government agencies
- Independently published studies by global health researchers
- Tabulated data reporting by national agencies (e.g., surveillance data)
- Secondary data available for integration and analysis by independent investigators

These types of data or data summaries give researchers concerned with global health opportunities to compare and contrast data across nations and regions. Information that is made available online in the form of a simple abstract of a study, which may have been undertaken in a specific part of the world for example, may start a chain of events that lead researchers down a path toward cooperation with other universities, think tanks, and government agencies. This type of collaboration can target and bring to bear interdisciplinary expertise around a specific health problem or environmental disparity (Bloom et al., 2006).

Newcomers to the world of global health, public health, environmental health, environmental design, landscape architecture, economics, the behavioral sciences, and many other disciplines would be well served by accessing some of the resources identified in Table 5-1. This table is a summary of some of the organizations that provide tabulated data and information resources around GHR that are easily accessible on the Internet and, at times, retrospective (secondary) data that can be fully downloaded and analyzed for cross-country comparative research. Such global information resources are best utilized if they help in decision-making processes, program evaluation, research, or policy formulation (Stansfield, Walsh, Prata, & Evans, 2006).

The importance of disseminating data and information for other researchers or practitioners to have available is best reflected in the US Centers for Disease Control and Prevention (CDC) *Morbidity and Mortality Weekly Report* (*MMWR*) publication. It serves as a weekly publication of national notifiable infectious diseases that reports new findings for other researchers to examine and scrutinize. The provisional data in the *MMWR* are used

TABLE 5-1 Sample of Global Agencies That Maintain Tabulated
or Secondary Data

Organization/Agency Name	Webpage Address (URL)
Bill and Melinda Gates Foundation	www.gatesfoundation.org/ default.htm
Canadian Institutes of Health Research	www.irsc.gc.ca
Centers for Disease Control and Prevention (CDC)	www.cdc.gov
Commonwealth Fund: International Health Policy & Practice	www.cmwf.org
Family Health International	www.fhi.org/en/index.htm
Fogarty International Center, National Institutes of Health	www.fic.nih.gov/ programs/index.htm
Global Forum for Health Research	www.globalforumhealth.org
Global Health Council	www.globalhealth.org
GlobalHealth.gov (U.S. Office of Global Health Affairs)	www.globalhealth.gov
GlobalHealthReporting.org	www.globalhealth reporting.org
Health Policy Monitor (Bertelsmann Stiftung)	www.hpm.org/index.jsp
International Association of Health Policy (IAHP)	www.healthp.org/index.php
International Federation of Pharmaceutical Manufacturers and Associations (IFPMA)	www.ifpma.org
International Health Economics Association (IHEA)	www.healtheconomics.org
Ipas (Protecting Women's Health)	www.ipas.org/english
John Snow, INC (JSI)	www.jsi.com/JSIInternet
Medical Care Development International (MCDI)	mcdi.mcd.org
Medicins Sans Frontieres (Doctors Without Borders)	www.doctorswithout borders.org
National Institutes of Health (NIH)	www.nih.gov
Office of U.S. Global AIDS Coordinator	www.state.gov/s/gac
Pan American Health Organization	www.paho.org
PATH	www.path.org
Population Council	www.popcouncil.org
Presidential Advisory Council on HIV and AIDS (PACHA)	www.pacha.gov
Research Triangle Park International (RTP)	www.rti.org
George Institute for International Health	www.thegeorgeinstitute.org

TABLE 5-1   Sample of Global Agencies That Maintain Tabulated
or Secondary Data *(continued)*

Organization/Agency Name	Webpage Address (URL)
Global Fund to Fight AIDS, Tuberculosis, and Malaria	www.theglobalfund.org/en
US Department of State	www.state.gov
United Nations	www.un.int
UNAIDS	www.unaids.org/en/default.asp
UNFPA (UN Population Fund)	www.unfpa.org
UNICEF (UN Children's Fund)	www.unicef.org
UNIFEM (UN Development Fund for Women)	www.unifem.org
US Agency for International Development (USAID)	www.usaid.gov
WHO information by country	www.who.int/countries/en
WHO regional office for Europe	data.euro.who.int/hfadb
World Health Organization (WHO)	www.who.int
WHO Statistical Information System	www3.who.int/whosis/menu.cfm
World Bank	www.worldbank.org
World Bank Group (data and research)	www.worldbank.org

Source: Kaiser Family Foundation (n.d.).

for program planning and evaluation, monitoring trends in incidence, and detecting disease outbreaks across the United States and its territories (CDC, 2006). This publication is made available online by the US government and is available electronically at no cost.

The *MMWR* is but one example that is readily available for public access and scrutiny. Apart from the availability of summary reports, global health researchers also have or are in need of access to a number of important Web sites. Such Web sites can serve to help narrow down or guide researchers in obtaining vital epidemiologic data or other data and information that can be downloaded, as in the form of tabulated data, and/or reanalyzed, as in the case of retrospective, secondary data.

There continues to exist many advantages in using epidemiologic data for secondary analysis (Sorensen, Sabroe, & Olsen, 1996). At times, the only data that researchers have available for global health studies is secondary data. Researchers concerned with global health issues need to consider, first and foremost, whether basic epidemiological data are already available for analysis or integration with other interdisciplinary secondary data sources in which it may be matched or linked.

As mentioned earlier, with the advent of the informatics revolution, global health researchers will be hard-pressed to not consider integrating diverse databases that may have been collected by others from inherently different disciplines (Bloom et al., 2006). Because of the global complexities surrounding individual, family, and community health, sophisticated models of secondary data analysis will continue to expand throughout the research community (Sorensen et al., 1996). Although secondary data may be in the form of survey research conducted by other researchers from other nations or in the same community or region, it may also be in the form of routinely collected public health surveillance data that tracks selected notifiable infectious and noncommunicable diseases and injuries.

Collecting the Data: Primary Data

Researchers have long played a pivotal role in the quality of life enjoyed throughout the world. If it were not for global health researchers willing to traverse oceans, jungles, deserts, mountains, and urban centers, the world would not be able to determine causes of diseases, injuries, and disabilities. The impact of the researcher on the world's well-being is virtually incalculable. What this means is that for up-to-date, state-of-the-art global health data to be made available, somewhere in the world a researcher concerned with global issues is working in the field, possibly in severe weather and placing themselves at risk, to collect data for subsequent analysis and reporting.

From the investigation of infectious disease outbreaks to the search for the origins of Ebola and HIV/AIDS, global health researchers have trekked far and wide around the planet to place themselves in the front lines of some of the most deadly and dangerous environments. Unlike secondary data, which has already been collected by someone else, new global health researchers interested in primary data collection may place themselves deep into an environment foreign to their normal standards of living. A new awareness throughout the world of global researchers is the recognition that certain diseases, such as HIV/AIDS, epilepsy, drug addiction, mental illness, and others carry with them a social stigma that not only affects the person with the disease but also challenges the researcher in being able to successfully access the population to be studied (Keusch, Wilentz, & Kleinman, 2006).

Regardless of the stigma or risk associated with a particular health or environmental problem, a global health researcher may need to realign his or her priorities to an area not well understood or not necessarily well recognized as a priority area of funding (Flory & Kitcher, 2004), as in the case of the 10/90 debate. The primary purpose of a researcher concerned about global issues is to answer his or her most basic research question. Once a researcher has come to terms with his or her priorities, he or she can begin seeking out answers to his or her research questions.

As mentioned, apart from the concerns of stigma associated with various diseases or conditions, a researcher is further challenged by needing to access research subjects in the local community. This can, at times, prove extremely difficult unless a researcher has gained indigenous, sometimes referred to as tacit, knowledge and expertise from local community members or other local researchers, such as nongovernmental organizations, which may have a long history in working with a specific population (Delisle, Roberts, Munro, Jones, & Gyorkos, 2005). Figure 5-2, for example, shows locally trained researchers in 2006 who served in multiple roles in the data collection process of a longitudinal

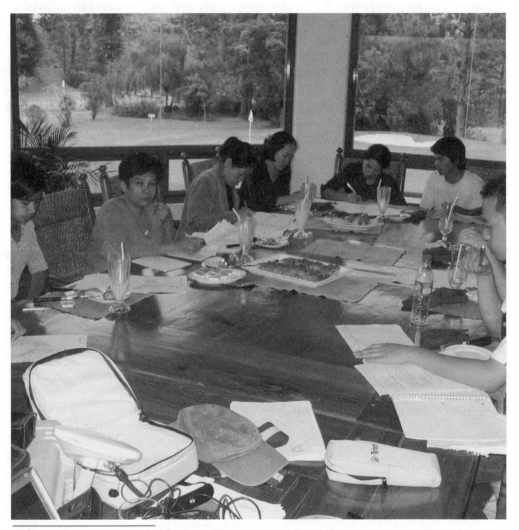

Figure 5-2 Filipino and Filipino-American researchers discussing research protocol readjustment.

research study currently underway by the authors of this chapter. Most of the researchers had training and were graduates of anthropology. Three of the researchers where from the United States and were of Filipino ancestry.

Flexibility is vital for GHR because people, places, and times do not necessarily follow standards consistent with one's home country, values, or place of business. What this means is that when conducting research from an international perspective, a seasoned or novice researcher must be willing to readjust their research protocol if the environment or situation changes. Otherwise, trying to follow a rigid and nonflexible data collection process may prove futile.

For example, when researchers of this chapter along with other members of their research team collected air quality data in the Philippines in 2004, original protocols needed to be changed and redesigned. This was due in part to changes in weather, environmental sickness of researchers caused by air pollution, urban land characteristics, and traffic patterns. Some of these factors were completely unforeseen, even though some of the principal research team members were from the region and could culturally identify with the environment. The more salient point is that global health research requires tenacity, flexibility, adaptability, and patience. Unlike clinical trials, where subjects and researchers follow strict protocols, field research is often more interdisciplinary in nature and requires—almost demands—a more inductive approach to each and every research design phase.

When global health researchers begin a primary data collection process, especially in a region of the world where research technologies and equipment are not readily available for acquisition or replacement, they need to ensure that they have all the necessary research equipment to carry out their study. Figure 5-3 illustrates the multiple data collection technologies used in the 2006 phase of the longitudinal field study undertaken by the authors of this chapter. The figure illustrates the many different types of scientific equipment used in conducting interdisciplinary field research, consisting of, but not limited to, Tremble Global Position System (GPS)/Geographical Information Systems (GIS) technology for geospatial mapping of street vendor sites and other environmental characteristics. Other equipment consisted of decibel meters, wind and temperature gauges, cameras, and a high-intensity receiving antenna. These technologies, while vital, are just part of the research tools some field researchers use in collecting environmental and health data and do not account for the fact that field researchers are also expected to take detailed field notes, develop surveys, or sketch physical characteristics of study sites.

Some of the most important challenges in conducting interdisciplinary global health primary data collection and field research are the need to ensure that the volumes of data collected are accurately merged and integrated into a high-quality database for later retrieval and analysis. The importance in data management becomes paramount to conducting a successful and scientifically valid and evidence-based research study.

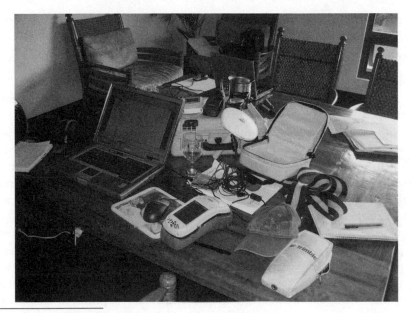

Figure 5-3 Interdisciplinary research equipment used for data collection.

Geographical Information Systems (GIS) in Global Health Research

Tabulated data or data still to be analyzed can be intimidating to most consumers of health statistics. Just the word *statistics* can bring tears to the eyes of many. The success of a GHR project may also lie in the ability of policy makers to understand the importance of the data visually. Neither numbers nor tables may make much sense to nonresearchers. Geographic information systems (GIS) can be a tool that clearly organizes the data so that it can be easily grasped and understood by even the most novice users of the information. GIS can serve as an ideal platform for data dissemination and reporting.

Geospatially mapping the location of diseases, populations, rivers, wells, buildings, sewage dumps, and many other types of environmental and cultural data characteristics may be vital towards an innovative understanding and tracking of diseases or environmental health hazards. The WHO, for example, provides a state-of-the-art GIS mapping capability on their Web site (see www.who.int/health_mapping/en/). GIS is nothing more than a graphic representation that serves as an interface between data and maps. Some of the more novel uses of GIS include the following:

- Determining geographical distribution or dispersion of diseases
- Analysis of spatial and temporal (time) trend data

- Visually overlapping other data such as health, topography, economics, demographics, and other characteristics important for analysis
- Observing structural intervention (e.g., mosquito nets relative to new cases of malaria or mosquito [vector] distribution over time)

Other important uses for GIS are in the expanding field of medical geography. Although GIS is a computer-aided database management system, medical geography incorporates concepts and methods for investigating health-related topics. Investigating geographic variations in global health has long been an interdisciplinary endeavor and brings into the equation the subdisciplines of geographical pathology, medical ecology and topography, geographical epidemiology, and other disciplines with interests in the geographical distribution of diseases relative to environmental and ecological issues (Meade & Earickson, 2000).

In summary, as GIS continues to expand its utility in the world of global health generally, and public health specifically, GIS mapping will take center stage as an emerging interdisciplinary technology that will become a useful tool for global health researchers who may or may not wish to collect primary data. GIS technology will not only serve the needs of primary researchers, but it can also serve as an access portal to tabulated or secondary data that can be placed into geospatial mapping programs for data visualization and reporting.

Conclusion

The need for a basic appreciation of some of the issues surrounding global health research has served to structure this chapter. Although many in the field of GHR may expect to see more detail in a chapter carrying the title of "Global Health Research," the purpose of this chapter was to provide an overview of some of the more pressing, actual hands-on issues that need to be considered when planning to undertake global health research, be it clinical, survey, or interventional. Before evidence-based practices, standards, and data can be made available more broadly and accepted more ubiquitously throughout the global community of researchers, greater attention needs to be directed and grounded in the world of GHR from an interdisciplinary framework.

References

Bloom, B. R., Michaud, C. M., La Montagne, J. R., & Simonsen, L. (2006). Priorities for global research and development of interventions. In D. T. Jamison et al. (Eds.), *Disease control priorities in developing countries* (pp. 103–118). New York: Oxford University Press and World Bank. Retrieved November 10, 2006, from http://www.dcp2.org/pubs/DCP

Centers for Disease Control and Prevention (CDC). (2006). *Morbidity and Mortality Weekly Report.* Retrieved November 24, 2006, from http://www.cdc.gov/mmwr/about.html

Delisle, H., Roberts, J. H., Munro, M., Jones, L., & Gyorkos, T. W. (2005). The role of NGOs in global health research for development. *Health Research Policy and Systems, 3,* 3.

Flory, J. H., & Kitcher, P. (2004). Global health and the scientific research agenda. *Philosophy and Public Affairs, 32*(1), 36–65.

Forti, S. (2005). *Building partnerships for global health research*. Canadian Coalition For Global Health Research. Retrieved November 18, 2006, from http://www.ccghr.ca/docs/toolkit/templates_e.pdf

Global Forum for Health Research. (2006). *The 10/90 gap—now*. Global Forum for Health Research. Retrieved November 5, 2006, from http://www.globalforumhealth.org

Hanney, S. R., Gonzalez-Block, M. A., Buxton, M. J., & Kogan, M. (2003). The utilisation of health research in policy-making: Concepts, examples and methods of assessment [Electronic version]. *Health Research Policy and Systems, 1*, 2.

Kaiser Family Foundation. (n.d.). *International health*. Retrieved November 29, 2006, from http://www.kaiseredu.org/research.asp?id=326

Keusch, G. T., Wilentz, J., & Kleinman, A. (2006). Stigma and global health: Developing a research agenda. *Lancet, 367*, 525–527.

Labonte, R., & Spiegel, J. (2003). Setting global health research priorities [Electronic version]. *British Medical Journal, 326*, 722–723.

Meade, M. S., & Earickson, R. J. (2000). *Medical geography* (2nd ed.). New York: Guildford Press.

Research!America. (2005). *Global health research investment by the United States: A special report*. Alexandria, VA: Research!America.

Sorensen, H. T., Sabroe, S., & Olsen, J. (1996). A framework for evaluation of secondary data sources for epidemiological research [Electronic version]. *International Journal of Epidemiology, 25*(2): 435–442.

Stansfield, S. K., Walsh, J., Prata, N., & Evans, T. (2006). Information to improve decision making for health. In D. T. Jamison et al. (Eds.). *Disease control priorities in developing countries* (pp. 1017–1030). New York: Oxford University Press and World Bank. Retrieved November 10, 2006, from http://www.dcp2.org/pubs/DCP

Uhlir, P. F., & Esanu, J. M. (2006). *Strategies for preservation of and open access to scientific data in China: Summary of a workshop*. National Research Council and Board on International Scientific Organizations. Washington, DC: National Academies Press.

World Health Organization (WHO). (n.d.). *Role of GIS in public health mapping*. Retrieved November 29, 2006, from www.who.int/health_mapping/en

Chapter 6

International Research Ethics

Jonathan B. VanGeest

Deborah S. Cummins

Research plays a pivotal role in addressing many of the global health issues identified in this text, including the large inequities that exist in global health and health care. To achieve its promise, however, research must be scientifically valid. Moreover, it must be rooted in sound ethical principles.

Broadly defined, ethics is the study of right behavior (Pojman, 1995; Singer, 1993). Ethics also seeks to delineate basic standards of conduct that are independent of personal opinions and feelings, social customs, or political and religious ideologies. Within the study of ethics, distinctions are often made between *theoretical ethics* (e.g., the study of general theories, concepts, or principles of ethics as well as articulation of standards of ethical behavior) and *applied ethics*, which examines the application of ethical theory or principles to a particular set of circumstances or issues. Although a detailed explanation of each is beyond the scope of this chapter, it is important to note that theoretical ethics are anchored in philosophy and theology and often deal with the larger questions of life, including questions about the existence of universal standards of ethical behavior. Applied ethics, on the other hand, are often discipline or subject specific, with questions and standards derived from lived experiences. Examples of applied ethics include nursing, medical, legal, and business ethics. The focus of this chapter is on the global application of research ethics, a branch of applied ethics that examines the ethical problems and dilemmas that arise during the conduct of research.

Research Ethics

The term *research ethics* refers to a range of ethically significant issues that often arise during the conduct of research—from fair distribution of authorship credit among members of a research team; to issues of plagiarism; to ensuring the confidentiality and integrity of data collection, analyses, and reporting; to responsible treatment of research subjects; to balancing the needs of subjects with a researcher's responsibility to society. In this chapter, we discuss ethical considerations that researchers face during the actual process of research, with special attention given to dilemmas that may arise in today's global environment. Although ethical dilemmas can arise across a range of issues, our focus is on the ethical treatment of human research subjects. Humans are routinely used in the development of new knowledge in the health sciences. Basic societal ethics demand that subjects be treated with a degree of respect and be protected from harm. These demands are mirrored in codes of professional ethics from the World Health Organization, World Medical Association, American Medical Association, American Nursing Association, and others addressing the welfare of human research participants. But research is a complicated process, with the protection of human subjects open to some interpretation, especially in international research where different norms, values, and ethical traditions intersect.

The Use of Human Subjects in Research

Human experimentation is defined as "any manipulation, test, or procedure of an experimental nature performed on a human being as part of a scientific or social science investigation" (Stern & Lomax, 1997). Common examples of studies involving the use of human subjects include clinical protocols to test new medications or treatment procedures as well as clinical psychiatry, sociology, and clinical psychology experiments performed inside or outside the clinical setting. There are a number of ethical considerations when human subjects are used in research, such as justifications for the use of placebo controls,[1] the adequacy of informed consent, subject risk versus benefits in areas of potential harm (e.g., embarrassment, privacy and confidentiality, pain and discomfort), and the selection of subjects into control and intervention groups (Beauchamp & Childress, 1996; Shamoo & Resnik, 2003; Stern & Lomax, 1997). These considerations, however, are not always readily apparent even to experienced researchers or may clash with the desired processes of inquiry. Not surprisingly, there have been documented cases of questionable research, including controversies involving the use of placebos, informed consent, and research on vulnerable populations, such as minorities, children, prisoners, and the mentally ill (Beecher, 1966; Beauchamp & Childress, 1996; Shamoo & Irving, 1993; Stern & Lomax, 1997).

The ethics of research became a more prominent issue during the Nuremberg war crimes trials that outlined atrocities committed by Nazi doctors and scientists on prisoners held in concentration camps (Shamoo & Resnik, 2003). Prior to World War II, the ethics of research was largely assumed, but many were shocked to learn of the nature of the experiments conducted on humans during the war years in the name of science. Examples included Dr. Josef Mengele's endurance experiments subjecting prisoners to high levels of electricity and radiation and his experiments to change eye color that often resulted in blindness. Other examples included hypothermia studies to see how long people could survive in freezing water, decompression studies examining human reactions to high-altitude flight, and vaccination and infection studies that intentionally

---

[1]In clinical trials, a test group of subjects receives the therapy being tested, and a control group receives a placebo (an inactive substance administered as if it were a therapy). The groups are then studied to determine if results from the test group exceed those from the control group.

exposed adults and children to diseases such as typhus, tuberculosis, malaria, scarlet fever, smallpox, and tetanus. After the trials, in an effort to prevent further abuses, the research community adopted the Nuremberg Code, the world's first international code governing research on human subjects. This was followed in 1964 by the Declaration of Helsinki, a statement of ethical principles developed by the World Medical Association to provide guidance for research involving human subjects. Briefly, the declaration made informed consent (voluntary consent of human subjects to participate in a study based upon an understanding of the facts and implications of participation) a central requirement of ethical research. It also stated that research should conform to accepted scientific principles and that concern for research subjects must always prevail over the interests of science and society.

Despite these established recommendations, research ethics has remained a contentious issue, and there have been instances where scientists have been criticized for failing to ensure the ethical conduct of their research, including many studies conducted in the United States. One oft-cited example is the Willowbrook hepatitis experiments (1956–1980) in which mentally retarded children were infected with the hepatitis virus in an effort to study the natural progression of the disease and to test the effectiveness of gamma globulin in preventing or treating the disease. The researchers justified their design by citing the endemic nature of the disease ("most" of the children at Willowbrook became infected within a year of admission) and the therapeutic benefits of the treatments offered the children in the study. There were serious questions, however, related to the adequacy of parental informed consent.[2] Another is the Tuskegee syphilis study (1932–1972) which took place in a public health clinic in Tuskegee, Alabama. In this study, 400 poor, mostly illiterate African-American males with untreated syphilis were enrolled in the experimental group to examine the natural progression of the disease. Subjects were not told they had syphilis (instead they were told that they had "bad blood"), did not give informed consent, and were not given medically proven treatments for the disease. Additional examples in the United States and elsewhere include the following:

- An Oregon state prison study (1963–1971) that exposed the testicles of 67 African-American prisoners to X-rays to determine the effects of radiation on sperm function
- Human radiation experiments that took place in the United States (1944–1974) that exposed adults and children to varying levels of radiation without their consent in an effort to examine the affects of radiation on health
- The Jewish chronic disease study (1964) that introduced live cancer cells into unsuspecting patients in an effort to learn more about the process by which the body rejects transplanted organs

---

[2]Questions were raised about how well parents understood the actual risks of their children becoming infected with hepatitis and whether they adequately understood the long- and short-term consequences of their children's involvement in the study.

Research Ethics in Today's Global Context

In today's global environment, attention is focused on research by groups in developed countries but carried out in developing countries, where requirements for review, approval, and oversight may be much less stringent. This is especially true of clinical trials involving human subjects, in which the intervention tested is unlikely to benefit citizens in the host country, either because of cost issues or because the healthcare infrastructure in that country can not support its distribution and use. The disparate availability of these interventions raises the ethical concern that the developed country may be exploiting a country that is resource poor and therefore more vulnerable (Caballero, 2002; Shapiro & Meslin, 2001; Silva, Sungar, Kleinstiver, & Rubin, 2006; Werner, 1999). This concern is heightened by increased participation of the private sector, particularly the pharmaceutical industry, in promoting research in less developed countries where they may enjoy significant regulatory and/or cost advantages. In addition, there is the ever-present question of whether it is ethically acceptable to conduct a trial in another country that you may not have been able to conduct in your own (because of more stringent review processes). Finally, the ethics of research is challenged by the many complex humanitarian emergencies (e.g., refugee settings, natural disasters, ethnic conflicts) occurring in developing countries worldwide (National Research Council, 2002). Although research is necessary to understand the causes and consequences of these emergencies, inherent difficulties in identifying potential harms related to research in these settings makes use of human subjects problematic.

Because of these issues, researchers in developed countries must take special care to ensure adequate justification for conducting research trials in developing countries, especially if the research is to be conducted in a region where the host population is especially vulnerable because of pervasive poverty, low health literacy (defined as a systematic lack of understanding the health issue under study), emergency conditions, lack of education, or the lack of familiarity with the research process. Researchers face a number of questions related to international research. They must be able to demonstrate a clear ethical imperative or rationalization for the research under consideration. They must also be ready to answer questions related to the application of relevant ethical standards governing the amount and/or type of research conducted.

A Closer Look: Clinical Trials in the Prevention of MTCT of HIV

The debate over global research ethics is illustrated by the controversies surrounding early clinical trials on the prevention of mother-to-child transmission (MTCT) of human immunodeficiency virus (HIV). As the name implies, MTCT is when an HIV-positive woman passes the virus on to her baby (either during pregnancy, labor and delivery, or when breast feeding). MTCT is a health problem globally, but is especially problematic in developing countries. In 2005 an estimated 700,000 children under 15 years of age became infected with HIV, mainly through mother-to-child transmission. Almost 90% of these

MTCT infections were in Africa. At the time of the clinical trials, MTCT of HIV could be significantly reduced through the use of a standard regimen of antiretroviral drugs and other interventions.[3] However, high antiretroviral costs (the cost of the standard anti-retroviral regimen was about $800, or upwards of 800 times the annual per capita allocation for health care in some developing countries), coupled with insufficient health delivery infrastructure in most African countries, placed treatment out of reach for a majority of the populations at risk. For these reasons, researchers began in the 1990s to test the efficacy of a short-term low-dose antiretroviral regimen in preventing perinatal HIV transmission using placebo-controlled clinical trials carried out in several technologically developing countries.[4]

The trials were criticized for what some considered an unethical use of a placebo (Lurie & Wolfe, 1997; Angell, 1997; Salvi & Damania, 2006). Specifically, these studies were accused of violating accepted international codes of research ethics because they did not provide subjects in the control group with a known effective therapy (e.g., the standard long-course antiretroviral therapy). Instead, controls were given no medication for preventing MTCT of HIV despite the already acknowledged proven therapeutic method for reducing perinatal transmission of HIV, a condition that might not be ethically acceptable in industrialized countries such as the United States where the standard treatment was readily available. Use of equivalency trials (comparing test subjects with a control group receiving the usual standard treatment) were also highlighted as a potential alternative to the use of placebo controls, as these allow researchers to examine whether the altered regimen is approximately as effective compared to the standard regimen (Lurie & Wolfe, 1997). Proponents of the studies, however, argued that a placebo was necessary in order to produce timely and truly meaningful results (Varmus & Satcher, 1997; Wendler, Emanuel, Reidar, & Lie, 2004).[5] More specifically, they argue that use of placebo-controlled trials provides definitive answers to questions about the efficacy of the short-term low-dose antiretroviral regimen in the very settings where—if successful—the intervention would be implemented.

---

[3]Clinical trials using a standard AZT drug regimen (i.e., administration of AZT orally during pregnancy, intravenously during delivery, and orally to the newborn infant) demonstrated a reduction of perinatal transmission of HIV by about 67%, from 25% to 8% (Connor et al., 1994; Sperling et al., 1996).

[4]The short-term low-dose regimen entailed a much lower (10%) dose of AZT administered to the mother for a shorter period of time. The regimen also did not include intravenous administration of AZT during delivery or the oral administration of AZT to the newborn infant (Levine, 1998b).

[5]Researchers note the difficulty of interpreting active-control research designs, including difficulty assessing benefit of the intervention against a possible placebo response (a positive medical response to taking a placebo often thought to be a physiological response to participating in a trial) or—in the case of the MTCT trials—the need to assess whether the affordable intervention is actually better than nothing (Emanuel & Miller, 2001; Levine, 1998b; Varmus & Satcher, 1997).

Reasonable Standard of Care Debate

At the heart of the debate over the appropriateness of the MTCT trials is the determination of what constitutes a "fair and reasonable standard of care" for subjects in developing countries who participate in clinical trials (Benatar & Singer, 2000; Emanuel & Miller, 2001; Landes, 2005; Shaffer et al., 2006; Wendler et al., 2004). The problem is that what constitutes a normal standard of care is not well defined or is subject to interpretation, a problem made clear in deliberations over the studies on the vertical transmission of HIV. On one end of the spectrum, researchers defending the use of placebo controls in developing countries argue that subjects are treated in accordance with the standard of care in those countries, which in light of the high costs of the standard AZT regimen (or the current highly active antiretroviral therapies [HAART] standard) actually consists of unproven regimens and/or no treatments at all. Others, however, suggest that this reasoning constitutes an unfair double standard with regard to the conduct of research globally, promoting the use of at-risk populations in resource-poor countries as research subjects (Landes, 2005; Lurie & Wolfe, 1997; Salvi & Damania, 2006). Still others, citing the ethical and methodologic complexities of clinical research, call for a middle ground in which use of placebo-controlled trials are permissible so long as the methodologic reasons for their use are compelling and that precise criteria (e.g., monitoring of subjects, explicit criteria for withdrawal of subjects from the study) are met to minimize the risks to subjects receiving the placebo (Emanuel & Miller, 2001).

Benatar and Singer (2000) and others have called for an expanded concept of usual standard of care that takes into account the nature of the study in question as well as specific social, economic, political, and cultural contexts in which it occurs. This would necessitate that international researchers develop a deeper understanding of, and consideration for, the country in which their research is taking place (Benatar & Singer, 2000; Emanuel & Miller, 2001; Resnik, 1998). To date, however, despite a recent amendment to the Declaration of Helsinki endorsing the universal application of a worldwide best standard of care, what constitutes a reasonable standard of care is still a matter of some controversy (Ehni, 2006; Hyder & Dawson, 2005; Lie, Emanuel, Grady, & Wendler, 2004; London, 2000).

Important Questions

Clearly the debate sparked by the conduct of the MTCT of HIV placebo-controlled trials within African and other developing countries has not ended. Similar debates are also ongoing in other areas of research, including international studies of effective treatments for arthritis, cardiovascular treatments, and antidepressant treatments for depression (Glasser, Clark, Lipicky, Hubbard, & Yusaf, 1991; Kahn, Warner, & Brown, 2000; Kavanaugh, 2005; Silva et al., 2006). These deliberations, however, have raised some very important and practical ethical questions that must be considered regardless of the area of study. Specifically, research must ask the following questions:

- What are the ethical justifications for the proposed study?

- When treatments are available (even treatments of undocumented or marginal benefit), what are the most appropriate comparison groups for studies of new interventions?

- Under what circumstances is it ethical to use placebos in case-control studies?

- What are the responsibilities and/or obligations of researchers to continue interventions/therapies for participants following the conclusion of a study?

Embedded within these questions are a number of ethical dilemmas that researchers often face when conducting global research involving human subjects (Shamoo & Resnik, 2003). First, there is the age-old ethical dilemma of the need to balance the individual good (well-being of individuals) against the welfare of society. Referring to the case discussed above, placebos may have enhanced the validity or social value of the research, but was it done at the expense of the rights and interests of those involved as subjects? A second and related dilemma relates to the assessment of the benefits and risks of the research. Researchers must weigh the potential risks and benefits to individual subjects against those of society, with the fielding of a study only justified when there is significant societal benefit *and* when individual subjects are at "minimal risk" of harm or discomfort (Box 6-1). Finally, researchers must weigh the actual burdens of research against the potential distribution of the benefits. This is especially important with research involving vulnerable subjects (e.g., women, children, the poor, and prisoners) and to the global conduct of research. For example, global research is often criticized in this regard because subjects in developing countries bear the burden of research, but seldom enjoy its benefits (again because the distribution of proven interventions is often prohibited because of cost and infrastructure issues).

Box 6-1   The Meaning of Risk

Risk is defined as the potential physical or psychological harm, discomfort, or stress caused by research participation. There are a wide range of risks associated with biomedical research, including risk to a subject's privacy and personal values, as well as the possible adverse physical or psychological health effects related to participating in clinical trials. The US federal regulations define "minimal risk" as being "the probability and magnitude of harm or discomfort anticipated in the research are not greater in and of themselves than those ordinarily encountered in daily life or during the performance of routine physical or psychological examinations or tests" (Misconduct in Science & Engineering, 1991).

Basic Principles

One approach towards resolving conflicts in these areas is to reexamine the basic ethical principles intended to guide research within today's global context. There are many important guidelines for the ethical conduct of research (Table 6-1). As noted, one of the most important is the Declaration of Helsinki. Other significant documents include the Belmont Report (National Commission, 1979) and the International Ethical Guidelines for Biomedical Research Involving Human Subjects (Council for International Organizations of Medical Sciences, 1993). Generally, these guidelines rest on three broad ethical principles: (1) *respect for persons* (autonomy and self-determination), (2) *beneficence* (maximizing benefits and minimizing harms), and (3) *justice* (including distributive justice with respect to the burdens and benefits of research). These principles are the cornerstone for regulations governing all clinical and nonclinical biomedical research involving individual subjects. Additionally, while these principles may be expressed somewhat differently in various global contexts, they are intended to be universal, transcending geographic, cultural, legal, and political boundaries.

Universal Requirements for Ethical Research

Within this larger framework, several authors have identified universal requirements or domains that provide the basis for determining whether research is ethical (Caballero, 2002; Emanuel, Wendler, & Grady, 2000; Levine, 1988a; Pimple, 2002; Shamoo & Resnik, 2003).

Respect for Persons
Researchers should respect the choices of autonomous individuals. Subjects incapable of making their own choices should be protected. Researchers should always respect the privacy, dignity, and rights of all research subjects and should take appropriate steps to ensure confidentiality. Researchers should also inform subjects of the results of clinical research and always work to maintain the welfare of subjects. *Informed consent* is a critical component of this requirement (Box 6-2).[6] Researchers should make every effort to ensure or document that subjects actually understand the study procedures, potential risks and benefits, alternatives to participation, and their full rights as study participants. Subjects must also be allowed to withdraw from a study for any time and for any reason. Also included in this requirement is the need to *protect vulnerable subjects*. Researchers must take extra precautions to avoid exploitation or harm when dealing with vulnerable subjects, especially research on subjects in resource-poor countries.

---

[6]Informed consent is so important to the ethical conduct of research that some authors list it as a separate or stand-alone requirement. See, for example, Emanuel et al. (2000) or Shamoo and Resnik, (2003).

TABLE 6-1   Selected Guidelines on the Ethical Treatment of Human Subjects

Guideline	Source	Year and Revisions	Comment
General			
Nuremberg Code	Nuremberg Military Tribunal	1947	Ten standards to which physicians must conform when carrying out experiments on human subjects
Declaration of Helsinki	World Medical Association	Adopted 1964 Amended 1975, 1983, 1989, 1996, and 2000	Declaration makes informed consent a central requirement of ethical research. Basis for implementation of the institutional review board (IRB) process
Belmont Report	National Commission for the Protection of Human Subjects of Biomedical and Behavioral Research	1979	Cornerstone of US federal regulations governing the protection of human subjects
International Ethical Guidelines for Biomedical Research Involving Human Subjects	Council for International Organizations of Medical Sciences in collaboration with the World Health Organization	Proposed 1982 Revised 1993 and 2002	Guidelines address issues of informed consent, standards for external review, and recruitment of participants.
Specific			
45 CFR Part 46	US Department of Health and Human Services	Adopted 1981. Current revision 2005	Embodies the ethical principles of the Belmont Report. Regulations apply to all research involving human subjects conducted or supported by the federal government.[†]

[†]Different countries have their own guidelines on the ethics of research. A compilation of international guidelines is available at http://www.hhs.gov/ohrp/international/HSPCompilation.pdf

(continues)

TABLE 6-1   Selected Guidelines on the Ethical Treatment of Human Subjects
(continued)

Guideline	Source	Year and Revisions	Comment
Health Insurance Portability and Accountability Act, Privacy Rule	US Department of Health and Human Services	2002	Standards for privacy of individually identifiable health information
Guidelines for Good Clinical Practice (GCP) for Trials on Pharmaceutical Products	World Health Organization	1995	Establishes globally applicable standards for the conduct of pharmaceutical trials involving human subjects
Good Clinical Practice: Consolidated Guidance	International Conference on Harmonisation of Technical Requirements for Registration of Pharmaceuticals for Human Use	1996	International ethical standard for designing, conducting, recording, and reporting clinical trials that involve the participation of human subjects
Declaration on Ethical Considerations Regarding Health Databases	World Heath Organization	2002	Declaration defines the appropriate uses and storage of patients' personal health information.
International Declaration on Human Genetic Data	United Nations Educational, Scientific, and Cultural Organization (UNESCO)	2003	International guidelines on collection and use of human genetic data

Value

Researchers should ensure that studies have value at either the individual or societal level. Specifically, for research to be ethical it must be significant (i.e., have the potential to lead to improvements in health and well-being), be generalizable to other settings or groups, and have practical applications. Vanderpool (1996) identifies two reasons why this requirement is important: (a) it necessitates responsible use of limited resources (e.g., research funding, facilities) and (b) it helps prevent the exploitation of research subjects. In short, it is never appropriate to involve human subjects in frivolous research. This

BOX 6-2 **Informed Consent**

Informed consent is the legal condition whereby a person consents to participate in a research study based upon their appreciation and understanding of the facts and implications of their participation. The right of potential research subjects to freely choose to participate is central to all of the international guidelines written for research on human subjects. The National Bioethics Advisory Committee (NBAC) (2001) identifies three types of disclosure that are central to the process of informed consent: (1) disclosure of risk, (2) disclosure of the use of placebos and randomization, and (3) disclosure of alternative treatments. These elements apply irrespective of different cultural standards that may exist related to the informed consent process (e.g., appropriateness of providing diagnoses, local barriers to use of placebos). The NBAC also recommends that researchers develop culturally appropriate ways to disclose information about their study, including testing participants' understanding following the informed consent process. Explicit disclosure requirements for studies conducted in the United States are found in the Federal Policy for the Protection of Human Subjects at 45 CFR 46.116(a), under the heading of "Basic Elements of Informed Consent."

requirement is also especially important with regards to research involving international collaborations.

Beneficence

This requirement specifies that researchers have an obligation to maximize the benefits of research to an individual or society while minimizing harm to participants (Beauchamp & Childress, 1996; Levine, 1988a). Clinical research, however, often involves a great deal of uncertainty with regard to potential risks and benefits. Thus, additional justification and oversight is required for research where there are no clearly identifiable benefits or when identified risks exceed potential benefits (as is often the case in many phase 1 clinical trials where efficacy of an intervention is not known). Researchers must also constantly monitor the research process and be willing to stop their protocol if harms become substantial compared to benefits. Similarly, if benefits greatly exceed the alternative (control), then randomization of subjects must also be stopped so that all participants can have access to the intervention.

Scientific Validity

This requirement simply states that for research to be ethical it must be methodologically sound. Researchers must have clearly defined and justifiable scientific objectives; design studies according to accepted principles, methods, and practices; and ensure that studies are feasible in application (Emanuel et al., 2000). Researchers should also work to eliminate all biases from their research protocols (e.g., sampling procedures, instrument design) and actively seek to identify and avoid conflicts of interest.

Justice

Researchers must ensure that research is fair. This is especially important with regards to subject selection (i.e., decisions about who will be included in the research, strategies for recruiting and selecting participants). Scientific goals of the study, not subject availability, must be the primary basis for determining who will be approached to participate and who will be excluded from the study. Researchers should also intentionally select subjects to minimize the risks and maximize the benefits of participation. For example, researchers should exclude from participation subjects deemed to be at elevated risk of harm. Similarly, if an intervention will likely benefit particular population subgroups (e.g., women, racial and ethnic minorities, children) researchers should make every effort to include these groups in the study. Included in this requirement is aforementioned concept of *distributive justice*; that researchers promote a fair and equitable distribution of the burdens and benefits of research across the different population subgroups and/or international partners involved in the study.

Tensions exist with regard to the application of these principles, with professional judgment critically important to the appropriate design and conduct of global research (Emanuel et al., 2000). Additionally, while intended to be universal, protection of human subjects still varies widely across countries, with interpretation and implementation of the guidelines and domains subject to adaptation to particular cultures, health conditions, and economic settings (Caballero, 2002; Shamoo & Resnik, 2003; Shapiro & Meslin, 2001). For these reasons, authors have suggested the following additional ethical requirements specifically for research performed in less-developed countries by scientists from developed countries (Caballero, 2002; Wendler et al., 2004).

Relevance to Local Situation

Researchers conducting global research need to establish that the conditions or therapies being studied are relevant to the country in which the studies are being carried out. By this standard, an investigation of a therapy that would never be available or affordable for citizens of the host country would not be ethical. Similarly, international studies that fail to address important health needs of communities in developing countries would be ethically suspect.

Host Community Benefit

Researchers must ensure that the host community receives a fair distribution of benefits from the study. This requirement makes explicit the aforementioned requirement of distributive justice within the context of international research. Specifically, if a community bears a higher level of risk with regard to a particular study, researchers must work to ensure that the host community receives a corresponding benefit from their participation. Additionally, in cases where risks and burdens are difficult to assess, researchers should provide additional benefits to the host community (e.g., development of health clinics, training of healthcare providers, community health screenings). Often these additional benefits are parallel but unrelated to the actual research being conducted (Caballero, 2002).

Host Community Nonmaleficence

Researchers need to make sure that international research conducted in a host community does not make subjects in that community worse off than they would be in absence of the study (Wendler et al., 2004). More specifically, a study must not interfere with an existing standard of care or the delivery of health care in the host community.

Applications of all of the identified requirements or domains are essential to the ethical design of global research. However, the last three are critically important in that they allow researchers to begin to address the fair and reasonable standard of care debate with regard to international trials involving human subjects (Wendler et al., 2004). Some contend that a total ban on research involving placebo controls (or even research with control subjects receiving less than a global standard for best care) may not be feasible, or in certain situations may even be counterproductive to the ethical treatment of subjects in developing countries (Varmus & Satcher, 1997; Wendler et al., 2004). Specifically, they contend that such a ban would prevent the study of agents or treatments that, while they may be more accessible to populations in the host country, are expected to be less effective than treatments based on the existing global standards for best care. Careful application of the ethical requirements, especially those related to host community relevance, benefit and nonmaleficence, however, would allow for such a study by ensuring that it is ethical, that it has the potential to benefit populations globally, and that human subjects receive sufficient benefits for their participation, both with regard to their actual study involvement (e.g., direct access to medications, treatments) as well as tangentially through the presence or conduct of the study within their communities. Ultimately, application of the ethical requirements makes certain that research is responsive in the long term to the health needs of the host country by facilitating access to interventions to the inhabitants upon completion of successful testing (Grady, 2006).

Applications: Another Look at Clinical Trials in the Prevention of MTCT of HIV

Studies of MTCT of HIV can again be used to illustrate. Wendler et al. (2004), in a review of outcomes of vertical transmission trials conducted between 1999 and 2000, illustrate how variability in placebo MTCT transmission rates may have led researchers relying solely on equivalence trials to conclude that the short-term low-dose antiretroviral regimen was not worth pursuing. More importantly, they indicate that these results were understood to be a realistic possibility even before the outset of the trials given the wide variations in HIV vertical transmission rates within the host communities. This suggested a priori a need for a placebo-controlled design capable of determining whether the short-term intervention was better than no treatment at all. Moreover, given the circumstances, decisions to use placebo controls could be supported by careful application of the ethical requirements outlined above.[7] This need was verified in the actual conduct of the trials, which resulted in transmission rates between 18.9% and 27.5% for the placebo group compared to rates between 9.9% and 18% for those receiving the short-term low-dose antiretroviral regimen; suggesting that the short-term treatment was indeed effective. In another example, they demonstrate how a ban on research involving placebo controls (or a ban on controls receiving less than the global standard for care) would have precluded studies on the use of nevirapine in preventing MTCT of HIV (Wendler et al., 2004). Nevirapine is a low-cost (hence more accessible) antiretroviral drug given to the mother orally during labor. Although less effective than some monotherapies, such as the long-course AZT therapy outlined above, or HAART (the drug does not protect against vertical transmission of HIV that occurs in utero), studies ultimately supported the efficacy of the drug as an economical way to reduce MTCT of HIV—dramatically improving HIV prevention in developing countries.

Protecting Human Subjects Globally: A Need for Oversight and Monitoring

Although important to resolving conflicts in global research, the requirements outlined above are necessary, but not sufficient, for research to be ethical. Said another way, it is important to understand that requirements do not constitute a simple prescription or formula for the protection of human subjects. Determining what is ethical still requires moral reasoning involving careful consideration of the potential benefits and harms specific to a particular research question or design, as well as the relevant social, economic, and political contexts within which the study will be carried out (Benatar & Singer, 2000; Resnik, 1998). Only by weighing and balancing the competing moral and scientific requirements can one develop realistic—and justifiable—conclusions regarding the ethics of a specific study. What the requirements do is to ensure appropriately informed discussion and (ultimately) decisions with regard to the ethical conduct of research involving human subjects. Professional judgment and expertise remain essential elements in this process. Also important is the need for independent review and oversight at the institutional level. Finally, and especially important with respect to global research, there should be community involvement in all phases of the research design, with special emphasis on processes for determination and disclosure of risks and benefits and informed consent.

Specifically, for a study to be successful (i.e., ethical), oversight is needed at multiple levels. The most basic levels involve both the researcher(s) and an independent review.

---

[7]For example, a cursory review suggests that the studies had potential societal value, given the high prevalence of MTCT of HIV in the host countries, and were methodologically sound. Additionally, the studies benefited from host community relevance, benefit, and did not make subjects prospectively worse off because of their participation (compared to existing standards of care in those communities).

Initially, in any project the research professional must bring to bear their individual expertise with regard to the subject under study and the appropriate research design. Professional judgment alone, however, is usually not enough, as professionals are often under competing interests or pressures (e.g., need for quality, timeliness, funding) that can distort the judgment of even the most well-intentioned investigators. Thus, additional oversight is provided through independent reviews to determine whether a project conforms to accepted human research regulations. Although independent reviews can be conducted by multiple agencies (e.g., funding agencies, research committees), in the United States, institutional review boards (IRBs) are typically used for this purpose.

An IRB is a group composed of at least five qualified members with varied backgrounds (with at least one member who must not be affiliated with the parent institution) that has been formally designated to review and monitor research in order to assure the protection of the rights and welfare of humans participating as subjects in research. Regardless of where the study is conducted, investigators supported by US federal monies are required to submit their research protocol to an IRB. Most institutions in the United States also require nonfederally funded research to be similarly reviewed. IRBs evaluate a proposed study in a number of areas, including its value, validity, fairness of selection criteria, risk-benefit ratios, and appropriateness of informed consent and confidentiality procedures (Shamoo & Resnik, 2003). Additionally, IRBs must carefully evaluate research involving vulnerable subjects (Table 6-2) and ensure that processes are in place for continual data and safety monitoring to protect human subjects.[8] For a study under review, an IRB has the authority to do the following:

- Approve, disapprove, or terminate research activities within its jurisdiction.
- Require modifications to the study protocols.
- Require that information about the study be given to participants.
- Require documentation of voluntary informed consent.

Under federal regulations, certain low-risk research categories are exempt from IRB review; however researchers still have ethical responsibilities to protect participants' rights.

Although important, research professionals or even IRBs are seldom able to fully consider the range of diverse social values, priorities, and concerns that can come into play in the conduct of international research. For these reasons, authors have begun to argue for additional community oversight (Lo & Bayer, 2003; Quinn, 2004; Strauss et al., 2001; Weijer & Emanuel, 2000), especially in the conduct of international research. This includes the use of community advisory boards (CABS) to improve not only the

---

[8]The US National Institutes for Health require that every clinical trial have provision for data and safety monitoring. Monitoring is required to determine safe and effective conduct and to recommend conclusion of the trial when significant benefits or risks have developed or when the trial is unlikely to be concluded successfully.

TABLE 6-2   Vulnerable Subjects

Population	Vulnerability	Recommendations/Guidelines
Children	Limited ability to comprehend the nature of the study or the implications of their participation	US regulations require IRBs to classify research on children based on their assessment of risk. Federally funded research categorized as having "greater than minor increase over minimal risk" is considered only under certain circumstances and must be reviewed by the Secretary of the Department of Health and Human Services. In such cases, permission and consent must be obtained from both parents if they have custody and are reasonably available, and assent of the child is required.
Mentally ill	Impaired decision-making capabilities hinder their ability to promote or protect their own interests.	Although extra protections for the mentally disabled are recommended, there is a lack of clarity in federal guidelines. Definition of acceptable risk for mentally ill subjects is usually a matter of interpretation by individual IRBs.
Prisoners	Potential for coercion based on their environment	Current US regulations allow prisoners to be involved in biomedical and behavioral research only if (1) the research is of minimal risk related to the causes and consequences of incarceration; (2) the study is of the prison as an institution; (3) the research is on the condition of prisoners; or (4) the research is therapeutic with potential benefits to the subjects. The risks involved must also be commensurate with risks that would be accepted by nonprisoner volunteers and selection of subjects within the prison must be fair to all prisoners and immune from intervention by prison authorities or prisoners.
Minorities	Historic vulnerabilities related to racism and prejudice exist. Minorities may also be subject to coercion because of poverty or literacy issues.	Regulations require equitable selection of minorities as research subjects. When conducting research involving minorities, investigators must pay attention to special vulnerabilities (e.g., additional vulnerabilities because of economic or educational disadvantage).

(continues)

TABLE 6-2   Vulnerable Subjects *(continued)*

Population	Vulnerability	Recommendations/Guidelines
		IRB-approved informed consent documents must also be available in English and other languages as appropriate and must account for the possibility of illiteracy. The role of cultural norms of subjects should also be addressed.
Pregnant women and human fetuses	Multiple vulnerabilities (e.g., ability to consent, risk to development) exist for both the mother and fetus.	US regulations do not allow pregnant women to participate in human clinical research projects unless: (1) the purpose of the activity is to meet the health needs of the mother, and the fetus will be placed at risk only to the minimum extent necessary; or (2) the risk to the fetus is minimal. Research involving pregnant women is permitted only if the mother and father are legally competent and both give consent. Father's consent need not be secured if (1) the purpose of the study is to meet the health needs of the mother; (2) his identity or whereabouts cannot be ascertained; (3) he is not reasonably available; or (4) the pregnancy resulted from rape.

partnerships between researchers and communities, but also the research quality and the relevance and usefulness of international research to host communities. Broad community participation is important in all phases of the research process (Lo & Bayer, 2003; Quinn, 2004; Strauss et al., 2001). However, CABS may be particularly important to informed consent, as they have the potential to identify cultural issues (e.g., deference to community leaders, age) that may complicate these processes (Lo & Bayer, 2003; Woodsong & Karim, 2005). CABS may also play a critical role in subject recruitment and study follow-up (Lo & Bayer, 2003; Strauss et al., 2001). Although vital, community oversight may be particularly challenging in the international context, where there may be limited understanding of basic research principles, wide variations of community government or representation, and large gaps in the social and educational backgrounds between researchers and their subjects. Thus, it is important for international researchers to intentionally invest in this area. Lo and Bayer (2003) suggest a number of steps to promote community partnerships, including efforts by research teams to promote partnerships through ongoing quality improvement efforts as well as team meetings designed to build and sustain such collaborations.

Despite some inherent difficulties, input and oversight from all three perspectives—research team members, institutional review boards, and communities—play important roles in the ethical evaluation of international research. Together, these partnerships are able to establish the scientific necessity or value of research in developing countries. They also provide a basis for the ongoing protection of the health and safety of participants, including those at significant risk of manipulation because of poverty, ignorance, health status, or other conditions. Finally, incorporating these three perspectives can lay the groundwork for more equitable distribution of the benefits of the research across the different countries involved.

Conclusion

Until host countries adopt human subject protections similar to those in developed countries, researchers involved in global research must actively promote the rights and safety of research participants. Identified universal requirements for ethical research—especially those related to host community relevance, benefit, and nonmaleficence—provide guidance in the determination of ethical research. Ultimately, although the design and execution of studies involving human subjects are the responsibility of all members of a research team, independent oversight remains critical to this process. Institutional review boards and community advisory boards, as they are specifically designed to protect the interests of vulnerable subjects, are important resources in the global protection of human subjects. Together, they can begin to address important ethical questions with regard to international research, such as those related to the appropriateness of placebo controls and the determination of a "fair and reasonable standard of care" for study participants.

Ultimately, it is important that research ethics not be considered as barriers to research, but an integral part of the process of planning, designing, and implementing studies involving human subjects. This is especially true in international research, where levels of trust and cooperation are influenced by complex and often contradictory cultural, political, economic, and historical factors. Given this situation, it is imperative that the design and execution of collaborative research be of the uppermost quality possible.

Case Studies[9]

Case Study 1: Responsibility to Community

The research institute has received a grant to study the effectiveness of a new vaccine developed at a large American university against a new strain of cholera found in

---

[9]Case studies were modified from existing case studies presented by the Program on Ethical Issues in International Health Research at the Harvard School of Public Health. Cases are fictional, but based on real events. Original case studies are available online at: http://www.hsph.harvard.edu/bioethics.

India and Bangladesh. Cholera (a watery diarrhea) has a mortality rate of over 30% in severe untreated cases; however, properly treated cases using oral rehydration therapy (ORT) and/or intravenous (IV) fluids effective in treating the fluid losses reduces the mortality rate to 5%. The cost of ORT is 1/50 of the IV treatment, and treatment can be carried out in simple treatment centers that are equipped only with cots, buckets, and fluid.

The vaccine will be given to children less than 5 years of age in a double-blind fashion with one group receiving the vaccine and the other a booster dose of tetanus toxoid. A government clinic services the community, a rural rice growing area 2 hours from Calcutta. The clinic is often short of medicines, equipment, and personnel. The placebo group is more likely to have cholera, and the institute feels that a treatment facility should be established in the field site to provide state-of-the-art care for all study participants with cholera and other diarrheas. The institute would provide the facility, the personnel, the equipment, and medicine free of charge to the community. Others have suggested that the government clinic be upgraded. The institute, however, would have no control over the selection of personnel or quality of care provided. The institute depends on grants and research awards to finance its activities.

At the present time, the vaccine costs $1.00 per dose and three doses are required; however, the cost could be reduced by 75% in the future. The government's annual per capita expenditure on health in this region is $5.00. Public health activists in Calcutta have raised a number of questions about the study: What is the institute's long-term commitment to providing health care to the community? How long should the institute be obligated to provide care? If the vaccine proves effective, will participants receive free doses? If so, for how long? Should all citizens of India and Bangladesh benefit from the results of the study, or will the vaccine be too costly for these countries?

Case Study 2: Informed Consent

A grant has been given by a US university to a research institute to conduct a double-blind study to evaluate the impact of periodic doses of high-dose vitamin A on the incidence of diarrhea and acute respiratory infections (ARI) in children less than 5 years of age in a community in an African country. Specifically, the study design calls for a high-dose vitamin A capsule or placebo to be administered every four months for one year to children from 6 months to 5 years. Morbidity (diarrhea and ARI) and mortality data would be measured weekly and blood samples would be drawn at 0, 6, and 12 months.

Investigators met briefly with the village chief and council and secured their approval. The next day, in accordance with the guidelines provided by the university's IRB, they began going from house to house to obtain signed informed consent from parents giving permission for their children to participate in the study. On the second day, they were summoned to the chief's house and politely informed that approval had already been given and it was unnecessary and unacceptable to seek individual signatures. When the researchers said that they were required by the grant to obtain signed informed consent forms, they were told that if they insisted on doing so they will be asked to leave the community.

How should this problem be handled by the research team? The donor? How critical is informed consent in this setting? Is informed consent culturally bound or is it a universal principal that can not be compromised?

Case Study 3: Testing a New Vaccine

A new vaccine against HIV appears promising; and the company, Highvax, now wishes to begin phase 3 trials in Bangkok, Thailand, where a cohort of intravenous drug users (IDU) with a high rate of HIV-1 has been identified. The study will be completed in 2 years. The vaccine will be provided free and the study will be carried out by the Thailand Health Institute. Highvax will cover the costs of the study, including the laboratory equipment necessary to conduct the studies. If successful, Highvax agrees to supply the vaccine free of charge to the addict population of Bangkok and at cost to the country of Thailand for 5 years. This will be a randomized double-blind prospective study with one group receiving the test vaccine and the other group receiving a placebo. All potential participants will be tested for HIV prior to being enrolled, with those identified as HIV+ referred for treatment. Study participants who convert to HIV+ during the study will be referred for standard treatment. Several boards have reviewed the study protocol and approved the study. Standard treatment in Thailand differs from standard treatment in the United States in that infections are treated but patients are not always given antiretroviral drugs, including monotherapies such as AZT or the newer HAART.

After the study has begun, an AIDS activist group condemns the study because it is not providing state-of-the-art care for individuals who convert to HIV+. The activists maintain that the reason that the study is being conducted in Thailand is because the triple therapy is not required, making it much less expensive than if the study was conducted in the United States. Highvax counters that to use the worldwide best standard of care would itself be unethical because it would be unsustainable in Thailand where physicians would be unfamiliar with the protocol and its potential side effects. Moreover, offering the best proven standard of care would be an unfair inducement to participate in the study; in essence functioning as a form of coercion to receive the new vaccine.

Is the study unethical because participants are not receiving the best care available in the world if they become HIV+? Would it be unethical to offer the worldwide best care even it was not available in Thailand (or available only to the wealthy)? Is there any compromise position that may be acceptable to both parties? Should a new vaccine be tested if it is unaffordable in the host country for wide distribution?

References

Angell, M. (1997). The ethics of clinical research in the third world. *New England Journal of Medicine*, *337*, 847–849.

Beauchamp, T. L., & Childress, J. F. (1996). *Principles of biomedical ethics*. New York: Oxford University Press.

Beecher, H. (1966). Ethics and clinical research. *New England Journal of Medicine, 274,* 1354–1360.

Benatar, S. R., & Singer, P. A. (2000). A new look at international research ethics. *BMJ, 321,* 824–826.

Caballero, B. (2002). Ethical issues for collaborative research in developing countries. *American Journal of Clinical Nutrition, 76,* 717–720.

Connor, E. M., Sperling, R. S., Gelber, R., Kiselev, P., Scott, G., O'Sullivan, M. J., et al. (1994). Reduction of maternal-infant transmission of human immunodeficiency virus type 1 with zidovudine treatment. *New England Journal of Medicine, 331,* 1173–1180.

Council for International Organizations of Medical Sciences (CIOMS). (1993). *International ethical guidelines for biomedical research involving human subjects.* Geneva, Switzerland: CIOMS.

Ehni, H. J. (2006). The definition of adequate care in externally sponsored clinical trials: The terminological controversy about the concept "standard of care." *Science and Engineering Ethics, 12,* 123–130.

Emanuel, E. J., & Miller, F. G. (2001). The ethics of placebo-controlled trials—a middle ground. *New England Journal of Medicine, 345,* 915–919.

Emanuel, E. J., Wendler, D., & Grady, C. (2000). What makes clinical research ethical? *Journal of the American Medical Association, 283,* 2701–2711.

56 Fed. Reg., Misconduct in science and engineering. 2286-90 (1991).

Glasser, S. P., Clark, P. I., Lipicky, R. J., Hubbard, J. M., & Yusuf, S. (1991). Exposing patients with chronic, stable, exertional angina to placebo periods in drug trials. *Journal of the American Medical Association, 265,* 1550–1554.

Grady, C. (2006). Ethics of international research: What does responsiveness mean? *Virtual Mentor, 8,* 235–240.

Hyder, A. A., & Dawson, L. (2005). Defining standard of care in the developing world: The intersection of international research ethics and health systems analysis. *Developing World Bioethics, 5,* 142–152.

Kahn, A., Warner, H. A., & Brown, W. A. (2000). Symptom reduction and suicide risk in patients treated with placebo in antidepressant clinical trials: An analysis of the Food and Drug Administration database. *Archives of General Psychiatry, 57,* 311–317.

Kavanaugh, A. (2005). Ethical and practical issues in conducting clinical trials in psoriasis and psoriatic arthritis. *Annals of Rheumatic Diseases, 65*(Suppl. II), ii46–ii48.

Landes, M. (2005). Can context justify an ethical double standard for clinical research in developing countries? *Global Health, 1,* 11–15.

Levine, R. J. (1988a). *Ethics and regulation of clinical research* (2nd ed.). New Haven, CT: Yale University Press.

Levine, R. J. (1988b). The "best proven therapeutic method" standard in clinical trials in technologically developing countries. *Journal of Clinical Ethics, 92,* 167–172.

Lie, R. K., Emanuel, E., Grady, C., & Wendler, D. (2004). The standard of care debate: The Declaration of Helsinki versus the international consensus opinion. *Journal of Medical Ethics, 30,* 190–193.

Lo, B., & Bayer, R. (2003). Establishing ethical trials for treatment and prevention of AIDS in developing countries. *BMJ, 327,* 337–339.

London, A. J. (2000). The ambiguity and the exigency: Clarifying "standard of care" arguments in international research. *Journal of Medical Philosophy, 25,* 379–397.

Lurie, P., & Wolfe, S. M. (1997). Unethical trials of interventions to reduce perinatal transmission of the human immunodeficiency virus in developing countries. *New England Journal of Medicine, 337,* 853–856.

National Bioethics Advisory Commission. (2001). Ethical and policy issues in international research: Clinical trials in developing countries (Vol. 1). Bethesda, MD: NBAC.

National Commission for the Protection of Human Subjects of Biomedical and Behavioral Research. (1979). *The Belmont report.* Washington, DC: US Department of Health, Education, and Welfare.

National Research Council. (2002). *Research ethics in complex humanitarian emergencies: Summary of a workshop.* Washington, DC: National Academies Press.

Pimple, K. D. (2002). Six domains of research ethics: A heuristic framework for the responsible conduct of research. *Science and Engineering Ethics, 8,* 191–205.

Pojman, J. (1995). *Ethics.* Belmont, CA: Wadsworth.

Quinn, S. C. (2004). Protecting human subjects: The role of community advisory boards. *American Journal of Public Health, 94,* 918–922.

Resnik, D. B. (1998). The ethics of HIV research in developing nations. *Bioethics, 12,* 289–306.

Salvi, V., & Damania, K. (2006). HIV, research, ethics and women. *Journal of Postgraduate Medicine, 52,* 161–162.

Shaffer, D. N., Yebei, V. N., Ballidawa, J. B., Sidle, J. E., Greene, J. Y., Meslin, E. M., et al (2006). Equitable treatment for HIV/AIDS clinical trial participants: A focus group study of patients, clinician researchers, and administrators in Western Kenya. *Journal of Medical Ethics, 32,* 55–60.

Shamoo, A. E., & Irving, D. N. (1993). Accountability in research using persons with mental illness. *Accountability in Research, 3,* 1–17.

Shamoo, A. E., & Resnik, D. B. (2003). *Responsible conduct of research.* New York: Oxford University Press.

Shapiro, H. T., & Meslin, E. M. (2001). Ethical issues in the design and conduct of clinical trials in developing countries. *New England Journal of Medicine, 345,* 139–142.

Silva, H., Sungar, E., Kleinstiver, S. J., & Rubin, R. H. (2006). Opportunities and challenges for clinical and cardiovascular research in Latin America. *American Journal of Therapeutics, 13,* 309–314.

Singer, P. (1993). *Practical ethics.* New York: Cambridge University Press.

Sperling, R. S., Shapiro, D. E., Coombs, R. W., Todd, J. A., Herman, S. A., McSherry, G. D., et al. (1996). Maternal viral load, zidovudine treatment, and the risk of transmission of human immunodeficiency virus type 1 from mother to infant. *New England Journal of Medicine, 335,* 1621–1629.

Stern, J. E., & Lomax, K. (1997). Human experimentation. In D. Elliott, & J. E. Stern (Eds.), *Research ethics: A reader.* Hanover, NH: University Press of New England.

Strauss, R., Sengupta, S., Quinn, S., Goeppinger, J., Spaulding, C., Kegeles, S. M., et al. (2001). The role of community advisory boards: Involving communities in the informed consent process. *American Journal of Public Health, 91,* 1938–1943.

Vanderpool, H. Y., (Ed.). (1996). *The ethics of research involving human subjects.* Frederick, MD: University Publishing Group.

Varmus, H., & Satcher, D. (1997) Ethical complexities of conducting research in developing countries. *New England Journal of Medicine, 337,* 1003–1005.

Weijer, C., & Emanuel, E. J. (2000). Ethics. Protecting communities in biomedical research. *Science, 289,* 1142–1144.

Wendler, D., Emanuel, E. J., Reidar, K., & Lie, M. D. (2004). The standard of care debate: Can research in developing countries be both ethical and responsive to those countries' health needs? *American Journal of Public Health, 94,* 923–928.

Werner, D. L. (1999). Imperialism, research ethics, and global health. *Journal of Medical Ethics, 25,* 62.

Woodsong, C., & Karim, Q. A. (2005). A model designed to enhance informed consent: Experiences from the HIV prevention trials network. *American Journal of Public Health, 95,* 412–419.

Appendix 6-A Selected Web-Based Resources on Research Ethics

Codes of Ethics

Nuremberg Code: www.ohsr.od.nih.gov/guidelines/nuremberg.html

Declaration of Helsinki: www.wma.net/e/policy/b3.htm

Belmont Report: www.ohsr.od.nih.gov/guidelines/belmont.html

International Ethical Guidelines for Biomedical Research Involving Human Subjects: www.fhi.org/training/fr/RETC/pdf_files/cioms.pdf

International Compilation of Human Subject Research Protections: www.hhs.gov/ohrp/international/HSPCompilation.pdf

World Health Organization Ethical Standards and Procedures for Research with Human Beings: www.who.int/ethics/research/en

Code of Federal Regulations (Title 45) for Protection of Human Subjects US Department of Health and Human Services: www.hhs.gov/ohrp/humansubjects/guidance/45cfr46.htm

Other Resources

Health Insurance Portability and Accountability Act (HIPAA): www.hhs.gov/ocr/hipaa

Bioethics resources on the Web/international ethical guidelines: www.bioethics.od.nih.gov

US Public Health Service Office of Research Integrity: www.ori.dhhs.gov

Guidelines for Good Clinical Practice (GCP) for Trials on Pharmaceutical Products: www.fda.gov/cder/guidance/959fnl.pdf

On Being a Scientist: www.newton.nap.edu/books/0309051967/html/index.html

National Institutes of Health Guidelines for the Conduct of Research Involving Human Subjects—The Gray Book: www.ohsr.od.nih.gov/guidelines/GrayBooklet82404.pdf

HRSA training module on protection of human subjects in biomedical research: www.hrsa.gov/humansubjects

American Journal of Bioethics online and other resources: www.bioethics.net

Chapter 7

Infectious Diseases from a Global Perspective

Timothy A. Akers, Barbara J. Blake, and Robert A. Hanson

Overview

The many complex issues surrounding infectious diseases include geography, environment, economics, population characteristics, transportation, and health condition, among others. During the past century, the race to combat infectious diseases has made great strides in saving millions of lives as nations become more developed through industrialization, advances in prevention and health promotion education occur, and pharmacological innovations are developed. Despite such advances, viral, bacterial, fungal, and parasitic diseases continue to cause a quarter of all deaths in the world. Moreover, this does not account for the impact of infectious diseases resulting in disabilities, devastated economies, demographic changes, and the social and physical environmental influences that can range from stigma felt by individuals living with HIV/AIDS to regions ravaged through vector control measures, such as the eradication of mosquitoes for malaria control.

As the world becomes smaller through air travel, population increases, and transnational commerce, existing and emerging infectious diseases (EID), or reemerging infectious diseases, continue to pose complex challenges and threats on systems of healthcare service delivery, regional and national policies, security, disease surveillance, and research infrastructure used for the tracking and intervention of new infectious disease cases. And, in an age of increased terrorism and zoonotic diseases—in which zoonoses account for two thirds of all infectious diseases that spread from animals to people—the need for understanding the complexities of the interdependence of nations and their health condition and systems is paramount if the spread of infectious diseases are to be prevented or controlled.

Because of the enormity of infectious diseases endemic to nations and regions and their complex etiology and pathology, this chapter is not intended to describe, characterize, and define the hundreds of viral, bacterial, fungal, or parasitic disease that coexist with humans throughout this world. Rather, for the sake of space and in the spirit of providing an overview of some of the more common infectious diseases that manifest themselves globally, this chapter will selectively describe what most domestic and international travelers encounter, and what nations routinely confront in their battle to coexist with their invisible neighbors. The first step in understanding global infectious disease is to narrow down what types of infectious diseases are the most commonly reported, encountered, or life threatening, and how one place in time can typify other areas in similar ways.

As of 2005, the World Health Organization reported that the leading causes of infectious disease deaths are HIV/AIDS, tuberculosis, malaria, pneumonia, and diarrheal diseases (World Health Organization [WHO], 2005a). Although these infectious diseases wreak havoc on nations, regions, and communities, it is best, at times, to also differentiate and distinguish between people and their environment, which takes into account a host of other devastating diseases. Moreover, it can be difficult to differentiate between people and their physical environment that may have led to the spread of an infection. But when examined systematically in the context of water, air, vector-borne transmissions, basic sanitation, and various prophylactic approaches, it becomes painfully clear how nations and people that neglect to follow or do not have the opportunity to follow basic prevention measures (fresh water, routine health education, or infrastructural resources), can lead to the spread of emerging and reemerging infectious diseases.

Historically

To paraphrase, one who forgets the past is doomed to relive it in the future. This saying is quite appropriate in the context of infectious diseases. As societies evolved from primitive hunters and gatherers towards larger civilizations, acute infectious diseases began to manifest as populations expanded outwards. When small, nomadic tribes began bartering resources between Asia and Europe, contact among these civilizations began increasing. Just within the past six centuries, the bubonic plague ("The Black Death"), which killed almost half of the European population, was carried by crusaders and merchant traders from central Asia to Western Europe. As time, travel, and migration progressed, we witnessed between the 1500s and 1600s, smallpox being carried by European migrants to the Americas, which further spread death and disease to the indigenous peoples of the New World. Although many historical examples can characterize the link between people and their environment, none is more telling then to examine how cholera spread throughout London in the 1800s. In the mid-1850s, Dr. John Snow, a physician in London, spent a great deal of time trying to convince colleagues that cholera was a waterborne disease. His assertion contradicted the current theory of the time that cholera, caused by the bacterium *Vibrio cholerae*, was transmitted through the air in the form of mists or miasmas. It was not until 1854 when he began mapping the location of all well water pumps and the location of every incidence of cholera that a pattern began to emerge. Through Dr. Snow's geospatial mapping of cholera incidences and deaths and the city's well water pumps, he was able to link the well on Broad Street, which tended to mix with the city's sewage system, to the cholera outbreak. It was through this evidence that Dr. Snow was able to persuade officials to remove the pump handle. Afterwards, cholera incidences were contained and decreased (Koch, 2005).

Another historical snapshot that links international travel and migration to infectious diseases, people, and their environment is best exemplified in the story of Mary Mallon, an Irish immigrant to the United States at the turn of the 1900s who eventually became known as "Typhoid Mary." Mary Mallon became the first healthy carrier of the typhoid bacterium *Salmonella typhi* in the United States. During this time, Mary Mallon was employed as a domestic cook where it was eventually determined that she infected over 53 people with the disease, in which three died. However, given the many years she worked as a cook in domestic settings it was never clearly determined just how many people became infected by her preparing their meals. As the typhoid bacteria were expelled through Mary Mallon's feces, it was improper hand washing that further spread the contamination through her food preparation (Turkington & Ashby, 1998).

The examples summarized reflect the nature of how global infectious diseases have spread between people and their environment. As we continue to examine the global infectious diseases most common throughout developed and developing nations, we begin seeing how the sciences of clinical and molecular epidemiology, virology, bacteriology, mycology, and public health can have global, regional, national, and local impact in the detection, prevention, or eradication of various infectious diseases.

People and Environment: Epidemiology and Regional Impact

One of the most effective methods for learning about infectious diseases from a global perspective is to examine, first and foremost, the epidemiology and ecology of the diseases that have the greatest impact on people and their physical and social environments. Changes in the ecological environment, such as agricultural development projects, reservoirs and dams, deforestation, floods, droughts, and other types of climatic changes, have resulted in the emergence or reemergence of diseases. Furthermore, changes in human demography and behavior have also influenced the epidemiological spread of cholera, malaria, typhoid, hepatitis, dengue fever, hepatitis, tuberculosis, and HIV, among others, resulting in the convergence between human and various pathogens (Armelagos, Barnes, & Lin, 1996). The following diseases described in this chapter are but a few examples of the more commonly known infectious diseases that have affected people and environments historically and to the present day.

Cholera

Although it is not easy at times to say which came first, the people or the pathogen, it is not difficult however to identify some of the possible causes of diseases. Cholera, for example, is one of the most common types of diseases that can be, for the most part, traced to people coming in contact with drinking water that has been contaminated by sewage. Common household flies have also been identified as carriers of the bacterium *Vibrio cholerae*. The effect of cholera is an acute intestinal infection caused by ingestion of contaminated food or water. Cholera is rarely transmitted by direct person-to-person contact. Cholera can spread when basic hygiene is inadequate and open-air food stands are located in potentially contaminated areas. The World Health Organization (WHO) states:

> Cholera remains a global threat and is one of the key indicators of social development. While the disease no longer poses a threat to countries with minimum standards of hygiene, it remains a challenge to countries where access to safe drinking water and adequate sanitation cannot be guaranteed. Almost every developing country faces cholera outbreaks or the threat of a cholera epidemic (WHO, 2006a).

In 2002, the WHO Global Task Force on Cholera Control was launched, and one of its priority areas clearly addresses "linking health and management of the environment in order to improve access to safe water for vulnerable populations and diminish incidence of waterborne diseases" (WHO, 2006a). This link between people and their environment is vital in helping to better understand how cholera can manifest regardless of a nation's level of development.

Dengue Fever (Arbovirus)

As the world continues to grow, urban landscapes expand, and as people continue traversing the global community, dengue fever is becoming an emerging disease with devastating impact on both the environment and the people. Case in point, while dengue fever is not new to the world stage, it is affecting over 2.5 billion people or two fifths (40%) of the world's population where the virus is transmitted. Dengue belongs to the Flaviviridae viral family and is a mosquito-borne infection that finds its home in predominantly the Southeast Asia and western Pacific nations, such as the Philippines, and in tropical and subtropical regions throughout the world. As urban areas and newly emerging urban environs continue to expand, the prevalence of dengue has now spread to more than 100 countries throughout Africa, the Americas, the Eastern Mediterranean, Southeast Asia, and the western Pacific (WHO, 2002).

The spread of dengue, while predominantly located in urban areas, is attributable to the vast amounts of still water stored throughout households and inadequate sewage disposal in densely populated regions. The need for developing better prevention and vector control measures may be linked, in part, towards developing better surveillance systems that can immediately track new cases in order to strengthen and recommend prevention strategies that impact and alter the behavior of individuals and households and community infrastructure.

Malaria *(Plasmodiums: falciparum, malariae, ovale, vivax)*

Malaria is one of the oldest known diseases and dates back before recorded history. The many different forms of malaria, noted above, are related to differing degrees of clinical disease severity, its individual reproductive life cycles, and treatment responses. Not unlike dengue, malaria is also transmitted by a mosquito bite. However, in contrast to dengue, malaria has devastated the African continent, especially the sub-Saharan region. The impact of malaria on the sub-Saharan and the eastern region specifically has also led many of those infected to become resistant to treatments, thereby resulting in patients needing combination therapies that are not as readily available and tend to be more expensive then their more abundant and inexpensive counterparts, such as chloroquine, quinine, and quinidine.

The greatest number and most vulnerable victims of malaria are children. They account for over 40% of the people that live in malaria-endemic countries throughout the world. This vector-borne disease infects between 300–500 million people annually, killing over 1 million each year, with 75% occurring in African children less than 5 years of age (WHO, n.d., "Roll back malaria").

Some of the best known prevention measures for malaria control are directed towards vaccine development, insecticides, prevention education, bed nettings, and bed nets that have been treated with insecticides. And, in a recent development, the WHO reports the establishment of new guidelines to reintroduce and support the "spraying of small amounts of DDT, or dichloro-diphenyl-trichloroethane, on walls and other surfaces inside homes in areas at highest risk of malaria" (McKay, 2006). This is an important development, apart from its many political and scientific debates, given the enormity of the problem through the world, especially in the African region. Aside from these various strategies, other challenges continue to manifest, such as drug resistance by both the vector and the parasite, which continues to be a major obstacle in the fight against malaria. However, therapies using a combination of medications have been shown to be efficacious in the treatment of malaria (Toure & Oduola, 2003; World Health Organization, n.d., "Roll back malaria").

Avian (Bird) Flu (H5N1)

As in the case of dengue and malaria, in which humans come in contact with mosquitoes, avian influenza, or commonly referred to as "bird flu," manifests its presence in birds, poultry, and some swine. The world community is seeing a new virus emerge as a front-runner to the war on infectious diseases. As humans and animals continue to mingle in close proximity to one another, viruses that were never thought to exist beyond their own animal species have started to cross the once unique barrier distinguishing animals from humans. Avian influenza is one such example. The epidemiology of the disease indicates that it is most prevalent in the Republic of Korea, Viet Nam, Japan, Thailand, Cambodia, Lao People's Democratic Republic, Indonesia, and China, with new infectious cases being reported currently.

Hong Kong, for example, on two separate occasions, experienced two major avian influenza outbreaks that jumped from chicken to humans. In 1997, 18 people became infected resulting in 3 deaths, while in 2003 there were 2 infections detected followed by 1 death. The epidemiological findings indicated that in 2003, a family traveled to the southern part of China where it is suspected that they acquired the virus (Turkington & Ashby, 1998; WHO, 2005b; WHO, 2006b). To contain the infection, Hong Kong's prevention response was to destroy millions of birds in order to limit its potential outbreak. Their approach may have served a valuable purpose and saved many lives. And when considering how to contain the spread, some theories for the prevention of avian influenza continue to recommend that uncooked infected poultry should not, nor their feces, come in contact with people or cooking surfaces. Properly prepared poultry dishes that are thoroughly cooked, following other basic sanitation (e.g., washing of hands, not sharing raw meat cooking utensils, avoiding cross-contamination) are all corrective measures to stave off further infections. The WHO recognizes that the risk for an avian pandemic is serious, and the world is ill prepared in developing responses to combat an eventual outbreak or to combat the potential human-to-human transfer.

West Nile Virus (Arbovirus)

West Nile virus belongs to the Flaviviridae viral family and is known to infect humans, birds, mosquitoes, horses, and other mammals (WHO, n.d.). In contrast to avian influenza, malaria, or dengue, West Nile does not discriminate in its choice of host. Birds of many varieties serve as its primary reservoir with mosquitoes being the transmission vector (Nash, Mostashari, Fine, Miller, O'Leary, Murray, et al., 2001). It is virulent enough to cross species, nations, and continents and has had a long history of traversing Africa, Eastern Europe, West Asia, and the Middle East. It was not until 1999 that the Western Hemisphere saw its first cases (West Nile Virus, n.d.). Since 1999, the virus, just within the North American continent, has accounted for 826 deaths and another 225,000 illnesses (Kilpatrick, Daszak, Jones, Marra, & Kramer, 2006). Not unlike some of the infectious diseases previously discussed, West Nile can also show few signs and symptoms but still spread illness and death. Depending on the variant of the virus, an infected person may be asymptomatic or have symptoms that can range from mild headaches to severe neurological affects or death. The best prevention measures are to limit exposure to mosquitoes and use various barrier protections (e.g., mosquito netting, insecticides, and mosquito repellants).

SARS (Severe Acute Respiratory Syndrome)

In February 2003, the World Health Organization identified for the 21st century its first emerging infectious disease officially named *severe acute respiratory syndrome* (SARS). SARS became recognized as a highly infectious disease that rapidly progressed across different environmental settings, from clinical to residential (Chan, Tang, & Hui, 2006). It is believed that SARS began its trek from the Guangdong Province, China, and later spread to Hong Kong, Viet Nam, Singapore, Taiwan, and eventually found its way to Canada and the United States. In midyear 2003, over 8,000 probable cases were reported in at least 26 countries, leaving in its wake over 700 deaths (Health Protection Surveillance Centre,

2005). Before it was eventually contained, SARS was characterized as a "superspreading event" because of its speed and spread internationally (WHO, 2004a). SARS is a novel coronavirus referred to as SARS-CoV which is mainly a respiratory pathogen. The reservoir for this pathogen has not been clearly identified, but it is speculated that a number of species can serve as host. SARS appears to be transmitted person-to-person through droplets expelled by way of coughing or sneezing. As an infected person touches their mouth, nose, or eyes, further spread can occur, as well by other means of contaminated surfaces (CDC, 2005a). In 2004, the WHO reported that the SARS epidemic had significant social and economic impact in highly affected areas as well as on the international travel industry. To date, it is still extraordinarily difficult to predict where it will reemerge in epidemic proportion.

Ebola (Hemorrhagic Fever)

Ebola—even the word evokes fear in scientists and healthcare workers alike—is part of the family of Filoviruses (see Figure 7-1). Currently, there is no standard treatment for the Ebola virus (CDC, 2002a). The Ebola virus kills up to 90% of the people who come in contact with the disease and presents extreme risk to healthcare workers, laboratory technicians, and scientists that come in contact with infected tissue, blood, feces, bodily fluids, infected patients, and nonhuman primates (Turkington & Ashby 1998). The origin of Ebola virus is still unknown. Its natural reservoir is yet to be determined. It has been theorized that the virus is zoonotic and has maintained its host in animals native to the African continent. Strains of the virus have been traced to the Democratic Republic of the Congo (formerly Zaire), Sudan, and the Ivory Coast (or, in French, *Côte d'Ivoire*). However, North America and Italy have also seen a unique strain of the filovirus. Within a US laboratory in Reston, Virginia, the filovirus transmitted through the air its deadly strain to

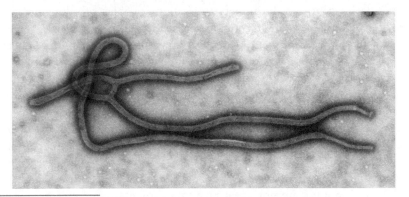

Figure 7-1 Transmission electron micrograph of the Ebola virus.

Source: CDC.

monkeys that were imported from the Philippines in 1989 (CDC, 2005b; WHO, 2004b). At the present, there is currently no standard treatment for Ebola hemorrhagic fever. Therefore, limiting exposure to vectors of transmission will serve to reduce an individual's risk of becoming infected. Although Ebola virus is extremely contagious, there still exists basic preventative practices, such as washing hands and wearing gloves and masks in an environment around infected patients or animals as well as in environments suspected of contamination.

As the environments in which people live, work, and play become more interdependent, infectious diseases, both old and emerging (or reemerging), will continue to mingle with how people coexist with their environment and those around them. Their behaviors will continue to have a significant impact in how infectious diseases are contained or spread. And, as medical, environmental, and behavioral sciences continue to advance and influence theory, practice, and policy, new levels of awareness will take center stage as expectations increase for individuals to take greater responsibility in how they, either unintentionally or intentionally, place others in danger, through such means as neglecting to practice basic sanitary hygiene, wash hands while preparing meals, or practice safer sex to avoid infecting others. Hepatitis, syphilis, tuberculosis, and HIV/AIDS are but a few examples that shift responsibility away from direct, physical environmental causation towards more individualized behavioral changes that take into account primary or secondary preventative measures which can help to effectively contain super spreading events.

Hepatitis A, B, and C

Hepatitis has many different variants, ranging from hepatitis A thru G. However, rather than focus on all variants of the hepatitis virus, we will narrow our focus to three of the more prevalent types. Viral hepatitis is a major global public health problem that has an ability to live both within and on animate and inanimate objects for long periods of time. When providing an overview of infectious disease, hepatitis A, B, and C serve as prime examples that distinguish between the behaviors people manifest and the environments they manipulate, regardless if referring to developed or developing nations. Hepatitis A (HAV) belongs to the Picornaviridae viral family and is a disease of filth. It can be characterized through the different methods in which people place others at risk for becoming carriers of infectious diseases, such as when poor sanitary conditions exist that result in the inadvertent transmitting of fecal matter to others because of the lack of basic hand washing or in unsanitary cooking areas (CDC, 2006). For example, the hepatitis A virus is spread from person to person by putting something in the mouth that has been contaminated with the stool of a person with hepatitis A. This type of transmission is called "fecal-oral." This is not uncommon at eating establishments and clinics, or amongst street vendors or household members who neglect to follow basic hygiene.

In contrasts to most other viruses, the hepatitis A virus can live for longer than a month on cooking surfaces, toys, utensils, and other surfaces where hands can become unsanitary. Hepatitis A, not unlike its other infectious disease counterparts, leaves an infected person few options because there does not exist, at present, any drug treatment. However, hepatitis A does have available a vaccine that can help prevent new infections, provided other basic hygiene is practiced that helps control its spread. Assuming a person is around someone who is infected with hepatitis A, there are certain segments of the population who are most susceptible: child care workers, sex partners of hepatitis A patients, close friends of infected school-age children, restaurant employees and patrons where someone handling food has hepatitis A, prison inmates, and unimmunized international commuters to developing countries (Turkington & Ashby, 1998).

Hepatitis B, unlike its HAV cousin that is the least dangerous and most common, is far more complex and has a longer incubation period and the acute phases are significantly more severe. The hepatitis B virus (HBV), which belongs in the Hepadnaviridae viral family, was historically or commonly referred to as "serum hepatitis" because it follows a blood-borne route. The virus is transmitted through blood, saliva that penetrates the skin (such as through a bite), semen, and vaginal fluids (Meers, Sedgwick, & Worsley, 1995). Transmission is most common among sex partners, intravenous drug users (IDU) who exchange needles, and others who share household hygiene implements that are carriers (e.g., razors, toothbrushes). Internationally, millions share a common connection in experiencing chronic HBV infection that begins with evidence of liver fibrosis and ends with liver cirrhosis, which destroys the livers ability to function. Hepatitis B is also the world's most common virus that causes liver cancer (Turkington & Ashby, 1998). Although there does exist a vaccine for HBV across all age groups, there does not exist medications available for recently acquired (acute) HBV infection for those not vaccinated (CDC, n.d.). However, for chronic hepatitis B infections in adults with evidence of active viral replication, there are a few medications that have shown promising outcomes and are considered the standard of care for the treatment of chronic HBV. To date, over 2 billion people throughout the world have been infected with the hepatitis B virus (HBV), in which more than 350 million have chronic (lifelong) infections, killing 1.2 million each year worldwide (WHO, 2000a).

As we progress down this milieu of infectious diseases, the world community is not only confronted with the more common types of HAV and HBV, but also the more mysterious type of viral hepatitis C (HCV), which belongs to the Flaviviridae viral family. The WHO reports that about 3% of the world's population, or some 180 million, are infected with HCV with an estimated 3 to 4 million persons newly infected annually. The virus is often referred to as a "viral time bomb." The virus has six known genotypes that span across all known continents. Genotype 1, which is found predominately in the United States, is the most difficult to treat with medication response rates of about 45–50%. Multiple drug regimens will be used in the near future to combat HCV, similar to those used to treat HIV. The main mode of transmission globally is primarily by direct contact with human blood products through the use of unscreened blood transfusion products and the reuse of needles and syringes that have not been adequately sterilized. Regardless of the status of a nation's level of development, the lack of standard protocols for sterilization of medical implements significantly increases the risk of HCV infections. In contrast to HBV, sexual transmission of HCV does occur, although far less frequently. Moreover, from a sociocultural perspective, behavioral practices that can infect the innocent may be due to the neglect of practitioners or artisans who fail to sterilize their tools for ear and body piercing, circumcision, and tattooing. And, in contrast to other forms of infectious diseases, HCV is not spread by sneezing, embracing or casual contact, coughing, food or water, or the sharing of eating utensils. Although no vaccine is yet developed, there are precautions that can help to reduce risk of spreading or contracting the hepatitis C virus, such as avoiding the sharing of lavatory paraphernalia (e.g., razors, toothbrushes). In addition, individuals who have multiple sex partners may place themselves or others at risk for acquiring or transmitting the virus (Meers et al., 1995; Merson, Black, & Mills, 2001; Turkington & Ashby, 1998; WHO, n.d.).

Syphilis (*Treponema pallidum*)

Syphilis is a systemic, sexually transmitted disease in which the WHO estimates that at least 12 million new cases occur worldwide annually (WHO, 2004c). Depending on the stage of the disease, syphilis can be characterized as primary, secondary, or tertiary. Syphilis is primarily transmitted through sexual contact or by means of congenital infection. Unlike some of the other infectious diseases previously discussed, primary syphilis can manifest an outward physical appearance by becoming visible as painless lesions, skin sores, and rashes. If untreated, systemic syphilis can lead to clinical signs of rash, fever, headaches and backaches, loss of appetite, among other signs. Or more severely, if left untreated and it progresses to a tertiary stage, complications can occur in the form of heart problems (aortitis), blindness (retinitis), and neurosyphilis (brain damage), which can eventually lead to central nervous system paralysis and/or insanity (Turkington & Ashby, 1998). In addition, having syphilis makes it easier for someone to contract the human immunodeficiency virus (HIV), the virus that causes acquired immunodeficiency syndrome (AIDS). Syphilis, fortunately in most cases, can be treated with penicillin; however, recent evidence of antibiotic resistance to penicillin by syphilis has decreased the effectiveness of this treatment worldwide. However, from an international perspective, there does not exist any treatment consensus because medical regimens and treatments vary by region (Long et al., 2006). Regionally, syphilis has no boundaries. Both developed and developing nations experience their own challenges around syphilis elimination and control. And, as of 1999, the largest regions throughout the world with the highest prevalence rate are Latin America, sub-Sahara Africa, and Southeast Asia (WHO, 2004d).

Tuberculosis (*Mycobacterium tuberculosis*)

Tuberculosis (TB) has often been considered a disease of poverty. The impact of TB globally has affected all borders, nations, and economic systems. TB is a respiratory disease that does not discriminate but rather spreads its acid-fast bacilli through the air by means of infected, aerosolized droplets from people who cough, sneeze, or talk with vigor.

Approximately 8 to 10 million new cases are reported globally each year (USAID, 2004; WHO, 2005b) with almost 2 billion people in the world, or one third of the world's population, infected with TB (CDC, 1999). Although TB is a preventable and curable disease, it continues to claim the lives of more than 1.7 million people annually (WHO, 2006c) and kills more people than any other infectious disease, with women having the highest TB mortality rate in the world. In 1993, the WHO declared tuberculosis a "global emergency" (WHO, 1994). As of 2004, the WHO estimates that the largest number of new TB cases occurred in Southeast Asia, thereby accounting for 33% of incident cases globally. However, notwithstanding these extraordinarily high numbers, the incidence per capita in sub-Saharan Africa is nearly twice that of Southeast Asia, resulting in nearly 400 cases per 100,000 population and almost three times higher than Southeast Asia with respect to mortality per 100,000 (WHO, 2006c).

Although strides have been made to try and stem the tide of TB globally, such as through strategies and initiatives resulting from the Global Partnership to Stop TB, the US CDC, USAID, the International Union Against Tuberculosis and Lung Disease, and the United Nations Millennium Development Goals, among other bodies (Dye, Maher, Weil, Espinal, & Raviglione, 2006), there have existed periods of resurgence, especially in the United States, which have been exacerbated by the onset of the HIV epidemic, increased TB cases attributable to foreign-born persons, and outbreaks of new infections in enclosed settings (e.g., healthcare facilities, correctional facilities, homeless shelters). The case rate among foreign-born persons currently residing in the United States, for example, is at least eight times higher than US-born persons (CDC, 2002b).

Given that TB is a preventable and curable disease, some of the more complex challenges (noting that cost and access for treatment continues to be a major factor, especially in developing nations and from a physical geography perspective), is working with patients who need directly observed therapy (DOT) to ensure they are responsible in adhering to their treatment regimen. Other major challenges confronting the global TB epidemic are directly linked to new cases of HIV/AIDS. Their infections coexist in most cases, and TB is used, at times, as a surrogate or proxy marker in helping to estimate the number of new HIV/AIDS case infections. This last section of the chapter will summarize HIV/AIDS, a disease that crosses all nations, races, ethnicities, religions, sexual orientations, ages, and economics.

Human Immunodeficiency Virus (HIV)/Acquired Immunodeficiency Syndrome (AIDS)

Globally HIV/AIDS has reached pandemic proportion. To date, the WHO estimates that over 65 million people have been infected with HIV, and AIDS has killed over 25 million people (see Figure 7-2). And, of the almost 40 million people living with HIV most are unaware that they are infected (UNAIDS, 2006). Although HIV seems to be slowing down globally, there are regions and countries throughout the world that continue to see skyrocketing HIV/AIDS case rates. A unique fact about the HIV virus is that it shares a

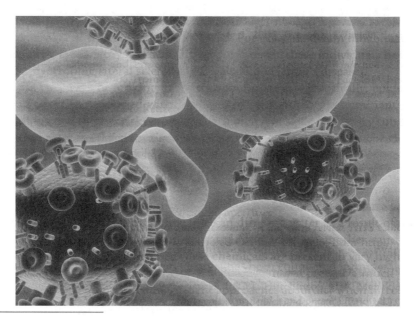

Figure 7-2   Artistic rendering of the HIV virus in the bloodstream.

Source: © Sebastian Kaulitzki/ShutterStock, Inc.

common characteristic with many other infectious diseases previous discussed—it is driven by behaviors, and it is preventable. Similar to Hepatitis B, HIV is transmitted through blood, semen, and vaginal fluids, and breast milk. The primary modes of transmission include unprotected sex and sharing of needles that contain infected blood; however, a mother can transmit it to her infant during childbirth or breast feeding.

Although significant resources are directed towards the development of treatments, such as in the case of highly active antiretroviral therapies (HAART), substantially fewer resources are set aside for HIV/AIDS prevention. In addition, as the epidemic shifts its transmission routes in other directions, as in the case of high-risk heterosexuals (as compared to sex between men and injection drug users), new prevention strategies that are evidence driven will need to take into account these varying characteristics, (UNAIDS, 2005).

Regionally and across individual nations, HIV prevention messages follow no consistency nor are they standardized where successful programs can be easily replicated. Rather, prevention intervention strategies vary across populations, interventions, communities, nations, and regions. Although these diverse characteristics are important in taking into account the subtle and unique qualities of an HIV endemic area, they also lack behavioral protocol that others can follow in similar situations. Such a protocol is not readily available to the global community around HIV/AIDS prevention. That is, the lack of evidence-driven prevention strategies further complicate the global community's ability to specifically identify which type of prevention strategy has the greatest impact (e.g., behavioral, structural,) in reducing risky behavior. For the most part, messages that emphasize "prevention works" (UNAIDS, 2005; UNAIDS, 2006) neglect, at times, to pragmatically understand that a prevention strategy's effectiveness may depend on whether an experimental or tested intervention shown to be effective in one setting, venue, or time period can be repeated successfully in another (Elford & Hart, 2003). For example, Thailand and Cambodia's highest modes of transmission have been through their sex workers, which their government's prevention strategy has been to promote condom usage by sex workers.

In Thailand, government and public health officials have successfully overcome the cultural and behavioral barriers related to the use of condoms by sex workers in the urban cities throughout the country; however, even more education and promotion is needed to reach the rural, border, and northern hill tribe populations. In Uganda, the government promoted the ABCs of HIV prevention, which meant to *Abstain, Be* faithful, use Condoms (Carey, 1999). Still, there are others that have discussed the debate as to whether an intervention works or does not (Cohen, 2003).

A need for designing an HIV/AIDS prevention intervention that meets at least minimum standards for transferability in a global community should take into account the following characteristics:

- The populations at risk
- The setting in which prevention services are being provided
- The prevention training of the provider
- The dosage and intensity of the prevention message
- The specific type of prevention intervention (e.g., one-on-one, community and street outreach, group level, intensive case management)

As alluded to previously, internationally, there still does not exist, to date, any prevention intervention classification system or taxonomy of prevention interventions that could be standardized to a population or region's unique characteristics (Akers & Hervey, 2003; Akers, Sowell, Blake, Taylor, & Bairan, 2004).

While the debate still continues about what works and what does not, the fact remains that many of the infectious diseases discussed above require, first and foremost, an individual to take responsibility in changing their individual behavior so as to protect others from harm. Such behaviors can range from sanitizing one's hands to wearing protective barriers during sexual contact. Whatever the method, it falls on the individuals to work within their environment to better combat current, emerging, or reemerging infectious diseases.

Interdisciplinary and Systemic Impact on Infectious Diseases

Thus far this chapter has set forth summary descriptions of the more common types of infectious diseases experienced globally. Their descriptive summaries serve as the foundation to more clearly understand how infectious diseases can be placed within the context of people and their environments. As described above, the transmission of certain types of infectious diseases may be attributable to environmental factors, such as if transmitted by way of vector or behavior. Whatever method of their transmission, one thing is certain: we exist in a world where new or emerging infectious diseases do not take years, decades, or centuries, but rather, hours, days, or weeks for superspreads to occur. A rapidly progressive field of study is gaining force across a wide scientific audience. The field of comparative medicine attempts to explain the obvious, symbiotic link between animal and human diseases, meaning zoonotic diseases, and the overall impact these infectious, omnipresent relationships have on our health system and the geographically unrestricted disease burden on a global scale.

During the past two decades, new infectious diseases are taking center stage, as in the case of HIV/AIDS, Ebola, and SARS. None of these diseases recognize geographical boundaries, especially with the advent of air travel. Moreover, as behaviors, technologies, sociopolitical and economic systems, and physical landscapes change, new ways of examining this complex milieu should be driven from an interdisciplinary perspective, especially in a world of emerging and reemerging infectious diseases (Becker, Hu, & Biller-Andorno, 2006; Lienhardt & Rustomjee, 2006).

As populations increase in urban areas, migration and demographic changes shift, environments become more congested, and residual waste byproducts increase—each placing humans or population centers at greater risk for becoming infected with deadly diseases—there continues to exist gaps in our knowledge in how best to integrate data systems that take into account physical environment, climate, disease, and human health (Colwell & Patz, 1998). From a physical environment perspective, how people interact with one another and their environment can serve as the driving force behind a range of infectious diseases and their impact in the spawning of new outbreaks, as in the case of road construction, wetland manipulation, deforestation, agricultural encroachment, irrigation and dam construction, and the degradation of coastal areas, among other activities (Patz et al, 2004).

These changes in the physical environment also share similar characteristics from a sociocultural perspective. That is, as political climates change globally, especially within developing nations experiencing unstable political, social, economic, and religious fragmentation, new leadership can emerge while old leaders may descend into factional, non-secular forms of retaliation. These various political changes can cloak themselves under zealous religious extremism and sectarian doctrine (Ursano, Norwood, & Fullerton, 2004). Certain infectious diseases have often been thought of as potential weapons of mass destruction, such as in the case of the Ebola virus, various forms of plague, SARS, dengue fever, and others (Fong and Alibek, 2005).

As we have seen, infectious diseases can bring about death in many forms. They may be intentional as in the case of biological terrorism; intentional as in the case of practicing unsafe sexual behaviors or neglecting to sanitize one's food preparation area; or unintentional, as in the case of vector-borne transmission. Whatever the mode of transmission or the intent, the fact remains that promulgating, controlling, preventing, or tracking infectious diseases requires an interdisciplinary and integrated system of disease tracking and data analysis.

Prevention Intervention Strategies

The need for developing prevention intervention strategies from an infectious disease perspective depend on whether the public health system has science behind the interventions it recommends. In other words, can infectious disease healthcare workers, scientists, policy makers, nongovernmental organizations, and community members speak with a level of confidence and assurance that a particular method to prevent the spread (or superspread) of an infectious disease is valid, efficacious, replicable, and most appropriate to its target population or environment? The need for answering these questions from a prevention intervention framework is essential, especially from behavioral, structural, or biomedical perspectives that blend both the art and science of the multilevel analysis of infectious diseases (Roux & Aiello, 2005). HIV/AIDS prevention intervention strategies, for example, are generally recognized as being effective. The problem however is the international community's inability to clearly and scientifically state some of the reasons why certain interventions work in some environs with various populations while others of similar characteristics do not. The best and most appropriate way in helping to determine whether various infectious disease intervention strategies work is to collect surveillance data and do research and evaluations that can help determine efficaciousness of an intervention or combination of interventions.

Surveillance, Research, and Evaluation: Three Sides of the Same Coin

A need exists for developing effective and comprehensive public health surveillance systems that can be shared or reported consistently across nations. Surveillance systems for infectious disease tracking are not generally viewed as research activities because their internal focus is on the routine collection of disease data. The CDC's definition of surveillance is "the ongoing systematic collection, analysis, and interpretation of outcome-specific data for use in the planning, implementation, and evaluation of public health practice" (Teutsch & Churchill, 2000).

The over 14 infectious diseases described in this chapter provide a snapshot of the types of scientific-based surveillance systems needed for international tracking. Although USAID, the UN, the WHO, and other international bodies that collect and disseminate infectious disease data provide surveillance, research, and evaluation services to the global community, more advanced forms of surveillance integration and data standardization is needed to significantly enhance these systems of tracking. Outcomes are more effectively determined when data are consistent, integrated, standardized, and systematically collected.

In theory, once infectious disease data are collected through surveillance systems, then patterns can be determined for more close examination through various research methodologies. Lastly, evaluation analysis can help determine whether an intervention is efficacious and achieving what it set out to accomplish, such as changing the behaviors of people and their environments. The most pressing problem, however, is that the international community of healthcare analysts needs high-quality data. But, as we often state, "As invalid as a statistic may be, it's valid if that is the only statistic available."

References

Akers, T. A., & Hervey, W. G. (2003). Why classification for HIV/AIDS prevention interventions? *Journal of the Association of Nurses in AIDS Care, 14*(4), 17–20.

Akers, T. A., Hervey, W. G., Sowell, R. L., Blake, B. J., Taylor, G. A., & Bairan A. (2004). A call for the development of a national standardized HIV/AIDS prevention intervention classification taxonomy. *International Conference on AIDS, 15*. Abstract No. ThPeC7484.

Armelagos, G. J., Barnes, K. C., & Lin, J. (1996). Disease in human evolution: The re-emergence of infectious disease in the third epidemiological transition. *Anthropology Outreach Notes*. Retrieved September 30, 2006, from http://www.nmnh.si.edu/anthro/outreach/anthnote/fall96/anthback.htm

Becker, K., Hu, Y., & Biller-Andorno, N. (2006) Infectious diseases—A global challenge. *International Journal of Medical Microbiology, 296*(4-5), 179–185.

Carey, M. P. (1999). Prevention of HIV infection through changes in sexual behavior. *American Journal of Health Promotion, 14*, 104–111.

Centers for Disease Control and Prevention. (n.d.). *Viral hepatitis B*. Retrieved November 7, 2006, from http://www.cdc.gov/ncidod/diseases/hepatitis/b/index.htm

Centers for Disease Control and Prevention. (1999). *The deadly intersection between TB and HIV*. Retrieved November 6, 2006, from http://www.cdc.gov/hiv/resources/factsheets/hivtb.htm

Centers for Disease Control and Prevention. (2002a). *Ebola hemorrhagic fever: information packet*. Retrieved September 27, 2006, from http://www.cdc.gov/ncidod/dvrd/spb/mnpages/dispages/Fact_Sheets/Ebola_Fact_Booklet.pdf

Centers for Disease Control and Prevention. (2002b). *The changing epidemiology of TB*. Retrieved November 6, 2006, from http://www.cdcnpin.org/scripts/tb/tb.asp#change

Centers for Disease Control and Prevention. (2005a). *Basic facts about SARS*. Retrieved September 27, 2006, from http://www.cdc.gov/ncidod/sars/factsheet.htm

Centers for Disease Control and Prevention. (2005b). *Questions and answers about Ebola hemorrhagic fever*. Retrieved October 21, 2006, from http://www.cdc.gov/ncidod/dvrd/spb/mnpages/dispages/ebola/qa.htm

Centers for Disease Control and Prevention. (2006). *Frequently asked questions about hepatitis A*. Retrieved September 2006, from http://www.cdc.gov/ncidod/diseases/hepatitis/a/faqa.htm

Chan, P. K. S., Tang, J. W., & Hui, D. S. C. (2006). SARS: clinical presentation, transmission, pathogenesis, and treatment options. *Clinical Science, 110*, 193–204.

Cohen, S. A. (2003). Beyond slogans: Lessons from Uganda's experience with ABC and HIV/AIDS. *The Guttmacher Report on Public Policy*, 6(5). Retrieved November 11, 2006, from http://www.guttmacher.org/pubs/tgr/06/5/gr060501.html

Colwell, R. R. & Patz, J. A. (1998). Climate, infectious disease and health: An interdisciplinary perspective. *American Academy of Microbiology*. Retrieved November 11, 2006, from http://www.asm.org/asm/files/ccpagecontent/docfilename/0000003767/climate%5b1%5d.pdf

Dye, C., Maher, D., Weil, D., Espinal, M., & Raviglione, M. (2006). Targets for global tuberculosis control. *International Journal of Tuberculosis and Lung Disease*, 10(4), 460–462.

Elford, J., & Hart, G. (2003). If HIV prevention works, why are rates of high risk sexual behaviour increasing among MSM? *AIDS Education and Prevention*, 15, 294–308.

Fong, I. W. & Alibek, K. (2005). Bioterrorism and infectious agents: a new dilemma for the 21st century (eds.). New York: Springer.

Health Protection Surveillance Centre. (2005). *Severe acute respiratory syndrome (SARS), updated guidelines for the global surveillance of SARS*. Retrieved October 21, 2006, from http://www.hpsc.ie/hpsc/A-Z/Respiratory/SARS/HealthcareProfessionals/File,1353,en.pdf

Kilpatrick, A. M., Daszak, P., Jones, M.J., Marra, P. P., & Kramer, L. D. (2006). Host heterogeneity dominates West Nile virus transmission. *Proceedings of the Royal Society*. Retrieved October 2, 2006, from http://nationalzoo.si.edu/Publications/ScientificPublications

Koch, T. (2005). *Cartographies of disease: Maps, mapping, and medicine*. Redlands, CA: ESRI Press.

Long, C. M., Klausner, J. D., Leon, S., Jones, F. R., Giron, M., Cuadros, J., et al. (2006). Syphilis treatment and HIV infection in a population-based study of persons at high risk for sexually transmitted disease/HIV infection in Lima, Peru [Electronic version]. *Sexually Transmitted Diseases*, 33(3), 151–155.

Lienhardt, C. & Rustomjee, R. (2006). Improving tuberculosis control: An interdisciplinary approach. *Lancet*, 367(9514), 949-950.

McKay, B. (2006, September 15). WHO calls for spraying controversial DDT to fight malaria. *Wall Street Journal*. Retrieved November 10, 2006, from http://online.wsj.com/public/article_print/SB115826757981263480-kG1hGbdcQnBmidFlPxJGz_hHAZs_20070915.html

Meers, P., Sedgwick, J., & Worsley, M. (1995). *The microbiology and epidemiology of infection for health science students*. London: Chapman & Hall.

Merson, M. H., Black, R. E., & Mills, A. J. (2001). *International public health: diseases, programs, systems, and policies*. Gaithersburg, MD: Aspen Publishers, Inc.

Nash, D., Mostashari, F., Fine, A., Miller, J., O'Leary, D., Murray, K, et al. (2001) The outbreak of West Nile virus infection in the New York city area in 1999 [Electronic version]. *New England Journal of Medicine*, 344(24).

Patz, J. A., Daszak, P., Tabor, G., Aguirre, A. A., Pearl, M., Epstein, J., Wolfe, N. D., Kilpatrick, A. M., Foufopoulos, J., Molyneux, D., & Bradley, D. J. (2004). Unhealthy Landscapes: Policy Recommendations on Land Use Change and Infectious Disease Emergence. *Environmental Health Perspective*, 112(10):1092-1098. Retrieved October 6, 2006, from http://www.pubmedcentral.nih.gov/articlerender.fcgi?artid=1247383

Roux, A. V. D. & Aiello, A. E. (2005). Multilevel analysis of infectious diseases. *Journal of Infectious Diseases*, 191, S25-S33.

Teutsch, S. M. & Churchill, R. E. (2000). *Principles and practices of public health surveillance* (2nd ed.). New York: Oxford.

Toure, Y. T., & Oduola, A. (2004). Malaria. *Nature*, 2, 276–277.

Turkington, C. & Ashby, B. (1998). *Encyclopedia of infectious diseases*. New York: Facts on File, Inc.

United Nations Programme on HIV/AIDS (UNAIDS). (2005). *AIDS epidemic update*. Retrieved November 11, 2006, from http://www.who.int/hiv/epi-update2005_en.pdf

United Nations Programme on HIV/AIDS (UNAIDS). (2006). *Report on the global AIDS epidemic.* Retrieved November 11, 2006, from http://www.who.int/hiv/mediacentre/news60/en/index.html

United States Agency for International Development (USAID). (2004). *Front lines: TB strikes 8 million worldwide annually.* Retrieved November 10, 2006, from http://www.usaid.gov/our_work/global_health/id/tuberculosis/news/frontlines_tbworld.html

Ursano, R.J., Norwood, A.E., & Fullerton, C.S. (2004). Bioterrorism: psychological and public health interventions (eds.). New York: Cambridge University Press.

West Nile virus. (n.d.). Retrieved October 2, 2006, from http://www.west-nile-virus-prevention.com

World Health Organization. (1994). *Framework for effective tuberculosis control: WHO Tuberculosis programme* [WHO/TB/94.179]. Retrieved November 10, 2006, from http://whqlibdoc.who.int/hq/1994/WHO_TB_94.179.pdf

World Health Organization. (2000a). *Hepatitis B.* Retrieved November 6, 2006, from http://www.who.int/mediacentre/factsheets/fs204/en

World Health Organization. (2000b). *Hepatitis C.* Retrieved November 6, 2006, from http://www.who.int/mediacentre/factsheets/fs164/en/index.html

World Health Organization. (2002). *Dengue and dengue haemorrhagic fever.* Retrieved October 1, 2006, from http://www.who.int/mediacentre/factsheets/fs117/en

World Health Organization. (2004a). *WHO SARS risk assessment and preparedness framework.* Retrieved September 28, 2006, from http://www.who.int/csr/resources/publications/CDS_CSR_ARO_2004_2.pdf

World Health Organization. (2004b). *Ebola haemorrhagic fever.* Retrieved October 21, 2006, from http://www.who.int/mediacentre/factsheets/fs103/en

World Health Organization. (2004c). *Sexually transmitted diseases diagnostics: Bulk procurement for syphilis tests.* Retrieved November 10, 2006, from http://www.who.int/tdr/publications/tdrnews/news72/syphilis_tests.htm

World Health Organization. (2004d). *Syphilis.* Retrieved November 10, 2006, from http://www.who.int/tdr/dw/pdf/dw6_2004.pdf

World Health Organization (2005a). Health and the Millennium Development Goals. Retrieved May 15, 2007, from http://www.who.int/mdg/publications/MDG_Report_08_2005.pdf

World Health Organization. (2005b). *Avian influenza.* Retrieved October 1, 2006, from http://www.who.int/topics/avian_influenza/en

World Health Organization (2005c). *WHO Report 2005: TB linked to HIV at alarming levels in Africa.* Retrieved November 5, 2006, from http://www.un.org/Pubs/chronicle/2005/issue2/0205p17.html

World Health Organization. (2006a). *The Global Task Force on Cholera Control.* Retrieved September 30, 2006, from http://www.who.int/topics/cholera/about/en

World Health Organization. (2006b). *Avian influenza ("bird flu")—Fact sheet.* Retrieved September 23, 2006, from http://www.who.int/mediacentre/factsheets/ avian_influenza/en

World Health Organization. (2006c). *Tuberculosis.* Retrieved November 10, 2006, from http://www.who.int/mediacentre/factsheets/fs104/en/index.html

World Health Organization .(n.d.). *Roll back malaria: Children and malaria.* Retrieved October 1, 2006, from http://www.rbm.who.int/cmc_upload/0/000/ 015/367/RBMInfosheet_6.htm

World Health Organization. (n.d.). *Roll back malaria: Malaria in Africa.* Retrieved October 1, 2006, from http://www.rbm.who.int/cmc_upload/0/000 /015/370/RBMInfosheet_3.htm

World Health Organization. (n.d.). *West Nile encephalitis.* Retrieved October 2, 2006, from http://www.who.int/vaccine_research/diseases/west_nile/en

Chapter 8

Global Use of Complementary and Alternative Medicine (CAM) and Treatments

Ping Hu Johnson

Introduction

In recent years, we have seen an increased interest in complementary and alternative medicine (CAM) and treatments in the United States. It appears to be a trend that more Americans are seeking holistic healthcare approaches and using natural products to treat their health problems, prevent diseases, and promote wellness. Although CAM is becoming increasingly popular, the conventional modern Western medicine remains predominant in the United States, and the majority of Americans still seek conventional medical care most of the time (Eisenberg et al., 2001). But outside of the United States, you will notice that what Americans considered CAM treatments and practices are considered traditional medicine and used by the majority of the global population (WHO, 1983). CAM treatments and practices have spread rapidly in the developed countries in the past decade (WHO, 2003).

CAM Defined: Complementary and Alternative *or* Traditional?

According to the World Health Organization (WHO, 2003) and the United States National Center for Complementary and Alternative Medicine (NCCAM, 2002), complementary and alternative medicine refers to a set of medical and healthcare systems, practices, and products that are not part of that country's own tradition and are not integrated into the dominant healthcare system. Based on this definition, it is clear that the conventional modern Western medicine and treatments are considered traditional in the United States. Also, what Americans considered to be CAM treatments and practices have mostly originated from other countries and cultures and are considered traditional medicine in those countries. WHO (2003) defines traditional medicine as the "knowledge, skills, and practices based on the theories, beliefs, and experiences indigenous to different cultures, whether explicable or not, used in the maintenance of health as well as in the prevention, diagnosis, improvement, or treatment of physical and mental illness."

Although the terms *alternative medicine* and *complementary medicine* have been used interchangeably in the literature, they mean different things. According to NCCAM (2002), alternative medicine is used *in place of* conventional medicine, and complementary medicine is used *together with* conventional medicine. Using a special diet to treat cancer instead of surgery, radiation, or chemotherapy recommended by a conventional doctor is an example of alternative medicine, while using aromatherapy to help lesson a patient's discomfort following surgery is an example of complementary medicine.

In this chapter, we use the term *CAM* to refer to the medical and healthcare systems, practices, and products that are not part of and not integrated into the dominant conventional modern Western healthcare system in the United States and industrialized countries. The term *traditional medicine* is used to denote the indigenous medical and healthcare systems, practices, and products that are used in countries other than the developed countries.

CAM in the United States

Unlike many countries in the world, allopathic medicine is the main stream medical practice and considered traditional medicine in the United States even though there had been Native American folk medical practices long before the early settlers migrated to the United States. In the past decade, we have seen an upsurge of CAM use in the United States due to the increasing demand from US consumers. Several surveys of nationally representative samples of US adults revealed that the proportion of adults who used at least one CAM therapy in a given year increased from 33.8% in 1990 to 42.1% in 1997 (Eisenberg et al., 1998) and 62% in 2002 (Barnes, Powell-Griner, McFann, & Nahin, 2004). CAM usage is even more prevalent among patients. It has been reported that up to 85% of patients used at least one form of CAM (Morris, Johnson, Homer, & Walts, 2000). According to the 2005 Institute of Medicine's *Report on Complementary and Alternative Medicine in the United States*, the use of CAM will continue to be present in the United States (Institute of Medicine, 2005).

Along with the increased popularity of CAM therapies come increased expenditures on CAM therapies and services. Based on the most current estimates, the total amount of money Americans spent on visits to CAM practitioners is estimated to have increased by approximately 45% between 1990 ($22.6 billion) and 1997 ($32.7 billion), and the amount of total out-of-pocket expense on CAM therapies and services was approximately $34.4 billion in 1997, which is comparable to the projected 1997 out-of pocket expenditures for *all* physician services (Eisenberg et al., 1998). Although those numbers are almost 10 years old, if we look at the significant increase in the number of people using CAM since 1997, it is reasonable to believe that the current expenditures on CAM have continued to expand.

With the increasing popularity and use of CAM, it is crucial that we understand the nature and extent of CAM use. Studies conducted in the past decade have identified the following people are more likely to use CAM:

- Women (Eisenberg et al., 1998; Barnes, et al., 2004)

- People with higher household income, almost certainly attributable to the reality that most CAM therapies are not covered by health insurance policies and require cash payments at the time of service (Eisenberg et al., 1998; Oldendick et al., 2000; Palinkas & Kabongo, 2000)

- Older adults (Barnes et al., 2004; Oldendick et al., 2000)

- Ethnic minorities (Barnes et al., 2004) and low-income individuals CAM (Barnett, Cotroneo, Purnell, Martin, Mackenzie, & Fishman, 2004; Dessio, Wade, Chao, Kronenberg, Cushman, & Kalmuss,, 2004)

- People with lower emotional role functioning and perceived general health (Palinkas & Kabongo, 2000)

- People who had been hospitalized in the last year, indicating that health status is a significant predictor of CAM utilization (Barnes et al., 2004)

- People with a holistic orientation to health and having had a transformational experience that changed their world view (Astin, 1998)

- People with certain health problems such as anxiety, back problems, headaches, chronic pain, and urinary tract problems (Astin, 1998)

The most common reasons that people were most likely to use CAM include the following:

- They believe CAM therapies integrated with conventional therapies would yield better results (54.9%).

- They thought trying CAM therapies would be interesting (50.1%).

- They were recommended by a medical professional (26%).

- They felt allopathic therapies were not effective (28%).

- They felt CAM therapies would be more cost-effective (13%) (Barnes et al., 2004).

- They believe CAM therapies can boost the immune system, treat cancer, and help them live longer (Astin, 1998).

Results from those studies indicate that the increasing prevalence of CAM use in the United States cannot be attributed to the perceived dissatisfaction with conventional medical care or caregivers or a societal rejection of allopathic medical care (Eisenberg et al., 2001). Such trends may indicate that more Americans have taken personal responsibility for their health and appreciate the choices they have between conventional and CAM care.

A recent survey of US adults demonstrates that when megavitamin therapy and prayer are included, 62.1% of US adults reported having used at least one CAM therapy in the past 12 months (Barnes et al., 2004). The frequencies of CAM use for each of the five domains are as follows, in order of prevalence:

- Mind-body therapies, including prayer—52.6%
- Any CAM therapies, excluding megavitamin therapy and prayer—35.1%
- Biologically based therapies, including megavitamin therapy—21.9%,
- Biologically based therapies, excluding megavitamin therapy—20.6%
- Mind-body therapies, excluding prayer—16.9%
- Manipulative and body-based therapies—10.9%
- Alternative medical systems—2.7%
- Energy therapies—0.5%

Among the specific CAM therapies used, the 10 most commonly used CAM therapies in a 12-month period are listed below (Barnes et al., 2004):

- Prayer specifically for one's own health (43% of US adults)
- Prayer by others for one's own health (24.4%)
- Nonvitamin, nonmineral, natural products (18.9%)
- Deep breathing exercises (11.6%)
- Participating in prayer group for one's own health (9.6%)
- Meditation (7.6%)
- Chiropractic care (7.5%)
- Yoga (5.1%)
- Massage (5.0%)
- Diet-based therapies (3.5%), and others

Although a large proportion of the US adult population use at least one of the CAM therapies, only 28–37% communicated the use to their doctors (Eisenberg et al., 2001). The most common reason for nondisclosure of CAM use was that patients believed "it was not important for their doctor to know," followed by "the doctor never asked," "it was not the doctor's business," and "the doctor would not understand." These views reveal a trend in the society of increased individual autonomy and personal responsibility for one's own health. In addition, among the US adults who reported seeing both a conventional doctor and a CAM provider in a given year, the majority (70%) saw a conventional doctor before or concurrent with their visits to a CAM provider, and 15% saw a CAM provider before seeing a conventional medical care provider. This presents an excellent opportunity for the conventional medical care providers to advise patients on the use or avoidance of certain CAM therapies. This also presents a challenge that conventional healthcare providers need to understand what the common CAM therapies are and whether they are safe or effective.

CAM in the World

Global Use of CAM

Throughout history, different cultures in different parts of the world have developed and used various types of traditional medicine or CAM. Countries in Africa, Asia, and Latin America have used traditional medicine for hundreds and thousands of years to meet their primary healthcare needs. In African countries, as much as 80% of the population uses traditional medicine for primary health care. In recent years, many forms of traditional medicine have been adapted by more and more developed countries and are considered complementary or alternative medicine (CAM) depending on how the traditional medicine is used (WHO, 2003).

In the last decade, we have seen a global increase in the use of traditional medicine (TM) and complementary and alternative medicines (CAM) in both developed and developing countries. Many types of traditional, complementary, and alternative medicines are playing a more and more important role in health care and healthcare reform worldwide (WHO, 2005). Several countries (China, the Democratic People's Republic of Korea, the Republic of Korea, and Vietnam) have fully integrated traditional medicine into their healthcare systems (WHO, 2003). Several other countries such as the United States are collecting standardized evidence on CAM therapies and encourage the integration of CAM into their mainstream medical care system. However, many countries have yet to collect and integrate standardized evidence on this type of health care.

The following facts will provide you with a better view of CAM's increased use and popularity:

- In China, traditional herbal preparations account for 30–50% of the total medicinal consumption.

- In Ghana, Mali, Nigeria, and Zambia, the first line of treatment for 60% of children with high fever resulting from malaria is the use of herbal medicines at home.

- WHO estimates that in several African countries traditional birth attendants assist in the majority of births.

- In Europe, North America, and other developed regions, over 50% of the population have used complementary or alternative medicine at least once.

- In San Francisco, London, and South Africa, 75% of people living with HIV/AIDS use TM/CAM.

- In Canada, 70% of the population has used complementary medicine at least once.

- In Germany, 90% of the population has used a natural remedy at some point in their life. Between 1995 and 2000, the number of doctors who had undergone special training in natural remedy medicine had almost doubled to 10,800.

- In the United Kingdom, annual expenditure on alternative medicine is $230 million.

- The global market for herbal medicines currently stands at over $60 billion annually and is growing steadily.

Source: WHO, (2005).

- About 80% of the world population uses traditional systems of medicines for primary health care and plants from the dominant component over other natural resources (Mukherjee & Wahile, 2006).

- There are more than 800 Chinese medicine pharmaceutical factories with an annual production of over 400,000 tons in more than 5000 drug varieties (Johnson & Johnson, 2002).

- In the United States, the proportion of adults who used some form of CAM therapy nearly doubled between 1990 (33.8%) (Eisenberg et al., 1998) and 2002 (62%) (Barnes et al., 2004).

- The US public spent between $36 billion and $47 billion on CAM therapies in 1997. Of this amount, between $12.2 billion and $19.6 billion was paid out of pocket (Center for Medicare and Medicaid Services, 1997).

- In Singapore, over 80% of the population has used some form of CAM in their lifetime (Koh, Ng, & Teo, 2004).

- In Brazil, up to 89% of the cancer patients used CAM (Samano et al., 2005).

Based on the above facts, it is clear that TM has maintained its popularity in developing countries and is used more frequently in developed countries. One reason for such a global expansion of TM and CAM use in industrialized world is their holistic approach to health and life, their belief in equilibrium between the mind, body and environment, their emphasis on health rather than on disease, and their treatment focus on the overall condition of the individual patient, rather than on the ailment or disease (WHO, 2005).

Major Forms of CAM

In response to the increasing demand for CAM, the U.S. Congress passed legislation to establish an office within the National Institutes of Health (NIH), the Office of Alternative Medicine (OAM), to investigate and evaluate potentially beneficial unconventional medical practices in 1992 (NIH, 2006a). This office was elevated to a center within NIH in 1999, known as the National Center of Complementary and Alternative Medicine (NCCAM) with the specific intent of exploring complementary and alternative healing practices in the context of rigorous science, to train CAM researchers, and to inform the public and health professionals about the results of CAM research studies (NIH, 2006a).

NCCAM classifies CAM into five major domains: alternative medical systems, biologically based therapies, manipulative and body-based methods, mind–body interventions, and energy therapies. Therapies in each of the five domains were developed over different time periods and have been used to deal with different health problems. Their therapeutic effects, efficacy, and side effects have been studied to different extents. Some CAM therapies are backed by scientific evidence of their safety and effectiveness, but most need to be examined for their safety, effectiveness, and efficacy (NCCAM, 2002).

Alternative Medical Systems

Alternative medical systems have complete systems of theory and practice and often evolved prior to and independently of the conventional biomedical approach used in the United States (NCCAM, 2002). They can be categorized into systems developed in oriental, Western, and other cultures. Systems developed in oriental cultures include traditional Chinese medicine and Ayurveda (traditional Indian medicine). Systems developed in Western cultures include homeopathic medicine and naturopathic medicine. Systems developed in other cultures include Native American, aboriginal, Middle Eastern, Tibetan, and South American medicine (Donatelle & Davis, 2005). This section will briefly introduce the more commonly practiced alternative medical systems.

Ayurvedic Medicine

Ayurvedic medicine (or Ayurveda) originated in India and has been practiced primarily in the Indian subcontinent for over 5000 years (Mukherjee & Wahile, 2006). Ayurveda medicine literally means "the science of life" with *ayur* meaning "life" and *veda* connoting "science" (White, 2000). This medicine is based on the Hindu belief that everyone is born in a state of balance within themselves and in relation to the universe (interconnectedness). You will experience good health if you have an effective and wholesome relationship with your immediate universe, and disease occurs when you are out of harmony with the universe. Ayurveda also believes in the body's constitution. "Constitution" is thought to be a unique combination of physical and psychological features and the way in which the body functions. Its characteristics are determined by three *doshas* (*vata*, *pitta*, and *kapha*). (For more information on the three doshas, read "What is Ayurvedic Medicine" by NCCAM at http://www.nccam.nih.gov). Each *dosha* is associated with a certain body type, a certain personality type, and a greater chance of certain types of illnesses. Therefore, the imbalance of *doshas*, the state of physical body, and mental or lifestyle factors increases a person's chances of developing certain types of diseases (NCCAM, 2005a).

To determine what is wrong with the person, an Ayurvedic practitioner seeks to identify the primary *dosha* and the balance of *doshas* by asking the person about his or her diet, behavior, lifestyle practices, and the reasons for the most recent health problem and symptoms the patient had; observing the person's teeth, tongue, eyes, skin, and overall appearance; checking the person's bodily sounds, urine, and stool; and feeling the person's pulse. The practitioner may prescribe diagnostic treatment to restore the balance of one particular *dosha*. Because of the emphasis on removing the cause of the disease, Ayurvedic doctors prescribe many changes in diet and lifestyle of the patient. After these changes have been made, the doctor will then prescribe a combination of therapies that may include herbs, metals, massage, yoga, breathing exercises, and meditation to balance the body, mind, and spirit (NCCAM, 2005a).

In India, Ayurvedic doctors are trained in a formal academic setting with 4 1/2 years of course work, a 1-year internship in Ayurveda, and advanced postgraduate training. Ayurvedic practitioners in the United States have various types of training. Some study Ayurveda after they are trained in Western medical or nursing schools. Others may have training in naturopathy either before or after their Ayurvedic training. Still others receive training in India. Students who complete their Ayurvedic training in India receive either a bachelor's or doctoral degree and may go to the United States or other countries to practice. Some practitioners are trained in a particular aspect of Ayurvedic practice, such as massage or meditation.

It is important to know that Ayurvedic medications have the potential to be toxic because of the high level of heavy metals (lead, mercury, and arsenic) used in Ayurvedic preparations (Saper et al., 2004; van Schalkwyk, Davidson, Palmer, & Hope, 2006). There is the potential for interactions between Ayurvedic treatments and other medicines. Tell your healthcare provider if you are using Ayurveda therapy and any associated dietary supplements or medications. If you are going to use Ayurvedic remedies, do so under the guidance of an experienced Ayurvedic practitioner. In the United States, there is no national standard for certifying Ayurvedic practitioners at the present time although some Ayurvedic professional organizations are working together to develop licensing requirements (NCCAM, 2005a). Consumers interested in Ayurveda should be aware that many persons claiming to practice Ayurvedic medicine have had little formal training in Ayurveda (White, 2000). For example, Ayurvedic services offered at spas and salons may not be provided by well-trained Ayurvedic practitioners. If you are interested in Ayurvedic treatment, you need to ask about the practitioner's training and experience and inform your healthcare provider about these Ayurvedic medications to ensure there is no conflict with medications or treatment prescribed by your conventional healthcare provider.

Homeopathic Medicine

Homeopathic medicine, also known as homeopathy, originated in Germany during the late 1700s by a physician, chemist, and linguist, Samuel Hahnemann. It was introduced to the United States in 1825 by a Boston-born doctor, Hans Burch Gram. Homeopathy holds the "similia principle" or "like cures like," "potentialization," and a concept that treatment should be selected based on a total picture of the patient including the patient's physical symptoms, emotions, mental state, lifestyle, nutrition, and other aspects (Ballard, 2000; Merrell & Shalts, 2002; Tedesco & Cicchetti, 2001).

The principle of "like cures like" considers that the symptoms are part of the body's attempt to heal itself and an appropriately selected homeopathic remedy will support this self-healing process (Scheiman-Burkhardt, 2001). The symptoms caused by a large dose of a substance can be alleviated by the extremely diluted small amount of the same substance. The concept of "potentialization" holds that systematically diluting a substance, with vigorous shaking at each step of dilution, makes the remedy more effective by extracting the vital essence of the substance. Homeopathy believes that even when the substance is diluted to the point where no single molecule exists in the remedy, the remedy may still be effective because the substance's molecules have exerted their effects on the surrounding water molecules (NCCAM, 2003a).

To determine the selection of homeopathic remedies, a homeopathic provider conducts an in-depth assessment of the patient during the patient's first visit. Based on how the patient responds to the remedy or remedies, the practitioner determines whether to prescribe any additional treatment.

In the United States, training in homeopathy is offered through diploma programs, certificate programs, short courses, and correspondence courses. Medical education in naturopathy includes homeopathic training. Most homeopathy in the United States is practiced along with another health practice for which the practitioner is licensed, such as conventional medicine, naturopathy, chiropractic, dentistry, acupuncture, or veterinary medicine when homeopathy is used to treat animals. In Europe, training in homeopathy is usually pursued as a primary professional degree completed after 3 to 6 years of formal training or as a postgraduate training for doctors.

Homeopathic remedies do not have to undergo any testing or review by the Food and Drug Administration (FDA) so some researchers question their effectiveness. Because they are extremely diluted solutions of natural substances that come from plants, mineral, or animals, and are given under the supervision of trained professionals, homeopathic remedies are considered safe and unlikely to cause severe adverse reactions (Dantas & Rampes, 2000). Although homeopathic remedies are not known to interfere with conventional drugs, you should discuss with your healthcare provider that you are considering using them. As with taking any medications, if you are taking a homeopathic remedy, you should contact your healthcare provider if your symptoms have not improved in 5 days and keep remedies out of reach for children. If you are a pregnant woman or nursing a baby, you should consult a healthcare provider before using any homeopathic remedies.

Naturopathic Medicine

Naturopathic medicine, or naturopathy, is an eclectic system of health care originating in Europe. Although many of its principles have been used in various healing traditions such as Chinese, Ayurvedic, Native American, and Hippocratic medicine for thousands of years, the term *naturopathy* was coined by a German-born doctor, John Scheel, in 1895 and was popularized by Dr. Benedict Lust, a hydrotherapist from Germany who in 1905 founded the American School of Naturopathy in New York. Because of the influence of various traditional healing principles, naturopathy has elements of complementary and conventional medicine to support and enhance self-healing processes and works with natural healing forces within the body.

The term *naturopathy* literally means "nature disease." Naturopaths seek to treat disease by stimulating an individual's innate healing capacities through the use of organic, nontoxic therapies such as fresh air, pure water, bright sunlight, natural food, proper sleep, water therapies, homeopathic remedies, herbs, acupuncture, spinal and soft-tissue manipulation, hydrotherapy, lifestyle counseling, and psychotherapy to heal ailments of body and mind (White, 2000). Naturopaths strive to treat the underlying cause of the condition and see illness as an opportunity to educate and empower patients to develop healthy lifestyles and to take responsibility for their lives.

Today, naturopathic medicine is practiced throughout Europe, Australia, New Zealand, Canada, and the United States. Naturopathic physicians are trained in the art and science of natural health care at accredited naturopathic medical schools. There are five major naturopathic schools in the United States and Canada that award naturopathic doctor (ND) degrees to students who have completed a 4-year graduate program that focuses on holistic principles, natural therapies, and an orientation to patients as partners in their own healing.

Traditional Chinese Medicine

Traditional Chinese medicine (TCM) has gained worldwide popularity. It seems to be foreign and mysterious to many in the Western world and yet, many Westerners are using it. TCM is a complete medical system that has diagnosed, treated, and prevented illness for over 2500 years. Inscriptions on bones and tortoise shells indicate treatments for health problems from 1500–1000 BC. The earliest TCM books date back to 221 BC (Johnson & Johnson, 2002). Korea, Japan, and Vietnam have developed their own unique versions of traditional medicine based on practices originated from China.

TCM is based on the ancient Chinese philosophical theory of *yin* and *yang*. In the TCM view, all of creation is born from the marriage of the two polar principles in the body, *yin* and *yang*, two opposing forces. The forces stand for earth and heaven, winter and summer, night and day, inner and outer, cold and hot, wet and dry, body and mind. Human beings, like everything else in the universe, have two opposite aspects, *yin* and *yang*, that are interrelated and interdependent (White, 2000). Interactions of *yin* and *yang* regulate the flow of *qi* (or vital energy) throughout the body. *Qi* is believed to regulate a person's mental, physical, spiritual, and emotional balance. If *yin* and *yang* become imbalanced, the flow of *qi* is disrupted and disease occurs (NCCAM, 2002).

TCM diagnosis involves taking a history; inspecting facial complexion, body build, posture, and motion; examination of the tongue and coating; listening to the sound of voice, respiration, and cough; smelling the odor of the patient; interrogating; and palpating the pulses. The TCM interrogation includes the "ten askings": One asks of chill and fever, two of perspiration, three asks of head and trunk, four of stool and urine, five of food intake and six of chest. Deafness and thirst are seven and eight, nine asks of past history and ten of causes. Experienced TCM practitioners can make a diagnosis based solely on the examination of the tongue and palpation of the pulse (Johnson & Johnson, 2002).

Based on the philosophy of TCM, the purpose of treatment is to restore *yin* and *yang* harmony. The TCM doctor uses acupuncture, *tui na* (Chinese massage, a more powerful and stronger form of massage than those practiced in the United States), herbal therapy, moxibustion (applying cones of herbal substances to the skin and igniting them to make smoke, or igniting a prepared strip of herbs to cause smoke and holding the smoking strip of herbs close to certain parts of the body), cupping (a small cup attached to the skin of the patient creating a vacuum after the heated air inside the cup cools), energetic exercises (e.g., *tai chi, qi gong*), and diet (adjusting the food based on its *yin* and *yang* properties) to recover and sustain health (Johnson & Johnson, 2002).

Traditionally, TCM practitioners are trained within the family. Typically, the father would train the son to be a TCM practitioner who would carry on and extend the rich firsthand experiences in TCM diagnosis and practices. Many such experiences were to be kept secret and within the family. Since 1949, the Chinese government has encouraged many of such family-trained TCM practitioners to share their secrete experiences. Many of them have been employed as clinical faculty members in various TCM colleges passing on their rich experiences in TCM. A modern TCM doctor typically receives 5 years of academic training in one of the TCM colleges in China or several Western countries. After 4 years of course work in basic science and TCM subjects, the TCM student completes a 1-year internship in a TCM hospital or a TCM department in a major comprehensive teaching hospital. Students who complete the formal academic training in TCM receive a bachelor's or doctoral degree. After they graduate from a TCM college, the TCM doctors can be employed by TCM hospitals or TCM departments in any comprehensive teaching hospitals where they receive advanced clinical training. Many TCM colleges in China also offer postgraduate training in TCM. It is rare to have a private TCM practice in China nowadays unless the TCM practitioner is trained by his father.

TCM is generally safe if it is used under the supervision of a well-trained and experienced TCM practitioner. It is important that you tell your healthcare provider if you are using any TCM treatment as some herbal preparations may interact with other medications you are taking.

Mind–Body Medicine

Mind–body interventions focus on the interactions among the brain, mind, body, and behavior as well as the powerful ways in which emotional, mental, social, spiritual, and behavioral factors directly affect health. The importance of mind in the development and treatment of diseases has been reflected in the diagnostic and healing approaches employed in traditional Chinese medicine and Ayurveda for thousands of years. The development of science and advancement of technology and medicine in the Western world starting in the 1500s and 1600s led to a separation of the physical body from the mind, the spiritual, and emotional aspects of the human being. In the 1920s, Walter Cannon revealed the direct relationship between stress and neuroendocrine responses in animals. Later in the 1950s, Hans Selye further identified the harmful effects of stress and distress on the human body. During World War II, physician Henry Beecher discovered that much of the pain suffered by the wounded soldiers could be relieved by saline injections. His later research indicated that as much as 35% of a therapeutic response to any medical treatment could be the result of a patient's belief, or the "placebo effect" (NCCAM, 2005b).

Currently, mind–body therapies represent a major part of the overall use of CAM by the public. In 2002, prayer for health reasons was used by 55% of the US adult population, and relaxation techniques (meditation, progressive relaxation, deep breathing exercises, yoga, etc.), guided imagery, biofeedback, and hypnosis, taken together, were used by approximately 40% of the population (Barnes et al., 2004).

Mind–body medicine employs many different techniques to enhance the mind's capacity to affect bodily function and symptoms. These techniques include patient support groups, cognitive-behavioral therapy, meditation, relaxation, hypnosis, *tai chi*, *qi gong*, prayer, mental healing, art, music, and dance. Some of them have become mainstream therapies, such as biofeedback, patient support groups, and cognitive-behavior techniques. Others are still considered as complementary and alternative (NCCAM, 2002).

Biologically Based Therapies

Biologically based therapies include natural and biologically based practices, interventions, and products such as herbs, whole diets, functional foods, animal-derived extracts, vitamins, minerals, fatty acids, amino acids, proteins, prebiotics and probiotics, and other dietary supplements.

Before manufactured drugs came into widespread use, herbal medicines had played an important role in human health. Reviewing the history of the development of medicines, we see that many herbal medicines were originally derived from foods, and many manufactured drugs were developed from medicinal plants. A single medicinal plant may be defined as a food, a functional food, a dietary supplement, or an herbal medicine in different countries, depending on the regulations applied to foods and medicines in each country. The influence of culture and history on the use of herbal medicines differs from country to country and region to region, and they still have a major impact on the use of herbal medicines in modern societies (WHO, 2005).

In the past two decades, we have seen a considerable increase in the interest in and use of dietary supplements. National surveys revealed that 40 to 46% of Americans reported taking at least one vitamin or mineral supplement at some time in a given month (Ervin, Wright, & Kennedy-Stephenson, 1999; Radimer, Bindewald, Hughes, Ervin, Swanson, & Picciano, 2004; Slesinski, Subar, & Kahle, 1995; Subar & Block, 1990). It is estimated that the sales of overall dietary supplements increased to $20.3 billion in 2005, of which nearly one fifth came from sales of herbs or botanical supplements in the United States (US Nutrition Industry, 2005).

Unlike dietary supplements, functional foods may claim specific health benefits because they may contain biologically active components such as polyphenols, phytoestrogens, fish oils, lycopene, and carotenoids that may provide health benefits beyond basic nutrition (NCCAM, 2004a; FDA, 2003). Examples of functional foods include tomatoes, kale, broccoli, blueberries, red grapes, green tea, soy, nuts, chocolate, and cranberries. Some manufacturers are creating "functional foods" by adding an ingredient to a certain food in order to enhance market appeal. Such food includes orange juice fortified with calcium, cancer-protective ketchup with lycopene, memory-boosting candy with ginkgo, relaxation-enhancing corn chips with kava-kava, and cholesterol-lowering margarines with plant stanol (Hoeger & Hoeger, 2006). In the last decade, we have seen a significant increase in the functional food market. Sales of functional foods increased from $11.3 billion in 1995 to about $16.2 billion in 1999 (NCCAM, 2004a).

Although whole diet therapy has been accepted for some health conditions, many unproven diets, especially for the treatment of obesity, have become very popular in recent years because of the increased prevalence of obesity among Americans. Popular diets have included the Atkins, macrobiotic, Pritikin, Ornish, Zone, South Beach, and others.

A major part of biologically based practices (i.e., herbal products), must be taken seriously. According to a recent national survey, one in four US adults used at least one non-vitamin, nonmineral, natural product in a given year for health reasons. Among those natural products, echinacea was used by 40.3% of the US adult population, followed by ginseng (24.1%), ginkgo biloba (21.1%), glucosamine with or without chondroitin (14.9%), St. John's wort (12%), fish oils/omega fatty acids (11.7%), and others (Barnes et al., 2004). Because of their widespread use, often for centuries, and because the products are "natural," many people assume dietary supplements are harmless. Unfortunately, this is not the case. Some herbal products have been proven to be harmful. For example, the herb "ma huang" (ephedra) is used in traditional Chinese medicine to treat respiratory congestion. In the United States, the herb was marketed as a dietary aid that led to at least a dozen deaths, heart attacks, and strokes. On April 12, 2004, the FDA banned the sale of dietary supplements that contain ephedra after it determined that ephedra posed an unreasonable risk to those who used it (FDA, 2004). Another example is that dietary supplements containing kava have been associated with liver-related injuries—including hepatitis, cirrhosis, and liver failure (FDA, 2002).

It is important to know that many plants are poisonous, some are toxic if ingested in large doses, others are dangerous when used with prescription or over-the-counter (OTC) drugs, and still others decrease the effect of the prescription or OTC drugs. One good example is the popular herbal remedy, St John's wort. It has been found to have significant negative drug interaction with Indinavir, a protease inhibitor used to treat HIV infection, and may potentially interact with prescription drugs used to treat conditions such as heart disease, depression, seizures, and certain cancers. It may also potentially interact with prescription drugs used to prevent conditions such as transplant rejection or pregnancy (oral contraceptives) (FDA, 2000). For warnings and safety information of dietary supplements, you can go to the FDA Warnings and Safety Information Web site at http://www.cfsan.fda.gov/~dms/ds-warn.html.

Manipulative and Body-Based Methods

Manipulative and body-based methods are based on manipulation and/or movement of one or more parts of the body. They include a heterogeneous group of CAM interventions and therapies such as chiropractic and osteopathic manipulation, massage therapy, *tui na*, reflexology, Rolfing, Bowen technique, Trager bodywork, Alexander technique, Feldenkrais method, and a host of others (NCCAM, 2004b). A recent survey of the US population suggests that 1 in 5 US adults received chiropractic manipulation in a given year, while nearly 1 in 10 received some form of massage therapy (Barnes et al., 2004). Among the domain of manipulative and body-based practices, chiropractic and message therapy are the most popular in the United States. For example, in 1997, US adults made an estimated 191,886 thousand visits to chiropractors and 113,723 thousand visits to massage therapists. Visits to chiropractors and massage therapists combined represented 50% of all visits to CAM practitioners. The remaining manipulative and body-based practices are sparser and are collectively used by less than 7% of the adult population (Eisenberg et al., 1998).

Manipulative and body-based therapies focus mainly on the structures and systems of the body, including the bones and joints, the soft tissues, and the circulatory and lymphatic systems. Some practices were derived from traditional medical systems, such as those from China, India, or Egypt, while others were developed within the last 150 years, such as chiropractic and osteopathic manipulation. Although many providers have formal training in the anatomy and physiology of humans, there is considerable variation in the training and the approaches of these providers both across and within therapies. For example, osteopathic and chiropractic practitioners, who primarily use manipulations that involve rapid movements, may have a very different treatment approach from massage therapists whose techniques involve slower applications of force. Despite this heterogeneity, manipulative and body-based practices share some common characteristics, such as the principles that the human body is self-regulating, has the ability to heal itself, and has body parts that are interdependent. Practitioners in all these therapies also tend to tailor their treatments to the specific needs of each patient (NCCAM, 2004b).

Chiropractic Medicine

Chiropractic medicine is a form of spinal manipulation, which is one of the oldest healing practices. Spinal manipulation was described by Hippocrates in ancient Greece. In 1895, Daniel David Palmer founded the modern profession of chiropractics in Davenport, Iowa. Based on his observations, he developed a chiropractic theory that believes the nervous system is the most important determinant of health and that most diseases are caused by spinal subluxations that respond to spinal manipulation (Ernst, Pittler, Stevinson, White, & Eisenberg,. 2001). Therefore, manipulations or adjustment of the spine is the core procedure used by chiropractic doctors who are also called chiropractors or chiropractic physicians. Manipulation is the passive joint movement beyond the normal range of motion, and chiropractic medicine prefers the term *adjustment* (NCCAM, 2003b).

Chiropractic training is a 4-year academic program consisting of both classroom and clinical instruction. At least 3 years of preparatory college work are required for admission to chiropractic schools. Students who graduate receive the Doctor of Chiropractic (DC) and are eligible to take the state licensure board examinations in order to practice. Some schools also offer postgraduate courses, including 2- to 3-year residency programs in specialized fields (NCCAM, 2003b).

In addition to manipulation, most chiropractors use other treatments such as mobilization, massage, and nonmanual therapies. Examples of nonmanual chiropractic treatments include:

- Heat and ice
- Ultrasound
- Electrical stimulation
- Rehabilitative exercise
- Magnetic therapy
- Mobilization, a technique in which a joint is passively moved within its normal range of motion
- Counseling (about diet, weight loss, and other lifestyle factors)
- Dietary supplements
- Homeopathy
- Acupuncture

Massage

Massage therapies manipulate muscle and connective tissue to enhance the function of those tissues and promote relaxation and well-being (NCCAM, 2002). Massage was first practiced thousands of years ago in ancient Greece, ancient Rome, Japan, China, Egypt, and the Indian subcontinent. In the United States, massage therapy first became popular and was promoted for a variety of health purposes starting in the mid-1800s, and interest in massage has increased since the 1970s (NCCAM, 2006a).

The term *massage therapy* covers a group of over 80 types of massage therapy practices and techniques. In all of them, therapists press, rub, and otherwise manipulate the muscles and other soft tissues of the body, often varying pressure and movement. They most often use their hands and fingers, but may use their forearms, elbows, or feet. Typically, the intent is to relax the soft tissues, increase delivery of blood and oxygen to the massaged areas, warm them, and decrease pain. Based on firsthand experience of receiving Chinese massage, a massage therapist trained in the United States indicated that massage therapies practiced in the United States today are much milder in their forces and different as compared to those practiced in traditional Chinese medicine.

To learn massage, most therapists attend a school or training program and a much smaller number receive training from an experienced practitioner. After they complete 500 hours of training, they can be certified to be massage therapists (NCCAM, 2006a).

> **BOX 8-1 Things You Should Know When Considering Massage Therapy**
>
> If you have one or more of the following conditions, do not use massage therapy:
>
> - Deep vein thrombosis (a blood clot in a deep vein, usually in the legs)
> - A bleeding disorder or taking blood-thinning drugs such as warfarin (Coumadin)
> - Damaged blood vessels
> - Weakened bones from osteoporosis, a recent fracture, or cancer
> - A fever
> - Any of the following in an area that would be massaged:
>   - An open or healing wound
>   - A tumor
>   - Damaged nerves
>   - An infection or acute inflammation
>   - Inflammation from radiation treatment

Massage therapy appears to have few serious risks if appropriate cautions are followed. A very small number of serious injuries have been reported, and they appear to have occurred mostly because cautions were not followed or a massage was given by a person who was not properly trained (NCAAM, 2006a). (See Box 8-1.)

If you have one or more of the following conditions, be sure to consult your healthcare provider before having massage:

- Pregnancy
- Cancer
- Fragile skin, as from diabetes or a healing scar
- Heart problems
- Dermatomyositis, a disease of the connective tissue
- A history of physical abuse

Side effects of massage therapy may include:

- Temporary pain or discomfort
- Bruising
- Swelling
- A sensitivity or allergy to massage oils

Energy Medicine

Energy medicine focuses on energy fields. They are of two types of energy fields: veritable and putative. The veritable energies employ mechanical vibrations (such as sound) and electromagnetic forces, including visible light, magnetism, monochromatic radiation (such as laser beams), and rays from other parts of the electromagnetic spectrum. They involve the use of specific, measurable wavelengths and frequencies to treat patients. For example, different degrees of heat produced by various heat lamps have been used in treating many disorders in China.

In contrast, putative energy fields (also called biofields) are believed to surround and penetrate the human body, but whose existence has yet to be measured. Therapies involving putative energy fields are based on the belief that human beings are permeated with a subtle form of energy, called *vital energy*. Energy medicine therapists assert that they can work with this subtle energy, see it with their bare eyes, and use it to cause changes in the physical body and influence health (NCCAM, 2005c).

Energy medicine practitioners believe that illness is caused by disturbances of the biofields. For instance, ancient Asian practitioners believed that the flow and balance of life energies are necessary for maintaining health and described tools to restore them over 2000 years ago. Many therapies in traditional Chinese medicine, such as herbal medicine, acupuncture, acupressure, moxibustion, and cupping, are believed to act by correcting imbalances in the internal biofield and by restoring the flow of *qi* through meridians to reinstate health. Some therapists are believed to emit or transmit the vital energy (external *qi*) to a recipient to restore health (Chen & Turner, 2004).

Examples of practices involving putative energy fields include Reiki and Johrei of Japanese origin and *qi gong* of Chinese origin. Each practice deals with the "healing touch" in which the therapist is purported to identify imbalances and correct a client's energy by passing his or her hands over the patient, and intercessory prayer in which a person intercedes through prayer on behalf of another. These approaches are among the most controversial of CAM therapies because neither the external energy fields nor their therapeutic effects have been confirmed by any biophysical means (NCCAM, 2005c). Yet, energy medicine is gaining popularity in the American marketplace and has become a subject of investigations at some academic medical centers. A recent national survey revealed that about 1% of the US adult population had used Reiki, 0.5% had used *qi gong*, and 4.6% had used some kind of healing ritual (Barnes et al., 2004).

Qi Gong

Qi gong is one type of energy therapy that supposedly can restore health. It has been practiced widely in China for over 2000 years. One study examined over 2000 records in *qi gong* therapy and found that *qi gong* has health benefits for conditions ranging from high blood pressure to asthma (Sancier & Holman, 2004). Several small randomized clinical trials have revealed the therapeutic effects of *qi gong* in improving psychological measures (Hui,

Wan, Chan, & Yung, 2006), reducing pain and long-term anxiety (Wu et al., 1999), heroin detoxification (Li, Chen, & Mo, 2002), and improving heart-rate variability (Lee, Kim, & Lee, 2005). However, no large clinical trials have been conducted.

Reiki

Reiki is an energy medicine practice that originated in Japan. Reiki means *universal life energy* in Japanese. Reiki believes that the patient's spirit and physical body are healed when spiritual energy is channeled through a Reiki practitioner. It is not fully known whether Reiki influences health and how it might do so. The National Center for Complementary and Alternative Medicine (NCCAM) is sponsoring studies to find out more about Reiki's effects, how it works, and diseases and conditions for which it may be most helpful (NCCAM, 2006b).

Therapeutic Touch

Therapeutic touch, another form of energy therapy, is derived from the laying on of hands. It is founded on several ancient healing practices. Since its introduction in 1972 by Dr. Dolores Krieger, RN, and Dora Kunz (The Nurse Healers, 2006), the use of therapeutic touch has increased significantly. A 1997 national survey found that about 4% of US adults used therapeutic touch in a given year and that nearly 40 million visits were made to therapeutic touch practitioners, ranking it fifth among the 16 CAM therapies assessed (Eisenberg et al., 1998).

It is believed that each person has a unique energy field (sometimes visible as an aura) that is simultaneously inside and surrounding the person's physical body. Therapeutic touch believes that for an individual to be healthy, the person's energy field must be flowing freely or balanced. A blockage or blockages in a person's energy field will prevent the free flow of energy, causing illness. Therapeutic touch is used to balance or retain the free flow of life energy in an individual and, therefore, restore good health (Brewer, 2006).

Therapeutic touch is a deliberately directed process during which a therapeutic touch practitioner moves his or her hands approximately 4 inches above the patient's body to detect the energy imbalance and repair any "holes" where the energy escapes from the body. During the process of restoring the energy balance, the practitioner assists the healing process.

To date, there has been little rigorous scientific research in this area although many small studies have suggested its effectiveness in a wide variety of conditions, including wound healing, osteoarthritis, migraine headaches, and anxiety in burn patients (NCCAM, 2005c). A meta-analysis of 11 controlled therapeutic touch studies found that 8 controlled studies had positive outcomes, and 3 showed no effect (Winstead-Fry & Kijekm, 1999). Another meta-analysis of research-based literature on therapeutic touch published in a 10-year period found that although therapeutic touch appears to have a positive, medium effect on physiological and psychological variables, no substantive claims can be made because of the limited published studies and problems with research methods that could seriously bias the reported results (Peters, 1999).

A recent review of 30 studies on therapeutic touch could not reveal any generalizable results (Wardell & Weymouth, 2004).

Due to the lack of well-designed research on the effects of therapeutic touch, we cannot determine efficacy of this therapy until sufficient scientific evidence becomes available. However, the therapist's individual attention and the passing of his or her hands over the patient's body may lead the patient to feel a sense of well-being (Brewer, 2006).

Research and Technology

Scientific evidence from randomized clinical trials is strong for many uses of acupuncture, some herbal medicines, and for some of the manipulative therapies (such as chiropractic and massage therapy) (WHO, 2003). There is an insufficient amount of valid and reliable randomized controlled data to demonstrate the mechanisms, efficacy, and applicability of most CAM approaches. In addition, many studies in CAM are flawed by insufficient statistical power, poor controls, inconsistent treatment, or lack of comparisons (Nahin & Straus, 2001).

Nevertheless, there exist significant challenges in research methods for CAM. The current model of research evaluation of CAM is based on that of Western medicine, (i.e., quantitative research methods) that cannot quantify the impact of profound traditional philosophy, culture, and religion. In this regard, qualitative research may be more appropriate. In the Western world, many researchers question the efficacy of many CAM therapies because "science has not provided sufficient evidence." However, it you take a look at the history, you will see that several traditional healing systems (e.g., traditional Chinese medicine and Ayurveda) have been practiced and used in treating diseases and promoting health for thousands of years. The long history of field-tested human experiments, long-term observations, and clinical trials has proved the value of those ancient healing systems.

It is possible that the currently available science and technology are unable to measure the effects of many CAM therapies, or it is possible we do not have the appropriate research methodologies available. As new knowledge is discovered and technologies are developed, it is possible that we will be able to detect the effects of many CAM therapies, especially those that have been practiced for thousands of years. The historical process of discovering the mind–body connection best illustrates this possibility. For example, the connection between the mind and body was first believed to be in existence in ancient times. Early technological advances (e.g., microscopy, the stethoscope, the blood pressure cuff, and refined surgical techniques) separated the mind from the physical body. The discovery of bacteria and antibiotics further dispelled the notion of belief influencing health. Later science discovered the link between the mind and the body. Nowadays, with functional magnetic resonance imaging (fMRI) and other modern technologies, we are able to confirm the connection between mind and body.

The US government has placed significant emphasis on CAM research. Research grants awarded by the National Center for Complementary and Alternative Medicine (NCCAM) more than doubled between 1999 and 2002 (see Figure 8-1) (NCCAM, 2003c).

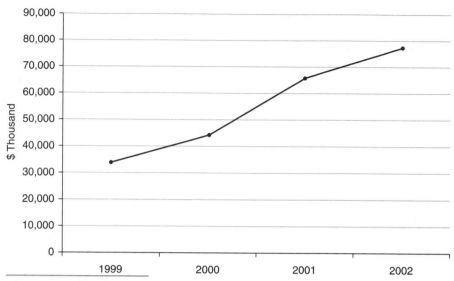

Figure 8-1 Total grants awarded by NCCAM: 1999–2002.

In recent years, NCCAM has supported studies in various therapies in each of the five major domains to different extents. It regularly examines and redefines its research priorities to fill gaps in the research, capitalize on emerging opportunities, and leverage resources. Currently, it has the following research areas of special interest:

- Anxiety and depression—Basic and preclinical research on CAM approaches
- Cardiovascular diseases—Preclinical and early phase clinical studies of CAM approaches to secondary prevention and management of hypertension, atherosclerosis, and congestive heart failure
- Ethnomedicine—Identification, description, and study of potentially valuable, vanishing traditional, or indigenous healthcare practices in geographic areas where there is little preservation
- Immune modulation or enhancement—Basic and preclinical studies of CAM approaches that may enhance or inhibit immune responses, including inflammation
- Inflammatory bowel disease and irritable bowel syndrome—CAM approaches to these conditions
- Insomnia—CAM approaches to primary and secondary insomnia
- Liver—CAM approaches to liver diseases
- Obesity and metabolic syndrome—CAM modalities, particularly mind–body treatments, as adjuvant therapies, especially with respect to the metabolic syndrome and type 2 diabetes

- Respiratory diseases—CAM approaches to prevention and treatment of infectious respiratory diseases

In addition to above areas, NCCAM continues to accept applications in areas not listed and encourages all investigators to discuss potential applications with relevant program officers (NCCAM, 2006c). With the support from the US government and many professional organizations along with the commitment and contributions from the scientists, we have made significant progress in CAM research in the last decade.

Biomedical science and technology have advanced CAM treatment and research significantly. For example, standardizing the "dose" of acupuncture through the use of an electrical apparatus to simulate the acupuncture needles makes quantitative research on acupuncture possible. Cells isolated and cultured in the laboratory have been used to study the effect of *qi* in TCM. Biomedical laboratory techniques have been used to assess the benefits of music (Chikahisa et al., 2006) and humor (Christie & Moore, 2005). Biopharmacology has contributed to the research on the effects of various herbal therapies on cancer (Richardson, 2001). Functional magnetic resonance imaging (fMRI) has been used to study the effects of acupuncture on the human brain among normal persons (Li et al., 2006) and among stroke patients (Li, Jack, & Yang, 2006), as well as to measure the effects of electroacupuncture versus manual acupuncture on the human brain (Napadow, Makris, Liu, Kettner, Kwong, & Hui, 2005).

In addition, information technology has been used to support collaborative research, monitor clinical trials, and to provide educational information to medical students, fellows, faculty, and community-based care providers who work with people and CAM (Monkman, 2001; Whelan & Dvorkin, 2003). The Internet has been used by NCCAM to disseminate authoritative information to the public and professionals (NCCAM, 2006c).

With the advancement of biomedical science, computer technology, and human genome, we can expect to see more applications of science and technology in CAM treatment and research. It is hoped that one day we will be able to provide scientific evidence that demonstrates the effects of the ancient traditional medicines.

Legal and Ethical Issues

Many countries face major challenges in the development and implementation of regulation for traditional, complementary, alternative, and herbal medicines. These challenges are related to the regulatory status, assessment of safety and efficacy, quality control, safety monitoring, and lack of knowledge about traditional, complementary, alternative, and herbal medicines by national drug regulatory authorities. In a recent WHO global survey on the national policies of traditional medicine and regulations of herbal medicines (WHO, 2005), it was found that only slightly over one third of responding WHO member countries reported having laws or regulations on traditional medicine or complementary alternative medicine (38% or 54 of 141 countries) and almost two thirds of responding member states (65% or 92 of 141) have laws or regulations on herbal medicines.

Although the United States and a few other countries did not participate in the WHO global survey on the national policy on traditional medicine and regulations of herbal medicines (WHO, 2005), the United States does not have a regulatory process to ensure the safety and efficacy of various CAM therapies at this time except for homeopathic remedies and dietary supplements. In 1938, the US Congress passed a law allowing homeopathic remedies to be regulated by the FDA in the same manner as nonprescription, over-the-counter (OTC) drugs. This means that people can purchase homeopathic remedies in any drug store without a prescription from a doctor. In addition, homeopathic remedies do not need to follow the US FDA's requirement for conventional prescription drugs and other OTC drugs. Specifically, FDA requires that all conventional prescription drugs must go through thorough testing and systematic review for their safety and effectiveness before they can be approved as prescription drugs. Only those prescription drugs that have been marketed as prescription medications for at least three years, have a relatively high use, and have not had any alarming adverse drug reactions and increased side effects during the time they were available as prescription drugs can be switched from prescription to OTC status. However, the FDA does require homeopathic remedies to meet certain legal standards for strength, quality, purity, and packaging (Junod, 2000).

The FDA regulates dietary supplements under a different set of regulations from those concerning conventional prescription and OTC drugs. Under the Dietary Supplement Health and Education Act of 1994 (DSHEA), dietary supplements are products (other than tobacco) intended to supplement the diet—they are not drugs. The dietary supplement manufacturer is responsible for ensuring that a dietary supplement is safe and the product label information is truthful and not misleading before it is marketed. The FDA is responsible for taking action against any unsafe dietary supplement products after they reach the market. Manufacturers of dietary supplements do not need to register their products with the FDA nor get FDA approval before producing or selling dietary supplements. This is different from other domestic and foreign facilities that manufacture, process, pack, or hold food for human or animal consumption in the United States that are required to register their facility with the FDA (2006).

In addition, a large proportion of patients who use CAM therapies do not inform their conventional doctors of their use. This combined with the possibility of adverse reactions with prescription drugs is placing the lives of many Americans in danger. Ethically, consumers have the right to use CAM therapies as a matter of autonomy, but they also have the duty not to harm themselves. Ethically, manufacturers must ensure their products are not harmful and have the claimed effect(s), but there are no laws or regulations that require manufacturers to prove that their products work as stated. When dealing with health and illness, ineffective products, although the products themselves are not harmful, may mask the signs and symptoms for accurate diagnosis, delay appropriate treatment, and jeopardize patients' lives. This, in effect, not only causes physical and emotional harm to patients, but costs the patients and the society money and resources.

To ensure patients' safety, CAM therapies must be evaluated with regard to safety and efficacy. The Federal Drug Administration has the ethical responsibility to take the lead

Box 8-2   Are You Considering Using CAM?

- Take charge of your health by being an informed consumer. Find out what scientific studies have been done on the safety and effectiveness of the CAM treatment in which you are interested.

- Decisions about medical care and treatment should be made in consultation with a healthcare provider and based on the condition and needs of each person. Discuss information on CAM with your healthcare provider before making any decisions about treatment or care.

- If you use any CAM therapy, inform your primary healthcare provider. This is for your safety and so your healthcare provider can develop a comprehensive treatment plan.

- If you use a CAM therapy provided by a practitioner, such as acupuncture, choose the practitioner with care. Check with your insurer to see if the services will be covered.

Source: NCCAM, 2006d.

Box 8-3   Key Issues to Consider When Selecting a CAM Practitioner

Selecting a healthcare practitioner is an important decision and can be the key to ensuring that you are receiving the best health care. The following key points are provided by the National Center for Complementary and Alternative Medicine (NCCAM) to assist you making a decision about selecting a CAM provider.

- If you are seeking a CAM practitioner, speak with your primary healthcare provider(s) or someone you believe to be knowledgeable about CAM regarding the therapy in which you are interested. Ask if they have a recommendation for the type of CAM practitioner you are seeking.

- Make a list of CAM practitioners and gather information about each before making your first visit. Ask basic questions about their credentials and practice. Where did they receive their training? What licenses or certifications do they have? How much will the treatment cost?

- Check with your insurer to see if the cost of therapy will be covered.

- After you select a practitioner, make a list of questions to ask at your first visit. You may want to bring a friend or family member who can help you ask questions and note answers.

- Come to the first visit prepared to answer questions about your health history, including injuries, surgeries, and major illnesses, as well as prescription medicines, vitamins, and other supplements you may take.

- Assess your first visit and decide if the practitioner is right for you. Did you feel comfortable with the practitioner? Could the practitioner answer your questions? Did the practitioner respond to you in a way that satisfied you? Does the treatment plan seem reasonable and acceptable to you?

Source: NCCAM, 2007b.

in this area. To protect the common good, there is a need to know not only what CAM can do for us, but what it can do *to* us. In addition, the US government has the ethical responsibility to develop specific regulations that require manufacturers of CAM devices, remedies, and dietary supplements to follow the requirement for devices and prescription drugs used in conventional medicine. Unless a device or remedy is proven to be safe and effective, no products should be allowed in the market. This may take a long time. Currently, there is intense debate in the US Congress regarding the 1994 DSHEA. Before such regulations are developed, approved, and implemented, we need to educate the consumers on how to select qualified CAM practitioners and therapies and how to evaluate

---

BOX 8-4   Important Questions to Ask the Practitioner You Select

- Ask what training or other qualifications the practitioner has. Ask about his or her education, additional training, licenses, and certifications. If you contacted a professional organization, see if the practitioner's qualifications meet the standards for training and licensing for that profession.

- Ask if it is possible to have a brief consultation in person or by phone with the practitioner. This will give you a chance to speak with the practitioner directly. The consultation may or may not involve a charge.

- Ask if there are diseases or health conditions in which the practitioner specializes and how frequently he or she treats patients with problems similar to yours.

- Ask if the practitioner believes the therapy can effectively address your complaint and if there is any scientific research supporting the treatment's use for your condition.

- Ask how many patients the practitioner typically sees in a day, and how much time he or she spends with each patient.

- Ask whether there is a brochure or Web site to tell you more about the practice.

- Ask about charges and payment options. How much do treatments cost? If you have insurance, does the practitioner accept your insurance or participate in your insurer's network? Even with insurance, you may be responsible for a percentage of the cost.

- Ask about the hours appointments are offered. How long is the wait for an appointment? Consider whether this will be convenient for your schedule.

- Ask about office location. If you are concerned, ask about public transportation and parking. If you need a building with an elevator or a wheelchair ramp, ask about them.

- Ask what will be involved in the first visit or assessment.

- Observe how comfortable you feel during these first interactions.

- Once you have gathered the information, assess the answers and determine which practitioner was best able to respond to your questions and may best suit your needs.

Source: NCCAM, 2007b.

CAM information from the Internet and other sources. The following bulleted points provide useful information offered by the National Center for Complementary and Alternative Medicine (NCCAM).

Box 8-5   10 Things to Know About Evaluating Medical Resources on the Web

The number of Web sites offering health-related resources grows every day. Many sites provide valuable information, while others may have information that is unreliable or misleading. This short guide contains important questions you should consider as you look for health information online. Answering these questions when you visit a new site will help you evaluate the information you find.

1. **Who runs this site?**
   Any good health-related Web site should make it easy for you to learn who is responsible for the site and its information. The National Center for Complementary and Alternative Medicine (NCCAM) Web site is clearly marked on every major page of the site, along with a link to the NCCAM homepage.

2. **Who pays for the site?**
   It costs money to run a Web site. The source of a Web site's funding should be clearly stated or readily apparent. For example, Web addresses ending in *.gov* denote a federal government-sponsored site. You should know how the site pays for its existence. Does it sell advertising? Is it sponsored by a drug company? The source of funding can affect what content is presented, how the content is presented, and what the site owners want to accomplish on the site.

3. **What is the purpose of the site?**
   This question is related to who runs and pays for the site. An "About This Site" link appears on many sites; if it's there, use it. The purpose of the site should be clearly stated and should help you evaluate the trustworthiness of the information.

4. **Where does the information come from?**
   Many health and medical sites post information collected from other Web sites or sources. If the person or organization in charge of the site did not create the information, the original source should be clearly labeled.

5. **What is the basis of the information?**
   In addition to identifying who wrote the material you are reading, the site should describe the evidence that the material is based on. Medical facts and figures should have references (such as to articles in medical journals). Also, opinions or advice should be clearly set apart from information that is "evidence-based" (that is, based on research results).

6. **How is the information selected?**
   Is there an editorial board? Do people with excellent professional and scientific qualifications review the material before it is posted?

(continues)

Box 8-5   10 Things to Know About Evaluating Medical Resources on the Web *(continued)*

7. **How current is the information?**

Web sites should be reviewed and updated on a regular basis. It is particularly important that medical information be current. The most recent update or review date should be clearly posted. Even if the information has not changed, you want to know whether the site owners have reviewed it recently to ensure that it is still valid.

8. **How does the site choose links to other sites?**

Web sites usually have a policy about how they establish links to other sites. Some medical sites take a conservative approach and don't link to any other sites. Some link to any site that asks, or pays, for a link. Others only link to sites that have met certain criteria.

9. **What information about you does the site collect, and why?**

Web sites routinely track the paths visitors take through their sites to determine what pages are being used. However, many health Web sites ask for you to subscribe or become a member. In some cases, this may be so that they can collect a user fee or select information for you that is relevant to your concerns. In all cases, this will give the site personal information about you. Any credible health site asking for this kind of information should tell you exactly what they will and will not do with it. Many commercial sites sell aggregate (collected) data about their users to other companies—information such as what percentage of their users are women with breast cancer, for example. In some cases they may collect and reuse information that is personally identifiable, such as your zip code, gender, and birth date. Be certain that you read and understand any privacy policy or similar language on the site, and don't sign up for anything that you are not sure you fully understand.

10. **How does the site manage interactions with visitors?**

There should always be a way for you to contact the site owner if you run across problems or have questions or feedback. If the site hosts chat rooms or other online discussion areas, it should tell visitors what the terms of using this service are. Is it moderated? If so, by whom, and why? It is always a good idea to spend time reading the discussion without joining in, so that you feel comfortable with the environment before becoming a participant.

Source: NCCAM, 2006e.

Ethical Issues Surrounding CAM Treatment and Research

The current clinical trials of acupuncture have examined its efficacy by administering a fixed course of treatment sessions based on biomedical diagnosis. This standardized approach conflicts with the traditional means of delivering holistic TCM treatments that are customized to the individual's level of strength or weakness of *yin* and *yang* (Hammerschlag, 1998). Similar ethical challenge exists in evaluating the effects of

Ayurvedic therapies that are determined based on the individual's constitution (Chopra & Doiphode, 2002). Homeopathic remedies are also highly individualized (White, 2000). Because many traditional medicines are deeply rooted in cultural traditions and religion, the interactions between the practitioner and the patient and the influence of the family, religion, and personal belief systems are important factors in the success of those traditional therapies. When patients are taken out of their traditional, social, and cultural context and placed in a scientifically controlled treatment environment, the question becomes, "Are we serving the best interest of our patients?"

With the current scientific research methods available, researchers continue to debate which research mythologies are most appropriate when conducting clinical trials of acupuncture (Hammerschlag, 1998). Some researchers argue against the use of placebo and sham controls (patients in control group receive no treatment or fake treatment), while others favor wait lists (patients receive the treatment once the study is completed) and standard care (patients receive routine care) designs. The former group believes withholding treatment to be inappropriate, and the latter group considers testing a treatment prior to demonstrating its efficacy against a placebo is just as inappropriate.

From these examples, we can see that there are many legal and ethical challenges in CAM treatment and research. It is hoped we will be able to meet these challenges as we learn more about CAM and develop more appropriate research methods.

Influences of Politics, Economics, Culture, and Religion

Politics—The Role of Government

Government has always played a major and an important role in CAM treatments and research. For example, the Indian government has begun systematic research of Ayurvedic practices since 1969. In China, TCM has gone through several waves of challenges and history. Between 1911 and 1949, the Chinese government embraced Western medicine with a goal to modernize the Chinese medical care system. This led TCM to go underground and nearly wiped out TCM. Since 1949, the new Chinese government has promoted the integration of Western and Chinese medicine, established major colleges of TCM, reprinted many older TCM works, and worked with WHO and other interested organizations and countries to promote TCM globally. In the last three decades, we have seen international training centers established in Beijing, Shanghai, Guangzhou, Nanjing, and Xiamen to train TCM personnel from all over the world, multiple TCM colleges established in many Western countries, and many cooperative research projects conducted between China and developed countries (Johnson & Johnson, 2002).

The influence of politics and government is significant in the United States. One politician, Senator Tom Harkin, played a key role in the establishment of the Office of Alternative Medicine (OAM) within the National Institutes of Health (NIH) in 1990 and the National Center for Complementary and Alternative Medicine (NCCAM) in 1999. Since the establishment of OAM and NCCAM, government funding for NCCAM has

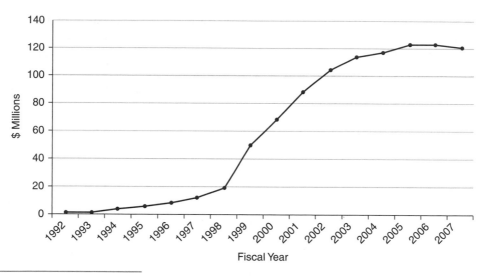

Figure 8-2 NCCAM funding appropriations history.

increased from $2 million in 1990 to $121 million in 2007 (Figure 8-2.). The support by the US government has allowed NCCAM to explore CAM practices in the context of rigorous science, train CAM researchers, and disseminate authoritative information to the public and professionals (NCCAM, 2007a; NIH, 2006b).

Worldwide, however, two thirds of the countries that participated in a WHO survey on national policy on traditional medicine and regulations of herbal medicines do not have such a national policy (68% or 96 of 141). Based on the definition provided by WHO (2005), a national policy on traditional medicine or CAM may include a definition of traditional medicine/CAM, provision for the creation of laws and regulations, consideration of intellectual property issues, and strategies for achieving the objectives of the policy. For those countries that do have such a national policy, most of them established it recently. Less than one third of the participating countries (28% or 40 of 141) reported having issued a national program on traditional medicine/CAM, slightly over half of the countries (53% or 75 of 141) reported having a national office in charge of traditional medicine/CAM, and 58 countries (41%) indicated having at least one national institute on traditional medicine, CAM, or herbal medicines (WHO, 2005). The United States did not participate in this survey.

The limited scientific evidence regarding the safety and efficacy of traditional medicine/CAM and the widespread use of traditional medicine/CAM worldwide makes it important for governments to do the following:

- Formulate national policy and regulation for the proper use of traditional medicine/CAM and its integration into national healthcare systems in line with the provisions of the WHO strategies on traditional medicines.

- Establish regulatory mechanisms to control the safety and quality of products and of traditional medicine/CAM practice.

- Create awareness about safe and effective traditional medicine/CAM therapies among the public and consumers.

- Cultivate and conserve medicinal plants to ensure their sustainable use.

Source: WHO, 2003.

Economics

The widespread use of traditional medicine and CAM in developing countries partially reflects the impact of the country's economy. Because traditional medicines and herbal medicine are cheaper and more accessible than Western medicine, many developing countries, especially those in Africa, Asia, and Latin America, use traditional medicine to help meet some of their primary healthcare needs of their citizens. It is estimated that up to 80% of the African population uses traditional medicine for primary health care (WHO, 2003). The poorer economic conditions in developing countries have limited access to modern Western medicine that is characterized by expensive consultations provided by doctors who are expensively trained, expensive procedures, expensive laboratory equipment, and expensive pharmaceuticals. One of the WHO's priorities is to promote safe and effective traditional medicine/CAM therapies to increase access to health care in developing countries (WHO, 2003).

In contrast, the economical conditions in developed countries have actually promoted the use of CAM. In developed countries, most CAM therapies are not covered by health insurance plans. Because of the better economies in the developed countries, people are better off and are financially able to pay out-of-pocket for various CAM services and treatments (Eisenberg et al., 1998; Oldendick et al., 2000; Palinkas & Kabongo, 2000).

Culture and Religion

The development of traditional medicines has been influenced by the different religious, cultural, and historic conditions in which they were first developed (WHO, 2005). For example, traditional Chinese medical care and practice are strongly influenced by Chinese tradition and religion including Confucian principles, Taoism, the theory of *yin* and *yang*, and Buddhism (Chen, 2001; Zhang & Cheng, 2000). The ideas from Hinduism, one of the world's oldest and largest religions, as well as ancient Persian thoughts about health and healing, formed the principles of Ayurveda. Mexican-American folk medicine, *Curanderismo*, mainly draws from the combination of Mayan and Aztec teachings and the Mexican heritage of Spanish Catholicism (Krippner, 1995).

Religious and cultural beliefs also influence the practice and use of traditional medical healings. Mexican-American healers often attribute an illness to an agent whose existence must be taken on faith because it cannot be detected with medical instruments. For instance, Mexican-American healers use prayers and songs to treat an illness caused by an inappropriate salute to an owl. This illness is characterized by heart palpitations, anxiety, sweating, and shaking. It is believed that this disease can lead to suicide if left untreated. Many Native American healings are considered spiritual in nature, and rituals and magic such as medicine wheels and sand paintings are used to treat such supernatural disorders. The Native American's imitative magic treatment is based on the belief that what happened to an image or drawing of a person did happen in reality (Krippner, 1995). Such beliefs were also prevalent among Chinese in the old times and still exist among many older Chinese nowadays.

Cultural beliefs significantly predict the use of traditional medical practices. For instance, in Chinese culture, it is believed that the mother loses a significant amount of *yang* during the delivery of a baby and must preserve any *yang* left so that *yin* would not be too strong. Therefore, a new mother must stay indoors for an entire month, regardless of the season, after delivering the baby, can not touch or eat anything cold (*yin*), can not take a bath, nor go outdoors without covering all of the exposed body parts to avoid cold air. All of those activities are considered *yin*, and the practices is believed to help promote *yang* and maintain *yin-yang* balance. If the new mother failed to follow those practices, her *yang* could not be restored and her *yin* would be too strong, which is believed to cause joint pain, lower back pain, loose teeth, and headaches later in her life. Also, ancient Chinese beliefs hold that animal organs correspond to human organs. If a particular human organ is weak, the same organ of an animal should be consumed. For example, a new mother is believed to have "weakened" blood caused by losing blood during and after the delivery, so she would eat cooked pig's blood to strengthen her own blood.

Developing and Developed Societies

Traditional medicine and CAM use is more prevalent in developing countries as compared to its use in developed countries. In India, Ayurveda has been the main healthcare system and is still used today by about two thirds of the rural population, which is 70% of the total population, to meet their primary healthcare needs (NCCAM, 2005a). In China, TCM is available to 75% of the areas in China and has been fully integrated into its health care system.

In contrast to the developing countries, the industrialized world uses traditional medicine and CAM as a choice because the number of well-educated and well-informed patients is increasing. They are attracted by the holistic and natural approaches employed by various CAM therapies. Well-educated and well-informed healthcare consumers want to become more involved in their overall health care, take a more natural and holistic approach to achieving personal well-being, and are willing to pay CAM therapies out of pocket (Astin, 1998; Eisenberg et al., 1998; Oldendick et al., 2000; Palinkas & Kabongo, 2000).

Case Study Examples

Homeopathic Remedy Treating Anxiety and Depression After Conventional Therapies Failed (Wember, 1997)

John had a relatively long history of depression. In the past, his anxiety and depression would dissipate over time after receiving psychotropic drugs. His present depression started a year ago caused by an incident at work where he felt betrayed. After he had taken six different antidepressant and antianxiety drugs and suffered from the side effects of the drugs, his depressive symptoms remained and he became more and more dysfunctional at work, to the point where he was on sick leave for the month prior to seeking homeopathic care. At the time he saw the homeopathic practitioner, he was extremely upset and still angry and aggressive. He received a single dose of Staphysagria lM. At the next appointment, three weeks later, he said he was "much better." His appetite had returned, and he had started to gain back the weight he had lost. He was calmer and sleeping better. He was working full time at home and would go back to the office that next week. He said, "I decided to change my priorities. I will do more things for myself and enjoy life a little more."

Homeopathy Treating Postpartum Depression (White, 2000)

A 28-year-old woman with postpartum depression revealed to her psychologist fantasies and impulses of throwing her 14-week-old daughter off of a cliff. Envying her friends without children and feeling distant and angry toward her husband as well as her infant, she was mired in a severe clinical depression that had been unresponsive to two trials of antidepressant medication. The psychologist referred the patient to a homeopath, a practitioner of the German-born form of medicine that uses a minute dose of an herb, plant, or other substance to effect healing, reportedly by stimulating a patient's "vital force." Within 4 days of beginning treatment with a remedy called *sepia*, the woman's depression lifted, and she began bonding with her infant. Homeopaths explain such rapid cures by saying that the energy of the remedy repairs the "leakage" in the patient's "energy balloon," created by particular traumas or life events. The specific remedy used in this case, sepia, made from the ink of the cuttlefish, reportedly is indicated when a woman is exhausted physically and emotionally from a myriad of responsibilities and work or from too many pregnancies, abortions, or miscarriages. A classic sign of its indication, according to homeopaths, is a person's indifference or aversion to loved ones. "The change was astounding!" her psychologist told the homeopath. "Now she loves the baby and is taking all kinds of photographs and videotapes of her child, and her marital relationship has improved considerably."

Traditional Chinese Medicine Treating Infertility

A Chinese couple in their early 30s went to see a TCM doctor hoping the TCM doctor could help them conceive a child. This couple had married for 3 years and gone through extensive clinical examination and laboratory tests including ultrasound. Nothing appears to be wrong with their reproductive organs and functions, but they just could not have a child. The TCM doctor checked the pulse, examined the tongue, and took the history from the couple. The TCM diagnose was that both the husband and the wife had *yin xu* (meaning weak *yin*) caused by weak "kidney," and he prescribed Chinese herbal medicine for the couple to strengthen the kidney, which would enhance *yin* and balance the *yin–yang* harmony. After 3 months of treatment, the wife was pregnant. The TCM doctor checked the wife's pulse at the 5 weeks of pregnancy and informed the wife that she was carrying a boy. Nine months later, a healthy baby boy was born to the couple. Now the baby boy is an 18-year-old college student.

Qi Therapy Used to Relieve Symptoms of Cancer in Terminally Ill Cancer Patient (Lee & Jang, 2005)

Jane suffered from late stage ovarian cancer and was experiencing unbearable abdominal discomfort and pain, depression, and fatigue. Four sessions of *qi* therapy on alternate days was given to Jane over a 7-day period. After 20 minutes of *qi* therapy, Jane experienced improvements in mood and alertness and a reduction in pain, anxiety, depression, discomfort, and fatigue, on both the first and last days of the interventions. Furthermore, the scores recorded on the last day for most symptoms were improved than those recorded on the first day. Although the result of this case study does not constitute conclusive evidence, the data suggest that *qi* therapy may have some beneficial effects on some symptoms of cancer.

References

Astin, J. A. (1998). Why patients use alternative medicine. *Journal of the American Medical Association, 279*, 1548–1553

Ballard, R. (2000). Homeopathy: An overview. *Australian Family Physician, 29*, 1145–1148.

Barnes, P. M., Powell-Griner, E., McFann, K., & Nahin, R. L. (2004). *Complementary and alternative medicine use among adults: United States, 2002. Advance data from vital and health statistics, No. 343.* National Center for Health Statistics. Retrieved August 20, 2005, from: http://www.cdc.gov/nchs/data/ad/ad343.pdf

Barnett, M. C., Cotroneo, M., Purnell, J., Martin, D., Mackenzie, E., & Fishman A. (2003). Use of CAM in local African-American communities: Community-partnered research. *Journal of the National Medical Association, 95*, 943–950.

Brewer, A. V. (2006). *Energy healing.* In J. Brewer, & K. King (Eds.), *Complementary and alternative medicine: A physician guide* [Electronic Book]. Retrieved September 20, 2006, from: http://medicine.wustl.edu/~compmed/cam_toc.htm

Center for Medicare and Medicaid Services. (1997). *National Health Expenditures Survey.* Retrieved March 20, 2005, from: http://www.cms.hhs.gov/statistics/nhe

Chen, Y. C. (2001). Chinese values, health and nursing. *Journal of Advanced Nursing, 36,* 270–273.

Chen, K. W., & Turner, F. D. (2004). A case study of simultaneous recovery from multiple physical symptoms with medical qigong therapy. *Journal of Alternative and Complementary Medicine, 10,* 159–162.

Chikahisa, S., Sei, H., Morishima, M., Sano, A., Kitaoka, K., Nakaya, Y., et al. (2006). Exposure to music in the perinatal period enhances learning performance and alters BDNF/TrkB signaling in mice as adults. *Behavioral Brain Research, 169,* 312–319.

Chopra, A., & Doiphode, V. V. (2002). Ayurvedic medicine. Core concept, therapeutic principles, and current relevance. *The Medical Clinics of North America, 86,* 75–89.

Christie, W., & Moore, C. (2005). The impact of humor on patients with cancer. *Clinical Journal of Oncology Nursing, 9,* 211-8.

Dantas, F., & Rampes, H. (2000). Do homeopathic medicine provoke adverse effects? A systematic review. *British Homeopathic Journal, 89,* S35–S38.

Dessio, W., Wade, C., Chao, M., Kronenberg, F., Cushman, L. E., & Kalmuss, D. (2004). Religion, spirituality, and healthcare choices of African-American women: Results of a national survey. *Ethnicity & Disease, 14,* 189–197.

Donatelle, R. J., & Davis, L. G. (2005). *Health: The Basics* (6th ed.). San Francisco, CA: Benjamin Cummings, Pearson Education, Inc.

Eisenberg, D. M., Davis, R. B., Ettner, S. L., Appel, S., Wilkey, S., Van Rompay, M., et al. (1998). Trends in alternative medicine use in the United States, 1990-1997: Results of a follow-up national survey. *Journal of the American Medical Association, 280,* 1569-1575.

Eisenberg, D. M., Kessler, R. C., Van Rompay, M. I., Kaptchuk, T. J., Wilkey, S. A., Appel, S., et al. (2001). Perceptions about complementary therapies relative to conventional therapies among adults who use both: Results from a national survey. *Annuals of Internal Medicine, 135,* 344–351.

Ernst, E., Pittler, M. H., Stevinson, C., White, A., & Eisenberg, D. (2001). *The desktop guide to complementary and alternative medicine.* Edinburgh, UK: Mosby.

Ervin, R. B., Wright, J. D., & Kennedy-Stephenson, J. (1999). Use of dietary supplements in the United States, 1988-94. *Vital and Health Statistics Series 11, Data from the National Health Survey, 244,* 1–14.

FDA (Food and Drug Administration). (2000). *Risk of drug interactions with St John's wort and Indinavir and other drugs.* Retrieved September 20, 2006, from http://www.fda.gov/cder/drug/advisory/stjwort.htm

FDA. (2002). *Consumer advisory: Kava-containing dietary supplements may be associated with severe liver injury.* March 25, 2002. Retrieved September 20, 2006, from http://www.cfsan.fda.gov/~dms/addskava.html

FDA. (2003). *Claims that can be made for conventional foods and dietary supplements.* Retrieved September 20, 2006, from www.cfsan.fda.gov/~dms/hclaims.html

FDA. (2004). *FDA announces rule prohibiting sale of dietary supplements containing ephedrine alkaloids effective April 12.* Retrieved September 20, 2006, from http://www.fda.gov/bbs/topics/NEWS/2004/NEW01050.html

FDA. (2006). *Dietary supplements overview.* Retrieved September 27, 2006, from http://www.cfsan.fda.gov/~dms/supplmnt.html

Hammerschlag, R. (1998). Methodological and ethical issues in clinical trials of acupuncture. *Journal of Alternative And Complementary Medicine, 4,* 159–171.

Hoeger, W. W. K. & Hoeger, S. A. (2006). *Principles and labs for fitness and wellness* (8th ed.). Belmont, CA: Thomson Wadsworth.

Hui, P. N., Wan, M., Chan, W. K., & Yung, P. M. (2006). An evaluation of two behavioral rehabilitation programs, qigong versus progressive relaxation, in improving the quality of life in cardiac patients. *Journal of Alternative and Complementary Medicine, 12,* 373–378.

Institute of Medicine. (2005). *Institute of Medicine report on complementary and alternative medicine in the United States.* Washington, DC: National Academies Press.

Johnson, P. H., & Johnson, R. D. (2002). *Looking to the East: The theory and practice of traditional Chinese medicine.* Paper presented at the 130th American Public Health Association (APHA) Annual Meeting, Philadelphia, Pennsylvania.

Junod, S. W. (2000). Alternative drugs: Homeopathy, Royal Copeland, and Federal Drug regulation. *Pharmacy in History, 42,* 13–35.

Koh, H. L., Ng, H. L., & Teo, H. H. (2004). A survey on knowledge, attitudes and usage of complementary and alternative medicine in Singapore. *Asia Pacific Biotech News, 8,* 1266–1270.

Krippner, S. (1995). A cross-cultural comparison of four healing models. *Alternative Therapies in Health and Medicine, 1,* 21–29.

Lee, M. S., & Jang, H. S. (2005). Two case reports of the acute effects of Qi therapy (external Qigong) on symptoms of cancer: Short report. *Complement Therapy in Clinical Practice, 11,* 211–213.

Lee, M. S., Kim, M. K., & Lee, Y. H. (2005). Effects of Qi-therapy (external Qigong) on cardiac autonomic tone: A randomized placebo controlled study. *International Journal of Neuroscience, 115,* 1345–1350.

Li, G., Jack, C. R., Jr., & Yang, E. S. (2006). An fMRI study of somatosensory-implicated acupuncture points in stable somatosensory stroke patients. *Journal of Magnetic Resonance Imaging, 24*(5), 1018–1024

Li, K., Shan, B., Xu, J., Wang, W., Zhi, L., Li, K., et al. (2006). Changes in FMRI in the human brain related to different durations of manual acupuncture needling. *Journal of Alternative and Complementary Medicine, 12,* 615–623.

Li, M., Chen, K., & Mo, Z. (2002). Use of qigong therapy in the detoxification of heroin addicts. *Alternative Therapies in Health and Medicine, 8,* 50–54, 56–59.

Merrell, W. C., & Shalts, E. (2002). Homeopathy. *Medical Clinics of North America, 86,* 47–62.

Monkman, D. (2001). Educating health professionals about how to use the Web and how to find complementary and alternative medicine (CAM) information. *Complementary Therapies in Medicine, 9,* 258.

Morris, K. T., Johnson, N., Homer, L., & Walts, D. (2000). A comparison of complementary therapy use between breast cancer patients and patients with other tumors. *American Journal of Surgery, 179,* 407–411.

Mukherjee, P. K., & Wahile, A. (2006). Integrated approaches towards drug development from Ayurveda and other Indian system of medicines. *Journal of Ethnopharmacology, 103,* 25–35.

Nahin, R. L., & Straus, S. E. (2001). Research into complementary and alternative medicine: Problems and potential. *British Journal of Medicine, 322,* 161–163.

Napadow, V., Makris, N., Liu, J., Kettner, N. W., Kwong, K. K., & Hui, K. K. (2005). Effects of electroacupuncture versus manual acupuncture on the human brain as measured by fMRI. *Human Brain Mapping, 24,* 193–205.

NCCAM (National Center for Complementary and Alternative Medicine). (2002). *Get the facts: What is complementary and alternative medicine (CAM)?* (NCCAM Publication No. D156). Retrieved September 27, 2006, from http://nccam.nih.gov/health/whatiscam/

NCCAM. (2003a). *Research report: Questions and answers about homeopathy* (NCCAM Publication No. D183). Retrieved September 20, 2006, from http://nccam.nih.gov/health/homeopathy/index.htm

NCCAM. (2003b). *Research report: About chiropractic and its use in treating low-back pain* (NCCAM Publication No. D196). Retrieved September 20, 2006, from http://nccam.nih.gov/health/chiropractic

NCCAM. (2003c). *NCCAM appropriations—Grants and direct operations.* Retrieved March 20, 2004, from http://www.nih.gov/about/almanac/organization/NCCAM.htm#appropriations

NCCAM. (2004a). *Back grounder: Biologically based practices: An overview* (NCCAM Publication No. D237). Retrieved September 20, 2006, from http://nccam.nih.gov/health/backgrounds/biobasedprac.htm

NCCAM. (2004b). *Back grounder: Manipulative and body-based practices: An overview* (NCCAM Publication No. D238). Retrieved September 20, 2006, from http://nccam.nih.gov/health/backgrounds/manipulative.htm

NCCAM. (2005a). *Back grounder: What is ayurvedic medicine?* (NCCAM Publication No. D287). Retrieved September 20, 2006, from http://nccam.nih.gov/health/ayurveda

NCCAM. (2005b). *Back grounder: Mind-body medicine: An overview* (NCCAM Publication No. D239). Retrieved September 20, 2006, from http://nccam.nih.gov/health/backgrounds/mindbody.htm

NCCAM. (2005c). *Back grounder: Energy medicine: An overview* (NCCAM Publication No. D235). Retrieved September 20, 2006, from http://nccam.nih.gov/health/backgrounds/energymed.htm

NCCAM. (2006a). *Massage therapy as CAM* (NCCAM Publication No. D327). Retrieved September on 20, 2006, from http://nccam.nih.gov/health/massage

NCCAM. (2006b). *Backgrounder—An introduction to Reiki* (NCCAM Publication No. D315). Retrieved June 20, 2006, from http://nccam.nih.gov/health/reiki

NCAAM. (2006c). *NCCAM facts at a glance.* Retrieved September 18, 2006, from http://nccam.nih.gov/about/ataglance

NCCAM. (2006d). *Get the facts: Are you considering using CAM?* Retrieved May 11, 2007, from http://nccam.nih.gov/health/decisions/index.htm

NCCAM. (2006e). *Get the facts: 10 things to know about evaluating medical resources on the web.* Retrieved May 11, 2007, from http://nccam.nih.gov/health/webresources

NCCAM. (2007a). *NCCAM funding: Appropriations history.* Retrieved May 10, 2007, from http://nccam.nih.gov/about/appropriations/index.htm

NCCAM. (2007b). *Get the facts: Selecting a complementary and alternative medicine (CAM) practitioner.* Retrieved May 11, 2007, from http://nccam.nih.gov/health/practitioner/index.htm

NIH (National Institutes of Health). (2006a). *The NIH almanac—Organizations: National Center for Complementary and Alternative Medicine.* Retrieved September 18, 2006, from http://www.nih.gov/about/almanac/organization/NCCAM.htm#appropriations

NIH. (2006b). *The NIH almanac—Appropriations.* Retrieved September 18, 2006, from http://www.nih.gov/about/almanac/appropriations/part2.htm

Oldendick, R., Coker, A. L., Wieland, D., Raymond, J. I., Probst, J. C., Schell, B. J., et al. (2000). Population-based survey of complementary and alternative medicine usage, patient satisfaction, and physician involvement. *Southern Medical Journal, 93,* 375–381.

Palinkas, L. A., & Kabongo, M. L. (2000). The use of complementary and alternative medicine by primary care patients. *Journal of Family Practice, 49,* 1121–1130.

Peters, R. M. (1999). The effectiveness of therapeutic touch: A meta-analytic review. *Nursing Science Quarterly, 12,* 52–61.

Radimer, K., Bindewald, B., Hughes, J., Ervin, B., Swanson, C., & Picciano, M. F. (2004). Dietary supplement use by US adults: Data from the National Health and Nutrition Examination Survey, 1999-2000. *American Journal of Epidemiology, 160,* 339–349.

Richardson, M. A. (2001). Biopharmacologic and herbal therapies for cancer: Research update from NCCAM. *Journal of Nutrition, 131,* 3037S–3040S.

Samano, E. S. T., Ribeiro, L. M., Campos, A. S., Lewin, F., Filho, E. S. V., Goldenstein, P. T., et al. (2005). Use of complementary and alternative medicine by Brazilian oncologists. *European Journal of Cancer Care, 14,* 143–148.

Sancier, K. M., & Holman, D. (2004). Commentary: Multifaceted health benefits of medical qigong. *Journal of Alternative and Complementary Medicine, 10,* 163–165.

Saper, R. B., Kales, S. N., Paquin, J., Burns, M. J., Eisenberg, D. M., Davis, R. B., et al. (2004). Heavy metal content of ayurvedic herbal medicine products. *Journal of American Medical Association, 292,* 2868–2873.

Scheiman-Burkhardt, Z. (2001). Homeopathic treatment in a polluted world. *Natural Life, 81,* 10–11.

Slesinski, M. J., Subar, A. F., & Kahle, L. L. (1995). Trends in use of vitamin and mineral supplements in the United States: The 1987 and 1992 National Health Interview Surveys. *Journal of the American Dietetic Association, 95,* 921–923.

Subar, A. F., & Block, G. (1990). Use of vitamin and mineral supplements: Demographics and amounts of nutrients consumed. The 1987 Health Interview Survey. *American Journal of Epidemiology, 132,* 1091–1101.

Tedesco, P., & Cicchetti, J. (2001). Like cures like: Homeopathy. *American Journal of Nursing, 101,* 43–49.

The Nurse Healers - Professional Associates International. (2006). *Therapeutic touch facts.* Retrieved September 21, 2006, from http://www.therapeutic-touch.org/newsarticle.php?newsID=18

U.S. Nutrition Industry. (2005). *Nutrition Business Journal's supplement business report 2005.* Retrieved September 20, 2006, from www.nutritionbusiness.com

van Schalkwyk, J., Davidson, J., Palmer, B., & Hope, V. (2006). Ayurvedic medicine: Patients in peril from plumbism. *The New Zealand Medical Journal, 119,* U1958.

Wardell, D. W., & Weymouth, K. F. (2004). Review of studies of healing touch. *Journal of Nursing Scholarship, 36,* 147–154.

Wember, D. (1997). The heart and soul of Homeopathy. *Journal of the American Institute of Homeopathy, 90,* 36–40.

Whelan, J. S., & Dvorkin, L. (2003). HolisticKids.org—Evolution of information resources in pediatric complementary and alternative medicine projects: From monographs to Web learning. *Journal of the Medical Library Association, 91,* 411–417.

White, K. P. (2000). psychology and complementary and alternative medicine. *Professional Psychology: Research and Practice, 31,* 671–681.

WHO. (1983). *Traditional medicine and health care coverage.* Geneva, Switzerland: WHO.

WHO. (2003). *Traditional medicine.* Retrieved September 17, 2006, from http://www.who.int/mediacentre/factsheets/fs134/en

WHO. (2005). *National policy on traditional medicine and regulations of herbal medicines: Report of a WHO global survey.* Retrieved May 12, 2007, from http://whqlibdoc.who.int/publications/2005/9241593237.pdf

Winstead-Fry, P., & Kijekm, J. (1999). An integrative review and meta-analysis of therapeutic touch research. *Alternative Therapies in Health and Medicine, 5,* 58–67.

Wu, W. H., Bandilla, E., Ciccone, D. S., Yang, J., Cheng, S. C., Carner, N., et al. (1999). Effects of qigong on late-stage complex regional pain syndrome. *Alternative Therapies in Health and Medicine, 5,* 45–54.

Zhang, D., & Cheng, Z. (2000). Medicine is a humane art. The basic principles of professional ethics in Chinese medicine. *The Hastings Center Report, 30,* S8–S12.

Chapter 9

Global Perspectives on Selected Chronic Cardiovascular Diseases

Bowman O. Davis, Jr.

Introduction

As people of the world saw their calendars roll over to a new millennium, few realized that the 21st century would be greeted differently by different human populations around the globe. Technologically developed, industrialized countries anxiously awaited the prospect of some undetected Y2K glitches that threatened to corrupt databases ranging from major financial institutions to individual home computers and jeopardize cherished financial security or personal convenience. Yet, individuals in developing nations saw the day as one of continuing poverty and struggle to acquire adequate nourishment and to survive disease. The dawn of the new millennium revealed a persistent disparity in relative prosperity among the diverse human populations of the world. Converted to US dollars, people of developed nations averaged approximately 18 times the per capita gross domestic product (GDP) of their developing nation counterparts (WHO, 1996).

In this age of global economic trade and global communication, the rapid spread of technology has not had equitable impact on everyone. Not only has there not been equitable sharing in technological advances and socioeconomic prosperity, but the assumption that all technological advances are good is subject to serious debate. Close examination reveals both positive and negative influences of technological advances. Paradoxically, as developed nations export beneficial advances in technology, including health care, they also export popular culture and lifestyles, such as alcohol and tobacco use, stressful work environments, sedentary life styles, and calorie-dense diets high in salt, sugar, and saturated fat that can have negative effects on the health of persons influenced by these trends. Disease burdens around the world often reflect this paradox. Developing nations struggle under the burden of infectious and communicable diseases, while socio-economically developed nations see their disease burden shift toward one of chronic and noncommunicable diseases. This shift is primarily due to the fact that infant mortality is decreased in the course of a country's economic development, and life expectancy at birth is increased sufficiently for chronic diseases to prevail. From the most developed nation to the least, the gap in average life expectancy can be as much as 37 years. Unfortunately, the path from developing to developed status leads through a transitional phase during which the disease burden on the population may be dual in nature where both infectious and chronic diseases are nearly equal in their mortality impact.

Accurately assessing the disease burden among populations around the world is a daunting task complicated by factors such as accounting for migratory segments of the population, inaccurate diagnoses of medical conditions, and inconsistent reporting and recording of disease incidences and causes of death. Within these constraints, the United Nations World Health Organization (WHO) collects and publishes in its annual *World Health Report* a yearly compilation of causes of death among its member states around the world. The availability of this comprehensive database reveals emerging trends in disease burdens and allows for analyses of health needs and of the effectiveness of healthcare measures, as well as for the redirection and prioritization of health care efforts and resources.

Specific methods are used to measure and characterize the overall health status of a given population and specific terminology is used to reference these data. For example, *prevalence* of a given disease is the total number of cases, both previously existing and newly diagnosed, present within a population at any given time. Whereas, *incidence* or *morbidity* refers to the number of new cases of a given disease reported each year. Finally, *mortality* rate reflects the actual deaths due to a specific, identifiable cause. For this discussion of chronic diseases, mortality rate is used as the index of disease burden within a population.

Demographic and Socioeconomic Transition

Biologists often represent the developmental status of a population by means of graphic "age pyramids," as shown in Figure 9-1. Growing populations have fertility rates greater than basic replacement levels (more than two offspring per female of reproductive age) and exhibit a typical upright pyramid with the number of individuals declining, primarily due to mortality, as they move vertically through the various age groups. Populations with fertility rates approaching replacement level show a loss of the pyramid shape as stability

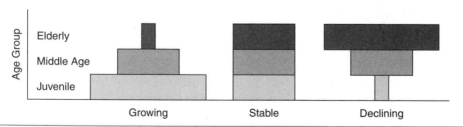

Figure 9-1 Population age structures.

is reached. However, if fertility rates drop below replacement levels, the age structure pyramid inverts as the population moves into decline. Human populations fit this model very closely, but to consider only age structure would give an incomplete picture with no insight as to the other aspects of population dynamics that might be causing the growth, decline, or stability.

The World Health Organization groups its member states by geographic regions and mortality strata to give a more complete picture of population status. Mortality strata range from *A*, very low child mortality and very low adult mortality, to *E* where child mortality is high and adult mortality is very high (Table 9-1). By these criteria, a majority of United Nations member states fall into the *developing* category with comparatively few having attained *developed* status. However, a cursory examination of Table 9-1 shows a progression of development from high mortality, developing nations with mortality strata of

TABLE 9-1 United Nations World Health Organization Member States Grouped by Geographic Regions and Mortality Strata

Mortality Stratum	Region	Developed Nations Member States	Developing Nations Low-Mortality Member States	High-Mortality Member States
(A) Very low child, very low adult	Americas	Canada, Cuba, USA		
	Europe	Andorra, Austria, Belgium, Croatia, Czech Rep., Denmark, Finland, France, Germany, Greece, Iceland, Ireland, Israel, Italy, Luxembourg, Malta, Monaco, Netherlands, Norway, Portugal, San Marino, Slovenia, Spain, Sweden, Switzerland, UK		
	West Pacific Region	Australia, Brunei, Dorussalam, Japan, New Zealand, Singapore		

(continues)

TABLE 9-1 United Nations World Health Organization Member States Grouped by Geographic Regions and Mortality Strata (continued)

Mortality Stratum	Region	Developed Nations	Developing Nations	
		Member States	Low-Mortality Member States	High-Mortality Member States
(B) Low child, low adult	Americas		Antigua, Barbuda, Argentina, Bahamas, Barbados, Belize, Brazil, Chile, Columbia, Costa Rica, Dominica, Dominican Rep., El Salvador, Grenada, Guyana, Honduras, Jamaica, Mexico, Panama, Paraguay, St. Kits, Nevis, St. Lucia, St. Vincent, Grenadines, Suriname, Trinidad, Tobago, Uruguay, Venezuela	
	Europe		Albania, Armenia, Azerbaijan, Bosnia/ Herzegovina, Bulgaria, Georgia, Kyrgyzstan, Poland, Romania, Slovakia, Tajikistan, Macedonia, Turkey, Turkmenistan, Uzbekistan, Yugoslavia	
	Mediterranean Region		Bahrain, Cyprus, Iran, Jordan, Kuwait, Lebanon, Lybia, Oman, Qatar, Saudi Arabia, Syria, Tunisia, United Arab Emirates	

(continues)

TABLE 9-1   United Nations World Health Organization Member States Grouped by Geographic Regions and Mortality Strata *(continued)*

Mortality Stratum	Region	Developed Nations Member States	Developing Nations	
			Low-Mortality Member States	High-Mortality Member States
	South East Asia		Indonesia, Sri Lanka, Thailand	
	Western Pacific Region		Cambodia, China, Cook Islands, Fiji, Kiribati, Laos, Malaysia, Marshall Islands, Micronesia, Mongolia, Nauru, Niue, Palau, New Guinea, Philippines, Rep. of Korea, Samoa, Solomon Islands, Tonga, Tuvalu, Vanualy, Viet Nam	
(C) Low child, high adult	Europe	Belarus, Estonia, Hungary, Kazakhstan, Latvia, Lithuania, Moldova, Russia, Ukraine		
(D) High child, high adult	Africa			Algeria, Angola, Benin, Burkina, Faso, Cameroon, Cape Verde, Chad, Comoros, Guinea, Gabon, Gambia, Ghana, Guinea-Bissau, Liberia, Madagascar, Mali, Mauritania, Mauritus, Niger, Sao Tome, Principe, Senegal, Seychelles, Sierra Leone, Togo

(continues)

TABLE 9-1 United Nations World Health Organization Member States Grouped by Geographic Regions and Mortality Strata (continued)

| Mortality Stratum | Region | Developed Nations | Developing Nations | |
		Member States	Low-Mortality Member States	High-Mortality Member States
(E) High child, very high adult	Americas			Bolivia, Ecuador, Guatemala, Haiti, Nicaragua, Peru
	Mediterranean Region			Afghanistan, Djibouti, Egypt, Iraq, Morocco, Pakistan, Somalia, Sudan, Yemen
	South East Asia			Bangladesh, Bhutan, Dem. Peoples Rep. of Korea, India, Maldives, Myanmar, Nepal
	Africa			Botswana, Burundi, Cen. African Republic, Congo, Cote d'Ivoire, Dem. Rep. of the Congo, Eritrea, Ethiopia, Kenya, Lesotho, Malawi, Mozambique, Namibia, Rwanda, South Africa, Swaziland, Uganda, Un. Rep. of Tanzania, Zambia, Zimbabwe

Note: Mortality strata: (A), very low child/very low adult; (B), low child/low adult; (C), low child/high adult; (D), high child/high adult; (E), high child/very high adult.

Source: Adapted from WHO (2002); Ezzati & Lopez (2004).

D and *E* through a group of countries transitioning in their mortality rates to a comparatively few states that have attained developed status. Thus, the mortality rates within child and adult age groups provide a useful index of a country's developmental status. Still the picture is incomplete without examining the underlying causes of death that contribute to these mortality data. Factors that impact a population's development, such as demographics, socioeconomics, culture, politics, and religion, must also be considered.

Although causes of death due to disease can be conveniently reduced to either infectious or chronic disease categories, the demographic and socioeconomic contexts within which these deaths occur are not as simply described. Demographically, a population can be described by certain characteristics such as age composition, immigration and emigration rates, fertility rate, life expectancy at birth, death rate, and so on. These properties are generally objective and quantifiable. However, they convey little about the actual lifestyles experienced by members of the population. Socioeconomic aspects of a population, such as per capita GDP, literacy rate, percent urbanization, and so on, give a better picture of the quality of life within the population. Interestingly, as populations transition from undeveloped or developing toward developed status, they undergo changes in both demographic and socioeconomic aspects that can be generally reflective of their stage of development and its characteristic causes of death.

It is important to emphasize the "generally reflective" descriptor here in order to avoid the pitfall of imposing stereotypic benchmarks on the progress of a population through its development. In reality, populations do undergo demographic and socioeconomic changes as they progress, but the characteristics of this developmental process are inevitably directed by geographical, political, cultural, and religious influences present within the population. Because these influences can be dramatically different from one population to another, each developing nation does so within its own unique set of circumstances. Therefore, each nation must be considered individually if a truly accurate assessment of its developmental progress is desired. It is not the purpose of this discussion to analyze in detail every aspect influencing this developmental transition in every country undergoing it. It is more important to begin with broader generalizations to develop an appreciation of the general complexities involved in the progression toward developed status.

It is important to realize the lack of universal application of every aspect of population transition. It is equally important to realize that there are complex interactions among the various demographic, socioeconomic, cultural, and political factors, many of which are poorly understood and appreciated. In a purely hypothetical example, fertility rate may be high in a rural, agricultural population where per capita income is low and access to medical care is limited. As a result, infant mortality is high and life expectancy is low. The high fertility rate is a positive factor in this population where large families are essential to maintain an agrarian lifestyle. However, high fertility rate in a different population would be a negative factor because it might increase child dependency stress on constituent families. Because literacy is of little perceived value, in this hypothetical population, literacy rates are low. Thus preventative healthcare measures are difficult to communicate, and resultant communicable disease avoidance is also low. Such a population would be vulnerable to infectious diseases circuitously making high fertility even more advantageous to offset disease losses. Cultural and religious factors can figure into the equation if they permit promiscuity, impose restrictions on family planning practices, or reinforce gender preferences of offspring. Such practices could keep family size large but with inequitable distribution of family resources to one gender. At the same time there may be increased risk of spreading infectious sexually transmitted diseases within and among family units.

Typically, high fertility and mortality combined with low income and literacy rates are characteristic of developing states. However, such a characterization does not address the population's stability. In fact, the population may be quite stable and in equilibrium with its geographic, demographic, cultural, and socioeconomic environment. The question then becomes one of humanitarian concern and whether or not to intervene in an attempt to raise the standard of living of individuals at the potential risk of disturbing the population's equilibrium.

Although the above example is purely hypothetical, it clearly illustrates that there can be no universal set of standards for assessing population development if the unique circumstances within which it is developing are not considered as well. With those precautionary notes emphasized, the following characterization of population transition will identify major transitional phases. It will also describe some of their demographic and socioeconomic characteristics with the understanding that they may not be universally applicable.

By applying the phases of demographic transition described by Lee and Chu (2000) as a basic framework and adding certain socioeconomic factors as appropriate, it is possible to generate a more descriptive model of population development within which the causes of death can be examined more specifically.

Beginning with a hypothetical, undeveloped population, the people are often widely dispersed in individual family units across a basically rural environment. With the primary livelihood being agriculture, the labor force is small and per capita income is low. Financial savings are virtually nonexistent since any family income is devoted to living essentials. Families often reside in primitive, unsanitary living conditions and are exposed to contaminated indoor air from fuels used for heating and cooking. Clean water for drinking and food storage capability may be inadequate as investment in infrastructure is minimal. Fertility rate is high but perinatal health care is substandard for both mothers and their children leading to an increased child mortality rate. Fertility rate may also be affected by the cultural preference for large families and the benefit of having large families to share the agricultural workload. Literacy levels are low since literacy has little perceived value in this agrarian lifestyle. The status of women in the population is often low with little incentive to improve either their literacy or their participation in the workforce. The combination of primitive living conditions, poor sanitation, illiteracy, and limited access to health care increases the prevalence of infectious diseases and results in a low life expectancy at birth because both child and adult mortality rates are high. With high fertility rates helping to offset the high mortality rates, the population may be transiently stable. However, it is extremely vulnerable to environmental disasters such as drought or infectious disease epidemics that could tip the delicate balance toward decline. Table 9-2 below compares selected nations from each WHO mortality stratum with regard to specific demographic and socioeconomic criteria for the decade from 1993 to 2003 where data were available. The contrast between the most and least developed states is apparent.

Phase One Transition: Reducing Child Mortality

The first phase of transition usually begins with a decline in child mortality. This decline may be the result of internal healthcare measures within the population structure or from external humanitarian efforts. Many developed nations export medical technology such as vaccination programs in an effort to reduce child mortality. The decline in child mortality increases the proportion of children in the population and raises the child

TABLE 9-2   Representative Demographic and Socioeconomic Data from Selected United Nations Member States of Each Mortality Stratum

Nation (Mortality Stratum)	Life Expectancy at Birth		Literacy Rate (Percent)		Fertility Rate (Children/ Adult Female)		Urbanization (Percent)		Per Capita GDP (US $)	
	1993	2003	1993	2003	1993	2003	1993	2003	1993	2003
USA (A)	76	77.3	99	99	2.1	2.1	76	—	23,240	—
China (B)	71	71.1	78	—	2.2	1.8	28	—	470	—
Russia (C)	68	64.6	99	—	1.5	1.2	77	—	2510	—
Sierra Leone (D)	43	34	21	—	6.5	6.5	34	—	160	—
Rwanda (E)	47	44.4	50	—	8.5	5.8	6	—	250	—

Source: Adapted from WHO (1995, 2004).

dependency stress on individual family units and on the population as a whole. This increased dependency stress can result in continued low per capita income with all of its consequences including continued low expenditure on healthcare practice and infrastructure. With minimal healthcare access and continued low literacy rates, infectious diseases remain as the primary cause of death among adults as life expectancy remains low. The rural, agrarian lifestyle persists, and the unsanitary living conditions and female status within the population show little change.

Phase Two Transition: Fertility Decline

In the second phase of transition, the most distinguishing feature is the beginning decline in fertility. A number of factors may influence this trend (Poston, 2000), and it may take two or three generations, or about 50 years, to go to completion. Completion is considered to be the attainment of a replacement level of about two children per reproductive female. For example, the People's Republic of China and Taiwan exist as examples of how socioeconomic and political factors can curtail fertility rate. In 1950, both China and Taiwan had fertility rates around six children per reproductive female. By 1995, both had declined to fertility levels below two. However, Taiwan's fertility decline resulted from voluntary reductions in family size as a possible result of socioeconomic development, whereas the decline in China was a result of combined socioeconomic development and government intervention in family planning (Poston, 2000).

Socioeconomically speaking, as livelihood gradually shifts from an agricultural base to one of an industrial or service labor force, large family size is no longer an asset and can be a liability. Under these conditions, adequate food can no longer be grown to feed a large family and most living essentials must now be purchased. To be competitive in the new work environment, literacy is of greater value than large family size. Literacy rate and educational level negatively correlate with fertility rate especially when the educational level of females is considered. Additionally, female value within the population may trend upward as more women move into the workforce, and this too can negatively impact fertility rate. During this phase, the labor force grows rapidly and contributes to an increased per capita income, assuming the economy grows sufficiently to provide jobs for the growing workforce. Because a workforce tends to locate close to a work source, migration from rural to urban environments may be evident. Urbanization of the population has a positive impact by increasing access to both education and health care and a negative impact on fertility as literacy improves. However, the shift from the physical labor of agriculture to the more stressful structured work environment can increase the mental stress on working adults. As actual work becomes more structured and less physically demanding, leisure time also increases and more sedentary life styles may become the norm.

Total dependency stress is low in this phase of transition as the generally healthy, middle-aged segment of the population predominates with very few dependent children and few dependent elderly members. With low dependency stress, financial savings may increase along with consumption as labor becomes more lucrative and the overall standard of living increases. Unfortunately, exposure to popular cultural promotions also increases as businesses perceive the population with its improving standard of living as a potential market for goods and services, some of which may be accompanied by behavioral practices and lifestyles that may not be conducive to good health. The glamorization of alcohol, tobacco, and drug use have negative impacts on health and longevity, as do readily available access to prepared foods dense in calories and high in salt, sugar, and fats substitute convenience for healthy diets. These dietary changes can increase the prevalence of obesity within a population having an increasingly sedentary lifestyle. Such lifestyle practices can exacerbate existing risk factors for chronic diseases, especially those of a cardiovascular nature. Thus, the mortality rates resulting from these chronic diseases increase at about the same time as, or even before, infectious diseases have been adequately controlled. In this case, socioeconomic improvement can change the nature of a population's overall disease burden instead of reducing it.

With increased per capita income, expenditure on healthcare services and infrastructure is now an affordable option. Easier access to improved health care further reduces mortality rates from infectious diseases and increases life expectancy. As life expectancy increases, individuals now live long enough to develop chronic diseases, especially if unhealthy lifestyles have become the cultural norm. In fact, the population may exhibit a time period where infectious and chronic diseases have a dual impact on mortality rates. Eventually, the population may progress beyond the dual disease burden stage toward one where chronic diseases predominate as the major cause of death. Figure 9-2 compares the relative mortality rates from infectious and chronic diseases from WHO geographic regions and mortality strata for the year 2000. Examination of these data shows a trend away from an infectious disease burden toward one of chronic diseases as the mortality stratum trends from *E* (high child, very high adult) to *A* (very low child, very low adult). Interestingly, the *D* mortality stratum of the geographic regions of Southeast Asia, Eastern Mediterranean, South America, and Eastern Europe shows a significant *dual* disease burden. Also important is the recognition that chronic diseases now account for more deaths worldwide than infectious diseases. This can be both a testament to the effectiveness of infectious disease eradication measures and an indication of the need to direct more effort toward the emerging chronic disease problem.

Phase Three Transition: Increasing Age Dependency

To appreciate the final phase of population development, selected aspects of the second phase must be considered as contributing to the major characteristic of third phase development, that of emerging age dependency. Increased life expectancy combined with the declining infant mortality and the shift to a more gender-diverse, urban labor force generates a comparatively large "balloon" of persons moving both into the labor force and into the older age strata of the population. As this ballooned middle-aged population stratum grows older, age dependency stress on the population increases. Interestingly, as

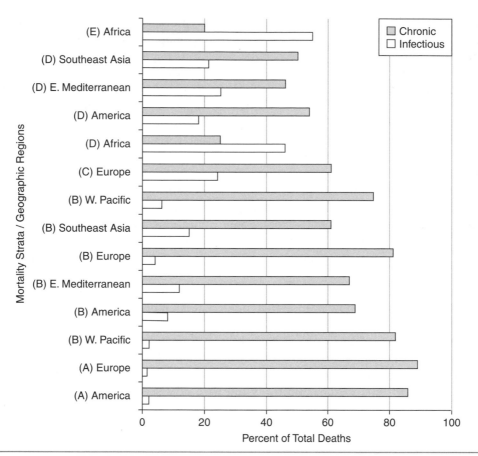

Figure 9-2 Comparison of deaths due to infectious versus chronic diseases by UN/WHO mortality strata and geographic regions for the year 2000.

Source: Adapted from WHO World Health Report (2001).

this aging occurs, the total dependency stress increases on the population until the total dependency stress is now similar to that of phase one. The only difference being that age dependency now replaces child dependency.

Age is a primary irreversible risk factor for chronic disease development, and the prevalence of these diseases inevitably increases within any aging population. The extent to which they increase in prevalence depends upon the number of risk factors occurring simultaneously. Unfortunately, a past history of substance abuse, tobacco and alcohol use, sedentary lifestyle, and unhealthy diet serves to exacerbate the chronic disease burden of the susceptible aging population segment. Additionally, the prolonged psychological stress of urban living and genetic predisposition, should it exist, can be contributing factors to the rise in chronic disease burden. This increase in chronic disease is particularly evident as an increase in cardiovascular disorders with ischemic heart disease and hypertension being the general manifestations.

Up to this point, hypothetical situations have been used to provide a basic awareness of the complexities of population development. They also provide a context within which to assess the importance of chronic disease burdens around the world. The next step in a logical progression is to examine in more detail the major contributing factors to this emerging global chronic disease burden.

The Underlying Role of Poverty

Although people around the world die from a variety of causes ranging from accidental deaths and political conflicts to infectious and chronic diseases, the age at which they die is somewhat more predictable. The old adage, "The rich die old while the poor die young," appears to have a factual basis. A contemporary application can be seen when the data previously presented in Table 9-2 are examined more closely. Nations with higher per capita GDPs also have longer life expectancies. This should come as no surprise, since a higher GDP leads to greater expenditure on healthcare infrastructure and greater individual access to health care. Interestingly, the table also shows a positive correlation between literacy rate and life expectancy. The impact of literacy can be seen across the entire age spectrum. Infant mortality is negatively correlated with literacy level for the obvious reasons that literate parents are more likely to be aware of disease prevention measures and to have the necessary personal income to access and practice them. For example, the WHO's Global Immunization Program, begun in 1974, helped to eradicate smallpox and increase the level of child immunization globally from 5 percent to 80 percent by 1995 (WHO, 1997). Although the reduction of childhood diseases was significant by the end of the last century, it was least effective in underdeveloped countries. This lack of child immunization combined with substandard or total absence of adequate peripartum care drives the child mortality rates high and drives life expectancy at birth low in developing nations.

In the middle and elderly age strata, the role of literacy is more individual as these age groups are less directly dependent upon care from others to protect them from diseases and unhealthy practices. Their receptivity to publicly communicated health warnings and their vulnerability to unhealthy cultural and lifestyle practices depends in part on their literacy level and the ease with which sound health practices can be communicated to them.

The WHO World Health Report (1995) devoted much of its narrative to the role of poverty in global mortality rates. In 1990, it was estimated that 20% of the world's human population lived in poverty. This estimate was accompanied by an observed 37-year gap in life expectancy between richer and poorer nations.

Poverty impacts longevity and subjects people to disease in a variety of ways: it destines people to drink unclean water and to live in unsanitary conditions; it forces people to breathe air polluted by industrial emissions as well as unclean fuels used for home heating and cooking; and it can be a contributing factor to mental stress, family unit disintegration, and substance abuse. More importantly, it excludes people from the educational process depriving them of the essential knowledge to prevent diseases that could be avoided by lifestyle changes. This educational deficiency leaves them with only cultural or religious practices for protection, which very often may not be adequate.

It is easy to make an erroneous leap in generalization by assuming that wealthier, industrialized nations are devoid of poverty. Conversely, a variant impact of poverty can be seen to be the result of industrialization. A developing industrial economy can entice people to migrate from rural to urban environments in search of higher income and a better lifestyle. However, the lack of adequate marketable skills or periods of economic depression can leave them stranded in isolated pockets of poverty within the urban environment. Similarly, it is a mistake to assume that everyone within a population will "catch the wave" of industrialization and be swept equally toward personal financial improvement. As America underwent industrialization during the 1800s and 1900s, some people in rural environments were not included in the transition. Although many migrated to the industrialized urban environments, some remained behind as did those in pockets of central Appalachia. In this geographic area, poverty rates approach 35% compared to the national rate of 14% (Phipps, 2006). Regardless of the circumstances that produced them, these pockets of poverty are not unique to either a rural or an urban environment and can be seen in both. Unfortunately, the people living in them, as with those in underdeveloped nations, may be subject to a dual threat from both infectious and chronic diseases.

The Chronic Disease Burden

Increasing life expectancy of a population has both positive and negative impacts on disease burden. Clearly, reducing child mortality and controlling infectious diseases to enable a longer life expectancy is, without doubt, a positive aspect. However, if a longer life expectancy increases the risk of developing chronic diseases, the population's disease burden is not eliminated but is just changed in character. The global average life expectancy has increased from 48 in 1955 to 66 in 1998 (WHO, 1998). But, averages can be misleading. As previously mentioned, the gap in life expectancy between the most and least developed nations can be as much as 37 years. This disparity is further reflected in the demographics of global mortality. In developed nations in 1995, only 1% of the total deaths occurred before age 5, while 77% occurred after age 65. In developing nations the statistics are reversed with 40% of deaths occurring before age 5 and only 16% after age 65. Infectious diseases, alone or in combination with chronic diseases, are still a concern in developing nations. But, developed nations with greater average life expectancies present a different mortality profile. As individuals within a population survive to adulthood and live longer, chronic diseases, which can be age dependent, emerge and prevail as the major cause of deaths.

Chronic diseases can occur with any organ system, but typically include a variety of malignancies, as well as respiratory, cardiovascular, renal, and neuropsychiatric disorders.

However, since renal and neuropsychiatric diseases combined account for only about 3% of the total deaths during any 1 year, the major emphasis here will be on cardiovascular diseases. Figure 9-3 illustrates the prevalence of these chronic diseases and their effects on mortality data for the decade between 1993 and 2003. Cardiovascular diseases far outweigh the distant second (neuropsychiatric) and third (renal disease). Interestingly,

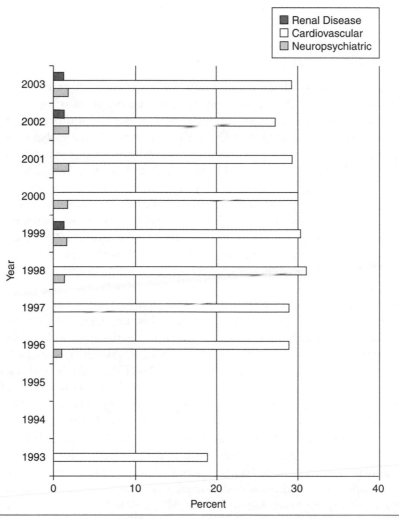

Figure 9-3 Percentage of total deaths due to selected chronic diseases among WHO member states.

Source: Data compiled from WHO World Health Reports (1995, 1996, 1997, 1998, 1999, 2000, 2001, 2002, 2003, 2004).

when available data were plotted, cardiovascular diseases could be seen to increase until the middle 1990s and remained high but relatively stable through the remainder of the observation period. During the same time interval, renal disease remained low in prevalence and unchanging while neuropsychiatric disorders, although low compared to cardiovascular disease, almost doubled in prevalence from 1996 to 2003. Although somewhat speculative, the prevalence of neuropsychiatric disorders may prove to be an index of societal stress experienced by a population.

The Cardiovascular Disease Burden

Cardiovascular disease (CVD) is a broad category of generally chronic diseases affecting the heart and blood vessels. This category includes conditions ranging from pericardial disorders, heart valve and rhythm abnormalities, elevated blood pressure values, and inflammatory disease states affecting the walls of arteries. From a global health perspective, detailed and specific diagnoses are not readily available, but generalized mortality data are. Such data again are collected by the WHO and grouped categorically into ischemic heart disease (diminished blood supply to the myocardium), cerebrovascular disease (cerebrovascular accident [CVA], stroke), and rheumatic heart disease. Synonyms for ischemic heart disease are commonly used within medical literature and require notation here to avoid confusion. These synonyms are coronary heart disease (CHD or coronary artery disease) and atherosclerotic coronary heart disease (ACHD). Data pertaining to the prevalence of these three major cardiovascular disorders are summarized in Figure 9-4 for the decade ending in 2003.

A cursory examination of the data reveals that ischemic heart disease and cerebrovascular strokes far exceed the prevalence of rheumatic heart disease, and their combined percentages accounted for about 25% of the total annual deaths worldwide by the end of the 1900s. Rheumatic heart disease is an acute inflammatory disorder that can follow a group A streptococcal (GAS) infection of the throat in 3–5% of these pharyngitis cases. During the acute inflammatory phase of the disease (rheumatic fever), valve leaflets of the heart can become inflamed and thicken from scar tissue formation. The diseased valves do not close properly leading to regurgitation (murmur) with the danger of congestive failure and death (Howson, Reddy, Ryan & Bale, 1998; Porth, 2005). Rheumatic heart disease is epidemiologically interesting because it is a chronic disease caused by an infectious microorganism that can be successfully treated with antibiotics when and where they are available. In developed, industrialized countries with access to antibiotic therapy, the prevalence of rheumatic heart disease dramatically declined in the last half of the 1900s. Although it ranked a distant third to ischemic heart disease and CVA globally, it was still responsible for 500,000 deaths worldwide in 1998 (WHO, 1998). Rheumatic heart disease can be part of the dual disease burden of developing nations where access to antibiotic therapy may be limited.

It is not just the prevalence of rheumatic heart disease that differs globally when the epidemiology of cardiovascular disease is examined. In fact, the mortality profile of major

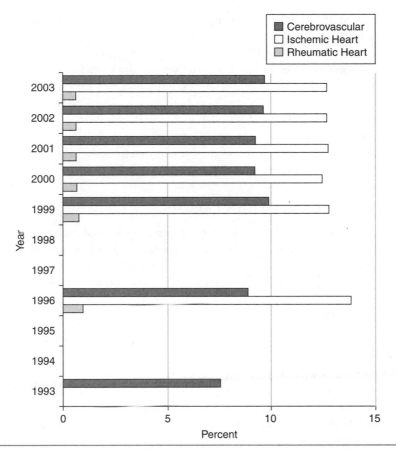

Figure 9-4 Percentage of total deaths due to selected cardiovascular diseases among UN/WHO member states.

Source: Data compiled from WHO World Health Reports (1995, 1996, 1997, 1998, 1999, 2000, 2001, 2002, 2003, 2004).

cardiovascular diseases differs with the particular country and its developmental status. In developed nations, CVD is the major cause of death within the populations, but the specific ranking of individual types of CVD shows atherosclerosis and hypertension to be the most prevalent. In developing states, CVD can be a part of the dual disease burden along with high mortality rates from a variety of infectious diseases. For example, rheumatic heart disease is the most prevalent CVD in Asia, but hypertension and related ischemic heart diseases prevail in the Americas, the Caribbean, and in more urbanized areas of Africa (Akinkugbe, 1990). This trend suggests that urbanization or the exposure to Western lifestyles may correlate positively with the prevalence of ischemic heart disease and cerebrovascular strokes.

Akinkugbe (1990) provided more supportive evidence of this trend. It has long been observed that blood pressure tends to rise with age in human populations. However, this age-dependent hypertension trend is not seen in developing populations of Africa that are isolated from Western influence and show relative freedom from known CVD risk factors. Among the examples cited for future study were the pygmies of northeastern Zaire, the bushmen of Botswana, and the Koma people of northeastern Nigeria. Additionally, a study of Kenyans showed a rise in blood pressure with migration into more urbanized areas of the country. Apparently, improvement in socioeconomic status along with exposure to Western lifestyle can yield a population within which the chronic disease profiles reflect an increased probability of developing cardiovascular disease.

Cardiovascular Disease Risk Factors

Factors that increase the risk of developing chronic cardiovascular disease may be demographic (age and gender), behavioral (lifestyle patterns), or genetic (familial). The presence of any given risk factor is considered to increase the likelihood of developing CVD, and the concurrence of multiple risk factors seriously compound this probability.

Chronological Age

Age, along with gender and familial inheritance, make up the irreversible risk factors predisposing individuals to develop CVD. Because CVDs are classed as chronic diseases, it is logical to expect them to increase in prevalence in the older age strata of a population. In fact, males above 45 years of age are at increased risk as are women older than 55 or having undergone premature menopause without exogenous estrogen (estradiol) replacement therapy (Porth, 2005). The gender differences in age susceptibility are poorly understood but may involve dietary and/or hormonal differences. For example, testosterone in males can mobilize body lipid reserves and increase blood lipid levels, while estrogen seems to protect against early onset of CVD and increase body fat stores. Female fertility depends in part upon adequate body fat stores, and the proportion of body fat to lean muscle mass increases in both sexes with advancing age.

Regardless of the underlying physiological mechanisms, phase two and phase three of population transition are characterized, in part, by increased life expectancy. This factor alone predisposes individuals to increased risk of CVD since individuals would now be living long enough to develop these chronic diseases. However, many transitional populations also develop unhealthy lifestyles, which expose them to multiple other risk factors in addition to simple aging.

Genetic Predisposition and Hyperlipidemia

Because lipids, including cholesterol and triglycerides, are insoluble in the water of blood plasma, they must be transported in minute chylomicron forms and in combination with water-soluble proteins as blood lipoproteins. These blood lipoproteins include the common low-density lipoproteins (LDL), which are high in fat and cholesterol components, and the beneficial high-density lipoproteins (HDL), which are high in protein including the cholesterol-destroying enzyme, cholesterol esterase. Additionally, a typical blood lipid profile includes metabolic intermediates such as very-low-density lipoproteins (VLDL) and intermediate-density lipoproteins (IDL) controlled also through metabolic activity of the liver. The processing of these lipid fractions involves metabolic pathways with enzymes or receptors that are produced by inherited genes of the human genome (Porth, 2005). Consequently, familial inheritance of hyperlipoproteinemia patterns constitutes a major irreversible risk factor for CVD.

Although familial inheritance is irreversible, unhealthy lipid profiles can often be controlled by medication. Yet, because of the cost of these medications, many developing populations do not have this option. Genetic predisposition is often compounded in its risk severity by dietary intake of saturated fats, trans fats, and cholesterol. These compounding factors are reversible with education regarding sound dietary practices. Again, developing populations may not have high literacy levels or may not have access to this dietary information. Making matters worse are the existence of cultural dietary preferences and societal pressures to resort to convenience foods, which may exacerbate the problem. Regardless of whether the high-risk blood lipid profile is caused by genetics or behavior, such a condition can predispose individuals to develop CVD, especially atherosclerosis.

Atherosclerosis is a type of *arteriosclerosis*, or "hardening of the arteries." Some arterial hardening is a normal consequence of aging. But, the often premature hardening due to atheromatous, fibrofatty, inflammatory lesions developing within and beneath the inner intimal layer of arteries leads to an acceleration of the sclerotization process. This inflammatory, atheromatous reaction in arteries can weaken the artery wall while occluding the vessel lumen and providing a site for platelet aggregation. Because atherosclerosis commonly affects the aorta, arteries of coronary circulation and the arterial supply to the brain, it can result in aneurysms as well as thromboembolic ischemic events leading to angina pectoris, myocardial infarction, transient ischemic attacks (TIA), or more serious cerebrovascular strokes (CVA). Clearly, genetic predisposition and/or diets rich in saturated fats and cholesterol can lead to a variety of cardiovascular and cerebrovascular disorders. The current trend for developing populations to adopt Western lifestyles with stressful, sedentary jobs and diets consisting mainly of convenience foods that are calorie rich with high salt, fat, and sugar content acts to exacerbate any genetic predisposition to develop CVD. Unfortunately, unhealthy lifestyles can act independently to increase the risk for CVD in individuals without an inherited risk.

Hypertension

Hypertension can be defined as a persistent increase in systolic and diastolic arterial pressures, and the condition can present as either *essential* or *secondary* elevations in blood pressure. Secondary hypertension results from some concurrent pathophysiological condition and is commonly seen in renal disease as a consequence of fluid and salt retention with resultant blood volume expansion. In contrast, essential hypertension is a chronic elevation of blood pressure, either systolic or diastolic, above 140/90 mm/Hg with no identifiable secondary cause. The actual causes of essential hypertension are unknown, but a number of risk factors, such as age, sodium retention, and anxiety, have been identified and correlated with the condition. However, anxiety seems to cause acute hypertensive episodes but has not been convincingly correlated with chronic hypertension (Porth, 2005).

Blood pressure is known to increase with age from an average of 50/40 mm/Hg at birth to about 120/80 mm/Hg by adolescence (Porth, 2005). Systolic pressure continues to increase slowly throughout life increasing the risk of cerebrovascular stroke in later life as high pulse pressure (systolic minus diastolic) stresses aging arteries. Because this phenomenon is not seen in isolated African populations distantly removed from Western influence, it could be speculated that lifestyle changes during population transition may be a contributing factor. People of African descent in developing or developed populations tend to show hypertension earlier in life, and they are statistically more susceptible to cardiovascular and renal damage compared to Caucasians. This observation is not completely understood and may have a genetic component. People of African descent do not respond readily to increased dietary sodium with an increased renal salt excretion (Porth, 2005). This tendency to retain salt may have had evolutionary survival value in a hot, sodium-deficient environment, but can have negative survival value in an environment with excessive dietary salt availability as exists with the convenience diets of many developed and some developing nations.

Nicholas, Agodoa, and Norris (2004) reported very little difference in prevalence of early-stage chronic kidney disease (CKD) among Caucasian, Hispanic and African people in the United States. However, people of African descent were twice as likely as Hispanics and four times more likely than Caucasians to progress to end-stage renal disease (ESRD). This racial/ethnic disparity in disease prevalence may reflect low levels of educational experience, income, and access to health care. Any or all of these factors could contribute to the observed high rates of prerenal disorders, such as hypertension and diabetes, in these minorities. These risk factors for ESRD can be controlled if detected and treated early, but both actions require educational awareness and adequate income for healthcare access.

Additionally, it is not uncommon to see several risk factors for hypertension occurring in the same individual. An example of this phenomenon, the insulin resistance syndrome (metabolic syndrome X), is a situation in which a cluster of risk factors occur simultaneously in one individual (Porth, 2005). For example, obesity and type 2 diabetes (noninsulin-dependent diabetes mellitus or NIDDM) lead to hyperinsulinemia. This elevated insulin level results in an increase in sympathetic nervous system activity, which, in turn, leads to an elevated heart rate and increased vasoconstriction. Because both cardiac output and peripheral resistance are increased simultaneously, blood pressure increases accordingly with hyperinsulinemia.

Dietary salt intake can affect blood pressure as well. High-sodium diets can expand blood volume through fluid retention and increase blood pressure. Since high-salt diets are usually high in either sodium or potassium, but rarely both, a high-sodium diet would likely be low in potassium. Low potassium can increase blood pressure, possibly by suppression of the rennin-angiotensin-aldosterone (RAA) mechanism (Porth, 2005).

Regardless of its causative factors, chronic hypertension is extremely dangerous for the simple reason that it is often asymptomatic and can exist for years undetected in persons without regular medical exams. Uncorrected elevated arterial blood pressure has negative impact on retinal, cardiac, cerebral, and renal blood vessels, as well as a direct effect on heart workload. Specifically, high blood pressure distends flexible vessel walls causing small lesions that predispose for the development of aneurysms and atheromatous plaque. Simultaneously high systemic arterial pressure increases the workload (afterload) on the left ventricle, leading to hypertrophy and, ultimately, ischemic heart disease. Myocardial ischemia evolves gradually as the enlarged muscle mass increases in its metabolic requirements for blood oxygen and nutrient delivery beyond that which the partially occluded vessels can provide. However, a sudden cardiac ischemic event (infarction) can occur should an embolus originating from an atheromatous artery totally block a smaller arterial branch of coronary circulation.

Finally, the increased renal perfusion as a result of elevated arterial blood pressure causes a concomitant increase in glomerular filtration. Chronically elevated glomerular filtration leads to an inflammatory thickening of the glomerular membrane and subsequent renal dysfunction or failure. Failing kidneys can expand blood volume by fluid retention and constrict arteries via activation of the RAA mechanism, both of which would increase pressure further and produce an unfavorable positive feedback situation leading to more progressive damage. Unfortunately, the large renal reserve in the human requires about 75% loss of renal capacity before symptoms appear. Consequently, both hypertension and its associated renal damage can progress unnoticed until serious damage is done.

It is not difficult to see how a transitioning population, which is experiencing a changing lifestyle with longer life expectancy, would be susceptible to marketing of convenience foods and might value a more leisurely life with a sedentary type of employment. Should these lifestyle modifications be accorded a high value in the changing culture, it is easy to understand the observed high levels of CVD and CVA in populations as they progress through the phases of transition.

Obesity

Obesity has become a major public health problem of global significance with its prevalence increasing in countries around the world regardless of their developmental status. The fact that obesity is currently responsible for twice as many deaths as malnutrition worldwide is not surprising since the global food supply has generally increased through enhanced productivity and distribution. Per capita daily food energy supply has increased from 2300 kcal in 1963 to 2720 kcal in 1995, and is projected to reach 2900 kcal by 2010 (WHO, 1998). This increased energy availability combined with a trend toward more sedentary urban lifestyles leads to a predictable increase in body fat storage.

By definition, obesity results when excess fat accumulates in adipose cells to the extent of endangering health. It is easier to define obesity than it is to quantify it. More specifically, at what point does energy storage as body fat cease to be an advantage and become detrimental to health given that there are cultural, racial, and gender differences that influence the perception of the ideal body type? In some cultures, excess body fat is viewed as an index of good health or prosperity. Strauss and Duncan (1998) found that even in the United States earned wages increased with body mass up to a peak within the normal BMI (body mass index) range and declined as the BMI range approached obesity. Racially, populations in colder climates tend normally to be shorter in stature with greater amounts of body fat serving physiologically for heat energy conservation. The human female tends to have a higher proportion of subcutaneous fat and, because of its role in body contouring, it can be considered a secondary sex characteristic. Physiologically, female fertility is dependent upon a certain amount of body fat, possibly ensuring adequate nutritional status to support dependent children. In the United States, minority females of African and Hispanic descent show a greater prevalence of obesity than do Caucasians (Porth, 2005). This observation suggests roles of genetics and socioeconomic status in the prevalence of obesity. Obesity is known to run in families, which indicates a genetic component of the disorder. Additionally, the diets consumed by lower-income individuals are often more dense in caloric content serving to increase the risk of obesity in lower socioeconomic strata. Thus, when people genetically predisposed to obesity occur in lower socioeconomic strata, the risk of developing obesity is compounded.

In light of these complicating factors, the WHO has attempted to quantify obesity by means of the body mass index (BMI) for which weight in kilograms is divided by height in meters squared to give a ratio value considered reflective of obesity level. By this standard, BMIs between 18.5 and 24.9 are considered normal and values greater than 30 represent obesity (WHO, 1998). However, caution must be exercised when applying these standards across racial and ethnic lines as the relationship between BMI and actual body fat varies with body build and may require adjustment for these variables. For instance, Americans of African and Polynesian descent have higher average BMIs, while Asians and Indonesians tend toward lower BMIs than Caucasians (Deurenberg, Yap, & van Staveren, 1998). Alternatively, it is important to realize that central fat (abdominal or upper-torso fat) is more indicative of health risk than is subcutaneous fat. This realization has led to the use of waist circumference or waist/hip circumference ratio as a measure of unhealthy obesity levels. These alternative indices correlate more closely with increased risk for CVD, and waist circumferences greater than 102 cm (40.2 in) for men and 88 cm (34.6 in) for women show substantially increased risk of obesity-related metabolic complications. From a health perspective, the risk of premature death more than doubles in a population when the mean BMI increases from 25 to 35 (Antipatis & Gill, 2001).

The primary reason for the effect of obesity on premature death involves the negative impact of excessive central fat on workload of the heart and on organ perfusion in general. Obese individuals with excessive central fat deposits are at greater risk of type 2 diabetes mellitus and hypertension leading to premature ischemic heart disease. It has been estimated that 2–3 mL of blood per minute is required to perfuse every 100 g of adipose tissue. This increased workload can lead to myocardial hypertrophy and increased heart muscle metabolism. Yet, the required increased blood supply through coronary circulation to support this increased metabolism may be impaired by premature atherosclerosis resulting from chronic hypertension, type 2 diabetes mellitus, and hyperlipidemia. This medley of pathophysiological disorders, which make up the metabolic syndrome X, are generally more prevalent in obese individuals. Additionally, general inflammation, indicated by C-reactive protein levels, is elevated with central obesity, and platelet aggregation is enhanced contributing further to vascular damage and increased risk of thrombotic events in obese individuals. Essentially, obesity in combination with hypertension become valid predictors of atherosclerotic cardiovascular disease that would predictably increase in prevalence in aging populations that have been chronically exposed to these risk factors (Tiengo & Avogaro, 2001).

The WHO/MONICA Project (Monitoring of Trends and Determinants in Cardiovascular Disease) collected data from randomly selected participants from different nations and found, with few exceptions, general increases in levels of obesity approaching epidemic status among UN member states over a 5-year observation interval during the 1980s. Mean BMI demonstrably increases with socioeconomic transition and is a greater problem in urban populations with more sedentary lifestyles. For each single point increase in average BMI, obesity prevalence increases by 5% within a population (Seidell, 2001). Obesity has been known to increase with age but now shows a progressively earlier age of onset increasing the time of chronic exposure for affected individuals and posing a significant child health problem. In developing populations, women were more frequently obese than men. Interestingly, men in developed countries were more likely to be obese than were either their female cohorts or males in developing countries (Antipatis & Gill, 2001; Gutzwiller, 1994). Apparently, socioeconomic status, which is reflective of income level, occupational physical activity, educational level, and place of residence, correlates with obesity prevalence. However, the correlations are not the same across different populations. In developed countries, these socioeconomic factors correlate negatively with obesity levels. But, in developing countries, the correlation is positive with early improvements in lifestyle appearing to increase obesity levels (Antipatis & Gill, 2001). This reverse correlation in developing countries may be reflective of exposure to Western culture with its convenience foods and sedentary lifestyles too early in their transition and before healthy lifestyles can be adopted. This same Western popular culture places more emphasis on the stereotypic "ideal" female body type than it does on that of males, which may help account for the gender difference in obesity observed in developed countries.

Because of the complex interactions among demographic, socioeconomic, cultural, and genetic factors that contribute to obesity prevalence, it may prove to be the most difficult CVD risk factor to control. Further complicating this control difficulty is the awareness that preventing obesity is easier than correcting it once it has developed. Preventing obesity requires early intervention with identification of at-risk individuals and subsequent application of preventive public health measures including educational awareness. Any control strategy becomes less likely to be effective as the number of obese individuals increases progressively over time, which will occur if the condition continues to appear at progressively earlier ages. Yet, without correction, the trend will only increase in negative economic impact through increasing healthcare costs and continued lost productivity.

Diabetes Mellitus

Diabetes mellitus, or sugar diabetes, is characterized by elevated blood sugar (hyperglycemia), increased urine output (polyuria) with excessive thirst, and glucose in the urine (glucosuria). It may have a variety of pathophysiological causes all related to either the availability of or the sensitivity to the hormone insulin from beta pancreatic islet cells. Type 1 diabetes, juvenile or insulin-dependent, is thought to result from insulin deficiency caused by autoimmune (type-1A) or idiopathic (type-1B) destruction of pancreatic beta cells. Type 2 diabetes (noninsulin-dependent diabetes, NIDDM) exhibits a range of pathophysiology from insulin resistance to insulin deficiency or a combination of the two. Type 2 diabetes is the most prevalent form (about 95% of total cases) and is part of the metabolic syndrome X risk factor for CVD. It is also the common form of diabetes occurring with obesity. The etiology of type 2 diabetes in obese people shows an initial resistance to insulin peripherally. This early resistance raises blood sugar level (hyperglycemia) and increases lipid lysis in adipocytes as an alternative energy source, which can lead to ketosis and ketoacidosis. Also, the elevated blood sugar increases beta cell secretion of insulin leading to hyperinsulinemia and can ultimately lead to loss of beta cell function. This hyperinsulinemia resulting from insulin resistance is an important factor in metabolic syndrome X and can lead to blood lipid abnormalities, hypertension, systemic inflammation with elevated C-reactive protein levels, and abnormal platelet aggregation. This cluster of pathophysiological signs predisposes people to atherosclerosis and ultimate ischemic heart disease and/or cerebrovascular stroke (Porth, 2005).

At this point, a dangerous disease sequela emerges. Obesity leads to peripheral insulin resistance and hyperglycemia, which, in turn, leads to hyperinsulinemia. Excess blood insulin levels lead to metabolic syndrome X culminating in CVD and/or CVA. Because central body fat increases with both advancing age and dietary caloric excess, it is reasonable to expect a higher prevalence of chronic cardiovascular and cerebrovascular diseases in populations in the second phase of transition as improvements in life expectancy and personal income occur. This would be particularly evident if changes in general lifestyle lead to unhealthy diets and more sedentary lives. Similarly, in phase three transition, where the proportion of elderly individuals increases, age-related obesity alone would be expected to increase the risk for CVD and CVA. Compound this trend with an earlier onset of obesity in the population age structure and risks for CVD and CVA can be chronically exacerbated.

Alcohol and Tobacco Use

Alcohol and tobacco use have long been correlated with chronic hepatic, gastrointestinal, respiratory, and cardiovascular diseases, but the detailed pathophysiology of their effects is poorly understood. Because alcohol and tobacco use are often seen in conjunction with obesity, hypertension, and diabetes, it is often difficult to separate true causes and effects. In fact, a major effect of alcohol and tobacco use is known to be the exacerbation of existing cardiovascular risk factors, and because of their addictive properties, they pose unique challenges for control efforts.

Alcohol consumption in excess of three drinks per day increases blood levels of cate-cholamines leading to increased blood pressure with systolic values being more dramatically affected. This effect becomes quite serious when seen in elderly or obese individuals with sedentary lifestyles and constitutes a significant health risk in these people. Alcohol decreases hepatic gluconeogenesis, a major mechanism of hepatic glucose production, and can lead to hypoglycemia. This effect is dangerous for people with diabetes who are on insulin therapy and at risk of hypoglycemia through their treatment regimens. Cerebrovascular stroke (CVA) risk increases with alcohol consumption because of three known physiological effects. First, cardiac arrhythmias, particularly atrial fibrillation (the "holiday heart" phenomenon), can transiently retard blood flow causing thrombi to form on the atrial walls or heart valve leaflets. Such thrombotic events give rise to emboli that can obstruct brain circulation causing a thromboembolic stroke. Secondly, the tendency for alcohol to exacerbate existing hypertension can contribute to accelerated atherosclerosis with resultant thromboembolic events. Finally, an enhanced effect on blood coagulation further increases thromboembolic risks (Porth, 2006; Massey & Amidon, 1998).

With chronic tobacco use, components of cigarette smoke may be toxic to the extent of causing inflammatory damage to vascular endothelium, increasing the likelihood of thrombotic events. Additionally, nicotine increases the incidence of vascular spasms while increasing plasma norepinephrine levels and lowering HDLs. These effects would predispose a smoker to hypertension, atherosclerosis, and CHD (Porth, 2006; Massey, 1998). In populations with a high underlying risk for cardiovascular disease, such as South Asia, India, and former USSR countries, tobacco consumption can serve to exacerbate their risk levels (Howson et al., 1998). Yet, tobacco use in the year 2000 was increasing with males in Russia and India (Ezzati & Lopez, 2004). These investigators also noted that in developed North America, male smoking was declining while increasing among females in the same WHO geographic region and mortality stratum.

The WHO World Health Report (1999) presented disturbing statistics on the prevalence of tobacco use globally. Estimates were that at the end of the 1900s about 4 million deaths per year were caused by tobacco use. This number was extrapolated to reach 10 million per year by 2030. It is easy to speculate that this mortality rate is primarily attributable to tobacco use in more developed nations since the per capita GDP would be high enough to permit significant tobacco use. In reality, smoking is increasing by 3.4% per year in developing countries, a level declared by the WHO as an epidemic. Because people in these developing nations must contend with infectious diseases as well, tobacco use and related chronic diseases may prove to be a significant part of their dual disease burden.

Because chronic diseases resulting from tobacco use can also be caused by other inherent or environmental risk factors, it is difficult to single out tobacco as the solitary causative agent. Consequently, it is difficult to get a reliable estimate of the true impact of tobacco use on health. Ezzati and Lopez (2000) attempted to factor out statistically any background disease rates caused by environmental factors other than smoking. They found that in developing countries cardiovascular diseases were the major smoking-attributable causes of death, representing 27.8% of total smoking-related deaths. Contrastingly, in developed countries, the cardiovascular deaths that were tobacco related jumped to 42.1%. The disproportionately high percentage of tobacco-related cardiovascular deaths in developed nations may be due to the fact that, in these populations, other risk factors for chronic diseases have been minimized by their level of socioeconomic development. A corollary to this conclusion might be that developing populations have to contend with both tobacco-related risks and with other chronic disease risks inherent in their developmental status.

Although tobacco use is increasing in developing nations, Table 9-3 shows an overall decline in developed nations, led primarily by trends in North America and Western Europe. This decline occurred after a peak in consumption in the early 1980s. This trend may reflect the efficacy of antismoking campaigns in developed nations in raising awareness of the hazards of smoking. Unfortunately, it may also reflect the recognition by tobacco manufacturers and marketers of the large potential market afforded by developing nations. As the per capita income in these developing nations increases and they are exposed to Western popular culture, they could be seen to represent an opportunity to extend tobacco sales.

After examining all these risk factors for cardiovascular disease, it is noteworthy that only chronological age and genetic inheritance represent *irreversible risks* over which indi-

TABLE 9-3   **Mean Per Capita Daily Cigarette Consumption Among UN/WHO Member States**

Status	1971	1981	1991
Developed	7.84	8.16	7.10
Developing	2.36	3.34	3.86

Source: Data compiled from WHO, 1999.

viduals have no control. The remaining risks, which are considered to be *behavioral* in nature, can be reduced or eliminated entirely by behavioral modification. To do so, however, requires first that people be made aware of potential health risks through education and, secondly, that they, through personal choice, avoid behaviors that predispose them to CVD. Unfortunately, these lifestyle behaviors can be acquired during adolescence or early adulthood leading to compounded problems. Adolescents and young adults often are perceived as being more susceptible to peer pressure and mass marketing of glamorized behaviors. They also may lack the experience and maturity to fully appreciate the risks that certain behaviors might pose since immediate negative effects of these behaviors rarely appear early in their indulgence. Additionally, alcohol, tobacco, and substance use can be psychologically and/or physiologically addictive making behavioral change in addicted individuals more difficult to achieve. Adopting these high-risk behaviors early in life increases the time of exposure as life expectancies increase within a population. In such situations, the unavoidable age risk factor eventually occurs in conjunction with the results of behavioral risks, leading to multiple risk factors and an increased probability of contracting chronic cardiovascular diseases.

Conclusions

At the beginning of this century, only 22% of the UN/WHO member states listed in Table 9-1 had attained developed status. More than 150 nations around the globe are in some phase of demographic or socioeconomic transition. Of these developing nations, 68 countries in Africa, the Americas, Southeast Asia, and the Eastern Mediterranean regions are experiencing high mortality levels at both ends of the population age strata. They contend with high child mortality and high adult mortality with generally low average life expectancies. Poverty is prevalent in these developing countries and is sustained by poor health and high fertility rates, both of which serve to keep per capita income low. Breaking this cycle of poverty is a meaningful goal of intervention efforts for this century. Interrupting this cycle requires an intervention stimulus to any or all of the following (Bloom, Canning, & Malaney, 2000):

- Income level
- Health status
- Fertility rate

Income Level Versus Health Status Improvements

It has long been known that economic and financial conditions affect access to food supply and have a direct impact on mortality. Child mortality is of particular concern because it correlates positively with high fertility rates, negatively with per capita income, and, where prevalent, it is seen to impede socioeconomic development. Prevalent childhood diseases and poor perinatal health care impact socioeconomic development by reducing the number of individuals surviving, thriving, and moving into the economically productive labor force of the middle-aged demographic strata. It would be logical to expect that improvements in economic status of a population would decrease child mortality and increase life expectancy through better living conditions and better access to health care. Although effective as a short-term emergency measure, financial aid alone without concomitant economic expansion is controversial and may be ineffective in some cases. Simple money infusion increases the cost burden on donor countries and has the inherent risk of being diverted by corrupt regimes away from targeted peoples. Additionally, a simple, short-term boost in economic activity can have the reverse effect of causing a surge in population growth, increasing dependency stress, and driving the population back to baseline per capita income levels. For an economic stimulus to have a long-term effect on the economic status of a population, it must involve sustainable measures that will perpetuate further economic growth.

Furthermore, Preston (1975) suggests that, during the 1900s, mortality became increasingly dissociated from economic level. This dissociation was occurring primarily because of the tendency for advances in medical care and health technologies to spread from developed nations to their lesser-developed neighbors. As a result of this trend, underdeveloped populations benefit by a reduction in mortality without having remarkable improvement in their per capita incomes. In these situations, mortality is more responsive to health interventions than it is to boosts in per capita income. When comparing per capita income with life expectancy in 30 countries during the 1930s and 1960s, Preston (1975) noted that average per capita incomes between $100 and $600 (in 1963 US dollars) showed dramatic increases in life expectancy. However, incomes above $600 showed little improvement in life expectancy.

It can be speculated that the observed initial economic-related improvements in life expectancy may have resulted from decreased rates of child mortality and other deaths caused by infectious disease. Because of the relative low cost of antibiotics and vaccines, child mortality and infectious diseases can be relatively inexpensively managed through minimal peripartum care, vaccination programs, and easy access to antibiotics. Thus, these initial improvements in life expectancy would require minimal financial resources. However, the chronic disease burden that inevitably occurs with an aging population of increasing life expectancy poses a different long-term problem requiring substantially more income for health management. For example, many chronic cardiovascular diseases cannot be cured in the traditional sense of the word. Instead, people afflicted with these chronic diseases undergo comparatively expensive health management regimens involving costly surgical procedures or expensive, long-term drug therapy. These treatment regimens may continue or recur throughout their life spans and can only extend their life expectancies within certain limits. Consequently, it may be that slight improvements in economic status are effective in minimizing the mortality from infectious diseases, but significantly larger economic expansion may be required to make the extended health management of chronic diseases affordable. Additionally, the simple ability to afford chronic disease management does not always guarantee a significantly longer life expectancy when compared to that of disease-free individuals.

Developed nations can and do export antibiotics, immunization vaccines, and other healthcare technologies as a humanitarian commitment to lesser-developed countries. Such exports should raise child survival rates and can give recipient populations a boost along the path of socioeconomic development. Within the context of typical population development, this practice should increase the number of people moving into the middle-aged labor force and eventually break the poverty cycle, providing sufficient income growth to manage the eventual chronic disease burden as the population ages. However, this scenario requires that the developing economy be growing at a rate capable of providing jobs for the growing labor force. Should this not be the case, the danger exists for subsequent generations to slip back into a low per capita income situation.

Further complicating the above scenario is the fact that, in addition to the export of medical technology, cultural practices may be exported as well. This potential activity is enhanced by the rapid growth of global communication. In an environment of expanding global communication, the improving lifestyles and personal income levels of developing nations may make them targets for marketing strategies undertaken to expand business consumer bases and overall profits. The impact of exporting these marketing strategies can be mixed. It may encourage people to strive toward better lifestyles through the pursuit of jobs that lead them to safer work environments and higher educational achievements. However, it can also result in the adoption of lifestyles that include less physical activity and greater dependence on convenience diets and other unhealthy behaviors. The combination of sedentary lifestyle with unhealthy diets and behaviors predisposes people to increased risk of chronic cardiovascular disease later in life as multiple risk factors begin to accrue along with normal aging. Moreover, as adoption of these unhealthy practices occurs progressively earlier in life, the greater will be the likelihood of developing chronic disease.

Tobacco use and obesity serve as examples of this trend. Tobacco-related deaths are at nearly equal levels of about 2.4 million per year in both developed and developing countries (Ezzati & Lopez, 2004). About 7% of the world's population have BMIs greater than 30, and obesity is occurring at earlier ages (Seidell, 2001). This increasing prevalence of obesity is occurring in both developed and developing countries and is likely related to unhealthy dietary practices in populations with increasingly more sedentary lifestyles.

Fertility Rate Improvements

Poston (2000) considered four specific factors to have influential effects on fertility: (1) advances in economic development through participation in a nonagricultural labor force; (2) improvement in general health conditions with reduction in infant mortality; (3) improvement in social conditions particularly in educational attainment; and (4) absolute and relative improvement in female status within the population. These four factors are not without interactions. For example, movement from an agricultural to an industrial labor force can generate higher per capita income. Higher incomes relate to better access to health care and education. Better education, especially among females, leads to improved female status within the population. Better education can also lead circuitously back to improved jobs and better health conditions. More affluent and better educated populations with improved health conditions show lower fertility rates as large families become more of a liability in a nonagrarian lifestyle. Thus, improvements in any or all of these factors should lead naturally to a decline in fertility. Such a decline in fertility correlates with elevated socioeconomic status and can contribute to breaking the poverty cycle of a developing population by relieving the child dependency stress while increasing per capita GDP.

All the fertility influences described above can occur naturally in the typical developmental process of a population. However, fertility declines can be accelerated over and above that which would occur naturally by governmental mandate as was done in the People's Republic of China (mainland China). In the 1970s China instituted a coercive fertility control program as discussed earlier in this chapter. Although it was successful in dropping the fertility rate below replacement levels, Taiwan was able to accomplish a similar reduction in fertility without direct government intervention. In Taiwan, the natural socioeconomic development process was effective in dropping fertility rate, presumably by affecting the perceived or actual economic costs and social value of children (Poston, 2000). Because both approaches were effective in reducing fertility rates below replacement levels, these examples illustrate how different social and political climates in two separate populations can produce similar outcomes.

Future Considerations

Even in developed countries, high prevalence levels of chronic diseases pose a significant economic threat through lost productivity from afflicted workers, along with increased healthcare costs. If this economic impact can be significant in developed market economies, it would be considerably more damaging to the fragile, fledgling economies of developing nations. Thus, a major problem confronting both developed and developing economies becomes one of deciding how to prioritize expenditures for chronic disease risk avoidance compared to that required for the expansion of healthcare infrastructure to sufficiently manage increasing levels of chronic disease. Both approaches require a significant, though not necessarily equal, financial commitment. Chronic health care has historically proven to be more costly than education. Regardless of the priority, the costs must come from the overall GDP generated through a population's economic activity, and its economy must be strong enough to withstand the added stress. As a larger percentage of GDP is diverted into risk management and health care for the chronically ill, less will be available for economic expansion, and the risk of economic stagnation or decline increases. The decision is not a simple one and, in reality, both probably will have to be dealt with simultaneously, and the combined actions will take a financial toll on a population's economy.

References

Akinkugbe, O. O. (1990). Epidemiology of cardiovascular disease in developing countries. *Journal of Hypertension, 8*(7): S233–S237.

Antipatis, V. J., & Gill, T. P. (2001). Obesity as a global problem. In P. Bjorntorp, (Ed.), *International textbook of obesity* (pp. 2–22). New York: John Wiley & Sons Ltd.

Bloom, D. E., Canning, D., & Malaney, P. N. (2000). Population dynamics and economic growth. In C. Y. Cyrus Chu, & R. Lee, (Eds.), *Population and development review: A supplement to volume 26* (p. 257). New York, Population Council.

Deurenberg, P., Yap, M., & van Staveren, W. A. (1998). Body mass index and percent body fat: A meta analysis among different ethnic groups. *International Journal of Obesity, 22,* 1164–1171.

Ezzati, M., & Lopez, A. D. (2004). Regional, disease specific patterns of smoking-attributable mortality in 2000. *Tobacco Control, 13,* 388–395.

Gutzwiller, F. (1994). Monitoring of cardiovascular disease and risk factor trends: Experiences from the WHO/MONICA project. *Annals of Medicine, 26*(1), 61–65.

Howson, C. P., Reddy, K. S., Ryan, T. J., & Bale, J. R. (1998). *Control of cardiovascular diseases in developing countries: Research, development, and institutional strengthening* (p. 237). Washington, DC: National Academy Press.

Lee, R., & Cyrus Chu, C. Y. (2000). Introduction. In C. Y. Cyrus Chu, & R. Lee, (Eds.), *Population and development review: A supplement to volume 26* (pp. 1–9). New York: Population Council.

Massie, B. M. (1998). Systemic hypertension. In L. M. Tierney, Jr., S. J. McPhee, & M. A. Papadakis (Eds.), *Current medical diagnosis and treatment* (pp. 429–447, 37th ed.). Stamford, CT: Appleton and Lange.

Massie, B. M., & Amidan, T. M. (1998). Heart. In L. M. Tierney, Jr., S. J. McPhee, & M. A. Papadakis (Eds.), *Current medical diagnosis and treatment* (pp. 333–348, 37th ed.). Stamford, CT: Appleton and Lange.

Nicholas, S., Agodoa, L., & Norris, K. (2004). Ethnic disparities in the prevalence and treatment of kidney disease. *Nephrology News and Issues, November,* 29–36.

Phipps, S. R. (2006). Settlement and migration. In R. Abramson & J. Haskell (Eds.), *Encyclopedia of Appalachia* (pp. 285–292). Knoxville, TN: University of Tennessee Press.

Porth, C. M. (2005). *Pathophysiology: Concepts of altered health states* (p. 1582, 7th ed.). Philadelphia: Lippincott Williams and Wilkins.

Poston, D. L. Jr. (2000). Social and economic development and the fertility transitions in mainland China and Taiwan. In C. Y. Cyrus Chu, & R. Lee (Eds.), *Population and development review: A supplement to volume 26* (pp. 40–41). New York: Population Council.

Preston, S. H. (1975). The changing relation between mortality and level of economic development. *Population Studies, 29,* 213–248.

Seidell, J. C. (2001). The epidemiology of obesity. In P. Bjorntorp (Ed.), *International textbook of obesity* (pp. 23–29). New York: John Wiley & Sons Ltd.

Strauss, J., & Duncan, T. (1998). Health, nutrition and economic development. *Journal of Economic Literature, 36*(June), 766–817.

Tiengo, A., & Avogaro, A. (2001). Cardiovascular disease. In P. Bjorntorp (Ed.), *International textbook of obesity* (pp. 365–377). New York: John Wiley & Sons Ltd.

World Health Organization (WHO). (1995). *World health report 1995: Bridging the gaps.* Geneva, Switzerland: Author.

WHO. (1996). *World health report 1996: Fighting disease, fostering development.* Geneva, Switzerland: Author.

WHO. (1997). *World health report 1997: Conquering suffering, enriching humanity.* Geneva, Switzerland: Author.

WHO. (1998). *World health report 1998: Life in the 21st century: A vision for all.* Geneva, Switzerland: Author.

WHO. (1999). *World health report 1999: Making a difference.* Geneva, Switzerland: Author.

WHO. (2000). *World health report 2000: Health systems: Improving performance.* Geneva, Switzerland: Author.

WHO. (2001). *World health report 2001: Mental health: New understanding, new hope.* Geneva, Switzerland: Author.

WHO. (2002). *World health report 2002: Reducing risks, promoting healthy life.* Geneva, Switzerland: Author.

WHO. (2003). *World health report 2003: Shaping the future.* Geneva, Switzerland: Author.

WHO. (2004). *World health report 2004: Changing history.* Geneva, Switzerland: Author.

WHO. (2005). *World health report 2005: Make every mother and child count.* Geneva, Switzerland: Author.

Chapter 10

Global Perspectives on Diabetes and Respiratory and Orthopedic Chronic Diseases

Janice Long, Betsy Rodriguez, and Carol Holtz

Introduction: The Global Burden of Chronic (Noncommunicable) Diseases

Globalization, which is the increasing interconnectedness of countries and the openness of borders to ideas, people, commerce, and finances, has both beneficial and harmful effects on the health of people worldwide. Historically, most of the attention has been given to control and treatment of infectious diseases, national security threats, provision of affordable medicines, and public policy changes for international trade and financial agreements. In contrast, the noncommunicable diseases, such as heart disease, lung disease, stroke, cancer, diabetes, and obesity, have been long neglected.

In 2003 there was an estimated 56 million deaths worldwide, of which 60% were caused by chronic noncommunicable illnesses. Only in Africa do communicable diseases cause more deaths than noncommunicable diseases. The highest rates of noncommunicable diseases are found in central and eastern European countries. Within the United States, chronic diseases today account for 70% of deaths of all Americans and for 75% of the total annual healthcare costs (Beaglehole & Yach, 2003).

Global prevalence of all leading chronic diseases is increasing, with the majority occurring in developing countries, and is projected to increase over the next two decades. Between 1990 and 2020, deaths from cardiovascular disease are expected to rise 120% for women and 137% for men. Chronic diseases are not simply replacing acute infectious diseases in developing countries, but are actually causing a double burden of disease (Porter, 2004).

New global alliances and funding have helped in research and treatment of many communicable diseases, particularly HIV/AIDS, malaria, tuberculosis, and vaccine-preventable diseases. Unfortunately, chronic diseases such as cardiovascular diseases, cancer, chronic respiratory diseases, and diabetes have been neglected, and now are part of the major global burden of diseases in all regions of the world except Africa. Chronic diseases in China and India are often overlooked. For instance in 2000, 2.8 million cardiovascular deaths occurred in China, and 2.6 million deaths occurred in India (Porter, 2004).

Causes of chronic noncommunicable diseases include an ageing population with lower fertility rates and increasing childhood survival. Global trade and marketing are promoting diets with higher proportions of saturated fats and sugars. In addition, tobacco use and decreased physical activity have led to atherosclerosis and many noncommunicable diseases. "Tobacco is the only consumer product, that when used as recommended by its manufacturers, eventually kills half of its regular users" (Beaglehole & Yach, 2003, p. 904).

Tobacco companies have had increasing difficulty in marketing their products in developed countries, but have been very aggressive in promotion of their products in developing countries. Diet patterns are changing in developing countries, which include more saturated fats and less natural complex carbohydrates, such as fruits and vegetables. In China the obesity rates in urban children ages 2–6 years increased from 1.5% in 1989 to 12.6% in 1997. By the year 2020, chronic diseases will become the leading contributors to early death and disability in many areas of the world because of increasing life expectancies. A nutrition transition including an increase in fat and sodium intake with a decline in complex carbohydrate consumption and reduced physical activity will lead to obesity in many developing countries. The falling price of vegetable fat and the rising price of dietary fiber from fruits and vegetables will also help facilitate these changes. The increasing consumption of fat as an energy source in the daily diet in China has greatly increased within all income classes from 1981 to 1993 (Beaglehole & Yach, 2003).

Tobacco consumption is increasing rapidly worldwide and has had, and will continue to have, a great health impact. Death rates from tobacco use are estimated to rise in India from 1.4% in 1990 to 13.3% in 2020, and during the same time frame, from 9.2% to 16% in China. Tobacco consumption is declining in developed countries but is significantly rising in developing countries. The tobacco industry is aggressively marketing in developing countries (Reddy & Srinath, 1999). Stated previously, reduction in lung cancer rates is due to the fall in tobacco consumption by men in developed countries as a result of dissemination of scientific research. However, in many European countries, in Asia, and in the Middle East, lung cancer is increasing, especially in women (Reddy, 1999; WHO, Integrated chronic disease prevention and control, 2005).

The effects of chronic diseases continue to be a major world problem. The poor are becoming more vulnerable to chronic diseases and have limited access to expensive technology and pharmaceuticals to cope with the increased demand. Epidemics of chronic disease are expected to shift from richer developed countries to poorer developing countries, and also from the rich to the poor within all countries. The globalization of knowledge and funds for prevention education and treatment of chronic diseases could help developing countries combat these burdens of disease. Investors from richer nations have concerns about the health and stability of their labor forces and consumer markets in developing countries. In addition, the globalization of travel can have a desirable effect in promoting better health throughout the world. For example, the American traveler who used to enjoy McDonald's hamburgers and Coca Cola in developing countries may later be seeking smoke-free airports and low-fat foods, with a newly acquired healthier lifestyle (Reddy, 1999).

Diets low in energy-dense foods (that are high in saturated fats and sugar) and high in fruits and vegetables, together with more active lifestyles, will help combat chronic diseases. The World Health Organization (WHO) and the Food and Agriculture Organization (FAO) gave new recommendations for governments to help decrease chronic diseases. These include reducing energy-rich foods high in saturated fat and sugar, cutting sodium in the diet, increasing fresh fruits and vegetables in the diet, and having moderate intensity physical activity for at least one hour per day. Alcohol consumption is also a global health issue; its use is directly related to cirrhosis of the liver, some cancers, and the majority of causes of violence and injuries (WHO, 2005).

Because of the increasing burden of chronic diseases, the United States faces a continuing financial and health crisis. It is most necessary to move from a palliative medical model of treating illness to one in which prevention is the greatest priority. Increases in funding plus investments in public health prevention programs are necessary to combat the ever-increasing numbers of people with chronic illnesses (Katz, 2004). In 2002 the WHO requested a global strategy on diet, physical activity, and health. This was a comprehensive approach to chronic disease prevention and control directed at governments.

Few chronic diseases take the toll on the world's population as seen in the burden of diabetes and asthma. These conditions are two of the most common chronic conditions affecting adults and children in every country. Lifestyles and environmental and social risk factors, many of which are controllable, contribute to the development or worsening of these chronic conditions despite advances in science and technology that make the conditions avoidable or controllable (Marmont & Wilkinson, 2002). Expert panels in both diabetes and asthma have made recommendations for diagnosis and treatment with guidelines and protocols available over the Internet in many languages.

Although there are numerous chronic global health issues that have significant worldwide concern, the authors have selected for this chapter the common global chronic diseases of musculoskeletal disorders, asthma, and diabetes. A diabetes intervention case study project for selected Latin American countries is also included.

Musculoskeletal Disorders

In both developed and developing countries the most frequent cause of disability severely affecting people's daily lives is musculoskeletal conditions. Although diseases that cause the greatest mortality get the most public attention, musculoskeletal diseases are the major cause of morbidity throughout the world. Longer life expectancy, with an increasing number of elderly in all population groups, has caused the increased prevalence of these disorders. Musculoskeletal conditions are very common worldwide and include more than 150 different diseases and syndromes. The main types are rheumatoid arthritis, osteoarthritis, osteoporosis, spinal disorders, major limb trauma, gout, and fibromyalgia. Limb trauma is increasing rapidly especially in developing countries due to road traffic accidents. Rheumatoid arthritis leads to work disability and limitation of movement after approximately 10 years from disease onset. Those diagnosed with musculoskeletal diseases frequently have difficulty with activities of daily living, such as eating, walking, toileting, and bathing. Forty percent of people over 70 years suffer from osteoarthritis of the knee, and of those having this disease, 80% have some degree of limitation of movement (Figure 10-1). Low back pain has reached worldwide epidemic proportions. In 1990 an estimated 1.7 million people had hip fractures caused by osteoporosis, and by 2050 the number of people affected will exceed 6 million worldwide. The greatest incidence of musculoskeletal disease is expected to be found in countries such as Brazil, Chile, China, Pakistan, the Philippines, India, Indonesia, Malaysia, Mexico, and Thailand. In the developed countries of the world, the United States, European countries, Japan, New Zealand, and Australia all have high rates (WHO, 2001).

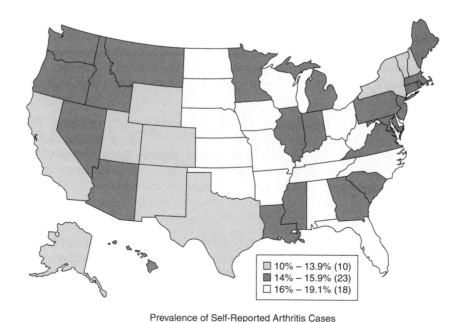

Prevalence of Self-Reported Arthritis Cases

Figure 10-1 Incidence of arthritis in the United States by location. Note: Parenthetical figures indicate numbers of states in each range.

Source: CDC.

The cost as reflected in treatment and loss of work resulting from musculoskeletal diseases can be staggering. Musculoskeletal diseases were the most expensive disease category in a Swedish cost-of-illness study, representing 22.6% of the total cost of illness. Within the United Kingdom work-related musculoskeletal disorders were responsible for 11 million days lost from work in 1995. These disorders are the second most common reason for consulting a doctor in many countries and result in up to 10-20% of all medical consultations. People infected with HIV often experience musculoskeletal symptoms secondary to the infection. Studies have demonstrated that 70% of patients with HIV/AIDS had bone, joint, or muscle involvement. Muscle disease in these patients can be a result of inflammation, infection, or related tumor growth. Although muscle pain can result at any phase of HIV, it generally comes during the later stages (Understanding the burden, 2001).

Major types of worldwide musculoskeletal conditions include the following (WHO, 2001):

- Rheumatoid arthritis—A chronic systemic disease that affects the joints, connective tissue, muscle, tendons, and fibrous tissue, with an onset mainly in the 20-40 year age range. It is a chronic disability causing pain and deformity.

- Osteoarthritis—A noninflammatory joint disease affecting the articular cartilage, associated with aging, and attacking stressed joints such as the knees, hips, finger joints, and lower back.

- Osteoporosis—A disease with reduction in bone mass resulting in fractures. This may be caused by genes, inadequate intake of calcium and Vitamin D, physical inactivity, or decrease in ovary function at menopause in women.

- Spinal disorders—Specific diseases of the spine, including trauma, mechanical injury, spinal cord injury, inflammation, infection, or tumors. These disorders may involve muscles, nerves, intervertebral disks, joints, cartilage, tendons, and ligaments.

- Severe limb trauma—Results from permanent disability from fractures, crushing injuries, dislocations, open wounds, amputation, and blood and nerve vessel injuries.

Rheumatoid Arthritis

Rheumatoid arthritis is the most frequent disability in the United States affecting more than 70 million people, or 1 out of every 3 adults. Costs in the United States include more than $16 billion annually. Another $80 billion is lost in productivity and wages as a result of pain and disability from this condition. Pain, together with functional limitations and dependence on others, is an increasing problem. It is a chronic, autoimmune, inflammatory disease of the joints with unknown etiology and no cure, characterized with periods of exacerbation (very active state) to remission (inactive state). Besides the physiological problems, it also may include psychological outcomes such as depression and anxiety (Chui, Lau, & Yau, 2004).

Twice as many women as men are affected by this disease. It mostly occurs in the United States and northern European countries, and more rarely in developing countries. Very few cases are found in Africa, but of those in African countries, more are found in urban areas. Smoking and obesity as well as family genetics are known risk factors (Woolf & Pfleger, 2003).

Many self-management programs have been established worldwide including in the United States, Australia, Canada, and England. These include relaxation techniques, exercise, joint protection, pain and stress coping strategies, and self-management skills. In Hong Kong, PRC, a community-based rehabilitation program offers knowledge and skill information. In a study examining a rheumatoid arthritis self-management program in Hong Kong, researchers found that the program of exercise, self-management skills, and communication with doctors enhanced positive self-help behavior and reduced visits to the general physician (Chui, Lau, & Yau, 2004).

Acupuncture therapy for rheumatoid arthritis is currently being tested in studies in Tel Hashomer, Israel. Acupuncture is a method of therapy in which thin needles are inserted into specific points (assisting energy flow), and for each treatment specific ones are manipulated. According to traditional Chinese medicine philosophy, illness results from an imbalance of energy flow, and the acupuncture needle insertions are connected to precise locations or "meridians" that are certain sites for channels of energy. In spite of the use of medications for treatment of rheumatoid arthritis, complementary medicine has been found to be very useful as a treatment for many patients. In the United States 26.7% of the population use some form of complementary medicine, such as acupuncture, for treatment for rheumatoid arthritis in addition to seeing a medical doctor for treatment (Zan-Bar, Aron, & Shoenfeld, 2004).

Many patients with rheumatoid arthritis who have muscle and joint pain are able to reduce their pain by doing physical exercise in heated pools. Since the 1960s Swedish patients with inflammatory joint disease have been prescribed intensive physiotherapy in a subtropical climate, called "climate therapy." The patients went to Mediterranean areas with warmer climates, which were proven to be far superior to outpatient treatment in Sweden. In a study in 1996, patients went to Tiberias, Israel's hot springs, for therapy for 4 weeks, staying in special hotels for treatments, and then returned to Sweden for continued outpatient care. Results indicated that the patients improved significantly after returning to Sweden, but then improvements were less after 3 and 6 months after returning (Hafstrom & Hallengren, 2003).

Osteoarthritis

Osteoarthritis is a disease in which there is a loss of articular cartilage within the synovial joints, which is associated with hypertrophy (thickening) of the bone. People with this disease often have joint pain, tenderness, limitation of movement, crepitus, and local inflammation. It can occur in any joint, but most often occurs in the hip, knee, joints of the hand, foot, and spine. This disease causes great pain and also loss of height as well as significant amount of bone fractures. Worldwide estimates for this disease are 9.6% for men and 18% for women, both genders being age 60 or greater. Research reveals that this condition is most prevalent in the United States and other European countries than elsewhere in the world, and the most commonly affected area is the knee (Chui, Lau, & Yau, 2004).

Osteoporosis

Osteoporosis is characterized by low bone mass and a deterioration of the bone tissue. This results in bone fragility and vulnerability to bone fractures. The bone mineral density is greater than 2.5 standard deviations below the mean bone mineral density of young women. In addition, osteopenia (low bone mass) is between 1 to 2.5 standard deviations below the mean bone mass of young adult women. Those affected often have hip, vertebrae, and forearm bone fractures. This disease most often occurs in postmenopausal Caucasian women, living in the northern parts of the United States. In the United Kingdom, 23% of women age 50 or older have osteoporosis. This disease affects more than 75 million people in Europe, Japan, and Latin and North America. In the United States alone, about 15% of the people have osteoporosis. The prevalence increases with age, and the condition is not reversible. Physical activity and adequate diet intake of especially calcium and Vitamin D are vital for maintaining healthy bones and preventing this disease (Chui, Lau, & Yau, 2004).

In Western Ontario, Canada, a medical study using leech therapy was found to be helpful in treating arthritis of the knee. Leech therapy was widely used in ancient times, but declined rapidly in Europe and the United States with the use of modern surgery and medicine. A polypeptide hirudin, an active substance in leech saliva was found to be effective for relieving pain in the knee in osteoarthritis (Michalsen, Klotz, Ludtke, Moebus, Spahn, & Dobos, 2003).

Hip Fracture

The National Center for Injury Prevention and Control states that 3–4% of older adults fall, causing greater that 400,000 hip fractures in the United States each year. Within this group 4% die during their initial hospitalization, and 10–35% die within the first year. Of those who do survive, many never regain their prefracture level of functioning. Most hip fractures result from underlying chronic musculoskeletal conditions, such as arthritis, osteoporosis, or a bone malignancy (CDC, 2004).

Diabetes

Diabetes has its name derived from the Greek word meaning "going through" and the Latin word, *mellitus*, which means "honey" or "sweet." This disease can be traced to the first century AD, when Aretaeus the Cappadocian described the disorder as a chronic affliction characterized by intense thirst and voluminous, honey-sweet urine (Porth, 2007). It is a devastating disease that affects nearly every system of the body. As a disorder of the metabolism of carbohydrates, proteins, and fats, diabetes mellitus results from alterations in insulin development and use in the body. Uncontrolled diabetes results from the inability of the body to affect the way glucose is transported into fat and muscle cells. Without the ability to move the glucose to the cells where it can be broken down into energy, the body is starved and fat and proteins are broken down. As a result, the effects of the disease can be seen across nearly all organs and functions of the body.

Types of Diabetes Mellitus

Diabetes is classified as type 1 diabetes, type 2 diabetes, or gestational diabetes. Types 1 and 2 affect both genders and gestational diabetes occurs only in pregnant women. Each type of diabetes has the characteristic of glucose elevation, but each differs in the type of population effected and treatment protocols.

Type 1 Diabetes

Type 1 diabetes is characterized by the destruction of the beta cells of the pancreas and is thought to be mediated by immune factors or may be idiopathic (Atkinson & Eisenbarth, 2001). Type 1 diabetes is rare in occurrence, affecting only about 5–10% of people within the United States and Europe. Most individuals with type 1 diabetes are thought to have the immune-mediated form of the condition (Porth, 2007). Type 1 diabetes has also been referred to as *juvenile diabetes* and occurs most often in young persons, but can occur at any age. The condition is characterized by the complete inability of the pancreas to produce insulin with resulting high blood glucose and muscle and fat cell catabolism. Without insulin administration, body cells will starve and die.

Type 2 Diabetes

Type 2 diabetes occurs when there is a decreased amount of insulin or the cells of the body are resistant to the insulin produced and a relative loss of insulin is present. Type 2 diabetes accounts for 90–95% of all persons with diabetes. Most people with type 2 diabetes are adults older than 40 years of age and have some degree of obesity. The symptoms of type 2 diabetes—fatigue, frequent urination, and slow healing sores—can be difficult to detect and often develop unnoticed for years before a person is diagnosed. As a result, persons with type 2 diabetes often learn they have the condition when they are diagnosed with a diabetes complication. Complications often found in type 2 diabetes include microvascular disorders that can cause visual loss, renal disease, or peripheral vascular disease. Although obesity and physical activity are the chief factors contributing to the condition, genetic links are also implicated.

Gestational Diabetes Mellitus

Defined by its name, gestational diabetes mellitus (GDM), occurs during pregnancy. It involves an intolerance to glucose that may be found in 2–14% of pregnancies (American Diabetes Association [ADA], 2004) and in particular those who have had a prior history of gestational diabetes, with a family history, are obese, had a high birth-weight baby in the past, or have had more than five pregnancies. With gestational diabetes early diagnosis is critical in addition to early intervention with careful medical management to prevent maternal and fetal complications (Masharani, Karam, & German, 2004). Treatment of GDM includes close monitoring for the mother and fetus and maintenance of low blood glucose levels in the mother with frequent maternal glucose monitoring.

In 1995 the World Health Organization estimated the prevalence rate of diabetes (all types) in participating countries to be approximately 135 million. The International Diabetes Federation (IDF) regions found a much higher increase in 2003 when the organization reported global estimates of 194 million people living with diabetes. Of those with diabetes, approximately 85–95% have type 2 diabetes in developed countries and an even higher rate of people in developing countries have this disease (International Diabetes Federation (IDF, 2003). Although type 1 diabetes is less frequent in global occurrence, there are variations among the patterns of prevalence of the condition. The prevalence of type 1 diabetes is higher in North America (0.25%), followed by Europe (0.19%). The IDF findings reported an even more worrisome fact that public awareness about diabetes is quite low (IDF, 2003).

At the current global growth rate of diabetes mellitus, the prevalence of the condition will increase to much more serious levels over the next two decades. The IDF reports projections for the global prevalence of diabetes by the year 2025 to approach 6.3% for adults between 20–79 years of age (IDF, 2003). Education and care interventions are needed to forestall the disease, most of which is influenced by lifestyle (IDF, 2003).

The highest regional prevalence of diabetes is seen in North America (NA) followed by Europe (EU) both in 2003 and as projected for 2025. The Southeast Asian (SEA) region has the highest prevalence of impaired glucose tolerance over all regions.

Age of Onset and Prevalence of Type 2 Diabetes

A younger population has more recently been identified with type 2 diabetes and is increasing in prevalence. It is thought that over the next 10 years, type 2 diabetes will become the predominant form of diabetes in the young in some ethnic groups worldwide (International Diabetes Federation Consensus Workshop, 2004). Mohan and colleagues (2006) reported that in 2005, in Chennai, India, the age-standardized prevalence of diabetes increased from 1989 to present by 72%. Of those who were from 40–49 years of age, 20% now have diabetes (Mohan et al., 2006). A study conducted by Tseng and colleagues (2006) found that incidences of diabetes in Taiwan increased across all age groups but was highest in the youngest groups (less than 35 years of age and including children). The study reported that obesity was an increasing problem particularly in the school children.

A study of over 10,000 in one region in the United Kingdom also found a rising prevalence of diabetes by age with the prevalence of diabetes in females increasing above that of males, beginning in the 30th year of age. Also noted in the study was a decrease of diabetes in those over 80 years of age (Morgan, Currie, Stott, Smithers, Butler, and Peters, 2000).

Another study conducted in Fukuoka, Japan, found that in men and women changes in lifestyle to a more Western diet and increases in dietary fat consumption were possible contributing factors to the increased prevalence of diabetes (Ohmura et al., 1993).

A study conducted in Italy was similar in results with increases in prevalence of type 2 diabetes, particularly in the older than 44-year-old groups, and was associated with increased rates of obesity. This suggests a lifestyle-related contribution to the burden of diabetes (Garancini et al., 1995). As a result of lifestyle behaviors that lead to obesity, many people worldwide are at high risk for the cascade of symptoms that often follows overweight and obesity and lead to diabetes. Obesity is one of the most difficult risk factors to change once it is present, so intervening before overweight occurs is the best measure for preventing diabetes in all age groups.

Treatment Recommendations

The cornerstone of treatment for diabetes has been the active participation in care by the individual who has the condition (ADA Task Force to Revise the National Standards, 2004). To assume responsibility for one's own care, a diagnosis must be made. With the findings of the IDF suggesting that one of the greatest barriers to treatment is the lack of the public's awareness of the disease, campaigns to educate the public must become the priority global intervention. Education on diabetic symptoms in concert with screening campaigns for those at risk for diabetes could offer a first stage of awareness to the populations of the world where diabetes or impaired glucose tolerance is most prevalent.

Early intervention with diabetes education and dietary and lifestyle adjustments before complications are present could provide for improved overall outcomes of the disease. Self-monitoring for blood glucose, a process that can easily be performed in the home, offers promise for individuals to manage their disease on a daily basis by knowing their blood sugar levels. Tests for the average blood glucose level over a 3-month period (hemoglobin A_1c or HbA_1c) are also available, though more costly. Research in the United Kingdom indicates that for type 2 diabetes, every 1 point reduction of the hemoglobin A_1c toward normal levels brings reductions in the risk for many of the complications that lead to the morbidity and mortality of diabetes (Stratton, Cull, Adler, Matthews, Neil, & Holman, 2006).

The ADA and the European Union-International Diabetes Federation (EUIDF) recognize that lifestyle changes alone are inadequate in the long term to achieve and maintain weight loss. Exercise and medical and nutrition adjustments are needed to attain the HbA_1c levels sought (Nathan et al., 2006). The ADA recommends that individuals try to maintain HbA_1c levels below 7.0%, and the European Union-International Diabetes Foundation recommends a level at or below 6.5%, which is closer to the normal level. Even with global advances in pharmacologic therapy included in current-day management, reduction and maintenance of near normal levels of glycemia have not been possible. The consensus of the ADA and the EUIDF supports the position that any reduction of HbA_1c offers a reduction in risk for the complications of diabetes. The complex nature of diabetes makes treatment quite problematic, and morbidity is particularly high in relationship to cardiovascular disease.

The United Kingdom Prospective Diabetes Study (Stratton et al., 2006), found that hypertension and glycemia have additive effects in the development of cardiovascular mortality, and that by treating both together, the cardiovascular risk for complications could be markedly reduced. Yet studies suggest that hypertension control is not consistently well achieved (Liebl, Mata, & Eschwege, 2002). Many factors must be considered in the treatment of diabetes, from socioeconomic implications and lifestyle factors to complex comorbid conditions that may accompany diabetes. Research is constantly underway to prevent diabetes and to reduce the seriousness of the complications. The greatest effect on diabetes outcome is thought to be in the prevention of the condition with changes in lifestyles that predispose individuals to the disease.

Cost of Diabetes Care

The concern for the world is not only in the human cost and loss of life, but also in the economic burden the disease causes. The evidence of this burden was reported by Koster, von Ferer, Ihle, Schubert, and Hauner (2006) as diabetes mellitus is a "public health issue of significant economic importance with a globally increasing prevalence . . . And one that has complications that contribute to long-term disease duration" (p. 1498). Studies from the United States and Europe suggest that the economic burden of diabetes is high (ADA, 1998; Liebl, Neiß, Spannheimer, Reitberger, Wagner, & Gortz, 2001). Age and type of treatment contribute to the overall cost of treatment, with the highest costs seen in the treatment of the complications of diabetes. As one of the most common global noncommunicable diseases, diabetes ranks as the fourth or fifth cause of death in developed countries (IDF, 2003). Complications from diabetes range from coronary artery and peripheral vascular disease, stroke, neuropathy, renal failure, to increased disability and reduced life quality and expectancy. This health issue "results in enormous health costs for virtually every society" (IDF, 2003, p. 7). Although it is important to remember that prevention of diabetes would contribute the greatest cost savings, prevention of complications through tight glycemic control and hypertension management is needed to reduce the economic burden of costly complications once diabetes is diagnosed.

Diabetes Prevention

With advances in transportation and technology, survival in the modern world is much different than that of years ago. Exercise has little by little been taken out of the daily life of the world's population. "In their struggle for longevity, modern-day humans are dying because of lack of physical exercise" (Erikssen, 2001, p. 571). Statistics support the fact that physical exercise is on a downward trend in the United States and in other developed nations (Snell & Mitchell, 1999). Automobiles carry people directly from the interior of their home to their destination, and parking lots for work and school often offer convenience for parking near the building entrances. Technology also has offered more advances in communication so that children and adults alike have access to friends and family via phones or the Internet, so the need to physically meet may be lessened. Even recreational activities in a virtual environment makes playtime something that occurs in a chair or on a sofa in the confines of the private residence, and running and playing are less often chosen as alternates as compared to the appeal of an online game or TV show. Fast food and vending machines with high-calorie, high-fat drinks and foods offer quick treats to all age groups and increase the diabetes risk, particularly for those who infrequently exercise.

Overweight in children is a growing worldwide concern gaining the attention of the World Health Organization (WHO) as the implications and severity of obesity are assessed in member countries (Schoenborn, Adams, & Barnes, 2002). In the United States, the Centers for Disease Control and Prevention (CDC) has placed the problem of obesity in the forefront of national efforts after studies and trends reveal that the burden of the condition on the US population is growing (Ogden, Flegal, Carroll, & Johnson, 2002). The National Health and Nutrition Examination Survey (NHANES) from 1988 to 1994 showed rates of overweight in children and adolescents at about 10%, rising to 14.4% by 1999–2000 and finally, the 2001–2002 survey findings indicated that 16% of children between 6–11 years of age were overweight (Hedley, Ogden, Johnson, Carroll, Curtin, & Flegal, 2004). The childhood overweight impact varies by US region, as evidenced by one study conducted in a rural region of a southern US state where risk for overweight was found to be 36.2% compared to the national rate at 31.2% (Lewis et al., 2006). These trends indicate a rapid growth in the prevalence of overweight in the United States and found that overweight is paralleled by a growing rate of chronic health conditions, particularly diabetes (Pickreign, 1997; Hedley et al., 2004).

Since 1990, physical inactivity has been among the leading risk factors for the global burden of disease, according to the Global Burden of Disease Study (Murray & Lopez, 1996). While many governments around the world are implementing laws to legislate smoking in public places as a deterrent to one of the health risks, legislating exercise would be very difficult to conceive and enforce in any country (Erikssen, 2001). In a unique move in the United States, a new law implemented in July 2006 charges public school systems with the responsibility of improving outcomes in child health through healthy food options in cafeterias and vending machines and through physical exercise programs while the child is in school (S. 2507). The hopes are that through interventions in public schools children can learn many healthy messages, and the future of diabetes in the United States will not be so grim.

Asthma

"When you cannot breathe—nothing else matters."
—American Lung Association

Asthma has been recognized as a burden on world populations for many years, but only in the last 15 years have guidelines for management been developed that offer evidence-based practice recommendations to providers in the management of the condition. Although asthma symptoms cannot be completely avoided, they can for the most part be controlled.

Definition

Asthma is a chronic episodic inflammatory disease of the airways that causes recurrent episodes of wheezing, breathlessness, chest tightness, and coughing, particularly at night or in the early morning (NHLBI, 2004). It is one of the most common diseases of childhood and often continues to afflict individuals throughout the lifespan. Asthma's symptoms result from the inflammation that occurs from environmental factors and results in airway hyperresponsiveness and airflow limitation (NHLBI, 2004). These symptoms are usually recognizable in advance of an impending exacerbation through the use of a peak flow meter that can be purchased and used in the home. Peak flow meters are available from several manufacturers and are marketed worldwide.

Diagnosis

Assessment of pulmonary function is important in the diagnosis of asthma both from the view of the medical history and pulmonary function. The medical history alone is inadequate as a diagnostic measure, and recommendations are for spirometry to diagnose the condition (NHLBI, 2004). Asthma is classified into categories of mild, moderate, and severe by the degree of symptom occurrences and treatment recommendations for the various levels. These recommendations can be found at www.nhlbi.nih.gov.

Three major factors occur in the airways that contribute to the symptoms of asthma. These symptoms may occur alone or in combination. The frequency and complexity of symptoms determines the degree of severity of asthma:

- Mucus plug formation—Changes in the airways occur once a trigger occurs and an immediate complex inflammatory response follows, resulting in a hypersecretion of mucus from the lining of the airway. The mucus formation also may form plugs of mucus that limit airflow further.

- Acute bronchoconstriction—Immune complexes are released as a result of the allergen/trigger that activates the asthmatic exacerbation. These immune complexes directly contract the smooth muscle of the airways. As a result of the narrowing of the airways from the smooth muscle contraction, the airways are narrowed and airflow limited (Marshall & Bienenstock, 1994).

- Airway edema—Airway wall edema limits the airflow through the airways even further resulting in diminished flow of air in asthma. The mucosa of the airway walls swell and become less compliant to changes in airflow.

Asthma Prevalence

In 2001, the disability-adjusted life years (DALYs) ranked asthma as the 25th leading worldwide cause of lost work. Asthma is generally less common in low-income countries than in high-income countries (Stewart, Mitchell, Pearce, Strachan, &Weilandon, 2001), and for developing countries, rates are lower on the DALY (Disability Adjusted Life Years) at .9, compared to other respiratory conditions such as tuberculosis, with rates on the DALY at 3.4 (GINA, 2004). Asthma ranks lower in developing countries also because it is a condition that is not likely to spread to other members of the population as compared to infectious respiratory conditions such as tuberculosis. The asthma DALY in India is 1.9, in sub-Saharan Africa it is 2.9, and in China it is 2.7 (Deen, Vos, Huttly, & Tulloch, 1999).

Asthma Treatment

The treatment of asthma includes controlling the environmental factors (triggers) that make asthma worse, pharmacologic therapy geared toward quick relief and long-term control of symptoms using a stepwise approach with self-management. By reducing the environmental factors that trigger an asthma episode, prevention of the numerous allergens is significant.

Triggers

Factors that create an exacerbation of asthma are known as *triggers*. Numerous environmental factors or triggers contribute to the development of asthma. They may be from an inhaled irritant or other sources or factors. The following includes some of the triggers.

Inhaled Factors

In developing nations, exposure to indoor air pollutants is responsible for over 1.6 million premature worldwide deaths accounting for about 3% of the global burden of disease (Ezzati, 2004). Biomass type fuels—sources such as wood, charcoal, crop residues, animal dung, and coal—are primary sources for cooking, heating, and other household needs, such as food preservation, in most developing countries. More than three billion people use these sources of energy, and the resulting pollutants cause chronic and acute conditions such as asthma and other respiratory conditions that affect the poor more often than individuals with higher socioeconomic conditions. Emissions of the pollutants are most worrisome when solid fuels are used in open or poorly ventilated stoves (Smith, Mehta, Maeusezahl-Feuz, 2004.

Although the effect of biomass fuels was found problematic as an exposure for asthma, the effect on pregnant women was particularly troubling. Two studies found an association between exposure to indoor air pollution during pregnancy and low birth weight. One study found that babies born to mothers who used wood for cooking indoors were 175 grams lighter than those born to mothers who used liquid petroleum, natural gas, or electricity (Mishra, Dai, Smith, & Mika, 2004).

Although stoves with improved ventilation have been developed to reduce the risk posed by burning the biomass type fuels, their use has not been widely accepted.

Preprocessing of biomass fuels poses hope for reductions in risk to offer cleaner burning of the fuels (Barnes, Openshaw, Smith, & van der Plas, 2002).

Tobacco smoke exposure ranks highest as an indoor air irritant that can trigger worsening symptoms of asthma (Leuenberger et al., 1994). People with known asthma should not smoke or be exposed to environmental smoke in any form because smoking reduces lung function, increases the need for medications, and increases missed days from work (Jindel, Gupta, & Singh, 1994). Infants of mothers who smoke have higher rates of infant and childhood asthma (Arshad, Bateman & Matthews, 2003).

In 2003, the World Health Organization reported that 1 in 10 adult deaths could be related to tobacco smoke and estimated that by the year 2030 that the number might be closer to 1 in 6. Health promotion activities and smoking cessation treatments for tobacco dependence are needed in most developing and developed countries. Although more than 30% of smokers try to quit at least annually, studies show that only 1–3% succeed without the help of smoking cessation programs or pharmaceutical support (Shafey, Dolwick and Guindon, 2003).

Other factors that contribute to the triggers for asthma include indoor dampness and humidity. At present, indoor dampness occurs within Nordic countries at a rate of 17–24%, within the Netherlands at a rate of 25%, and within Canada at a 37% rate. Home indoor dampness can often be detected from signs of water leakage or visible mold on walls, floors, or ceilings (Masoli, Fabian, Holt, & Beasley, 2004)

Another factor that must be considered is the common house dust mites and animal and cockroach allergens that are triggers that can cause an exacerbation of asthma. House dust mites are universal in areas of high humidity (most areas of the United States are included), but are not usually present at high altitudes or dry climates unless moisture is added to the indoor atmosphere (NHLBI, 2004). Dust mites can be found in high concentrations in pillows, mattresses, carpets, upholstered furniture, clothes, and stuffed toys. Pet dander comes from all warm-blooded pets including small rodents and birds. These animals produce dander, urine, and feces that can cause allergic reactions (Swanson, Agarwal, & Reed, 1985). Molds and fungi are present in moist humid environments and homes that have dampness problems. Children who live in homes where there are high humid conditions are at greater risk for respiratory conditions such as asthma (Cuijpers, Swaen, Wesseing, Sturmans, & Wouters, 1995).

Factors where individuals have regular exposure, such as in a work setting, may worsen the condition. Exposure to fluorides and other respiratory irritants are suggested as environmental agents that can result in asthma (Taiwo et al., 2006). In Australia and New Zealand asthma was found among workers in aluminum smelters and is referred to as "potroom" asthma. Individuals who had exposure improved in pulmonary function once they were removed from the potroom worksite; however, the longer the worker had been exposed, the lower the level of improvement. Studies offered hope as preventive measures were identified that reduced the development of the condition in the worksite (Arnaiz, Kaufman, Daroowalla, Quigley, Farin, & Checkoway, 2003).

Pharmacologic Treatments for Asthma

Pharmacologic management of asthma is broken into two components—relievers and controllers. Medications for relieving the symptoms of asthma through inhalers include products that relax and open the airway to improve the movement of air and are short term in their action. Controller medications are long term in action and include steroids and nonsteroidal medications that must be taken on a regular basis to be effective. Medications for treating asthma can be costly, and they may not be available in developing countries. Immunotherapy may be considered when specific allergens are present and cannot be avoided. Allergens such as grass or trees can pose as a major irritant for asthma (NHLBI, 2004)

Cost of Asthma Treatment

The cost of management varies by the severity and extent of the exacerbation and whether hospitalization is needed or if self-management can be used to control episodes of the disease. Some episodes require emergency room visits, but they are successfully treated and hospitalization is not required. More severe exacerbations may require hospitalization and costs are correspondingly higher. Through the use of the peak flow meter, which is a lower-cost alternative to pulmonary function tests, individuals in low-income countries could be provided with a measure of evaluation to offer early intervention preventing serious exacerbations. A group of lower-priced generic drugs, by oral and inhalation routes of administration, can keep the cost to the government-provided health services to a minimum. With lower-cost asthma medications, a greater benefit could be realized for the population who suffer with asthma.

The Global Initiative for Asthma recommends that countries identify low-cost drugs that can be made available for those who suffer with asthma. Otherwise, the cost of treatment for countries where the health of the population falls on the government will be far greater than can be provided. The report found that as much as 30% of the entire expenditure for health in a country would have to be spent on asthma medication alone if only 5% of the population had asthma, and the cost of asthma treatment was in the range of US$30 (GINA, 2002). Guidelines for medications should include what is available as well as what is affordable for treatment of asthma.

Preventing Limb Amputations: A Diabetes Intervention Case Study Involving Working Across Borders in Latin America (Five Andean Countries: Bolivia, Ecuador, Perú, Colombia and Venezuela)

Introduction: Ways of Working Across Boundaries

There are, of course, many ways of entering the multifaceted issue of "working across boundaries." This case study raises some issues for discussion about establishing partnerships to improve a health system in order to avoid or prevent leg amputations among people with diabetes in five Andean countries in Latin America, and explores some of the philosophical and practical pitfalls encountered in a project that attempts to implement a prevention protocol for foot care with healthcare professionals working in the primary care level. In this case study the researchers examine what is probably the most difficult of the boundaries to work across: the boundary between "foreign" and local knowledge.

The project had its roots in a discussion amongst Peruvians and Latin American health care professionals and other Latin Americans with diabetes who held leadership positions in the International Diabetes Federation (IDF) for the Central, South America, and the Caribbean Region (IDF-SACA region). The conceptualization of the project took place after the implementation of the First Diabetes Awareness workshop in Perú, which was developed to address the lack of awareness of diabetes and its complications in this country. As a result of the workshop, Perú developed the first diabetes awareness action plan. This versatile action plan contained global strategies that can be applied at all levels—from local to international—and that can be adapted to suit various target audiences. The action plan targets several sectors, such as the government, the social civil force, people with diabetes, associations, and academia. The plan addressed the diabetic needs of Perú in raising awareness of diabetes for everyone working towards improvements in diabetes education, treatment, and care. Conclusions for the workshop in Peru pointed out the need to develop cross-collaboration among countries to strengthen the health system at the primary care level. The priority was the reduction and prevention of foot amputations among people with diabetes. The idea evolved to birth the Eje Vascular Andino Project or EVA project. Five Andean countries committed to develop, implement, and evaluate the *Eje Vascular Andino (Eva)* Andean Vascular Axis, Program for Prevention and Early Diagnosis of the Diabetic Foot, in the five countries (Bolivia, Ecuador, Perú, Colombia, and Venezuela) of the Andean Community of Nations.

The EVA project was an initiative targeting primarily people with diabetes and also health professionals at the primary healthcare level.

Goal and Purpose of the Project

The goal of the project was to prevent lower-extremity amputations in people with diabetes in primary health care units. Another goal of the EVA project was to unite Bolivia, Colombia, Ecuador, Perú, and Venezuela in working together as well as in collaboration with the IDF-SACA region. This was done to increase the awareness of foot care and to improve the knowledge and skills of foot care for healthcare providers and people with diabetes.

The purpose of the project was to increase the number of patients who receive interventions to prevent lower leg injuries following clinical foot care protocol. The objectives of this program were to decrease the rate of lower-extremity complications in people with diabetes through efforts of prevention and to decrease the rate of amputations in people with diabetes who already have neurological and vascular complications through early and effective intervention in the levels of primary health care.

Therefore, the EVA objectives guides a process to:

- Identify people with a "foot at risk."

- Provide education to healthcare providers, patients, and their relatives on how to take better care of the foot and to avoid foot complications based on the concept of "train the trainers" with the expectation that capacity will be built to promote early detection and treatment on any lesion or significant sign or symptom of foot problems.

- Promote awareness for people with diabetes on how to avoid foot complication and amputations.

Partners involved in EVA were member associations of the IDF from the Andean region, the ministries of health in each country, the Pan American Health Organization (PAHO), and the Word Diabetes Foundation, which was the sponsor. The EVA project had a timeframe of 1 year—from August 2005 to October 2006.

Problematic Situation Addressed by the Project

Diabetes mellitus (DM) is a growing problem worldwide and is a costly burden to both individuals and to society as a whole. Morbidity and mortality of DM is due, for the most part, to the complications associated with the disease. Of all the complications associated with diabetes, the diabetic foot presents the most alarming figures; approximately 15% of all the people who have diabetes mellitus developed an ulcer in the foot or leg during the course of their disease. The magnitude of these figures reveals that more than 25% of the hospital admissions of people with diabetes in the United States and Great Britain are related to foot problems.

The "diabetic foot" is defined as all injuries that people with diabetes present in the lower extremities. The most serious consequence of the diabetic foot is a lower-extremity amputation. Various data indicate that anywhere from 60–83% of all lower-extremity amputations occur in people with diabetes. It is well established that the pattern of ulceration, infection, and gangrene precedes a great majority of leg amputations in the diabetic. In other cases it is the lack of healing of an ulcer that leads to serious complications in the person with diabetes. Given that foot complications cause from 40% to 70% of all lower extremity amputations (International Working Group on the Diabetic Foot, 1999), it is presumed that if ulceration is avoided through an adequate prevention strategy that begins with educating the person with diabetes and screening for risk factors in every person with diabetes, the objectives of this project will be in the process of being achieved.

An amputation can be prevented in a person with diabetes. The factors responsible for foot lesions can be avoided through correct training of the patient. Furthermore, early diagnosis and adequate treatment of injuries can maintain proper foot function in most patients, thus avoiding a large number of amputations. Multidisciplinary strategies for all people with diabetes are recommended, not only for people who have complications. IDF's International Consensus of the Diabetic Foot relates that there are five basic steps for prevention:

- The regular inspection and examination of the foot and footwear
- The identification of the high-risk patient
- The education of the patient, family, and healthcare providers
- Appropriate footwear
- The treatment of nonulcerative pathology

In addition to educating the patient and healthcare professional in foot care, a focused effort is made towards improving diabetes control because well-controlled diabetes is related to better quality of life and survival. Available information suggests that diabetes care in Latin America and the Caribbean is suboptimal. Barbados, Trinidad and Tobago, Tortola, and the British Virgin Islands participated in a collaborative study on the quality of diabetes care in the public health services. In general, 37% of patients in Tortola, 61% in Trinidad and Tobago, and 47% in Barbados were found to have poor glycemic control. The examination of feet and eyes was found in less than 20%, and 9% of patients, respectively (Gulliford, Alert, Mahabir, 1996). Similar results have been reported in other countries in Latin America and the Caribbean, such as Jamaica and Chile.

An evaluation of the quality of care carried out by PAHO and supported by the Declaration of the Americas on Diabetes (DOTA) in Bahamas, St. Lucia, and Jamaica, identified gaps in the care provided to people with diabetes. This study was an audit of medical records and showed that 67% of the patients had inadequate glycemic control (fasting glucose of 8 mmol/L or more) and that only 25% had a registered foot examination (Pan American Health Organization, 2004).

Relevance of the Project

In the Andean region of South America, diabetes is a growing problem. In Bolivia (1998), the prevalence of diabetes in adults over 25 years of age was 7.2% (Barceló, Daroca, Rivera, Duarte, & Zapata, 2001). The International Diabetes Federation (IDF) estimates that the prevalence of DM in the adult population in Peru, Venezuela, and Colombia is 5.1%, 5.2%, and 4.3% respectively (Diabetes Atlas, 2003). If some specific areas of the countries are considered, the rates are higher; for example, Bolivia has a prevalence of higher DM in cities of rapid growth such as Santa Cruz (with 10.7% prevalence) and Cochabamba (with 9.4%). A study in Bogotá, Colombia, found a prevalence of 7% (Aschner, King, Triana de Torrado, & Rodríguez, 1993).

The complications of diabetes are costly not only in terms of loss of physical abilities, but also in terms of financial costs to the patient and health system. Long hospital stays, amputations, and other care for the diabetic foot result in high costs. The IDF reports that in developing countries, the care of the diabetic foot can reach 40% of the available healthcare resources (Aschner et al., 2005).

Keeping in mind the high prevalence of diabetes in the Andean region and the evidence showing the high incidence of amputations in people with diabetes, it is timely to approach the problem of the diabetic foot in this region. This project intends to prevent lower-extremity amputations in people with diabetes in primary healthcare units by increasing the number of patients who receive actions to prevent lower-extremity injuries, according to clinical protocol.

The evidence shows that it is possible to achieve this objective; 49–85% of all the problems associated with the diabetic foot can be avoided by prevention strategies (Bakker & Riley, 2005). Brazil is a great example of the success of diabetic foot interventions. In Brasilia, the capital of Brazil, a project was implemented called the Diabetic Foot Saving Project. In this project, nurses received training in basic foot care. As a result of this project, the rate of major amputations was reduced by 90%.

PAHO's VIDA (Veracruz Initiative for Diabetes Awareness) project demonstrated that the training of health workers in diabetic foot care increased the proportion of patients who receive a foot examination from 47% to 96% and of patients who receive foot care education from 32% to 75% (Barceló, 2005). In addition to these examples, several countries in Latin America and the Caribbean have developed programs and materials for the prevention of foot complications. Implementation of a project to decrease lower-extremity complications and amputations in people with diabetes in the Andean region of South America is needed at this time.

The Challenge

Diabetes is a serious chronic disease. In 2003, the global prevalence of diabetes was estimated at 194 million. This figure is predicted to reach 333 million by 2025 as a consequence of longer life expectancy, sedentary lifestyle, and changing dietary patterns. Although many serious complications, such as kidney failure or blindness, can affect individuals with diabetes, the complications of the foot take the greatest toll. Of all lower-extremity amputations, 40–70% is related to diabetes. In most studies, the incidence of lower leg amputation is estimated to be 5–25/100,000 inhabitants/year; among people with diabetes, the figure is 6–8/1,000.

Lower-extremity amputations are usually preceded by a foot ulcer in people with diabetes. The most important factors related to the development of these ulcers are peripheral neuropathy, foot deformities, minor foot trauma, and peripheral vascular disease. The spectrum of foot lesions varies in different regions of the world due to differences in socioeconomic conditions, standards of foot care, and quality of footwear.

The diabetic foot is a significant economic problem, particularly if amputation results in prolonged hospitalization, rehabilitation, and an increased need for home care and social services. Approximately 3–4% of all people with diabetes have a foot problem and use 12–15% of the healthcare resources. The average cost for primary healing in the United

States has been estimated to be between US$7,000 and US$10,000. The direct cost of an amputation associated with the diabetic foot is estimated to be between US$30,000 and US$60,000. The estimated cost for three years of subsequent care ranges from US$43,000 to US$63,000—mainly from the increased need for home care and social services. The corresponding cost for individuals with primary care has been estimated to be just over US$16,000 and go as high as nearly US$27,000. In addition to these costs, there are indirect costs due to loss of productivity to consider. If cost estimates are broadened to include the costs to the individual and loss of quality of life, then the total estimated cost of the diabetic foot in the United States is about US$4 billion a year.

Foot complications are one of the most serious and costly complications of diabetes. However, through a care strategy that combines prevention, the multidisciplinary treatment of foot ulcers, appropriate organization, close monitoring, and the education of people with diabetes and healthcare professionals, it is possible to reduce amputation rates by between 49% and 85%. It is this objective that should motivate the advocacy work of those fighting to make a difference for those living with diabetes around the world. It is imperative that there is an increase in worldwide awareness among healthcare providers at all levels and that there is a reduction in the unnecessary suffering that foot complications can bring.

The Journey

An advisory team was organized, consisting of members of the ministries of health of the participating countries, the PAHO/WHO representative offices of each country, with the support and supervision of PAHO Washington, the related scientific societies (of endocrinology, diabetes, vascular surgery), the associations of people with diabetes in each of the participating Andean countries as well as the IDF-SACA (South America/Central America) region of IDF who provided the endorsement. The principal role of the advisory board was to provide general coordination and oversight to the project. The advisory board monitored the fulfillment of the project's objectives.

A clinical protocol for the management and prevention of the diabetic foot was developed. This protocol was based on the International Consensus of the Diabetic Foot and other available materials and was reviewed by the advisory team and experts in the foot such as the *Fédération Internationale des Podologues* (FIP).

The project protocol for the management and prevention of the diabetic foot was based on a protocol developed and tested by the International Consensus of the Diabetic Foot, known as the *"Practical Guidelines on the Management and the Prevention of the Diabetic Foot,"* which was published in 1999 by the International Working Group on the Diabetic Foot (IWGDF). This effort was headed by Dr. Karel Bakker under the Declaration of the Americas (DOTA). The protocol that the EVA project used is a combination of the existing protocols adapted to the reality and circumstances of the Andean countries.

Training was provided for primary healthcare staff such as physicians, nurses, nursing assistants, and health promoters in performing the clinical foot exam according to the established protocol. The training was conducted in at least 10 primary care units in each country. The diabetes educators from the EVA project carried out the training (Betsy Rodríguez and Dr. Elizabeth Duarte). These educators offered an international workshop for representatives from each country, and then the country trained the healthcare professionals in their respective countries. The cities and units were selected based on the incidence and prevalence of diabetes as well as the recommendations from the ministries of health of the participating countries and the opinions of PAHO and the Andean Health Organization Hipólito Unanue Agreement, Andean Community (ORAS-CONHU).

The final selection of sites was the responsibility of the head of the advisory team, in accordance with the group members: representatives from the ministries of health of the participating countries, PAHO representatives in each country with the support and supervision of PAHO-Washington, the ORAS-CONHU, the related scientific associations (of endocrinology, diabetes, vascular surgery), associations of people with diabetes, and the endorsement of the IDF-SACA region.

Both public and private health facilities were targeted. In the Andean region, people with diabetes are treated in both sectors. For example, a patient could go to a public hospital in a city for treatment, but the follow-up of the same patient occurs in a private clinic or in a health center in a rural area. For this reason, all the health personnel needed to be trained (public and private).

Information related to foot care was transmitted through the community health workers to the people with diabetes who attend the clinics or units. In addition, self-care and self-control of people with diabetes was promoted, for which collective training activities were carried out in the health facilities, in the communities, as well as individual talks during the consultation. Educational materials on self-care of the foot were distributed. Additional materials addressing the selection of footwear and methods for glycemic control was also developed and distributed both during collective and individual activities.

The head of the project in each country was responsible for monitoring the implementation of the project in their respective country.

The project consisted of four components:

- Delivery of care services for the lower extremity—The objective that was pursued was that all people with diabetes receive at least one annual foot exam that follows the guidelines in the clinical foot care protocol. The fulfillment of the standards was confirmed through audits of clinical files, direct observation, and through satisfaction surveys of users of the services.

- Education in diabetic foot care for the health team—This component ensured that the medical staff that serves people with diabetes has and practices the knowledge of clinical evaluation and management of the lower limbs. In addition, the objective is that they know how to transmit information to their patients. The knowledge was evaluated through file audits and personal tests.

- Promotion of self-care and self-control of the lower limbs in diabetic patients—This component implied developing the patients' capacity to carry out self-examination of their foot, selection of adequate footwear, and basic hygienic measures. To do this, the health team was trained, especially the community health care, so that they can transmit knowledge and organize support groups in the communities.

- Referral system for the lower limb at risk—having established standards and treatment protocols for the care and control of the lower limbs in people with diabetes, the objective of this component was to guarantee the monitoring at the level of follow-up received care by the people who are at risk for lower extremity problems. This activity was carried out through the evaluation of the referral and counterreferral system. The clinical personnel were instructed about the system of referral at the second level and the operation of the counter referral at the first level was coordinated with the second level.

- Implementation of a treatment protocol for the diabetic foot—The International Consensus of the Diabetic Foot will be reviewed and a protocol and forms will be selected to be implemented in the health facilities. Subsequently, workshops on dissemination of the protocols and published forms will be made, so that each establishment begins to use them. Prior to the utilization of the protocols, the establishments will be supplied with the paperwork and the instruments necessary for foot evaluation in people with diabetes

The Discovery

The following table summarizes the current status and the expected outcomes.

TABLE 10-1 Current Status and Expected Outcome for the EVA Project	
Current Situation in Five Andean Countries: Bolivia, Perú, Ecuador, Venezuela, Colombia	**Expected Outcomes from the EVA Project**
• The number of people with diabetes who have a lower limb examination is less than 10%.	• 90% of people with diabetes under care will undergo a clinical examination of the legs.
• There is no technical monitoring of the implementation of standards and protocols of treatment for the lower limbs of patients with diabetes.	• A standing clinical diabetic protocol for care is followed in the primary care units.
	• The care personnel have technical capability to conduct the lower-extremity examination.

(continues)

TABLE 10-1 Current Status and Expected Outcome for the EVA Project
(continued)

- Nonexistence of promotion of self-care and self-control of lower extremities in the people with diabetes
- Deficient monitoring of the referral and counterreferral system of the lower limbs at risk in people with diabetes

- 90% of the people with diabetes know how to carry out the self-examination of the foot and know the importance of the risk factors such as adequate footwear, metabolic control, and hygiene.
- Establish an efficient patient referral system at the primary and secondary levels and have a counterreferral system functioning adequately.

The Implementation

- Implementation of a treatment protocol for the diabetic foot—The International Consensus of the Diabetic Foot will be reviewed and a protocol and forms will be selected in order for it to be implemented in the health facilities. Subsequently, workshops on dissemination of the protocols and published forms will be made so that each establishment begins to use them. Prior to the utilization of the protocols, the establishments will be supplied with the paperwork and the instruments necessary for foot evaluation in people with diabetes.

- Training of health workers in the management of the foot of people with diabetes—A training workshop (or workshops) for health workers will be held in each country, in which they will be taught to follow the treatment protocols and complete the screening, clinical assessment and risk management forms. There will be an audit of the clinical files of patients with diabetes, in which the utilization of the corresponding administrative paperwork will be monitored (e.g., adequate completion of the forms, the fulfillment of the protocols, and the quality of care). The QUALIDIAB/Qualisoft auditing instrument may be used for this audit. It has proven to be an effective, reliable tool in past interventions.

- Training people with diabetes in the management and control of their feet—Training activities will be carried out in the health facilities and in the communities. They will be directed to people with diabetes and their family members (those responsible for their care) and to health promoters, with the objective of learning to identify risk in the feet. To do this, techniques to use the monofilament and the self-exam form will be taught. The students will also learn to identify signs of risk in the feet in order to activate the healthcare system to the found physical condition.

- Implementation of referral and counterreferral system—The referral system will be reviewed and made known to the healthcare personnel. A record of references that are sent and received will be kept, as well as the response to the reference. Furthermore, compliance with the recommendations that are received in the counterreferral will be monitored, both in the health facility and in the community. The primary healthcare staff training will include details of the referral and counterreferral system.

The Evaluation

- Implementation of a treatment protocol for the diabetic foot—The measurement indicators for this activity will be the following:
  - Reproduction and dissemination of the protocol of treatment of the diabetic foot
  - Reproduction and dissemination of the diabetic foot screening form
  - Reproduction and dissemination of the diabetic foot evaluation form
  - Reproduction and dissemination of the form for risk management according to foot categories for people with diabetes
- Training of the health workers in the management of the foot of people with diabetes—The measurement indicators for this activity will be the following:
  - Files with paperwork for the evaluation and management of the patients with diabetes with the corresponding forms
  - Forms adequately filled out by the medical staff
  - Files that register the fulfillment of the treatment protocol
  - Patients with diabetes whose feet have been evaluated in accordance with risk control guides
- Training people with diabetes in the management and control of their feet—The indicators to measure this activity will be the following:
  - Patients who are examined by health promoters
  - Health promoters who adequately identify risks in the feet of people with diabetes.
  - People with diabetes who self-identify conditions of risk in their feet
  - People with diabetes whose family members collaborate in foot care
  - Health promoters that have been trained by the establishment
  - Patients with diabetes trained by the establishment

- Implementation of referral and counterreferral system—The indicators to measure will be the following:
  - Health facilities that meet the reference criteria
  - Health facilities that monitor the references
  - Degree of relevance of the sent reference
  - Fulfillment of the reference in the community
  - Number of received cases referred and counterreferred in the establishments

Results

It is expected that this project will be implemented in at least 10 primary care units in each country. At least 3 or 4 training sessions were held; during each training session, at least 50 people will be trained. A minimum of 300 people attend each clinic, therefore, the aim is to reach 3000 patients per country.

Members of the advisory team will have a role as coordinators in each of the project's activities. The advisory team will be in constant communication with the persons responsible for executing the project's activities in each of the countries. The advisory team will also appoint two people (official and substitute) for the coordination with the 10 health units in each country.

Conclusions

Regardless of differences in social protection policies from country to country, it is possible to note some common characteristics. These include:

- Some services are provided by the ministry of social security and others by the ministry of health.
- Institutional arrangements vary in terms of duties and rights according to the bargaining power of the labor group involved.
- Centralization of the social services system results in inefficient service delivery and poor quality services.
- Low coverage by a social security system provides uneven coverage across regions and income classes and excludes workers in the informal sector.
- A complex and intricate power structure is dominated by such powerful stakeholders as politicians, bureaucrats, labor leaders, private providers, international suppliers of healthcare inputs, and insurance companies

Despite these common features, health care in Latin America is provided through a wide range of organizational forms of delivery. The EVA project is an attempt to be a partial approach to the reality in these five countries.

EVA National Context

The international context of the Andean region is key to this particular project. Although the five countries share many similarities, there are also many differences in terms of the national status of diabetes. At the moment, whereas Peru has a National Diabetes Law and Bolivia is working toward improving quality of care in diabetes, Ecuador and Venezuela do not have any well-known diabetes program. Colombia can serve as a model for the other countries given that it has a well-established program and many prestigious diabetes experts.

Sustainability

The commitment of the governments through their ministries of health in a joint effort with the scientific societies will give sustainability to this project. Moreover, the fact of having duly trained health workers and periodic evaluations will result in a program fully integrated into the public and private health systems, ensuring the long-term sustainability of the treatment of people with diabetes. The material that is developed for this program will be widely disseminated and the advisory team will support the ministries of health and scientific societies throughout the duration of this program.

The Andean community is a subregional organization with international legal status formed by Bolivia, Colombia, Ecuador, Peru, and Venezuela, and is made up of the organizations and institutions of the Andean Integration System (Sistema Andino de Integración; ASI). It relies on the Andean Health Agency Hipólito Unanue Agreement (Organismo Andino de Salud Convenio Hipólito Unanue, ORAS-CONHU). This agreement is an institution of subregional integration, belonging to the Andean Integration System, whose objective is to coordinate and support the efforts that the member countries carry out, individually or collectively, for the improvement of the health of its people.

It coordinates and promotes actions designed to improve the level of health of its member countries, giving priority to cooperation mechanisms that promote the development of subregional systems and methodologies. In that same sense, it coordinates similar actions that are aimed at the same objectives with other subregional, regional, and international agencies.

Located in South America, the five Andean countries bring together 120 million inhabitants over 4,710,000 km^2. The Andean Integration System is the set of bodies and institutions that closely work together and whose actions are directed toward achieving the same objectives: to intensify the Andean subregional integration, to promote its external influence, and to strengthen the actions related to the process.

In April 2006 in Lima, Perú, the First Workshop on Diabetes Awareness of the Declaration of the Americas on Diabetes (DOTA) took place. This event was co-sponsored by the General Secretariat of the Andean Community and had the participation of representatives from Bolivia and Ecuador in addition to the host country, Perú.

In view of the success of the event and the expectations that have arisen, with the intention of maintaining the work in diabetes as the Andean group of nations, the EVA project has created a strategic alliance that will operationally articulate the work with each ministry of health of the Andean countries for the purpose of improving the living conditions of the people with diabetes and decreasing and/or avoiding the incidence of complications, especially the diabetic foot.

References

ADA (American Diabetes Association) Task Force to Revise the National Standards. (1995). National standards for diabetes self-management education programs. *Diabetes Educator, 21,* 189–193.

American Diabetes Association (ADA). (1998). Economic consequences of diabetes mellitus in the US in 1997. *Diabetes Care, 21,* 296–309.

ADA. (2004). Gestational diabetes mellitus. *Diabetes Care Supplement, 1,* 88–90.

Arnaiz, N. O., Kaufman, J. D., Daroowalla, F. M., Quigley, S., Farin, F., & Checkoway, H. (2003). Genetic factors and asthma in aluminum smelter workers. *Archives of Environmental Health, 58*(4), 197–200.

Arshad, S., Bateman, B., & Matthews, S. (2003). Primary prevention of asthma and atopy during childhood by allergen avoidance in infancy: A randomized controlled study. *Thorax, 58,* 489–493.

Aschner, P., King, H., Triana de Torrado, M., & Rodríguez, B. M. (1993). Glucose intolerance in Colômbia: A population-based survey in an urban community. *Diabetes Care, 16*(1), 90–93.

Atkinson, M. A., & Eisenbarth, G. S. (2001). Type 1 diabetes: New perspectives on disease pathogenesis and treatment. *Lancet, 358,* 221–229.

Bakker, K, & Riley P. (2005). El año del pie diabético. *Diabetes Voice, 50*(1), 11–14.

Barceló, A., Daroca, M. C., Rivera, R., Duarte, E., & Zapata, A. (2001). Diabetes in Bolivia. *Pan American Journal of Public Health, 10*(5), 318–322.

Barnes, D., Openshaw, K., Smith, K., & van der Plas, R. (2002). *What makes people cook with improved biomass stoves? A comparative international review of stove programs* (World Bank Technical Paper No. 242. Energy Series). Washington, DC: The World Bank.

Beaglehole, R., & Yach, D. (2003). Globalisation and the prevention and control of noncommunicable disease: The neglected chronic disease of adults. *Lancet, 362,* 903–908.

CDC. (2004). *Chronic disease prevention.* Retrieved June 13, 2005, from http://www.cdc.gov/programs/chronic.htm

Child Nutrition and WIC Reauthorization ACT of 2004. (2005). S. 2507. Retrieved February 11, 2006, from http://www.cbo.gov/ showdoc.cfm?index=5518&sequence=0

Chui, D., Lau, J. S. K., & Yau, I. T. Y. (2004). An outcome evaluation study of the Rheumatoid Arthritis Self-Management Programme in Hong Kong. *Psychology, Health & Medicine, 9*(3), 286–291.

Cuijpers, C. E., Swaen, G. M., Wesseing, G., Sturmans, F., & Wouters, E. F. (1995). Adverse effects of the indoor environment on respiratory health in primary school children. *Environment Research, 68,* 11–23.

Deen, J. L., Vos, T., Huttly, S. R. A., & Tulloch, J. (1999). Injuries and noncommunicable diseases: Emerging health problems of children in developing countries. *Bulletin of the World Health Organization, 77*(6), 518–524.

Diabetes Atlas. (2003). (2nd ed.). Brussels, Belgium: International Diabetes Federation.

Erikssen, G. (2001). Physical fitness and changes in mortality: The survival of the fittest. *Sports Medicine, 31*(8), 571–576.

Ezzati, M. (2004). Indoor air pollution and health in developing countries. *Lancet, 366,* 104–106.

Finnish Institute of Occupational Health. (2003). *Musculoskeletal disorders: A global concern.* Retrieved June 29, 2005, from http://www.ttl.fi/Internet/English/Information/Electronic+journals/Asian-Pacific+Newslett

Garancini, M. P., Calori, G., Ruotolo, G., Manara, E., Izzo, A., Ebbli, E., et al. (1995). Prevalence of NIDDM and impaired glucose tolerance in Italy: An OGTT–based population study. *Diabetologia, 38,* 306–313.

GINA (Global Initiative for Asthma). (2002). *Global strategy for asthma management and prevention* (NHLBI/WHO Workshop Report No. 95-3659). Bethesda, MD: National Institutes of Health, National Heart Lung and Blood Institute.

Gulliford, M. C., Alert, C. V., & Mahabir, D. (1996). Diabetes care in middle-income countries: A Caribbean case study. *Diabetic Medicine, 13,* 574–581.

Hafstrom, I., & Hallengren, M. (2003). Physiotherapy in subtropic climate improves functional capacity and health-related quality of life in Swedish patients with rheumatoid arthritis and spondylarthropathies still after 6 months. *Scandinavian Journal of Rheumatology, 32,* 108–113.

Hedley, A., Ogden, C., Johnson, C., Carroll, M., Curtin, l., & Flegal, K. (2004). Prevalence of overweight and obesity among US children, adolescents, and adults (1999–2002). *Journal of the American Medical Association, 291*(23), 2847–2850.

International Diabetes Federation (IDF). (2003). *Diabetes atlas. Executive summary* (2nd ed.). Retrieved August 8, 2007, from http://www.eatlas.idf.org/webdata/docs/Atlas%202003-Summary.pdf

International Diabetes Federation Consensus Workshop. (2004). Type 2 diabetes in the young: The evolving epidemic. *Diabetes Care, 27,* 1798–1811

International Working Group on the Diabetic Foot. (1999). *International consensus on the diabetic foot.* Brussels, Belgium: International Diabetes Federation

Jindel, S. K., Gupta, D., & Singh, A. (1994). Indices of morbidity and control of asthma in adult patients exposed to environmental tobacco smoke. *Chest, 106*(3), 746–749.

Katz, D. (2004). The burden of chronic disease: The future is prevention [Electronic version]. *Public Health Research, Practice, and Policy, 1*(2), 1.

Koster, I., von Ferber, L., Ihle, P., Schubert, I., & Hauner, H. (2006). The cost burden of diabetes mellitus: The evidence from Germany—the CoDIM Study. *Diabetologia, 49,* 1498–1504.

Leuenberger, P., Schwartz, J., Ackermann-Liebrich, U., Blaser, K., Bolognini, G., Bongard, J. P., et al. (1994). Passive smoking exposure in adults and chronic respiratory symptoms (SAPALDIA Study). Swiss Study on Air Pollution and Lung Disease in Adults, SAPALDIA Team. *American Journal of Respiratory Critical Care Medicine, 150*(5 Pt 1), 1221–1228.

Lewis, R.D., Meyer, M.C., Lehman, S.C., Trowbridge, F. L., Bason, J. J., Yurman, K. H., et al. (2006). Prevalence and degree of childhood and adolescent overweight in rural, urban, and suburban Georgia. *Journal of School Health, 76*(4), 126.

Liebl, A., Mata, M., & Eschwege, E. (2002). Evaluation of risk factors for development of complication sin Type II diabetes in Europe. *Diabetología, 45,* S23–S28.

Liebl, A., Neiß, A., Spannheimer, A., Reitberger, U., Wagner, T., & Gortz, A. (2001). Costs of type 2 diabetes in Germany. Results of the Code-2 study. *Dutsch Medical Wochenschr, 126,* 585–589.

Marmont, M., & Wilkinson, R. G. (Eds.). (2002). *Social determinants of health.* London: Oxford Press.

Marshall, J. S., & Bienenstock, J. (1994). The role of mast cells in inflammatory reactions of the airways, skin and intestine. *Current Opinions in Immunology, 6,* 853–859.

Masharani, U., Karam, J. H., & German, M. S. (2004). Pancreatic hormones and diabetes. In F. S. Greenspan, & D. G. Garner (Eds.), *Basic and clinical endocrinology* (pp. 658–746, 7th ed.). New York: Lange Medical Books/McGraw-Hill.

Masoli, M., Fabian, D., Holt, S., & Beasley, R. (2004). The global burden of asthma. Developed for the global initiative for asthma. *Allergy, 59*(5),469–478.

Michalsen, A., Klotz, S., Ludtke, R., Moebus, S., Spahn, G., & Dobos, G. (2003). Effectiveness of leech therapy in osteoarthritis of the knee. *Annals of Internal Medicine, 139*, 724–730.

Mishra, V., Dai, X., Smith, K. R., & Mika, L. (2004) Maternal exposure to biomass smoke and reduced birth weight in Zimbabwe. *Annals of Epidemiology, 14*, 740–747.

Mohan, V., Deepa, M., Deepa, R., Shanthirani, C. S., Farooq, S., Ganesan, A., et al. (2006). Secular trends in the prevalence of diabetes and impaired glucose tolerance in urban South India—the Chennai Urban Rural Epidemiology Study. (CURES-17). *Diabetologia, 49*, 1175–1178.

Morgan, C. L., Currie, C. J., Stott, N. C. H., Smithers, M., Butler, C. C., & Peters, J. R. (2000). Estimating the prevalence of diagnosed diabetes in a health district of Wales: The importance of using primary and secondary care sources of ascertainment with adjustment for death and migration. *Diabetic Medicine, 17*, 141–145.

Murry, C., & Lopez, A., (Eds.).(1996). *The global burden of disease*. Cambridge, MA: Harvard University Press.

Nathan, D. M., Buse, J. B., Davidson, M. B., Heine, R. J., Holman, R. R., Sherwin, R., et al. (2006). Management of hyperglycaemia in type 2 diabetes: A consensus algorithm for the initiation and adjustment of therapy. *Diabetologia, 49*, 1711–1721.

NHLBI (National Heart, Lung, and Blood Institute). (2004). *Global initiative for asthma. (GINA). Global strategy for asthma management and prevention* (NHLBI/WHO Workshop Report No. 02-3659). Bethesda, MD: NLBHI.

Ogden, C. L., Flegal, K. M., Carroll, M. D., & Johnson, C. L. (2002). Prevalence and trends in over-weight among US children and adolescents, 1999–2000. *Journal of the American Medical Association, 288*(114), 1772–1773.

Ohmura, T., Ueda, K., Kiyohara, Y., Kato, I., Iwanoto, H., Nakayama, K., et al. (1993). Prevalence of type 2 (non-insulin dependent) diabetes mellitus and impaired glucose tolerance in the Japanese general population: The Hisayama study. *Diabetologia, 36*, 1198–1203.

Pan American Health Organization. (2004). Institutional response to diabetes and its complications (Unpublished report). Washington, DC: PAHO.

Pickreign, J. (1997). Update: Prevalence of overweight among children, adolescents, and adults—United States, 1988–1994. *Morbidity & Mortality Weekly Report, 46*(9), 198–202.

Porter, D. (2004). *Chronic diseases need global health attention. Journal of the American Medical Association* and archives journals Web site. Retrieved June 18, 2005, from http://www.eurekalert.org/pub_releases/2004-06/jaaj-cdn052704.php

Porth, C. M. (2007). *Essentials of pathophysiology: Concepts of altered health states*. Philadelphia: Lippincott Williams & Wilkins.

Reddy, K., & Srinath, R. (1999). Chronic disease epidemics in developing countries: Can we telescope transition? *Chronic Disease Epidemics*. Retrieved June 18, 2005, from http://www.medguide.org.zm/diseases/chrondis.htm

Schoenborn, C. A., Adams, P. F., & Barnes, P. M. (2002). *Body weight status of adults: United States, 1997–98. Advance data from vital and health statistics 330*. Hyattsville, MD: National Center for Health Statistics.

Shafey, O., Dolwick, S., & Guindon, G. (2003). *Tobacco control country*. Retrieved May 28, 2007, from http://www.wpro.who.int/NR/rdonlyres/437C3114-24FE-45CA-9A62-8E119BC66CC6/0/TCCP2.pdf.

Smith, K. R., Mehta, S., & Maeusezahl-Feuz, M. (2004). Indoor air-pollution from household solid fuel use. In M. Eszzati, A. D. Lopez, A. Rodgers, & C. J. L. Murray (Eds.), *Comparative quantification of health risks: Global and regional burden of disease attributable to selected major risk factors* (pp. 1435–1493). Geneva, Switzerland: World Health Organization.

Snell, P. G., & Mitchell, J. H.. (1999). Physical inactivity—an easily modified risk factor? *Circulation, 100*, 2–4.

Stewart, A. W., Mitchell, E. A., Pearce, N., Strachan, D. P., & Weilandon, S. K. (2001). The relationship of per capita gross national product to the prevalence of symptoms of asthma and other atopic disease in children. *International Journal of Epidemiology, 30*, 173–179.

Stratton, I. M., Cull, C. A., Adler, A. I., Matthews, D. R., Neil, H. A. W., & Holman, R. R. (2006). Additive effects of glycaemia and blood pressure exposure on risk of complications in type 2 diabetes: A prospective observational study (UKPDS 75). *Diabetologia, 49*, 1761–1769.

Swanson, M. C., Agarwal, M. K., & Reed, C. E. (1985). An immunochemical approach to indoor aeroallergen quantitation with a new volumetric air sampler: Studies with mite, roach, cat, mouse, and guinea pig antigens. *Journal of Allergy & Clinical Immunology, 76*, 724–729.

Taiwo, O. A., Sircar, K. D., Slade, M. D., Cantley, L. F., Vegso, S. J. L, Rabinowitz, P. M., et al. (2006) Incidence of asthma among aluminum workers. *Journal of Occupational and Environmental Medicine, 48*(3), 275–282.

Tseng, C. H., Tseng, C. P., Chong, C. K., Huang, T. P., Song, Y. M., Chou, C. W., et al. (2006). Increasing incidences of diagnosed type 2 diabetes in Taiwan: Analysis of data from a national cohort. *Diabetologia, 49*, 1755–1760.

Understanding the burden of musculoskeletal conditions. (2001). [Electronic version]. *British Medical Journal, 322*, 1079–1080.

WHO. (2001). *WHO and the Bone and Joint Decade. The global economic and healthcare burden of musculoskeletal disease.* Retrieved June 11, 2005, from www.boneandjointdecade.org

WHO. (2005). *Integrated chronic disease prevention and control.* Retrieved June 18, 2005, from http://www.who.int/chp/about/integrated_cd/en

Woolf, A., & Pfleger, B. (2003) Burden of major musculoskeletal conditions. *Bulletin of the World Health Organization, 81*(9), 646–656.

Zan-bar, T, Aron, A., & Shoenfeld, Y. (2004). Acupuncture therapy for rheumatoid arthritis. *APLar Journal of Rheumatology, 7*, 207–214.

Chapter 11

Overview of Cancer for Allied Healthcare Professionals: A Public Health Perspective

*Linda G. Alley, Temeika L. Fairley, Cheryll Cardinez, and Paran Pordell**

Introduction

The fight to eliminate cancer as a major health problem extends around the world (American Cancer Society [ACS], 2007). Although better prevention, early detection, and advances in treatment have helped some developed nations lower their incidence and mortality rates for certain types of cancers, in most parts of the world cancer is a growing problem (ACS, 2007a). Worldwide, the number of new cancer cases is expected to grow by 50% to a total of 15 million by the year 2020 (Stewart & Kleihues, 2003), with 10 million deaths per year expected by 2020 (ACS, 2007a). According to *The Cancer Atlas*, the global epidemic of cancer is shifting from developed to developing nations (Mackay, Jemal, Lee, & Parkin, 2006), where about 85% of the world population resides (ACS, 2007a).

This chapter is written from a public health perspective, to acquaint allied healthcare professionals with important issues and concepts related to cancer and cancer patient care, both within the United States and in other parts of the world. The four sections address: (a) key cancer and public health concepts and definitions; (b) cancer prevention; (c) early detection, screening, and education; and (d) cancer care considerations, including treatment, survivorship, palliative care, and end-of-life care. Efforts have been made throughout the chapter to highlight cancer-related topics that undergraduate students and healthcare professionals in a variety of disciplines are likely to encounter early in their careers. Global perspectives are also provided to highlight both the similarities of some issues as well as different challenges that countries throughout the world encounter in addressing cancer. For the reader's consideration, an urgent call for healthcare actions that must be taken worldwide—if any major reductions in deaths and disability from cancer are to be realized—is also outlined.

---

*The findings and conclusions in this report are those of the authors and do not necessarily represent the views of the Centers for Disease Control and Prevention.

To obtain more in-depth information and details on the cancer-related topics presented in this chapter, readers are encouraged to refer to the numerous high-quality national reports, guidelines, books, journal articles, and other current documents cited here. We also highlight the Web sites of key national organizations and other helpful online resources. The Web sites of respected organizations are valuable resources because they are frequently updated to reflect the almost constant changes in state-of-the-art knowledge about cancer.

Key Cancer and Public Health Concepts and Definitions

Cancer and the Comprehensive Cancer Control Approach

An often-cited definition of cancer is provided by the American Cancer Society (2007a): "Cancer is a group of diseases characterized by uncontrolled growth and spread of abnormal cells" (p. 1). Over 100 different diseases are covered by the term *cancer*, and each of these diseases has a unique profile in terms of the population at risk, symptoms, and prognosis (Curry, Byers, & Hewitt, 2003). If the spread of abnormal cells is not controlled, it can lead to death of the individual affected. Cancer can be caused by external factors (tobacco, chemicals, radiation, and infectious organisms) and internal factors (inherited mutations, hormones, immune conditions, and mutations that occur from metabolism); these causal factors, acting together or in sequence, may initiate or promote the development of a cancer (ACS, 2007a). A period of 10 or more years often passes between exposure to such factors and the onset of detectable cancer (ACS, 2007a). The resulting time period between cancer development, detection, diagnosis, treatment, and possible progression can be quite long, ranging from months to decades, depending on cancer type.

For this reason, cancer prevention and control efforts must take a coordinated, long-term perspective (McKenna, Taylor, Marks, & Koplan, 1998). The comprehensive cancer control (CCC) process was developed to support the long-term perspective. Through this process, a community pools resources to reduce the burden of cancer by reducing risk, facilitating early detection, ensuring better treatment, and enhancing survivorship; these efforts, in turn, encourage healthy lifestyles, promote recommended cancer screening guidelines and tests, increase access to high-quality cancer care, and improve quality of life for cancer survivors (Centers for Disease Control and Prevention [CDC], 2006a). An excellent example of a far-reaching public health-oriented collaboration is the National Comprehensive Cancer Control Program (NCCCP) which is supported by the Centers for Disease Control and Prevention (CDC). The CDC's NCCCP is a national collaborative initiative that seeks to create the necessary conditions for dramatically reducing the burden of cancer incidence and mortality and improving the quality of life for cancer survivors (Black, Cowens-Alvarado, Gershman, & Weir, 2005).

In the United States, the NCCCP conducts its work by supporting the development and implementation of state CCC plans (Black, Cowens-Alvarado, Gershman, & Weir,

2005). Since 1998, the number of member CCC programs participating in NCCCP has grown from 6 to 63; currently, member programs include all 50 states and the District of Columbia, 6 tribes and tribal organizations, and 6 United States Associated Pacific Islands/Territories (CDC, 2007a). The CDC's Division of Cancer Prevention and Control works with national organizations, state health agencies, and other key groups to develop, implement, and promote effective cancer prevention and control practices within the NCCCP. Internationally, cancer prevention and control initiatives are taking place on each continent. Canada, China, France, and Chile are currently implementing national cancer control programs. According to the World Health Organization (WHO), the basic principles of cancer control include the following (WHO, 2006a):

- Leadership
- Involvement of stakeholders
- Creation of partnerships
- Responding to people's needs
- Decision making
- Applying a systematic approach
- Seeking continuous improvement
- Planning and implementing cancer control using a stepwise approach

Cancer Burden

Burden refers to the size of a health problem in a specified area, measured by several statistics, such as incidence, mortality, rates, and prevalence, as well as other indicators such as cost, morbidity ("any departure from physiological or psychological well-being") (Mackay, Jemal, Lee, & Parkin, 2006, p. 17), and risk factors (Stewart & Kleihues, 2003; Black, Cowens-Alvarado, Gershman, & Weir, 2005). Knowledge of the burden of a disease can help determine where investments in time, money, and other resources may be most effective in reducing the burden. ACS's *Worldwide Cancer Burden Report* (2006b) described the factors that contribute to the burden in developed countries versus those that contribute to the burden in developing countries. Contributing factors include regional differences in age structure, prevalence of major risk factors, availability of detection services, and completeness of reporting data to cancer registries. The 2007 Institute of Medicine (IOM) report on cancer control opportunities in low- and middle-income countries provides an excellent review of the significant burden of cancer in both low- and middle-income countries and major opportunities for such countries to achieve better cancer control (including cancer planning, cancer prevention and early detection/screening, cancer management, and psychosocial support for patients and families) (Sloan & Gelband, 2007).

As shown by the body of literature on cancer prevention, we have had for the last 10 years the knowledge needed to reduce the burden of cancer in the United States by about 50% (Harvard Center for Cancer Prevention, 1997; Black, Cowens-Alvarado, Gershman, & Weir, 2005). However, this knowledge has not been translated into systematic action across the country, and the failure to take this step presents a major challenge to current CCC efforts (Black, Cowens-Alvarado, Gershman, & Weir, 2005). With regard to the global cancer burden, the 2006 *Cancer Atlas* (Mackay, Jemal, Lee, & Parkin, 2006) defines the burden within the context of brief discussions of three related topics outlined below: the risk of getting cancer, the incidence of major cancers worldwide, and geographical diversity in the risks of developing cancers.

The Risk of Getting Cancer

Cancer risk is commonly expressed either as lifetime risk (the probability that one will develop or die from cancer over the course of one's lifetime) or relative risk (a measure of the strength of the relationship between risk factors and a particular cancer) (ACS, 2007a). Although anyone can develop cancer, most cases occur in adults who are middle-aged or older, since the risk of being diagnosed with cancer increases as people age (ACS, 2007a). The most common cancers involve epithelial tissues (linings of the airways, gastrointestinal, and urinary systems); the risk of developing these types of cancer increases rapidly with age, as does the overall risk of cancer (Mackay, Jemal, Lee, & Parkin, 2006). "Cancer develops when a sequence of mutations occurs in critical genes in one cell of the body, as a result of exposure to carcinogens, such as tobacco, infectious organisms, and chemicals, and internal factors such as inherited mutations, hormones, and immune conditions. Cumulative exposure to such agents increases with time, so that the probability of cancer increases as we age" (Mackay, Jemal, Lee, & Parkin, 2006, p. 42). Although all cancers involve the malfunction of genes that control cell growth and division, only about 5% of all cancers are strongly hereditary, in that an inherited genetic alteration confers a very high risk of developing one or more specific types of cancer (ACS, 2007a). In children, leukemias and cancers of connective tissue are more common than epithelial tissue cancers (Mackay, Jemal, Lee, & Parkin, 2006). More information regarding the differences between childhood and adult cancers can be found in the discussion section of the 2007 IOM report on cancer control (Sloan & Gelband, 2007).

Worldwide, most cancers can be linked to a few controllable factors, including tobacco use, poor diet, lack of exercise, and infectious diseases (ACS, 2007a; Curry, Byers, & Hewitt, 2003), all of which are discussed in the section on prevention, below. Tobacco use is the number one cause of cancer and the number one cause of preventable death throughout the world (Mackay, Eriksen, & Shafey, 2006; ACS, 2007a), and reduction in tobacco use offers the greatest opportunity to reduce the global incidence, morbidity, and mortality of cancer (Curry, Byers, and Hewitt, 2003). In fact, all cancers caused by cigarette smoking and heavy use of alcohol could be prevented completely (ACS, 2007a). The most important modifiable risk factors (i.e., risk factors that can be changed), as outlined by the

2006 *Cancer Atlas*, include an unhealthy diet (high in saturated fats with an insufficient intake of fresh fruits and vegetables), physical inactivity, infections with viruses or bacteria that cause cancer, and ultraviolet radiation exposure; other modifiable risk factors are alcohol use, occupational exposures to carcinogens such as asbestos and secondhand tobacco smoke (also referred to as passive smoking), socioeconomic status, environmental pollution, obesity, food contaminants, and ionizing radiation (Mackay, Jemal, Lee, & Parkin, 2006). Modifying some risk factors requires individual behavior changes, while modifying other risk factors requires changes at the population level (e.g., by employers or communities); often, improvement in risk factors is best accomplished by employing both individual and population level efforts (Mackay, Jemal, Lee, & Parkin, 2006).

Incidence of Major Cancers Worldwide

Cancer incidence refers to the number of newly diagnosed cases of cancer that occur in a defined population during a specified period of time, such as a year (Mackay, Jemal, Lee, & Parkin, 2006; Menck & Bolick-Aldrich, 2007). The term *cancer incidence rate* is the rate at which new cases occur in a population and is calculated by dividing the number of new cases that occur during a specified time period by the total number of people who were at risk for the given cancer in the defined population; this rate is generally expressed as the number of cancers per 100,000 people (Mackay, Jemal, Lee, & Parkin, 2006; Menck & Bolick-Aldrich, 2007). Cancer incidence is distinguished from another common term, *cancer prevalence*, which refers to how many cases of a particular cancer there are in a defined population at a given point in time (Hutchison, Menck, Burch, & Gottschalk, 2004).

The most common cancers worldwide are lung, breast, colorectal, stomach, and prostate (Mackay, Jemal, Lee, & Parkin, 2006). Liver cancer is the most common cancer for men in several African countries, although Kaposi sarcoma is the most common cancer in 13 of these African countries that are severely affected by the HIV/AIDS epidemic. Either breast or cervical cancer is the most common malignancy for women in almost all countries, except for in some East Asian countries, where stomach cancer is more frequent (Mackay, Jemal, Lee, & Parkin, 2006). The cancer that causes the most deaths worldwide is lung cancer, followed by stomach and liver cancer, although the pattern is quite different in males and females (Mackay, Jemal, Lee, & Parkin, 2006). Cancer affects all races, ethnicities, genders, and ages. The cancers that are common in developing countries are those that have a poor prognosis, including cancers of the lung, stomach, liver, and esophagus (Mackay, Jemal, Lee, & Parkin, 2006).

Geographical Diversity

The risk of developing different cancers varies widely by world region, as noted by the examples that follow. Studies of migrants or populations who move from one location to another confirm that differences in the risk of various cancers are largely environmental in origin (not due to ethnic or genetic differences) and especially are a product of different lifestyles (Mackay, Jemal, Lee, & Parkin, 2006). Liver cancer incidence reflects the prevalence of infection by hepatitis viruses, especially hepatitis B virus. Esophageal cancer rates are high in east Africa and Asia, including China and Central Asia, while testicular cancer is rare in African and Asian men (Mackay, Jemal, Lee, & Parkin, 2006). Although it is not rare anywhere in the world, breast cancer is primarily a disease of affluent countries (Mackay, Jemal, Lee, & Parkin, 2006). In contrast, the burden of disease from cervical cancer is highest in the poorer southern countries in Africa, Latin America, and South and Southeast Asia (Sloan & Gelband, 2007). Worldwide, lung cancer is the most common cancer, both in terms of new cases and of deaths; about 80% of cases in men and 50% in women are caused by tobacco smoking (Mackay, Jemal, Lee, & Parkin, 2006). The 2006 ACS report on the worldwide cancer burden illustrated and briefly described international variations in cancer incidence and mortality for the most common cancers (i.e. lung, female breast, colon and rectum, stomach, prostate, liver, and cervical) in both economically developed and developing regions of the world (ACS, 2006b). The bacterium *Helicobacter pylori* (*H. pylori*) is a major cause of stomach cancer, which is poorly responsive to treatment (Sloan & Gelband, 2007). The prevalence of *H. pylori*, as well as that of stomach cancer, has declined dramatically without targeted measures in much of the world; this suggests the possibility of developing interventions for geographic regions where *H. pylori* is not declining, which includes most low-income countries (Sloan & Gelband, 2007; Mackay, Jemal, Lee, & Parkin, 2006).

In the United States, cancer overall is the second leading cause of death, exceeded only by heart disease (ACS, 2007a). One of every four deaths in the United States is due to cancer (ACS, 2007a), and the American Cancer Society estimates that in 2007, close to 1.5 million Americans will receive a new diagnosis of invasive cancer and over a half million Americans will die of this disease—more than 1500 people a day (ACS, 2007a). The 2007 new cancer case estimate does not include carcinoma in situ (noninvasive cancer) of any site (except for urinary bladder cancer) or the more than 1 million cases of basal and squamous cell skin cancers expected to be diagnosed in 2007. Men in the United States are most often diagnosed with or die from prostate, lung, and colorectal cancers, whereas women are most often diagnosed or die from female breast, lung, and colorectal cancers (United States Cancer Statistics Working Group [USCSWG], 2006). Incidence rates for cervical cancer have decreased steadily over the past 20 years, as Papanicolaou test (also referred to as the Pap test) screening, discussed later in the section on early detection and screening, has become more common (ACS, 2007a). There are variations in incidence and mortality by race and ethnicity and by geographic area in the United States (ACS, 2006a). This may be the result of regional differences in exposure to known or unknown risk factors such as sociodemographic population characteristics (e.g., age, race and ethnicity, geographic region, urban or rural residence), use of screening activities, health-related behaviors (e.g., behaviors related to tobacco use, diet, physical activity), exposure to cancer-causing agents, or cancer registry operations factors (e.g., completeness and timeliness of data collection; specificity in coding data collected for various cancer sites) (CDC, 2005a; Devesa, Grauman, Blot, Pennello, & Hoover, 1999; Howe, Keller, & Lehnherr, 1993).

Cancer Mortality

Cancer mortality refers to "the numbers of deaths from cancer that occur in a population during a specified period of time" (Mackay, Jemal, Lee, & Parkin, 2006, p. 17). Mortality rate refers to the rate at which deaths occur in a population and is calculated by dividing the number of deaths that occur during a specified period of time by the number of people at risk for the given cancer in the specified population (Mackay, Jemal, Lee, & Parkin, 2006; Menck & Bolick-Aldrich, 2007). Overall, the probability of an individual dying from cancer during his or her lifetime does not differ appreciably between the developed and developing world (Mackay, Jemal, Lee, & Parkin, 2006). At the same time, although the risk of getting cancer is higher in the developed world, cancers in the developing world are more fatal (Mackay, Jemal, Lee, & Parkin, 2006).

To give the reader a sense of the complexity of how mortality data are collected and used, a brief discussion of considerations related to this important cancer measure is provided. Data on cancer deaths are compiled in accordance with World Health Organization (WHO) regulations. The WHO specifies that member nations classify and code causes of death in accordance with the current version of the *International Classification of Diseases,* which is version 10 (ICD-10) (WHO, 1992). The ICD 10 manual provides detailed classification of diseases, as well as definitions, tabulation lists, the format of the death certificate, and the rules for coding cause of death (WHO, 1992), to try to ensure uniformity of data collection. Tabulations of cause-of-death statistics are based solely on the underlying cause of death and are selected from the conditions entered by the physician in the cause-of-death section of the death certificate (WHO, 1992). The accuracy of this information, reported by the physician, influences cancer mortality statistics.

Vital statistics in the United States are available from the National Vital Statistics System (NVSS), which operates within CDC's National Center for Health Statistics (NCHS). The NVVS is the oldest and most successful example of intergovernmental sharing of public health data. Vital statistics data are provided through state-operated registration systems and are based on vital records filed in state vital statistics offices. Legal responsibility for the registration of vital events rests with the individual states. Through its Vital Statistics Cooperative Program, the CDC cooperates with state vital statistics offices to develop and recommend standard forms for data collection and model procedures to ensure uniform registration of the events monitored by the NVSS (USCSWG, 2006).

The Expanding Role of Cancer Registries

Cancer registries serve as important links between high-quality cancer data collection and high-quality patient care. Despite the enormous contributions made by registries, registry staff often work in fairly low-visibility positions in clinical settings, so healthcare professionals working in hospitals may be unaware of the time- and labor-intensive, highly technical, and very valuable work of these cancer surveillance leaders. Thus, highlights of cancer registries and the registration process are provided here. Cancer registries are data collection systems that assess the occurrence and characteristics of reportable cancers, and they are designed for the collection, management, and analysis of data on persons who have been diagnosed with cancer (Hutchison, Menck, Burch, & Gottschalk, 2004). The organized and systematic cancer registration process involves the collection of five items in the fundamental data set: (a) occurrence of cancer, (b) type of cancer (site, morphology, and behavior), (c) extent of disease at the time of diagnosis (stage), (d) types of treatment received by the patient, and (e) treatment outcomes (survival) (Hutchison, Menck, Burch, & Gottschalk, 2004). Cancer registries exist in a wide range of settings and function within varying organizational structures, such as hospitals, physicians' offices, radiation facilities, freestanding surgical centers, research centers, and pathology laboratories (USCSWG, 2006; Hutchison, Menck, Burch, & Gottschalk, 2004). The status of cancer registration in other countries is addressed by Menck (2004).

Cancer registries may collect details of new cancer cases and their follow-up, either for a defined population (e.g., a geographical area; a particular cancer diagnosis) or for a hospital (Mackay, Jemal, Lee, & Parkin, 2006). Registries that seek to collect and maintain data on all possible patients within a defined geographic area (such as a state, province, or city) are referred to as population-based (Hutchison, Menck, Burch, & Gottschalk, 2004). Because the reader of this book may hear the term *cancer registry* in the course of daily business, two main types of registries are briefly noted here. Hospital-based cancer registries provide detailed information about cancer patients receiving care at the hospital, the nature of their tumors (including the precise histological types and stage of disease), treatment received, and the outcome of the disease to date (Mackay, Jemal, Lee, & Parkin, 2006). Central cancer registries collect cancer information from more than one facility (typically including hospitals, as well as other healthcare facilities such as radiation therapy clinics) and consolidate multiple reports from the various facilities on a single patient into one record (Hutchison, Menck, Burch, & Gottschalk, 2004). If a patient has multiple primary cancers, special attention is given so that this information is properly captured. Hospital and central registries are unified in a synergistic and complex effort to help reduce the burden of cancer through the common use of cancer patient data (Menck, Deapen, Phillips, & Tucker, 2007).

Two national cancer data surveillance systems from which a healthcare provider will find useful publications when seeking updated United States cancer statistics are the Surveillance, Epidemiology, and End Results Program (SEER) and the National Program of Cancer Registries (NPCR). The SEER is a federally funded program of the National Cancer Institute, comprising 18 population-based cancer registries in various parts of the United States (NCI, 2007c). The member registries have been included based on their ability to operate and maintain a high-quality reporting system and for their epidemiologically significant population subgroups; some of the member registries are state based, some are based in urban communities, and one is a rural part of one state (NCI, 2007c). The SEER covers approximately 26% of the United States population. Established in 1973, SEER includes population-based information on stage of disease at diagnosis and patient survival data. It is the only comprehensive source of population-based information in the United States that includes stage of cancer at the time of diagnosis and patient survival data (NCI, 2007c). The National Program of Cancer Registries (NPCR) is the federally funded CDC program that currently supports central registries and promotes the use of high-quality registry data in 45 states, 3 territories, and the District of Columbia. Established in 1995, NPCR covers 96% of the United States population (CDC, 2007b; Intlekofer & Michaud, 2007). The NPCR data collected by state cancer registries enable public health professionals to understand and address the cancer burden more effectively in their states; the NPCR data are critical to planning state-specific cancer control activities that meet to the needs of residents of the participating NPCR states. Each year, CDC and NCI combine their high-quality cancer incidence data, from the NPCR and SEER, respectively, to produce an important set of official federal cancer statistics, in collaboration with the North American Association of Central Cancer Registries (NAACCR). The resulting collaborative effort, the annual *United States Cancer Statistics* report, provides state-specific, regional, and national data for cancer cases diagnosed for a single year (USCSWG, 2006). Current cancer statistics are available on the United States Cancer Statistics (USCS) Web site at http://www.cdc.gov/nccdphp/publicationsaag/dnpa2006_text.htm (CDC, 2007c).

When registries first came into use about six decades ago, they focused primarily on describing cancer patterns and trends and sometimes calculating survival. In the last 20 years, the roles of registries have been significantly expanded to play an increasingly important role in planning and evaluation of cancer control activities and in improving the care of individual cancer patients (Parkin, 2006; Menck, Deapen, Phillips, & Tucker, 2007; Hutchison, Menck, Burch, & Gottschalk, 2004; Mackay, Jemal, Lee, & Parkin, 2006). Cancer registries serve as the "eyes and ears" of cancer control around the world, and the statistics they produce are essential in planning and evaluating activities of comprehensive cancer control programs (Mackay, Jemal, Lee, & Parkin, 2006). Some cancer registries continue to follow patients throughout their lifetimes to identify those who have recurring cancer or a second cancer, have received additional treatments, have had progression or remission of disease, and/or have died (Clive, 2004).

Cancer registries also have increasingly important public health and research functions (Mackay, Jemal, Lee, & Parkin, 2006). For example, NPCR cancer registry data were recently used in a multistate patterns of care (PoC) research study to assess the completeness and quality of NPCR cancer registry data collected in seven participating states and to determine the extent to which guidelines-based, stage-specific treatments were provided to patients with specific cancer diagnoses residing in those states (McDavid, Schymura, Armstrong, Santilli, Schmidt, Byers, et al., 2004; Intlekofer & Michaud, 2007).

Such studies provide information that can be used to continue to improve the quality of NPCR registry data and to identify groups of patients (e.g., by age, race, ethnicity) who may be receiving less than adequate care. Such work can thereby help researchers and clinicians develop a better understanding of treatment disparities and ways to correct them. Obtaining high-quality data—which is at the core of cancer registry surveillance work—is an important step toward motivating action to reducing the burden of cancer, whether through prevention, screening, treatment, and/or survivorship-related activities (Black, Cowens-Alvarado, Gershman, & Weir, 2005). In other parts of the world, cancer registries are very active and experienced in some countries while still developing in others. The reader is referred to interesting references that trace the development of registries in other countries over the last 60 years (Parkin, 2006; Mackay, Jemal, Lee, & Parkin, 2006; Menck, 2004). The International Association of Cancer Registries (IARC) has a global membership and sponsors a variety of publications, including an every-five-years publication in collaboration with IARC, entitled *Cancer Incidence in Five Continents*. This publication contains statistical data from all the best-quality registries worldwide (Mackay, Jemal, Lee, & Parkin, 2006).

Cancer Costs

"The costs of cancer pose an economic burden on both the individual and society," (Mackay, Jemal, Lee, & Parkin, 2006, p. 57), regardless of the country being considered. Although data limitations do not allow for a worldwide comparison of the economic costs of cancer (Mackay, Jemal, Lee, & Parkin, 2006), the 2006 *Cancer Atlas* published data from selected countries and described the diverse and significant costs incurred for selected cancers. Three categories of cost domains especially relevant to cancer that are often discussed in the literature include: *direct costs*, including both medical costs (e.g., hospitalizations and treatments) and associated nonmedical costs (e.g., transportation to hospital or physician's office); *indirect costs*, such as time spent seeking medical care or economic productivity lost due to premature death; and *intangible/ psychosocial costs*, such as pain, suffering, or grief (Brown & Yabroff, 2006). Interestingly, Mackay and colleagues (2006) noted that cancer prevention may be the best way to save money for many countries, given that the costs associated with cancer continue to increase.

Not surprisingly, in the United States, the costs of cancer are staggering and continuing to rise. The National Heart, Lung, and Blood Institute (NHLBI) estimated the overall annual cost of cancer in 2006 to be $206.3 billion (NHLBI, 2006). All of these costs are likely to increase because of the anticipated growth and aging of the United States population (USCSWG, 2006). Lack of health insurance and other cost barriers prevent many Americans each year from receiving optimal health care; almost 1 million US citizens (6% of the population) are unable to obtain needed medical care due to cost, according to 2004 data from the National Health Interview Survey (ACS, 2007a).

Cancer Prevention

This section focuses on concepts and definitions related to the broad area of cancer prevention, which includes key actions such as reducing tobacco use and exposure to secondhand smoke; maintaining optimal nutrition, physical activity, and body weight; and minimizing exposure to infectious disease agents. These actions will contribute to reducing the global cancer burden over the long term. Prevention, sometimes described as primary prevention, refers to activities directed toward avoiding the occurrence of disease (Menck & Bolick-Aldrich, 2007). Prevention represents the most beneficial population-based public health approach to reducing morbidity and mortality from cancer. Its ultimate goal is to promote health and potentially eliminate disease risk. Cancer prevention strategies generally address known risk factors such as exposure to infectious agents, environmental carcinogens, and specific lifestyle behaviors, while some risk factors, such as age, gender, and genetic predisposition, cannot be altered. Public health measures that incorporate prevention strategies are meant to benefit people at the individual, community, and environmental levels. In addition to the key topics covered in this section, the 2007 IOM report on cancer control opportunities (Sloan & Gelband) discusses other important cancer causes and risk factors, thus providing more useful information for the new healthcare professional.

Reducing Tobacco Use and Exposure to Secondhand Smoke

Tobacco is the only consumer product proven to kill more than half of its regular users and is responsible for about 5 million deaths worldwide every year (Mackay, Eriksen, & Shafey, 2006), with the burden being roughly equal in developed and developing nations. Cigarette smoking and other forms of tobacco, which collectively are the largest single contributor to cancer mortality, are responsible for a large and growing global public health burden (Sloan & Gelband, 2007). Cigarettes are the most common method of consuming tobacco throughout the world, with the exception of chewing tobacco in India and possibly kreteks (clove-flavored cigarettes) in Indonesia (Mackay, Eriksen, & Shafey, 2006). For the interested reader, *The Tobacco Atlas* (Mackay, Eriksen, & Shafey, 2006) provides useful descriptions and illustrations of 11 types of tobacco products used in various parts of the world.

By the year 2025, tobacco use is expected to become the leading cause of death and disability worldwide, killing more than 10 million people every year (Mackay, Eriksen, & Shafey, 2006). Further, if today's efforts to curb tobacco use are not successful, tobacco will kill 650 million of its current users, about 10% of the current total world population (Mackay, Eriksen, & Shafey, 2006). As of 1999, enough evidence had accrued to support smoking as a cause of eight cancers: lung, laryngeal oral, pharyngeal, esophageal, bladder, kidney, and pancreatic (Curry, Byers, & Hewitt, 2003). By 2003, sufficient evidence was available to: (a) implicate smoking as a cause of cancers of the colon, stomach, and cervix, and leukemia, as well as a probable cause of liver cancer, and (b) associate smoking with an increase in the risk of developing aggressive forms of prostate cancer (Curry, Byers, & Hewitt, 2003).

The complex topics of health consequences of smoking, current mortality worldwide from smoking, and the benefits of smoking cessation were discussed in detail in the 2007 IOM report on cancer control opportunities (Sloan & Gelband, 2007). The biggest single impact on cancer worldwide will be made solely by reducing tobacco use (Mackay, Jemal, Lee, & Parkin, 2006). Substantial health benefits steadily accrue for smokers who quit, with the cessation of tobacco use reducing the risk of many cancers over time (Curry, Byers, & Hewitt, 2003). Passive smoking, also known as exposure to secondhand smoke or environmental tobacco smoke, causes a variety of adverse health effects in nonsmokers, and the growing evidence about the health risks of passive smoking has led to a ban on smoking in public areas in many countries (Mackay, Jemal, Lee, & Parkin, 2006). However, such bans are not sufficient to protect people from harm caused by exposure to tobacco smoke (Mackay, Jemal, Lee, & Parkin, 2006), prompting considerations of many interventions and policy changes worldwide, to decrease tobacco use and thereby protect nonsmokers from passive smoking (Sloan & Gelband, 2007), as well.

The Framework Convention on Tobacco Control (FCTC), described as a pillar in tobacco control, is the world's first internationally binding, global health treaty designed to reduce noncommunicable diseases (Mackay, Jemal, Lee, & Parkin, 2006; WHO, 2003a; WHO, 2006a). The FCTC includes provisions for both *demand reduction of tobacco* and *supply reduction of tobacco*, along with the evidence of the impact of the key interventions. The key provisions of the framework are related to: (a) advertising, sponsorship, and promotion, (b) packaging and labeling of tobacco products, (c) protection from exposure to tobacco smoke, and (d) illicit trade in tobacco products (Sloan & Gelband, 2007). The IOM report outlines explicit interventions to *reduce the demand for tobacco* including: (a) tobacco taxation, (b) restrictions on smoking, (c) provision of health information and counteradvertising, (d) bans on advertising and promotion, and (e) smoking cessation treatments. Further, the report identified the main interventions to *reduce the supply of tobacco,* which are: (a) the control of smuggling, (b) price increases, (c) nicotine replacement therapy, and (d) a package of interventions other than nicotine replacement therapy (Sloan & Gelband, 2007). From a global health perspective, the most important step toward decreasing the burden of cancer relative to tobacco is ratification of the FCTC by as many countries as possible, at which time they will be obligated to adopt its provisions (Sloan & Gelband, 2007). It is encouraging and instructive to note that experts believe that interventions to reduce tobacco use will have much broader benefits beyond the reduction of tobacco-related cancers, resulting in significant decreases in other illnesses, as well, such as cardiovascular and respiratory diseases (Sloan & Gelband, 2007).

Maintaining Optimal Nutrition, Physical Activity, and Body Weight

Nutrition, physical activity, and body weight have been linked to almost one-third of all cancer deaths (Byers, Nestle, McTiernan, Doyle, Currie-Williams, Gansler, et al., 2002).

Diet, activity levels, and body weight are interrelated, and research suggests that these three factors act in complex ways to either promote or reduce the risk of cancer (Sloan & Gelband, 2007; CDC, 2006b). In fact, some studies suggest that the state of nutrition and extent of physical activity, along with level of alcohol consumption, may be the most important modifiable causes of cancer or cancer risk (Mackay, Jemal, Lee, & Parkin, 2006). Almost 10% of cancer death in low- and middle-income countries are attributable to the risk factors of poor diet, being overweight or obese, and physical inactivity, all three of which could be the focus of interventions (Sloan & Gelband, 2007).

Worldwide, diet may be the most important modifiable cause of cancer: diet-related factors account for about 30% of cancers in developed countries and 20% in developing countries and, thus, may be the most important modifiable causes of cancer (Mackay, Jemal, Lee, & Parkin, 2006). A poor diet has been linked to several cancers, with the most consistent evidence linking consumption of large amounts of fruits and vegetables with a lower risk of developing cancers of the colon and rectum, lung, stomach, esophagus, mouth, and pharynx (World Cancer Research Fund & American Institute for Cancer Research, 1997; Curry, Byers, & Hewitt, 2003; Sloan & Gelband, 2007).

Alcohol intake is related to the quality of one's diet. Avoidance of heavy alcohol consumption may decrease risk of cancers of the oral cavity, pharynx, larynx, esophagus, liver, and breast, with the risk varying by cancer site but increasing for all sites with greater alcohol consumption (Sloan & Gelband, 2007). With respect to cancers of the breast, colon, rectum, and aerodigestive tract, there is a clear dose-response relationship; even moderate levels of alcohol consumption may slightly increase cancer risk (Curry, Byers, & Hewitt, 2003). Alcohol consumption is an established cause of cancers of the mouth, pharynx, larynx, esophagus, liver and breast, with risk increasing substantially with intake of more than two drinks per day (ACS, 2007a). For the interested reader, considerable similarities between the problem of excessive alcohol use and the problem of tobacco use have been identified, along with potentially powerful strategies related to reducing individual consumption and to provide public education about the harmful effects of these substances on health.

Physical activity, the second factor discussed here, is closely associated with nutrition and body weight factors. Regular physical activity, defined as bodily movement produced by the contraction of skeletal muscle that significantly increases energy expenditure (Casperson, 1989), is known to lower the risk of cancers of the colon and breast and, possibly, endometrial cancer as well (Curry, Byers, & Hewitt, 2003). Physical activity improves health, reduces the risk of acquiring certain cancers, and benefits cancer survivors with respect to reducing depressive symptoms. Engaging in regular physical activity allows the body to function more efficiently while complementing healthy dietary practices.

Over the last 14 years, more than 200 population-based studies have linked work, leisure, and household physical activities to cancer risk. Research investigating a possible relationship between physical activity and cancer has focused largely on cancer of the colon, endometrium, testes, prostate, lung, and breast. Numerous studies have demonstrated an association between physical activity and colon and breast cancers (Batty &

Thune, 2000; Shephard & Futcher, 1997; Colditz, Cannuscio, & Frazier, 1997; McTiernan, Ulrich, Slate, & Potter, 1998). No significant association has been found between physical activity and decreasing the risk of developing rectal, lung, or prostate cancer (Batty & Thune, 2000; Martinez, Giovannucci, Spiegelman, Hunter, Willett, & Colditz, 1997; Lee, 2003; World Cancer Research Fund & American Institute for Cancer Research, 1997).

It has been proposed that engaging in regular physical activity positively influences insulin, prostaglandin, and bile acid levels in the body and affects growth and proliferation of cells within the colon as well as boosts immune function (McTiernan, Ulrich, Slate, & Potter, 1998; McKeown-Eyssen, 1994; Giovannucci, 1995; Martinez, Heddens, Earnest, Bogart, Roe, Einspahr, et al., 1999). These substances may also reduce bowel transit time, which ultimately decreases the duration of contact between cancer-causing substances in digestive by-products (fecal matter) and the colonic mucosa (Batty & Thune, 2000). Participating in high levels of physical activity throughout the lifespan seems to impart the greatest protection (Lee, Gourley, Duffy, Esteve, Lee, & Day, 1989; Kune, Kune, & Watson, 1990). A study of Harvard University alumni males found that men who were moderately active at two assessments were 48% less likely to develop colon cancer than their inactive male counterparts (Lee, Paffenbarger, & Hsieh, 1991). Furthermore, data from at least two prospective studies pointed out that men and women can lower their colon cancer risk by engaging in moderate physical activity such as brisk walking or stair climbing for an hour daily (Giovannucci, 1995; Martinez, Giovannucci, Spiegelman, Hunter, Willett, & Colditz, 1997).

Engaging in regular physical activity is associated with a reduced risk of breast cancer in premenopausal and postmenopausal women in part because it may decrease the collective exposure to cyclic estrogens and progesterone as well as influence energy balance (Thune, Brenn, Lund, & Gaard, 1997). A woman's breast cancer risk is largely dependent on the amount of estrogen circulating in her body (Willett, 2000; Hankinson et al., 1995). Some studies have taken the importance of lifelong physical activity one step further by investigating the engagement of regular physical activity in childhood and whether or not it affects breast cancer risk. Engaging in regular physical activity may result in delayed menarche or a delay in the onset of regular ovulatory menstrual cycles, which may decrease lifelong risk for breast cancer (Willett, 2000).

Body weight, the third factor discussed here, is closely associated with the nutrition and physical activity factors. Having excess body weight—either by being overweight or obese—is a national public health crisis in the United States affecting all age groups, races and ethnicities, and both sexes. Obesity is caused primarily by a combination of a sedentary lifestyle that lacks physical activity and excessive consumption of high-calorie, high-fat, low-nutrient foods. Overweight and obesity both increase the risk of colon, breast (postmenopausal), endometrial, kidney, and esophageal cancers, and may also be linked to pancreatic, ovarian, and gall bladder cancers (NCI, 2004; IARC, 2002a). Calle, Rodriguez, Walker-Thurmond, & Thun (2003) estimated that 14% to 20% of all deaths from cancer are attributable to overweight or obesity in adults age 50 years and older. In the United States, nearly 59 million adults are obese and close to 9 million young people (ages 6 to19) are considered overweight in the United States (CDC, 2004a).

Obesity and overweight are distinguished from each other, as follows: Obesity is defined as having a body mass index (BMI) greater than or equal to 30.0, while being over-weight is defined as having a BMI between 25.0 to 29.9. The BMI is defined as weight in kilograms divided by height in meters squared (kg/m^2) (Garrow & Webster, 1985). Some experts have estimated that if American adults balanced energy input and output more effectively through practices of eating healthy foods containing less fat and engaging in regular physical activity, therefore maintaining a body mass index (BMI) below 25 throughout their lives, the nation could steer clear of more than 900,000 cancer deaths per year (Calle, Rodriguez, Walker-Thurmond, Thun, 2003).

The United States is clearly faced with an epidemic that must be addressed at every stage of life, primarily by modifying eating habits and regularly engaging in physical activity. Although diet and physical activity are clearly documented as very important determinants of cancer, interventions that are known to have a substantial effect on diet and exercise habits are not well established in high-income countries (Sloan & Gelband, 2007). The WHO report entitled *Global Strategy on Diet, Physical Activity, and Health* makes a series of recommendations related to establishing stronger evidence for policy, advocating for policy changes, fostering stakeholder involvement, and developing a strategic frame-work tailored for specific countries (WHO, 2004; Sloan & Gelband, 2007). From a global perspective, highly consistent evidence indicates that excessive calorie intake in relation to level of physical activity increases the risk of many cancers and that this is the second most important avoidable cause of cancer mortality in many countries after cigarette smoking (Willett, 2006).

Minimizing Exposure to Infectious Disease Agents

Worldwide, almost 18% of cancer is caused by infections (Mackay, Jemal, Lee, & Parkin, 2006); the main implicated infectious disease agents are mentioned here. *Helicobacter pylori*, which is estimated to cause close to 6% of the world's cancers, increases the risk of stomach cancer, especially in developing countries (Mackay, Jemal, Lee, & Parkin, 2006). One proposed hypothesis is that *H. pylori* causes chronic inflammation of and damage to the gastric mucosa, with the resulting infection placing an individual at three to six times greater risk for developing gastric cancer (Stewart & Kleihues, 2003; Sepulveda & Graham, 2003).

The human papillomavirus (HPV), a common sexually transmitted virus, causes all cer-vical cancers as well as most of the rarer cancers of the anus and about half of cancers of the external genitalia; to a lesser extent, HPV also causes cancers of the month and oropharynx and possibly also respiratory cancers (Mackay, Jemal, Lee, & Parkin, 2006; CDC, 2006c). Nearly all cases of cervical cancer are caused by persistent infection with cer-tain oncogenic strains of HPV; although 90% of women infected with HPV will clear their infections with no intervention, HPV will persist in the remaining 10% who make up the population at risk of cervical cancer (Bosch & Munoz, 2002; Sloan & Gelband, 2007; CDC, 2006e). Despite the established role of HPV in the development of cervical cancer, screening rates for HPV are low. Stewart and Kleihues (2003) found that the major barrier to cervical cancer prevention is not being screened at all. Recently, both GlaxoSmithKline (GSK) and Merck & Co., Inc. have each developed vaccines to prevent infection with the most prevalent types of HPV associated with cervical cancer—types 16 and 18 (associated with 70% of cervical cancers), and both vaccines have shown complete efficacy in preventing persistent infection by HPV types 16 and 18 (Sloan & Gelband, 2007). In addition, the Merck vaccine is also designed to protect against HPV types 6 and 11, the most common agents of genital warts (Sloan & Gilband, 2007).

Chronic infection with either hepatitis B virus (HBV) or hepatitis C virus (HCV), both of which are common, increases the risk of liver cancer 20 fold or more (Mackay, Jemal, Lee, & Parkin, 2006). Together these two infections are responsible for more than 85% of the liver cancer in the world (Mackay, Jemal, Lee, & Parkin, 2006). It is estimated that more than one-third of the world's population is infected with hepatitis B. Hepatitis C virus infection is the most common chronic blood-borne viral infection in the United States (CDC, 2006c). Sloan and Gelband (2007) noted that HBV vaccines have been available for 20 years and are not expensive; yet, they are still not being used in areas with some of the highest liver cancer rates. Increasing the worldwide coverage and usage of the hepatitis B virus vaccine has the potential to save lives now and in the future and to build cancer control capacity in geographic areas where it is currently limited (Sloan & Gelband, 2007; CDC, 2006d). There is currently no vaccine available to prevent hepatitis C transmission. Finally, the Epstein-Barr virus, the human immunodeficiency virus (HIV), and the human herpesvirus-8 are each responsible for about 100,000 new cancer cases each year, while the schistosomes, human T-cell lymphotropic virus type I, and the liver flukes are infectious organisms that less frequently cause cancer (Mackay, Jemal, Lee, & Parkin, 2006).

As noted throughout this section on prevention, positive changes in lifestyle factors have the potential to reduce a large proportion of cancer burden (Curry, Byers, & Hewitt, 2003). Also, the 2003 IOM report on reaching the potential for timely cancer prevention and early detection noted that although specific research methods and results of analyses related to cancer prevention and early detection activities vary, the studies are all remarkably consistent in pointing to the potential benefits of reducing tobacco use, improving nutrition, increasing physical activity, maintaining a healthy body weight, keeping alcohol consumption at low to moderate levels, and getting screened regularly for cancer (Curry, Byers, & Hewett, 2003). For health professional-oriented summaries of current data on prevention for particular disease sites, the reader is referred to NCI's *Physician Data Query (PDQ) Comprehensive Cancer Database* series of detailed summaries (NCI, 2007a). Most of the *PDQ* prevention summaries are also available in patient versions, written in easy-to-understand, nontechnical language.

Early Detection, Screening, and Education

This section focuses on concepts and definitions related to the critically important area of early detection. Early detection is the complementary strategy to cancer prevention. The two core components of early detection of cancer are screening and education (Mackay, Jemal, Lee, & Parkin, 2006; Curry, Byers, & Hewitt, 2003; Gullatte, Phillips, & Gibson, 2006). The two primary strategies for early detection are: (a) early diagnosis, often triggered by the patient's discovery of early signs and symptoms, leading to an appointment with a healthcare provider, and (b) screening of asymptomatic and apparently healthy individuals to detect precancerous lesions or an early stage of cancer, leading to referral for diagnosis and treatment (WHO, 2006a). One of the principal ways to reduce deaths from cancer is to ensure that people seek medical help for suspicious symptoms and that they use screening programs where they are available (McCaffery, Wardle, & Waller, 2003).

More than 16 million new cancer cases and 10 million deaths are expected by 2020, and 70% of these deaths will occur in developing countries (ACS, 2006b). A high proportion of cancers that are relatively curable in developed countries (because the cancers are screened for and, thus, are detected early) are detected only at advanced stages in developing countries (because the cancers are not subjected to screening early) (WHO, 2006b). Variation in cancer burden in developed and developing countries may result in part from differences in access to effective screening and treatment programs. For example, cervical cancer is the most commonly diagnosed cancer among women in developing countries that lack organized screening programs. However, cervical cancer accounts for only 4 percent of cancers in women in well-developed countries where cervical cancer screening is widespread (ACS, 2006b).

The burden of cancer is high worldwide, despite the fact that many cancers are preventable. The prognosis is generally better and treatment usually more successful if the disease is detected and treated early (WHO, 2006b). For example, 70–80% of deaths caused by cervical cancer can be reduced with the implementation of screening programs and adequate patient follow-up (ACS, 2006b; Kitchener, Castle, & Cox, 2006). In the United Kingdom, this translates into at least 1,000 lives per year among a population of 50 million (Parkin, 1991; Abwao, Green, Sanghvi, Tsu, & Winkler, 1998). Declining death rates for many cancers in developed nations prove that cancer can be controlled with aggressive intervention worldwide.

Failure to implement proven methods of cancer prevention and control leads to avoidable disease and death (Curry, Byers, & Hewitt, 2003). One of the principal ways to reduce deaths from cancer is to ensure that people seek medical help for suspicious symptoms and that they use screening programs where they are available (McCaffery, Wardle, & Waller, 2003). Studies have shown that diagnosing and treating cancer in its early stages and implementing early detection programs are the most cost-effective means of reducing the burden of cancer (Groot, Baltussen, Uyl-de Groot, Anderson, & Hortobagyi, 2006; Pignone, Rich, Teutsch, Berg, & Lohr, 2002).

General Principles Governing the Introduction of Early Detection Programs

The implementation of early detection programs requires considerable resources. Education and screening programs generally involve costs to the individual (in terms of time spent, distance traveled, cash payments for detection and diagnosis), as well as to the health services providers (staff subsidies for detection and diagnosis, treatment, and follow-up), and sometimes may be associated with undesired harm (WHO, 2002). For these reasons, population-level screening programs should be undertaken as a component of early detection only where their effectiveness has been demonstrated, where resources (e.g., personnel, equipment) are sufficient to cover at least 70% of the target group, where facilities exist for confirming diagnoses and for treatment and follow-up of those with abnormal results, and where prevalence of disease is high enough to justify the efforts and cost of screening (WHO, 2003b). Because the implementation of screening programs is of such importance to the control of cancer around the world, considerable attention has been given to implementation of the process and related procedures. The International Union Against Cancer (UICC) has established a general set of principles governing the introduction of screening programs (Miller, Chamberlain, Day, Hakama, & Prorok, 1990; Prorok, Chamberlain, Day, Hakama, & Miller, 1984). These principles are the basis for decisions regarding screening program implementation in both developed and developing nations worldwide:

1. The disease should be an important health problem—the disease should be common and the cause of substantial mortality and/or morbidity.

2. The disease should have a detectable preclinical phase.

3. The natural history of the condition should be known.

4. The disease should be treatable, and there should be a recognized treatment for lesions identified during treatment.

5. The screening test should be acceptable and safe.

Screening

The fundamental tenet of screening for cancer is that finding the disease before symptoms develop enables detection at a less advanced stage and that the institution of treatment at that time will produce improved health outcomes (Curry, Byers, & Hewitt, 2003; Zapka, 2003). Several cancers are amenable to screening and early diagnosis: oral cavity, nasopharynx, stomach, colorectal, melanoma and other skin cancers, breast, cervix, ovary, urinary, bladder, and prostate (WHO, 2002). Specific screening mechanisms have been developed to detect most of these cancers; however, their inclusion in national and international population-level screening programs is contingent upon evidence that they are safe and also acceptable (i.e., efficacious at reducing cancer burden). Numerous national and international organizations and entities have released guidelines on cancer screening, including those proposed by the American College of Surgeons, American Academy of Family Physicians, the US Preventive Services Task Force (USPSTF), and the American Cancer Society, to name a few (Zoorob, Anderson, Cefalu, & Sidani, 2001). Most developed and medium-resource countries have programs and/or national policies for cervical cancer screening (cytology tests) and breast cancer screening (mammography); however, few have programs and policies for colorectal cancer screening, specifically, the fecal occult blood test (FOBT), sigmoidoscopy, and colonoscopy (ACS, 2006b).

To be widely effective, education and screening should be accessible to all members of the population at risk. However, there are indications that minority ethnic groups, people living in deprived areas, and those with less education are prevented from accessing services (Chiu, 2003). Disparities in access to early detection resources contribute to differences in cancer burden. This is a challenge for people living in developed as well as developing countries. In the United States, issues of health disparities that plague the cancer community are, in part, associated with access to cancer screening and follow-up care. Programs such as the National Breast and Cervical Cancer Early Detection Program (NBCCEDP), created in 1991 by the CDC, were implemented to help improve access to cancer screening for at-risk populations (CDC, 2005b). Lack of access to screening and care in developing countries is caused primarily by the lack of available resources for noncommunicable diseases and fragile health infrastructures (Sloan & Gelband, 2007). Thus, considerable attention must be given to implementing cancer screening programs in developing nations.

Studies show that primary care physicians do not always comply with cancer screening guidelines (Young & Ward, 1999). One reason is that recommendations for cancer detection and screening are often fragmented in the sense that they are developed by various medical organizations, which may make decision making more difficult as far as which recommendations to follow (Zoorob, Anderson, Cefalu, & Sidani, 2001). There are numerous national and international guidelines on cancer screening, each of which may update the recommendations for each cancer to reflect new research findings, new literature reviews, and expert opinions, adding to the confusion.

Screening for Breast Cancer

Breast cancer is the most common malignancy affecting women, with more than one million cases occurring worldwide annually (Althuis, Dozier, Anderson, Devesa, & Brinton, 2005). Even though half of the global breast cancers are diagnosed in the developing world, they account for 75% of total deaths from disease (Stewart & Kleihues, 2003). This pattern is worsening, with incidence rates increasing as much as 5% each year (Stewart & Kleihues, 2003). Affluent societies have the highest incidence rates (WHO, 2002). Societal influences on cancer risk are not limited to citizens of these countries whose families have been in the country for many years. Rates of breast cancer in immigrant communities are affected, as well. Studies of migrant populations have revealed that when women migrate from low-risk to high-risk regions, the migrant populations acquire the rates of the host country after two or three generations (Ziegler, Hoover, Pike, Hildesheim, Nomura, West, et al., 1993; John, Phipps, Davis, & Koo, 2005). In some regions, including North America, Western Europe, and Australia, breast cancer mortality rates have started to decline, mainly due to improvements in early detection and treatment. When regular mammography screening occurs among women aged 50 to 64 years, breast cancer mortality is reduced by 30% to 40% (Taplin, Ichikawa, Yood, Manos, Geiger, Weinmann, et al., 2004). Five-year survival rates are higher than 70% in most developed countries (WHO, 2002). The public health impact of breast cancer has been acknowledged by members of the international community, many of whom have implemented population-based mammography screening programs (WHO, 2005).

In the United States, reduction of breast cancer mortality has been a public health priority since the mid-1980s; although evidence of success in achieving this goal has only appeared recently (ACS, 2006b). However, a recent study by Breen and colleagues (2007), using data from CDC's National Health Interview Survey, found a decline in mammography rates in United States women, particularly in the age group most likely to benefit from screening. While reasons for this troubling development remain unclear, researchers speculated that it could be due to factors such as increasingly long waiting times to get appointments, waning fears about breast cancer, the drop in hormone use after menopause, and the ongoing debate over the benefits and risks of screening mammograms.

Because breast cancer is characterized by systemic dissemination, presentation of symptoms and diagnosis may not occur until the disease is advanced or metastatic. Screening tests for breast cancer include clinical breast examination and mammography (i.e., an X-ray examination of the breast); regular, monthly breast self-examination is also encouraged (Marsden, Baum, & Sacks, 1998). Mammography is the primary screening tool for early detection because it can detect the tumor before it is felt or causes symptoms. This screening tool is associated with a reduction of up to 30% in breast cancer mortality (Kerlikowske, Grady, Rubin, Sandrock, & Ernster, 1995; IARC, 2002b). Worldwide, population-based screening for breast cancer occurs primarily through mammographic examination, at prescribed intervals, of all women of a specified age range (WHO, 2003b). Each country determines the specific age range and appropriate screening interval for its program. At the minimum, programs worldwide screen all women 50 or more years of age every one to three years. Screening of women ages 40 to 49 is performed in several developed countries (e.g., United States, Australia, and Sweden). Genetic testing for breast cancer involves a blood test that looks for mutation within the BRCA1 and BRCA2 genes (breast cancer-associated tumor suppressor genes). These tests are usually reserved for women at high risk for breast cancer. Breast cancer risk is higher among women with a family history of breast or ovarian cancer (ACS, 2007c).

Population screening for breast cancer by mammography should only be considered in countries that (a) have high rates of breast cancer, (b) can afford the high technology cost, and (c) have the skilled professionals required (Sikora, 1999). As of 1995, at least 22 countries had established national, subnational, or pilot population breast cancer screening programs (Ballard-Barbash, Klabunde, Paci, Broeders, Coleman, Fracheboud, et al., 1999). In general, these countries have access to the basic resources (i.e., equipment, trained personnel, media campaign resources) needed to implement and maintain successful breast cancer screening programs. Implementation of breast cancer screening programs should reduce the proportion of women who are diagnosed with late-stage cancer because screening should identify cancers before they progress to late stage.

Screening for Cervical Cancer

Cervical cancer is the second most commonly diagnosed cancer and the third leading cause of cancer death in women worldwide (ACS, 2006b). In developing countries, cervical cancer is the leading cause of cancer death (Ferlay, Bray, Pisani, & Parkin, 2004). Over 83% of new cervical cancer cases and deaths occur in the developing part of the world, including 68,000 cases in Africa, 77,000 in Latin America, and 245,000 in Asia (ACS, 2006b; Howson, Harrison, & Law, 1996). Although developing nations are reporting increasing cervical cancer rates, most developed countries have reported a decline in cervical cancer incidence and mortality in the last 30 years (WHO, 2003b). This decline suggests that the cervical cancer burden could also be reduced worldwide by applying current knowledge (Ponten, Adami, Bergstrom, Dillner, Friberg, Gustafsson, et al., 1995).

Cervical cancer is one of the most preventable and treatable cancers (Schiffman, Brinton, Devesa, & Fraumeni, 1996). When detected in the earliest stage, the 5-year survival rate for cervical cancer is 92% (ACS, 2007b). The prevention and early detection of cervical cancer is accomplished largely through timely screening using the Pap test, which identifies abnormal (cancerous or precancerous) cell changes in the cervix and is considered the gold standard. The importance of being screened regularly for cervical cancer cannot be underestimated in that once detected at a regional or distant stage (stage III or IV), the cervical cancer survival rate is estimated at less than 10% (Perez, Grigsby, Nene, Camel, Galakatos, Kao, et al., 1992). Estimates suggest up to 80% of cervical cancer can be prevented if comprehensive screening programs are made available (Sankaranarayanan, Budukh, & Rajkumar, 2001). Population-based screening programs using the Pap test were initiated in British Columbia in 1949, in regions of Norway in 1959, and Scotland in 1960. Many developed countries now have cervical cancer screening programs. However, the Pap test is not practical in all settings as it requires a trained cytologist, laboratory facilities, and multiple clinical visits (Abwao, Green, Sanghvi, Tsu, Winkler, 1998).

Cervical cancer screening programs vary in how they are organized, in the degree to which they are based on public versus private health care, whether the program is systematic or population-based or opportunistic (based upon self-presentation), the age range of the women to whom screening is offered, the recommended interval between successive screenings, and the follow-up and management of women found to have cervical abnormalities (WHO, 2002). Adequate screening programs in developing countries are sparse due to lack of resources and infrastructure to support the programs. Often, Pap test programs in developing countries are limited to women attending primary care, ante-natal, gynecology, and family planning clinics in urban areas, with no organized efforts either to encourage testing for high-risk women or to ensure that those found to have abnormal smears receive follow-up and treatment (Sankaranarayan, Budukh, & Rajkumar, 2001). Fortunately, more cost-effective screening methods are gaining promi-nence in resource-poor settings. These include visual inspection using either acetic acid (VIA) or Lugol's iodine (VILI) and DNA testing for HPV in cervical cell samples (Goldie, Gaffikin, Goldhaber-Fiebert, Gordillo-Tobar, Levin, Mahe, et al., 2005). HPV is an impor-tant causal agent of cervical cancer, and testing of women at high risk of HPV infection could prove beneficial, as infection with oncogenic (high-risk) types of HPV (16 or 18) is associated with aggressive forms of cervical cancer (Schiffman, Brinton, Devesa, & Fraumeni, 1996). Although current HPV tests may be cost prohibitive for developing nations, developed countries are considering implementation of these tests as an adjunct to cytological screening (i.e., Pap test).

Screening for Colon and Rectal Cancers
Cancer of the colon and rectum are rare in developing countries but are the second most frequent types of malignancy in affluent societies (WHO, 2003b). Reducing the number of deaths from colorectal cancer depends on detecting and removing precancerous col-orectal polyps, as well as detecting and treating the cancer in its early stages (Pignone, Saha, Hoerger, & Mandelblatt, 2002). Colon and rectal cancers are one of the few internal cancers that are amenable to early detection, that is, prevention by detection of preclinical lesions. Colorectal cancer screening allows clinicians to detect cancer at an early stage and possibly prevent cancer from occurring through the identification and removal of prema-lignant adenomas, some of which can progress to colorectal cancer (Alberts, Martinez, Hess, Einspahr, Green, Bhattacharyya, et al., 2005). Although a small proportion of col-orectal cancers occur among those with a genetic or family history of the disease (Lindor, 2004; Kinzler & Vogelstein, 1996), the primary objective of colorectal cancer screening is to detect the 90% of cases of colorectal cancer that occur sporadically, most of these in patients above the age of 50 (WHO, 2003b). The approved screening tests for colorectal cancer are the fecal occult blood test (FOBT), endoscopy (flexible sigmoidoscopy and colonoscopy), and double-contrast barium enema. The FOBT is currently considered the optimal screening strategy in terms of cost-effectiveness. It is currently the only colorectal cancer screening test that has been tested in randomized controlled trials. This test iden-tifies persons at risk, though falling short of being definitive for cancer (Rennert, Rennert, Miron, & Peterburg, 2001). Endoscopy, either using a colonoscope or a flexible sigmoido-scope, is the most definitive means of detection (Kavanagh, Giovannucci, Fuchs, & Colditz, 1998; Lieberman, 1997; Winawer, 1993). Endoscopy also allows for sampling of tissues and interventional procedures such as polyp removal.

Screening techniques for colorectal cancer have been widely available in developed nations like the United States for some time, yet are considerably underutilized (CDC,

1999). Currently, patient compliance with colorectal cancer screening and follow-up recommendations regarding endoscopy is poor as the procedure is costly and generally unpopular with the public. Screening recommendations for colorectal cancer vary by country. Japan, Germany, and the Czech Republic recommend the use of FOBT, while the Scandinavian countries and the United Kingdom recommend screening with primary sigmoidoscopy (WHO, 2003b).

Screening for Prostate Cancer

Prostate cancer is the most commonly diagnosed cancer among males and the second leading cause of cancer mortality (ACS, 2006b). Prostate cancer generally develops slowly, and the risk for the disease increases with age. Early detection of prostate cancer is feasible and yet subject to controversy, since the capacity to detect early disease can reduce mortality rates but may result in overtreatment for the individual patient, with substantial cost to society (Dennis & Resnick, 2000). Nonmonetary costs to the patients (e.g., irreversible side effects of some treatments, such as impotence and incontinence) must be weighed against the expected benefits of treatment, given that the cancer may be slow growing (NCI, 2007b). Screening for prostate cancer using the digital rectal examination (DRE) is often recommended; however, DRE is not a sensitive screening test for early detection. Other screening tests include the prostate-specific antigen (PSA) test and transrectal ultrasound. The PSA test, a screening test used to detect elevated PSA (a protein) levels in the blood, was widely introduced in the United States with initial major increases in incidence of the disease and a subsequent reduction. Prostate cancer screening efficacy is currently under review by numerous organizations. It is not yet clear if any of these screening modalities reduce the mortality from the disease, and experts in major medical organizations disagree on the specifics of prostate cancer screening recommendations. Currently, the USPSTF believe that there is insufficient research evidence to recommend either using or abstaining from using PSA and DRE as prostate cancer screening modalities (USPSTF, 2002). Early detection for prostate cancer often hinges on joint decisions to screen for disease made by clinicians and patients. The American Urological Association (AUA) recommends screening for specific groups of men (American Urological Association [AUA], 2000). They also add that deciding whether or not to be screened for prostate cancer is a personal decision that should be made by each patient after consulting with his physician and becoming informed of the advantages and disadvantages of early detection and treatment options (AUA, 2003). Although multiple organizations in the United States recommend prostate cancer screening for certain groups, the international cancer control community does not formally do so (WHO, 2002).

Public and Healthcare Professional Education

The strategy of early diagnosis for cancer control can be promoted by increasing awareness among health professionals and the public (WHO, 2003b). Increased education and awareness among physicians, allied healthcare workers, and the general public in developing countries, in addition to increased availability of effective therapy, could have a major impact on the cancer incidence, mortality, and survival (WHO, 2006b; Ponten, Adami, Bergstrom, Dillner, Friberg, Gustafsson, et al., 1995); Jayant, Nene, Dinshaw, Budukh, & Dale, 1998). Public health education campaigns teach people to recognize early signs of the disease and urge them to seek prompt medical attention. Health professionals, especially primary health workers who are at the forefront of the initial contact between possible cancer patients and the medical care system, should be trained to identify suspicious cases and refer them for rapid diagnosis (WHO, 2002). Professional education is essential to the proportion of primary healthcare workers whose initial training may have only exposed them to advanced and often untreatable cancers. Further, it may be necessary to improve accessibility to trained healthcare workers who are competent in performing the necessary examinations (including female health workers for women) (WHO, 2002).

Education is particularly important in developing countries, where insufficient resources limit the availability of screening programs (ACS, 2006b). For example, the cancer control program of Kerala, India, developed an early detection program emphasizing education followed by diagnosis. Access to advanced technology and expensive screening methods is limited in this region. The cancer control program in Kerala trained over 12,000 cancer control volunteers in 85 villages to promote awareness of cancer and detect early signs of disease, to advocate and motivate people to undergo diagnostic screening test and therapy, and to extend financial support. Institution of the program resulted in cancers being diagnosed at an earlier stage than before the program was in place (WHO, 2003b). Cancer education programs, such as the Kerala program, can educate people to recognize the early signs and symptoms of cancer and emphasize the fact that cancer diagnosed early is more likely to be treatable and respond to effective treatment. These efforts can also promote public awareness of early signs of certain cancers (e.g., oral cavity, larynx, colon, rectum, skin, breast, cervix, urinary bladder, and prostate) as well as proper follow-up with healthcare providers, if individuals experience unexplained symptoms (WHO, 2006b).

In summary, early detection of cancer is part of a wider strategy that includes diagnosis, treatment of the condition detected, and follow-up. These components must work together in order to produce the desired outcomes (e.g., decreased mortality). Cancer screening or education programs in the absence of suitable treatment and follow-up will fail. When deciding whether to implement such programs, policy makers and cancer control planners should factor in the impact of the cancer burden in the population and the cost-effectiveness of such programs. For interested readers, up-to-date health professional-oriented summaries containing current screening and detection information are available online from the NCI *PDQ (Physician Data Query) Comprehensive Cancer Database* for many of the common cancers, such as lung, colorectal, breast, and prostate, as well as less common cancers (NCI, 2007a). These summaries contain current information related to screening and detection for particular disease sites, the levels of evidence for the statements included in the summaries, and the significance of and evidence of benefit for the stated positions included in the summaries; supporting references to current literature are also offered. Most of the screening and detection summaries are also available in patient versions that are written in easy-to-understand, nontechnical language (NCI, 2007a).

The health infrastructure of each country also affects the implementation of screening and detection programs. Early detection of cancer undoubtedly contributes to increased disease burden. Thus, more resources to support the health services infrastructure may be required to address the additional disease burden. Decisions to implement early screening and detection programs should be evidence-based and take into account the public health importance of the specific cancer, characteristics of early-detection tests, efficacy and cost-effectiveness of early detection, personnel requirements, and the level of development of health services in a given setting.

Cancer Care Considerations

Cancer Treatment

Employing effective treatment is the single most important strategy to ensure optimal life following a cancer diagnosis, and advances in treatments have enhanced survival for many patients (Mackay, Jemal, Lee, & Parkin, 2006). According to the NCI, although (a) approximately one-third of all cancers are avoidable through lifestyle changes and early detection, and (b) enough information is available to permit the early diagnosis and effective treatment of *another* one-third of cancer cases, millions of cancer cases worldwide still cannot currently be prevented or cured; thus, new and effective treatments must urgently be sought (NCI, 2006). According to WHO, the primary goals of cancer treatment, depending on extent of disease and other key variables, are: (a) cure, (b) prolongation of useful life, and (c) improvement of quality of life (WHO, 2002). A primary aim for treatment is multidisciplinary management, which is more effective than sequential independent management of patients; further, combined modality approaches result in more cures and improved organ and function preservation (WHO, 2002).

The main methods of treatment for cancer are surgery, radiotherapy, and chemotherapy (including hormonal manipulation), with each of the three effecting cures in certain cancers (WHO, 2002). Biologic therapy and targeted therapy are additional important treatments (ACS, 2007a). The three principal modes of therapy may be given alone or in combination for best success, depending upon key patient-related considerations (Stewart & Kleihues, 2003). For detailed information on various therapies and rehabilitation considerations, refer to recently published documents on state-of-the-art treatments, immediate side effects, possible long-term and late appearing side effects, and which treatments are best suited for particular cancers (e.g., ACS, 2007a; Stewart & Kleihues, 2003; WHO, 2002; NCCN, 2007; NCI, 2007a).

The reader is also referred to two key, continuously updated national sources for cancer treatment information: the National Comprehensive Cancer Network (NCCN) *Clinical Practice Guidelines in Oncology* and the NCI *PDQ (Physician Data Query) Comprehensive Cancer Database*. The NCCN *Clinical Practice Guidelines* are a recognized standard for clinical policy in the oncology community, providing easy access to continually updated guidelines based upon evaluation of scientific data integrated with expert judgment (NCCN, 2007). Also included in the NCCN *Clinical Practice Guidelines* are clinical trials information, which are available in versions tailored for patients, clinicians, and industry. Interested readers can also access the NCCN *Drugs and Biologics Compendium and Cancer Resource Lines* (NCCN, 2007). The adult treatment and pediatric treatment summaries contained in the NCI *PDQ* cancer information summaries contain evidence-based summaries of prognostic and treatment information for the major types of cancer in both adults and children, as well as for unusual childhood cancers in the pediatric summaries. The NCI *PDQ* also houses the world's most comprehensive cancer clinical trials registry, containing more than 5000 abstracts on open, active, and approved clinical trial protocols (NCI, 2007a). Both the NCCN and the NCI *PDQ* are available online. Innovative approaches that use the main treatment methods in novel ways are continually under development; thus, studying up-to-date literature is invaluable in learning about state-of-the-science approaches to treating cancer. A reported 30% of cancer patients worldwide use complementary and alternative medicine (Mackay, Jemal, Lee, & Parkin, 2006). Complementary and alternative medicine *PDQ* summaries are available for review by health professionals; these summaries contain background information about the treatments, a brief history of their development, information about their proposed mechanism(s) of action, and information about relevant laboratory, animal, and clinical studies (NCI, 2007a). Similar summaries written for patients use language for nonexperts and include glossary links to scientific terms (NCI, 2007a). A recent review of medical and psychological concerns of cancer survivors following cancer treatment and barriers to care (Stewart & Kleihues, 2003) and coping with cancer concerns and resources (NCCN, 2007; NCI, 2007a) are also instructive.

Worldwide, prompt treatment of one-third of cancer cases is possible where resources and access to patients allow (WHO, 2002). Particularly in developed parts of the world (e.g., in northern and western Europe and the United States), advances in treatment modalities (such as improved forms of chemotherapy) have increased survival for many patients (Mackay, Jemal, Lee, & Parkin, 2006). However, achieving the treatment goal related to prompt care is hampered by poor availability of treatments and delays in seeking cancer care, both of which contribute to lower survival rates in many developing countries (WHO, 2002). The WHO urges that all countries of the world develop and implement well-conceived, well-managed national cancer control programs; policies in such programs should promote treatment and follow-up guidelines for each stage of specific cancers, and data should be collected that allow measurement of the success of the treatment policy. The close link between early detection and treatment is emphasized as an important aspect of such programs (WHO, 2002). Even in developed nations, problems in accessing treatment care can vary according to the patient's geographic location, socioeconomic status, and age (Mackay, Jemal, Lee, & Parkin, 2006).

Considering the treatment issue from another perspective, WHO recommends that treatment guidelines emphasize the importance of avoiding the offering of curative therapy when a cancer is incurable; in such situations, patients with incurable cancers should be offered palliative care instead (WHO, 2002). The WHO (2002) also emphasizes the importance of guarding against neglecting early detection and palliative care in favor of treatment-oriented approaches, regardless of whether these treatment approaches are cost-effective or whether they improve patients' quality of life.

Survivorship, Palliative Care, and End-of-Life Care

More people are surviving cancer and living longer because of advances in early detection, treatment, and supportive care options (Hewitt, Greenfield, & Stovall, 2006; Wingo, Howe, Thun, Ballard-Barbash, Ward, Brown, et al., 2005). Currently, cancer is often experienced as a chronic illness (Foley & Gelband, 2001), and the patient may require specialized care for months and often years; such care may involve a range of professional services that extends beyond the discipline of oncology (Stewart & Kleihues, 2003). Unfortunately, improvements in the development and delivery of symptom control throughout all stages of cancer and in other aspects of palliative care needed in the late stages of cancer have not kept pace with the medical advances that have allowed people to live longer (Foley & Gelband, 2001). However, given the fast growing and avid interest of many healthcare providers, patients, and the general public in the topics of survivorship, palliative care, and end-of-life care—with the emphasis on achieving high levels of comfort and quality of life—these comfort-oriented healthcare topics are emerging as subjects equal in importance to more cure-oriented topics.

Allied healthcare professionals, such as nurses, physician assistants, physical and occupational therapists, and dieticians, will benefit from developing a working knowledge of survivorship, palliative care, and end-of-life care issues, all of which are pertinent to understanding the patients' and families' experience of cancer. Knowledge in these three areas can inform healthcare providers' clinical practice and thereby improve their ability to administer high quality care to patients. Because allied healthcare professionals working in both inpatient and outpatient settings routinely spend many hours each day in service to cancer patients, these skilled healthcare providers often have invaluable and in-depth knowledge of the everyday problems and needs of cancer patients and their families. Armed with up-to-date knowledge about the issues that patients and families face, healthcare professionals can add meaningful information to the patients' care plans and thereby improve care for patients.

In the three sections that follow, a brief overview of the three broad topics of survivorship, palliative care, and end-of-life care are presented, along with definitions of selected terms and a short description of key issues. National and international reports, position papers, and guidelines cited throughout are key references that can provide detailed discussions of the topics included herein for the reader needing more information.

Survivorship

The risk of developing cancer in one's lifetime is more than one in three; as a result, each of us is likely to experience cancer or know someone who has survived cancer (Hewitt, Greenfield, & Stovall, 2006). More than 10 million people in the United States are living with a history of cancer (ACS, 2007a; Reuben, 2006), with this number representing a tripling of the number of survivors since 1971 (Hewitt, Greenfield, & Stovall, 2006). Cancer survivors constitute 3.5% of the US population (Travis, Rabkin, & Brown, 2006), and 65% of cancer survivors are expected to live at least 5 years after diagnosis (ACS, 2006a). From an international perspective, more than 25 million people throughout the world are cancer survivors, and the number grows daily (NCI, 2006). Although most people eventually die from their cancer, treatment advances are allowing many patients with cancer to live much longer than ever before, with periods of adaptation to cancer as a chronic disease (Foley & Gelband, 2001).

Interest in cancer survivorship, as well as maintaining a high quality of life throughout the course of an experience with cancer, is rising among healthcare providers, patients, families, and the general public (Riddle & Boeshaar, 2006; Kolata, 2004). Not surprisingly, the terms *cancer survivor* and *cancer survivorship* have different meanings to different people (Reuben, 2006), and how to refer to this growing population has stirred some controversy (Hewitt, Greenfield, & Stovall, 2006). Some controversy continues as to who should be considered a survivor. For the purpose of this discussion, a survivor definition, supported by CDC, NCI, and the National Coalition for Cancer Survivorship, is useful: An individual is considered a cancer survivor from the time of diagnosis through the balance of his or her life; family members, friends, and caregivers are also affected by the survivorship experience and are therefore included in this definition (CDC, 2004b). The following definition of survivorship care provides further context within which to consider the survivor's experience during this time period: survivorship care is a distinct phase of care for cancer survivors that includes four components: (a) prevention and detection of recurrent and new cancers and of late effects; (b) surveillance for cancer spread or recurrence, or second cancers; (c) intervention for consequences of cancer and its treatment; and (d) coordination between specialists and primary care providers to ensure that all of the survivor's health needs are met (Hewitt, Greenfield, & Stovall, 2006). This fourth component likely has great appeal to the readers who are multidisciplinary health professionals. A thoughtful, detailed, and well-developed plan of coordinated care created by a multidisciplinary team can ensure that the survivorship plan will be as high quality as the earlier, intense plan that guided the diagnosis and treatment phases of care.

Physical, psychosocial, employment-related, educational, financial, and legal issues may affect cancer survivors across the lifespan (Reuben, 2004). Indeed, the diagnosis and treatment of cancer is a threat to a person's physical, psychological, social, spiritual, and economic well-being (CDC, 2004b). The Lance Armstrong Foundation (LAF) distinguishes between living *with* cancer, which refers to the experience of receiving a cancer diagnosis and any treatment that may follow, living *through* cancer, which refers to the extended stage following treatment, and living *beyond* cancer, which refers to posttreatment and long-term survivorship (CDC, 2004b). Although these distinctions are meant to signify the experience of survivorship as a progression, the process is unique for each patient, and movement from one phase to the next may not be clearly delineated (CDC, 2004b), adding to the complexity of providing comprehensive care for cancer survivors.

Securing effective, long-term care is an important strategy for ensuring optimal living following a cancer diagnosis. There is also growing agreement among healthcare providers and cancer patients and their families that the transition from active treatment to the posttreatment period is critical to the cancer patient's long-term health (Hewitt, Greenfield, & Stovall, 2006). In addition, cancer survivors need lifelong care to monitor for and treat late effects of cancer therapies, recurrences, and second cancers, and to address psychosocial, nutritional, rehabilitation, and other needs that may arise years after treatment ends (Reuben, 2006). Although the medical and psychological effects of cancer and its treatment have been recognized for many years, survivorship has only recently come to be recognized as a distinct phase of the cancer trajectory (Hewitt, Greenfield, & Stovall, 2006). Despite the heartening fact that present cancer survivors number at more than 10 million in the United States—which is a direct result of advances in diagnosis and treatment—these successes have come at a cost: nearly 75% of people who survive cancer live long enough to develop significant sequelae, in the form of late-appearing or long-term side effects (Haylock, Mitchell, Cox, Temple, & Curtiss, 2007).

Various follow-up care guidelines (e.g., covering screening, evaluation, psychosocial services) to assist healthcare providers in delivering care to survivors have been proposed as a result of advances in knowledge of how to manage conditions that arise in this patient group. In addition, as people with cancer live longer as a result of improved access to effective screening, diagnosis, and treatments (making cancer a chronic condition in many cases), another issue that has begun to generate an increased amount of attention is how to produce and use comprehensive guidelines that adequately address the possible long-term and late effects of a particular cancer diagnosis and treatment (Hewitt, Greenfield, & Stovall, 2006). Although no specific care guidelines are widely accepted and followed in clinical settings, the President's Cancer Panel (Reuben, 2006) urges the acceleration of efforts to develop and disseminate survivorship follow-up clinical guidelines that are based on the best available evidence (including best practices and expert opinions) until the evidence base is further developed through targeted outcomes and related research. The NCI strives to improve the quality and delivery of cancer care throughout the world by publishing documents that outline best practices for doctors, nurses, and other healthcare providers who interact directly with cancer patients and their families (NCI, 2006). Another major issue that continues to be addressed by the president's cancer panel is improving access to care and insurance coverage for healthcare services needed by survivors (Reuben, 2004).

Healthcare professionals who want to remain abreast of the dynamic and fast-developing process for creating guidelines for survivorship care are referred to the in-depth discussion by Haylock and colleagues regarding their work in progress called "Prescription for Living," a template that provides clinicians with a concise guide to treatment and follow-up care planning while also offering survivors a guide for planning healthful lifestyles (Haylock, Mitchell, Cox, Temple, & Curtiss, 2007). An important theme repeated throughout the current survivorship literature is that the care of survivors encompasses the entire cancer control continuum, from prevention, detection, diagnosis, and treatment, through what some refer to as a survivorship phase, with end-of-life care completing the continuum (Pollack, Greer, Rowland, Miller, Doneski, Coughlin, et al., 2005).

Palliative Care

In the last 50 years, there have been amazing advances in the treatment and early detection of a few types of cancer and at least modest gains in many others; yet, the reality is that half of all patients diagnosed with cancer today will die of their disease within a few years (Foley & Gelband, 2001). "The imperative in cancer research and treatment has been, understandably, an almost single-minded focus on attempts to cure every patient at every stage of disease" (Foley & Gelband, 2001, p. 9). Unfortunately, however, in our society's aggressive pursuit of cures for cancer, symptom control and comfort care have been neglected (Foley & Gelband, 2001). Recent literature suggests that acute care settings generally focus primarily on curative treatments and remain ill-equipped to provide palliative care (Wingo, Howe, Thun, Ballard-Barbash, Ward, Brown, et al., 2005). At the same time, however, there is growing recognition of the importance of symptom control and other aspects of palliative care, from diagnosis through the dying process (Foley & Gelband, 2001). Further, there is growing realization that "patients should not have to choose between treatment with curative intent or comfort care. There is a need for both, in varying degrees, throughout the course of cancer, whether the eventual outcome is long-term survival or death" (Foley & Gelband, 2001, p. 9).

Multiple definitions of palliative care highlight the complexity inherent in the term. The *National Action Plan for Cancer Survivorship: Advancing Public Health Strategies,* jointly produced by CDC, the Lance Armstrong Foundation, and other partners, defines palliative care, in accordance with the NCI, as follows: "Care given to improve the quality of life of patients who have a serious or life-threatening disease. Also called comfort care, supportive care, and symptom management" (CDC, 2004b, p. 65). Palliative care is also defined as "treatment of symptoms associated with the effects of cancer and its treatment" (Hewitt, Greenfield, & Stovall, 2006, p. 481). The WHO defines palliative care in cancer as the "active total care of patients whose disease is not responsive to curative treatment" (cited in Foley & Gelband, 2001) and additionally specifies that many aspects of palliative care are appropriate and applicable early in the course of the illness, in conjunction with active, anticancer treatment (WHO, 2002). Palliative care may begin at the time of a cancer diagnosis and increase in amount and intensity, as needed, throughout the course of a patient's illness until death (Foley & Gelband, 2001).

New healthcare professionals and those in training must keep the following in mind as they develop their clinical skills relative to palliative care: the WHO has emphasized that palliative care should not be relegated to the last stages of care; rather, the principles of palliative care should be applied as early as possible in the course of a chronic disease such as cancer (WHO, 2002). "Palliative care is an approach that improves the quality of life of patients and their families facing the problem associated with life-threatening illness, through the prevention and relief of suffering by means of early identification and impeccable assessment and treatment of pain and other problems," including those in the physical, psychosocial, and spiritual realms (WHO, 2002, p. 84).

The World Health Organization's position is that at all stages of disease, the patient needs comprehensive care, and a patient with a disease that will eventually be fatal requires good palliative care from the time of diagnosis forward; further, comprehensive care should proceed concurrently with anticancer treatment, whether with curative or palliative intent (Stewart & Kleihues, 2003). Treating symptoms is of the utmost importance, as symptoms influence not only quality of life but also the course of disease (WHO, 2002). From a global perspective, the relevance of palliative care is seen in the fact that in developing countries, the proportion of cancer patients requiring palliative care is at least 80% (WHO, 2002). The WHO asserts that global improvements in palliative care do not depend so much upon the creation of specialized palliative care services separate from mainstream health care, but rather "upon the permeation of the whole health care system by the principles of palliative care" (Stewart & Kleihues, 2003, p. 299). In addition, because palliative care can be provided relatively simply and inexpensively, such services should be made available in every country (Stewart & Kleihues, 2003).

In its recommendation to member governments, the WHO stated that any national cancer control program should address the needs of its citizens for palliative care. Within such a program, six major skills sets that comprise complete palliative care include: (a) communication, (b) decision making, (c) management of complications of treatment and the disease, (d) symptom control, (e) psychosocial care of patient and family, and (f) care of the dying (Foley & Gelband, 2001). Some of these skills, such as communication, decision making, and psychosocial care of patient and family, are important throughout the trajectory of illness, while other skills emerge and recede in importance at different times. Physical symptoms of cancer can be both acute and chronic, can occur at various times throughout the disease trajectory, and may include pain, fatigue, nausea, hair loss, and others, depending on the cancer site and the types of treatments being used (CDC, 2004b).

The WHO also outlined three specific issues that must be addressed in the context of palliative care of any patient: (a) relief of major symptoms in all stages of disease, especially cancer-related pain relief; (b) comprehensive care of patients who are close to death; and (c) support for the family during the course of the illness and after the patient's death (cited in Stewart & Kleihues, 2003). Pain relief, along with management of other symptoms through every stage of cancer and its treatment, is a major concern for survivors and their caregivers (CDC, 2004b). Particular attention is given here to the issue of pain because of its common occurrence in all countries throughout the world. Considerable evidence in the healthcare literature indicates that inadequate treatment of pain is a frequent and neglected problem, even in technologically advanced countries with adequate resources and specialist palliative care services (Stewart and Kleihues, 2003; WHO, 2002; Hill, 1990; Max, 1990). The WHO has asserted that freedom from cancer pain must be regarded as a human rights issue, and unrelieved pain in cancer patients is unacceptable because it is generally avoidable with proper treatment (WHO, 2002). This chapter's authors emphasize that the necessity to have simple and yet still excellent national pain management policies and procedures in place is especially critical when one considers that in some countries, successful palliation may be all the treatment that is available to cancer patients. Furthermore, even in technologically advanced countries, good pain management (which, in part, relies on having an excellent pain policy and associated procedures in place in the healthcare organization) is often one of the most important aspects of cancer care.

Although precise information on the prevalence of cancer-related pain is lacking, numerous surveys spanning a 22-year period have continued to show that moderate to severe pain is experienced by 30–50% of patients with active disease and/or receiving treatment and by 60–90% of patients with advanced disease (ACS, 2007a; Deschamps, Band, & Coldman, 1988; Foley & Sundaresan, 1985; Weissman, Dahl, & Joranson, 1990). The needed analgesics to relieve most cancer-related pain have been available for decades, and 85% of cancer patients could currently have satisfactory relief using only simple, inexpensive, "low-technology" oral analgesics (Grossman & Nesbit, 2004; Sloan & Gelband, 2007), with the remaining 15% of patients achieving satisfactory relief using more sophisticated pain control measures (Grossman & Nesbit, 2004; Cleeland, 1990). Healthcare professionals should have a basic understanding of the three-step analgesic ladder—also referred to as the WHO Pain Relief Ladder—and should be familiar with commonly used pain rating scales that give healthcare professionals simple tools to use in communicating clearly with patients regarding pain levels; multiple current resources (e.g., Sloan & Gelband, 2007; NCCN, 2007; ACS, 2007a) are available as resources on these topics. Barriers to cancer pain relief are well described and documented in the literature. Key barriers include inadequate knowledge, inadequate pain assessment, healthcare provider attitudes, patient and family misconceptions, lack of availability of appropriate medications, restrictive laws and regulations and their enforcement, and community barriers, particularly in relation to the use of strong and weak opioid pain relievers (Stewart & Kleihues, 2003; ACS, 2007a; NCCN & ACS, 2005; NCI, 2007a). In addition to opioids, a variety of nonopioid analgesics and other adjuvant medications, as well as noninvasive and invasive medical techniques, can also play essential roles in helping patients achieve adequate pain relief. For more complete information on descriptions and selection of the proper pain relief measures, the reader is referred to the current pain references cited in this section.

Pain experts over the last 20 years have suggested that implementation of a well-developed, organizational policy approach to managing patients' pain, one that fosters setting optimal pain management goals, making good pain management a priority, and accepting accountability for adequately relieving pain, could be instrumental in changing clinical practice patterns and building institutional commitment to improving pain management (Alley, 2001; Gordon, Dahl, & Stevenson, 2000; Pasero, Gordon, McCaffery, & Ferrell, 1999). Consistent with this deliberate organizational commitment, optimal management of pain would require adequate infrastructure (e.g., sufficient personnel, facilities, drugs) and effective methodology (e.g., modes of drug delivery; dose adjustment by the patient) (Stewart & Kleihues, 2003). Neither the formal and effective organizational commitment to pain relief nor the necessary infrastructure is routinely in place in most healthcare settings.

From a global perspective, quality-of-life outcomes such as adequate pain relief and freedom from nausea are universally accepted as valuable (NCI, 2006), although these outcomes are often not fully achieved. Conceptually, quality of life encompasses not only the physical aspects of well-being but also includes the cognitive, spiritual, emotional, and social aspects of life; further, it is important to note that a "good" quality of life as viewed by a cancer patient in central Africa may be very different from that as defined by a cancer patient in the suburbs of an American city (NCI, 2006).

End-of-Life Care

A key aspect of palliative care for dying patients is end-of-life care. At the end of life, only a few people (i.e., less than 10%) die suddenly and unexpectedly (Emanuel, Ferris, von Gunten, & Von Roenn, 2006). Most people (i.e., more than 90%) die after a long period of illness, with gradual deterioration until an active dying phase at the end (Field & Cassel, 1997). Thus, providing end-of-life care is an important responsibility for all health professionals caring for patients at this stage of life; for such providers, there is an established (albeit, growing) body of knowledge to guide this care (Twycross & Lichter, 1998; Ferris, von Gunten, & Emanuel, 2003; Ellershaw & Ward, 2003).

End-of-life care is defined as "care provided during the period of time in which an individual copes with declining health from an ultimately terminal illness" (Hewitt, Greenfield, & Stovall, 2006, p. 478). The goal of end-of-life care is to achieve the best possible quality of life for cancer patients by controlling pain and other symptoms and addressing psychological and spiritual needs (CDC, 2004b). The CDC/Lance Armstrong Foundation *National Action Plan for Cancer Survivorship* posits that "end-of-life care affirms life and regards dying as a normal process, neither hastening nor postponing death while providing relief from distress and integrating psychological and spiritual aspects of survivor care" (CDC, 2004b, p. 4).

For at least a decade, end-of-life care has been a prominent healthcare issue, and both patients and healthcare professionals have been advocating for improvements (AMA, 1996; Holland & Chertkov, 2001). Recently, the end of life has begun to capture the attention of the public health community, as end of life has three characteristics of other public health priorities: high burden, major impact, and a potential for preventing suffering associated with illness (Rao, Anderson, & Smith, 2002). However, most clinicians have received little or no formal training in managing the dying process or death, and families usually have even less experience and knowledge in these areas (Emanuel, Ferris, von Gunten, & Von Roenn, 2006). Although key principles of end-of-life care are well discussed in the literature, established standards of care are not universally followed, especially in institutional settings, where almost 85% of Americans die (Rummans, Bostwick, & Clark, 2000). There are challenges to ensuring good end-of-life care and a comfortable death in institutions whose cultures are not focused on end-of-life care (Ferris, Hallward, Ronan, & Billings, 1998).

People with cancer suffer from a variety of symptoms at all stages of disease and its treatment, though symptoms are most frequent and severe in advanced stages (Foley & Gelband, 2001). Much of the current suffering could be alleviated if available symptom control measures were used more widely (Foley & Gelband, 2001). It is unclear as to whether the trend toward aggressive care in acute care hospitals is in response to patient care preferences or to the culture of acute care hospitals (Wingo, Howe, Thun, Ballard-Barbash, Ward, Brown, et al., 2005). In either case, allied health professionals can improve the services they provide by understanding the barriers throughout the healthcare and medical research systems that stand in the way of the delivery of effective palliative care and end-of-life care to cancer patients where and when they need it. These barriers, as well as conclusions and recommendations to address the barriers, are outlined in the 2001 IOM report entitled *Improving Palliative Care for Cancer* (Foley & Gelband, 2001).

Particularly in the United States, healthcare experts agree that a major barrier to adequate palliative care has been the institutionalization of a healthcare system that focuses on either active therapy or palliative or hospice care and does not allow for the appropriate interface between these two approaches (Foley & Gelband, 2001; Lynn & O'Mara, 2001; Holland & Chertkov, 2001; Payne, 2001). Hospice care is widely considered to be the most substantial innovation to serve the dying, although many end-of-life patients, even in the technologically advanced United States, do not receive hospice care (Foley & Gelband, 2001). The term *hospice* has at least three somewhat different uses that can be confusing and even misleading (Field & Cassel, 1997); thus, the three common uses are briefly listed here. First, a hospice may be a discrete site of care in the form of an inpatient hospital or nursing home unit or a freestanding facility. Secondly, a hospice may be an organization or program that provides, arranges, and advises on a wide range of medical and supportive services for dying patients and their families and friends, with care based in the patient's home. The third and most culturally sweeping meaning of hospice refers to an approach to caring for dying patients that is based on clinical, social, and spiritual principles (Field & Cassel, 1997). To gain a better understanding of issues related to evaluating the adequacy of end-of-life care, the reader is directed to the detailed IOM report entitled *Approaching Death* (Field & Cassel, 1997), which offers a blueprint for change at the global level in end-of-life care practices (Stewart & Kleihues, 2003).

Noteworthy Compilations of Cancer Information

High quality cancer-related reports, guidelines, books, journal articles, and online resources have been cited throughout this chapter. Of special note, the following are examples of resources providing compilations of information that have, in addition to the typical narrative text format, additional helpful features. *The Cancer Atlas* (2006), jointly produced by ACS, CDC, and UICC, uses graphic and colorful atlas map formats for making visual points relative to each 2-page topic. The atlas also provides a detailed timeline on the history of cancer starting 70–80 million years ago up to the present, tables of risk factors for cancers in various countries, extensive statistics on cancer, indexed by country, information on sources used in the figures, tables, and graphs, and a listing of useful contacts at WHO headquarters and regional offices, WHO cancer programs, and key cancer organizations, indexed by specific countries (Mackay, Jemal, Lee, & Parkin, 2006).

The latest edition of the groundbreaking report, *The Tobacco Atlas,* produced by ACS, gives shape and meaning to statistics about tobacco use and control. *The Tobacco Atlas* uses full-color maps and graphics to illustrate a wide range of tobacco issues, revealing similarities and differences between countries and exposing behavior of tobacco companies, all in a user-friendly format (Mackay, Eriksen, & Shafey, 2006). This small volume addresses in a succinct yet detailed manner the following: types of tobacco use; prevalence of tobacco use among various populations (including health professionals!) and smoking health risks; the costs of tobacco; and an overview of the tobacco trade and the promotion of tobacco. The atlas also details numerous activities underway to curtail, ban, or otherwise limit tobacco usage and availability. Finally, the National Comprehensive Cancer Network (NCCN) *Clinical Practice Guidelines in Oncology* (NCCN, 2007) and the NCI *PDQ (Physician Data Query) Comprehensive Cancer Database* (NCI, 2007a) are noted for their highly interactive Web sites, with continuously updated content available on an impressive number of cancer-related topics and attention given to the available evidence-based sources. In addition to summaries on adult and pediatric treatments, the NCI *PDQ Comprehensive Cancer Database* also provides useful summaries on topics that are not as widely covered, such as genetics, complementary and alternative medicine, and supportive care.

Conclusions

Throughout this chapter, we have introduced the public health perspective on key cancer and cancer patient care issues, both within the United States and in other parts of the world. The goal of this chapter has been to provide allied healthcare professionals with knowledge of key cancer-related topics in order to improve the quality of health services provided to oncology patients. This chapter also has discussed the common as well as the different challenges faced by developed and developing countries of the world as they work to decrease cancer-related morbidity and mortality. Although predicted increases in the number of new cases of cancer is mostly due to a steadily increasing proportion of elderly people in the world, the increase will be even greater if current levels of smoking and the high prevalence of unhealthy lifestyles persist (Mackay, Jemal, Lee, & Parkin, 2006).

All of the issues discussed in this chapter provide useful background information for both healthcare providers and public health professionals who are providing patient services and/or conducting research with an eye toward improving some aspect of cancer care. Regardless of future advances in high-technology medicine, any major reduction in deaths and disability from cancer will come from efforts directed toward cancer prevention, not from cancer cures (Mackay, Jemal, Lee, & Parkin, 2006). Thus, one of the primary goals of this chapter has been to raise awareness of the importance of cancer prevention activities and to promote cancer prevention efforts among new healthcare providers, with a major focus placed on patient and professional education. If successful, such cancer prevention efforts could result in 2 million lives per year being saved by 2020, and 6.5 million lives per year by 2040 (Mackay, Jemal, Lee, & Parkin, 2006). At the same time, we encourage allied health professionals to consider well and use effectively the principles of palliative care and high quality survivorship discussed in the chapter. At any point in the disease trajectory, all healthcare professionals—who are in any way involved with clinical services to people with cancer—can enhance the care provided to such individuals and their families by advocating for the delivery of high quality services to meet their basic—and essential—oncology care needs.

References

Abwao, S., Green, P., Sanghvi, H., Tsu, V., & Winkler, J. L. (1998). *Prevention and control of cervical cancer in the east and southern Africa region: Meeting report.* Seattle, WA: PATH.

Alberts, D. S., Martinez, M. E., Hess, L. M., Einspahr, J. G., Green, S. B., Bhattacharyya, A. K., et al. (2005). Phase III trial of ursodeoxycholic acid to prevent colorectal adenoma recurrence. *Journal of the National Cancer Institute, 97*, 846–853.

Alley, L. G. (2001). The influence of an organizational pain management policy on nurses' pain management practices. *Oncology Nursing Forum, 28*, 867–874.

Althuis, M. D., Dozier, J. M., Anderson, W. F., Devesa, S. S., & Brinton, L. A. (2005). Global trends in breast cancer incidence and mortality 1973-1997. *International Journal of Epidemiology, 34*, 405–412.

American Cancer Society (ACS). (2006a). *Cancer facts and figures 2006.* Atlanta, GA: Author.

American Cancer Society (ACS). (2006b). *The worldwide cancer burden report.* Atlanta, GA: Author.

American Cancer Society (ACS). (2007a). *Cancer facts and figures 2007.* Atlanta, GA: Author.

American Cancer Society (ACS). (2007b). *Cancer reference information: What are the key statistics about cervical cancer?* Retrieved July 16, 2007, from http://www.cancer.org/docroot/CRI/content/CRI_2_4_1X_What_are_the_key_statistics_for_cervical_cancer_8.asp

American Cancer Society (ACS). (2007c). *Cancer reference information: What are the risk factors for breast cancer?* Retrieved July 11, 2007, from http://www.cancer.org/docroot/CRI/content/CRI_2_4_2X_What_are_the_risk_factors_for_breast_cancer_5.asp

American Medical Association (AMA). (1996). Good care of the dying. *Journal of the American Medical Association, 275*, 474–478.

American Urological Association (AUA). (2000). Prostate-specific antigen (PSA) best practice policy. *Oncology, 14,* 267–280.

American Urological Association (AUA). (2003). *Prostate cancer awareness for men. A doctor's guide for patients based on the PSA best practice policy.* Linthicum, MD: Author.

Ballard-Barbash, R., Klabunde, C., Paci, E., Broeders, M., Coleman, E. A., Fracheboud, J., et al. (1999). Breast cancer screening in 21 countries: Delivery of services, notification of results and outcomes ascertainment. *European Journal of Cancer Prevention, 8,* 417–426.

Batty, D., & Thune, I. (2000). Does physical activity prevent cancer? Evidence suggests protection against colon cancer and probably breast cancer. *British Medical Journal, 321,* 1424–1425.

Black, B. L., Cowens-Alvarado, R., Gershman, S., & Weir, H. K. (2005). Using data to motivate action: The need for high quality, an effective presentation, and an action context for decision-making. *Cancer Causes and Control, 16*(Suppl. 1): 15–25.

Bosch, F. X. & Munoz, N. (2002). The viral etiology of cervical cancer. *Virus Research, 89*(2): 183–190.

Breen, N. A., Cronin, K., Meissner, H. I., Taplin, S. H., Tangka, F. K., Tiro, J. A., et al. (2007). Reported drop in mammography: Is this cause for concern? *Cancer, 109*(12), 2405–2409.

Brown, M. L., & Yabroff, K. R. (2006). Economic impact of cancer in the United States. In D. Schottenfeld & J. F. Fraumeni (Eds.), *Cancer Epidemiology and Prevention* (3rd ed.). Oxford, England: Oxford University Press.

Byers, T., Nestle, M., McTiernan, A., Doyle, C., Currie-Williams, A., Gansler, T., et al. (2002). American Cancer Society guidelines on nutrition and physical activity for cancer prevention: Reducing the risk of cancer with healthy food choices and physical activity for cancer prevention. *CA: A Cancer Journal for Clinicians, 52,* 92–119.

Calle, E. E., Rodriguez, C., Walker-Thurmond, K., & Thun, M. J. (2003). Overweight, obesity, and mortality from cancer in a prospectively studied cohort of U.S. adults. *New England Journal of Medicine, 348,* 1625–1638.

Casperson, C. J. (1989). Physical activity epidemiology: Concepts, methods, and applications to exercise science. *Exercise Sport Science Review, 17,* 423–473.

Centers for Disease Control and Prevention (CDC). (1999). Screening for colorectal cancer—United States, 1997. *Morbidity & Mortality Weekly Report, 48,* 116–121.

Centers for Disease Control and Prevention (CDC). (2004a). *Physical activity and good nutrition: Essential elements to prevent chronic diseases and obesity.* Retrieved August 16, 2004, from http://www.cdc.gov/nccdphp/aag/aag_dnpa.htm

Centers for Disease Control and Prevention (CDC). (2004b). *A national action plan for cancer survivorship: Advancing public health strategies.* Atlanta, GA: Centers for Disease Control and Prevention and the Lance Armstrong Foundation.

Centers for Disease Control and Prevention (CDC). (2005a). *Behavioral risk factor surveillance system operational and user's guide. Version 3.0.* Atlanta, GA: Author.

Centers for Disease Control and Prevention (CDC). (2005b). *National Breast and Cervical Cancer Early Detection Program: Summarizing the first 12 years of partnerships and progress against breast and cervical cancer.* Atlanta, GA: Author.

Centers for Disease Control and Prevention (CDC). (2006a). *National Comprehensive Cancer Control Program—2007 fact sheet.* Retrieved August 6, 2007, from http://www.cdc.gov/cancer/ncccp/about.htm

Centers for Disease Control and Prevention (CDC). (2006b). *Division of Nutrition and Physical Activity, Behavior Risk Factor Surveillance System (BRFSS) statistics.* Retrieved August 2, 2007, from http://www.cdc.gov/nccdphp/dnpa/physical/stats/index.htm

Centers for Disease Control and Prevention (CDC). (2006c). *National hepatitis C prevention strategy, hepatitis C infection in the U.S.* Retrieved September 5, 2006, from http://www.cdc.gov/ncidod/diseases/hepatitis/c/plan/HCV_infection.htm

Centers for Disease Control and Prevention (CDC). (2006d). *Genital HPV infection—CDC fact sheet.* Retrieved September 12, 2006, from http://www.cdc.gov/std/HPV/STDFact-HPV.htm

Centers for Disease Control and Prevention (CDC). (2006e). *HPV and HPV vaccine: Information for healthcare providers, August 2006.* Retrieved September 29, 2006, from http://www.cdc.gov/std/HPV/STDFact-HPV-vaccine-hcp.htm

Centers for Disease Control and Prevention (CDC). (2007a). *National Comprehensive Cancer Control Program (NCCCP).* Retrieved April 30, 2007, from http://www.cdc.gov/cancer/ncccp

Centers for Disease Control and Prevention (CDC). (2007b). *National Program of Cancer Registries (NPCR).* Retrieved May 30, 2007, from http://www.cdc.gov/cancer/npcr

Centers for Disease Control and Prevention (CDC). (2007c). *United States cancer statistics.* Retrieved April 30, 2007, from http://www.cdc.gov/cancer/npcr/uscs

Chiu, F. L. (2003). *Inequalities of access to cancer screening: A literature review. NHS Cancer Screening Programmes. Cancer Screening Series No 1.* Retrieved October 10, 2006, from http://www.cancer-screening.nhs.uk/ publications/cs1.pdf

Cleeland, C. S. (1990). Pain assessment. *Advances in Pain Research and Therapy, 13,* 287–291.

Clive, R. E. (2004). Introduction to cancer registries. In C. L. Hutchinson, H. R. Menck, M. Burch, & R. Gottschalk. (Eds.), *Cancer registry management principles and practice* (2nd ed.). Alexandria, VA: National Cancer Registrars Association, Inc.

Colditz, G. A., Cannuscio, C. C., & Frazier, A. L. (1997). Physical activity and reduced risk of colon cancer: Implications for prevention. *Cancer Causes Control, 8,* 649–667.

Curry, S. J., Byers, T., & Hewitt, M., (Eds.). (2003). *Fulfilling the potential of cancer prevention and control.* Washington, DC: The National Academies Press.

Dennis, L. K. & Resnick, M. I. (2000). Analysis of recent trends in prostate cancer incidence and mortality. *Prostate, 42,* 247–252.

Deschamps, M., Band, P. R., & Coldman, A. J. (1988). Assessment of adult cancer pain: Shortcomings of current methods. *Pain, 32*(2), 133–139.

Devesa, S. S., Grauman, D. J., Blot, W. J., Pennello, G. A., & Hoover, R. N. (1999). *Atlas of cancer mortality in the United States, 1950–1994.* Bethesda, MD: National Cancer Institute.

Ellershaw, J., & Ward, C. (2003). Care of the dying patient. *British Medical Journal, 326,* 30–34.

Emanuel, L., Ferris, F. D., von Gunten, C. F., & Von Roenn, J. H. (2006). *The last hours of living: Practical advice for clinicians.* Retrieved October 10, 2006, from http://www.medscape.com/viewprogram/5808

Ferlay, J., Bray, F., Pisani, P., & Parkin, D. M. (2004). *GLOBOCAN 2002 cancer incidence, mortality, and prevalence worldwide.* IARC scientific publications No. 5, ver. 2.0. Lyon, France: IARC Press.

Ferris, T. G., Hallward, J. A., Ronan, L., & Billings, J. A. (1998). When the patient dies: A survey of medical housestaff about care after death. *Journal of Palliative Medicine, 1,* 231–239.

Ferris, F. D., von Gunten, C. F., & Emanuel, L. L. (2003). Competency in end of life care: The last hours of living. *Journal of Palliative Medicine, 6,* 605–613.

Field, M. J., & Cassel, C. K. (Eds.). (1997). *Approaching death: Improving care at the end of life.* Washington, DC: National Academy Press.

Foley, K. M., & Gelband, H. (Eds.). (2001). *Improving palliative care for cancer, report by the Institute of Medicine and National Research Council* Washington, DC: National Academy Press.

Foley, K. M., & Sundaresan, N. (1985). Supportive care of the cancer patient: Management of cancer pain. In V. T. Devita, S. Hellman, & S. A. Rosenberg (Eds.), *Cancer—principles and practice of oncology* (2nd ed., pp. 1940–1961). Philadelphia: Lippincott.

Garrow, J. S. & Webster, J. (1985). Quetlet's index (W/H^2) as a measure of fatness. *International Journal of Obesity, 9,* 147–153.

Giovannucci, E. (1995). Insulin and colon cancer. *Cancer Causes & Control, 6,* 164–179.

Goldie, S. J., Gaffikin, L., Goldhaber-Fiebert, J. D., Gordillo-Tobar, A., Levin, C., Mahe, C., et al. (2005). Cost-effectiveness of cervical-cancer screening in five developing countries. *New England Journal of Medicine, 353,* 2158–2168.

Gordon, D. B., Dahl, J. L., & Stevenson, K. K. (2000). *Building an institutional commitment to pain management* (2nd ed.). Madison, WI: University of Wisconsin-Madison, UW Board of Regents.

Groot, M. T., Baltussen, R., Uyl-de Groot, C. A., Anderson, B. O., & Hortobagyi, G. N. (2006). Costs and health effects of breast cancer interventions in epidemiologically different regions of Africa, North America, and Asia. *Breast Journal, 12*(Suppl. 1), S81–S90.

Grossman, S. A. & Nesbit, S. (2004). Symptom management and palliative care. In M. D. Abeloff, J. O. Armitage, J. E. Niederhuber, M. B. Kastan, & W. G. McKenna (Eds.), *Clinical oncology.* Philadelphia: Elsevier Inc.

Gullatte, M. M., Phillips, J. M., & Gibson, L. M. (2006). Factors associated with delays in screening of self-detected breast changes in African-American women. *Journal of the National Black Nurses Association, 17,* 45–50.

Hankinson, S. E., Willett, W. C., Manson, J. E., Hunter, D. J., Colditz, G. A., Stampfer, M. J., et al. (1995). Alcohol, height, and adiposity in relation to estrogen and prolactin levels in postmenopausal women. *Journal of the National Cancer Institute, 87,* 1297–1302.

Harvard Center for Cancer Prevention. (1997). Summary. *Cancer Causes and Control, 8*(Suppl. 1), S50.

Haylock, P. J., Mitchell, S. A., Cox, T., Temple, S. V. & Curtiss, C. P. (2007). The cancer survivor's prescription for living. *American Journal of Nursing, 107*(4), 58–70.

Hewitt, M., Greenfield, S., & Stovall, E., (Eds.). (2006). *From cancer patient to cancer survivor: Lost in transition.* Washington, DC: The National Academies Press

Hill, C. S. (1990). Relationship among cultural, educational, and regulatory agency influences on optimum cancer pain treatment. *Journal of Pain and Symptom Management, 5,* S37–S45.

Howe, H. L., Keller, J. E., & Lehnherr, M. (1993). Relation between population density and cancer incidence, Illinois, 1986–1990. *American Journal of Epidemiology, 138,* 29–36.

Holland, J. C., & Chertkov, L. (2001). Clinical practice guidelines for the management of psychosocial and physical symptoms of cancer. In K. M. Foley & H. Gelband (Eds.), *Improving palliative care for cancer, report by the Institute of Medicine and National Research Council.* Washington, DC: National Academy Press.

Howson, C. P., Harrison, P. F., & Law, M., (Eds.). (1996). *In her lifetime: Female morbidity and mortality in sub-Saharan Africa.* Washington, DC: National Academy Press.

Hutchison, C. L., Menck, H. R., Burch, M., & Gottschalk, R. (Eds.). (2004). *Cancer registry management: Principles and practice* (2nd ed.). Dubuque, IA: Kendall/Hunt Publishing Company.

International Agency for Research on Cancer (IARC). (2002a). *IARC handbooks of cancer prevention: Weight control and physical activity.* Lyon: IARC Press.

International Agency for Research on Cancer (IARC). (2002b). IARC Working Group on the Evaluation of Cancer Prevention Strategies. *Handbooks of cancer prevention:* Vol. 7. *Breast cancer screening.* Lyon, France: IARC Press.

Intlekofer, R., & Michaud, F. (2007). The National Program of Cancer Registries. In H. R. Menck, L. Deapen, J. L. Phillips, & T. Tucker (Eds.), Central cancer registries: Design, management and use (2nd ed., pp. 357–369). Dubuque, IA: Kendall/Hunt Publishing Company.

Jayant, K., Nene, B. M., Dinshaw, K. A., Budukh, A. M., & Dale, P. S. (1998). Survival from cervical cancer in Barshi registry, rural India. *IARC Scientific Publications, 145,* 69–77.

John, E. M., Phipps, A. I., Davis, A., & Koo, J. (2005). Migration history, acculturation, and breast cancer risk in Hispanic women. *Cancer Epidemiology Biomarkers & Prevention, 14,* 2905–2913.

Kavanagh, A. M., Giovannucci, E. L., Fuchs, C. S., & Colditz, G. A. (1998). Screening endoscopy and risk of colorectal cancer in United States men. *Cancer Causes & Control, 9,* 455–462.

Kerlikowske, K., Grady, D., Rubin, S. M., Sandrock, C., & Ernster, V. L. (1995). Efficacy of screening mammography. A meta-analysis. *Journal of the American Medical Association, 273,* 149–154.

Kinzler, K. W. & Vogelstein, B. (1996). Lessons for hereditary colorectal cancer. *Cell, 87,* 159–170.

Kitchener, H. D., Castle, P. E., & Cox, J. T. (2006). Chapter 7: Achievements and limitations of cervical cytology screening. *Vaccine, 24*(Suppl. 3), S63–S70.

Kolata, G. (2004, June 1). New approach about cancer and survival. *New York Times,* pp. A1, A14.

Kune, G. A., Kune, S., & Watson, L. F. (1990). Body weight and physical activity as predictors of colorectal cancer risk. *Nutrition and Cancer, 13,* 9–17.

Lee, H. P., Gourley, L., Duffy, S. W., Esteve, J., Lee, J., & Day, N. E. (1989). Colorectal cancer and diet in an Asian population—A case control study among Singapore Chinese. *International Journal of Cancer, 43,* 1007–1016.

Lee, I. M. (2003). Physical activity and cancer prevention: Data from epidemiological studies. *Medical Science Sports Exercise, 35,* 1823–1827.

Lee, I. M., Paffenbarger, R. S., Jr., & Hsieh, C. (1991). Physical activity and risk of developing colorectal cancer among college alumni. *Journal of the National Cancer Institute, 83,* 1324–1329.

Lieberman, D. (1997) Endoscopic screening for colorectal cancer. *Gastroenterology Clinics of North America, 26,* 71–83.

Lindor, N. M. (2004). Recognition of genetic syndromes in families with suspected hereditary colon cancer syndromes. *Nature Clinical Practice Gastroenterology & Hepatology, 2,* 366–375.

Lynn, J., & O'Mara, A. (2001). Reliable, high-quality, efficient end-of-life care for cancer patients: economic issues and barriers. In K. M. Foley & H. Gelband (Eds.), *Improving palliative care for cancer, report by the Institute of Medicine and National Research Council.* Washington, DC: National Academy Press.

Mackay, J., Eriksen, M., & Shafey, O. (2006). *The tobacco atlas* (2nd ed.). Atlanta, GA: American Cancer Society.

Mackay, J., Jemal, A., Lee, N. C., & Parkin, D. M. (2006). *The cancer atlas.* Atlanta, GA: American Cancer Society.

Marsden, J., Baum, M., & Sacks, N. P. M. (1998). Hormone replacement therapy in women with previous breast cancer. *Trends in Endocrinology and Metabolism, 9,* 32–38.

Martinez, M. E., Giovannucci, E., Spiegelman, D., Hunter, D. J., Willett, W. C., & Colditz, G. A. (1997). Leisure-time physical activity, body size, and colon cancer in women. Nurses' Health Study Research Group. *Journal of the National Cancer Institute, 89,* 948–955.

Martinez, M. E., Heddens, D., Earnest, D. L., Bogart, C. L., Roe, D., Einspahr, J., et al. (1999). Physical activity, body mass index, and prostaglandin E2 levels in rectal mucosa. *Journal of the National Cancer Institute, 91,* 950–953.

Max, M. B. (1990). Improving outcomes of analgesic treatment: Is education enough? *Annals of Internal Medicine, 113,* 885–889.

McCaffery, K., Wardle, J., & Waller, J. (2003). Knowledge, attitudes, and behavioral intentions in relation to the early detection of colorectal cancer in the United Kingdom. *Preventive Medicine, 36,* 525–535.

McDavid, K., Schymura, M. J., Armstrong, L., Santilli, L., Schmidt, B., Byers, T., et al. (2004). Rationale and design of the National Program of Cancer Registries' breast, colon, and prostate cancer patterns of care study. *Cancer Causes and Control, 15,* 1057–1066.

McKenna, M. T., Taylor, W. R., Marks, J. S., & Koplan, J. P. (1998). Current issues and challenges in chronic disease control. In R. C. Brownson, P. L. Remington, & J. R. Davis (Eds.), *Chronic disease epidemiology and control*. Washington, DC: American Public Health Association.

McKeown-Eyssen, G. (1994). Epidemiology of colorectal cancer revisited: Are serum triglycerides and/or plasma glucose associated with risk? *Cancer Epidemiology Biomarkers & Prevention, 3,* 687–695.

McTiernan, A., Ulrich, C., Slate, S., & Potter, J. (1998). Physical activity and cancer etiology: Associations and mechanisms. *Cancer Causes & Control, 9,* 487–509.

Menck, H. R. (2004). Cancer registries in other countries. In C. L. Hutchinson, H. R. Menck, M. Burch, & R. Gottschalk. (Eds.), *Cancer registry management principles and practice* (2nd ed.) Alexandria, VA: National Cancer Registrars Association, Inc.

Menck, H. R. & Bolick-Aldrich, S. (2007). Glossary of terms and concepts. In H. R. Menck, L. Deapen, J. L. Phillips, & T. Tucker (Eds), *Central cancer registries: Design, management and use* (2nd ed., pp. 421–439). Dubuque, IA: Kendall/Hunt Publishing Company.

Menck, H. R., Deapen, D., Phillips, J. L., & Tucker, T. (Eds.). (2007). Central cancer registries: Design, management and use (2nd ed.). Dubuque, IA: Kendall/Hunt Publishing Company.

Miller, A. B., Chamberlain, J., Day, N. E., Hakama, M., & Prorok, P. C. (1990). Report on a workshop of the UICC project on evaluation of screening for cancer. *International Journal of Cancer, 46,* 761–769.

National Cancer Institute (NCI). (2004). *Cancer facts. Obesity and cancer.* Retrieved August 6, 2007, from http://cis.nci.nih.gov/fact/pdfdraft/3_risk/fs3_70.pdf

National Cancer Institute (NCI). (2006). *NCI international portfolio: Addressing the global challenge of cancer.* (Publication No. 06-6650). Bethesda, MD: Author.

National Cancer Institute (NCI). (2007a). *PDQ (Physician Data Query) comprehensive cancer database.* Retrieved April 26, 2007, from http://www.cancer.gov/ cancertopics/pdq/cancerdatabase

National Cancer Institute (NCI). (2007b). *Treatment choices for men with early-stage prostate cancer: Thinking about treatment choices.* Retrieved July 18, 2007, from http://www.cancer.gov/ cancertopics/prostate-cancer-treatment-choices/page3

National Cancer Institute (NCI). (2007c). *Overview of the SEER Program.* Retrieved July 12, 2007, from http://seer/cancer.gov/about

National Comprehensive Cancer Network (NCCN). (2007). *National Comprehensive Cancer Network (NCCN) clinical practice guidelines in oncology.* Retrieved April 25, 2007, from hppt://www.nccn.org.

National Comprehensive Cancer Network (NCCN) & American Cancer Society (ACS). (2005). *Cancer pain: Treatment guidelines for patients (Ver. II).* Atlanta, GA: ACS.

National Heart, Lung, and Blood Institute (NHLBI). (2006). *NHLBI fact book, fiscal year 2005.* Bethesda, MD: Author.

Parkin, D. M. (1991). Screening for cervix cancer in developing countries. In A. B. Miller, J. Chamberlain, N. E. Day, M. Hakama, P. C. Prorok (Eds.), *Cancer screening.* Cambridge, UK: Cambridge University Press.

Parkin, D. M. (2006). The evolution of the population-based cancer registry. *Nature Reviews Cancer, 6,* 603–612.

Pasero, C., Gordon, D. B., McCaffery, M., & Ferrell, B. R. (1999). Building an institutional commitment to improving pain management. In M. McCaffery & C. Pasero (Eds.), *Pain: Clinical manual* (2nd ed.). St. Louis: Mosby.

Payne, R. (2001). Palliative care for African Americans and other vulnerable populations: Access and quality issues. In K. M. Foley & H. Gelband (Eds.), *Improving palliative care for cancer, report by the Institute of Medicine and National Research Council.* Washington, DC: National Academy Press.

Perez, C. A., Grigsby, P. W., Nene, S. M., Camel, H. M., Galakatos, A., Kao, M. S., et al. (1992). Effect of tumor size on the prognosis of carcinoma of the uterine cervix treated with irradiation alone. *Cancer, 69,* 2796–2806.

Pignone, M., Rich, M., Teutsch, S., Berg, A. O., & Lohr, K. N. (2002). Screening for colorectal cancer in adults at average risk: A summary of the evidence for the U.S. Preventive Services Task Force. *Annals of Internal Medicine, 137,* 132–141.

Pignone, M., Saha, S., Hoerger, T., & Mandelblatt, J. (2002). Cost-effectiveness analyses of colorectal cancer screening. *Annals of Internal Medicine, 137,* 96–104.

Pollack, L. A., Greer, G. E., Rowland, J. H., Miller, A., Doneski, D., Coughlin, S. S., et al. (2005). Cancer survivorship: A new challenge in comprehensive cancer control. *Cancer Causes & Control, 16* (Suppl. 1): 51–59.

Ponten, J., Adami, H. O., Bergstrom, R., Dillner, J., Friberg, L. G., Gustafsson, L., et al. (1995). Strategies for global control of cervical cancer. *International Journal of Cancer, 60,* 1–26.

Prorok, P. C., Chamberlain, J., Day, N. E., Hakama, M., & Miller, A. B. (1984). UICC workshop on evaluation of screening programmes for cancer. *International Journal of Cancer, 34,* 1–4.

Rao, J. K., Anderson, L. A., & Smith, S. M. (2002). End of life is a public health issue. *American Journal of Preventive Medicine, 23,* 215–220.

Rennert, G., Rennert, H. S., Miron, E., & Peterburg, Y. (2001). Population colorectal cancer screening with fecal occult blood test. *Cancer Epidemiology Biomarkers & Prevention, 10,* 1165–1168.

Reuben, S. H. (2004). *Living beyond cancer: Finding a new balance, President's Cancer Panel, 2003–2004 annual report.* Bethesda, MD: National Cancer Institute.

Reuben, S. H. (2006). *Assessing progress, advancing change, President's Cancer Panel, 2005–2006 annual report:* Bethesda, MD: National Cancer Institute.

Riddle, B. L., & Boeshaar, D. K. (2006). Event driven data set for cancer surveillance. *Journal of Registry Management, 33,* 57–62.

Rummans, T. A., Bostwick, J. M., & Clark, M. M. (2000). Maintaining quality of life at the end of life. *Mayo Clinic Proceedings, 75,* 1305–1315.

Sankaranarayanan, R., Budukh, A. M., & Rajkumar, R. (2001). Effective screening programmes for cervical cancer in low- and middle-income developing countries. *Bulletin of the World Health Organization, 79,* 954–962.

Schiffman, M. H., Brinton, L. A., Devesa, S. S., Fraumeni, J., Joseph, F. (1996). Cervical cancer. In D. Schottenfeld & J. Fraumeni (Eds.), *Cancer epidemiology and prevention.* New York: Oxford University Press.

Sepulveda, A. R. & Graham, D. Y. (2003). Role of *Helicobacter pylori* in gastric carcinogenesis. *Hematology Oncology Clinics of North America, 17,* 505–523.

Shephard, R. J. & Futcher, R. (1997). Physical activity and cancer: How may protection be maximized? *Critical Reviews in Oncogenesis, 8,* 219–272.

Sikora, K. (1999). Developing a global strategy for cancer. *European Journal of Cancer, 35,* 24–31.

Stewart, B. W. & Kleihues, P. (2003). *World cancer report.* Lyon, France: IARC Press.

Sloan, F. A., & Gelband, H. (2007). Cancer control opportunities in low- and middle-income countries. Washington, DC: The National Academies Press.

Taplin, S. H., Ichikawa, L., Yood, M. U., Manos, M. M., Geiger, A. M., Weinmann, S., et al. (2004). Reason for late-stage breast cancer: Absence of screening or detection, or breakdown in follow-up? *Journal of the National Cancer Institute, 96,* 1518–1527.

Thune, I., Brenn, T., Lund, E., & Gaard, M. (1997). Physical activity and the risk of breast cancer. *New England Journal of Medicine, 336,* 1269–1275.

Travis, L. B., Rabkin, C. S., & Brown, L. M.(2006). Cancer survivorship—genetic susceptibility and second primary cancers: Research strategies and recommendations. *Journal of the National Cancer Institute, 98*, 15–25.

Twycross, R., & Lichter, I. (1998). The terminal phase. In D. Doyle, G. W. C. Hanks, & N. MacDonald (Eds.), *Oxford textbook of palliative medicine* (2nd ed.). Oxford, England: Oxford University Press.

US Cancer Statistics Working Group (USCSWG). (2006). *United States cancer statistics 2003 incidence and mortality*. Atlanta, GA: Centers for Disease Control and Prevention *and* National Cancer Institute.

US Preventive Services Task Force (USPSTF). (2002). Screening for prostate cancer: Recommendations and rationale. *Annals of Internal Medicine, 137*(11), 915–916.

Weissman, D. E., Dahl, J. L., & Joranson, D. E. (1990). Oral morphine for the treatment of cancer pain. *PPO Updates, 4*(6), 1–8.

Willett, W.C. (2000). Diet and cancer. *Oncologist, 5*, 393–404.

Willett, W. C. (2006). Diet and nutrition. In D. Schottenfeld, & J. F. Fraumeni, Jr. (Eds.), *Cancer epidemiology and prevention*, (3rd ed. pp. 405–421). New York: Oxford University Press.

Winawer, S. J. (1993). Colorectal cancer screening comes of age. *New England Journal of Medicine, 328*, 1416–1417.

Wingo, P. A., Howe, H. L., Thun, M. J., Ballard-Barbash, R., Ward, E., Brown, M. L., et al. (2005). A national framework for cancer surveillance in the United States. *Cancer Causes and Control, 16*, 151–170.

World Cancer Research Fund and American Institute for Cancer Research (WCRF). (1997). *Food, nutrition, and prevention of cancer: A global perspective*. Washington, DC: American Institute for Cancer Research.

World Health Organization (WHO) (1992). *International statistical classification of diseases and related health problems* (10th Rev.) Geneva: Author.

World Health Organization (WHO) (2002) *National cancer control programmes. Policies and managerial guidelines* (2nd ed.). Geneva: Author.

World Health Organization (WHO). (2003a). *Framework convention on tobacco control*. Retrieved March 15, 2007, from http://www.who.int/tobacco/framework/WHO_FCTC_english.pdf

World Health Organization (WHO). (2003b). *World cancer report*. Geneva: Author.

World Health Organization (WHO). (2004). *Global strategy on diet, physical activity and health*. Retrieved April 15, 2007, from http://www.who.int/dietphysicalactivity/goals/en

World Health Organization (WHO). (2005). *Fifty-eighth World Health Assembly, resolution WHA58.22, cancer prevention and control*. Geneva: Author.

World Health Organization (WHO). (2006a). *Cancer control: Knowledge into action. WHO guide for effective programmes*. Geneva: Author.

World Health Organization (WHO). (2006b). *Non-communicable diseases: Cancer*. Retrieved October 10, 2006, from http://www.emro.who.int/ncd/cancer-detection.htm

Young, J. M. & Ward, J. E. (1999). Strategies to improve cancer screening in general practice: Are guidelines the answer? *Family Practice, 16*, 66–70.

Zapka, J. (2003). A framework for improving the quality of cancer care: The case of breast and cervical cancer screening. *Cancer Epidemiology Biomarkers & Prevention, 12*, 4–13.

Ziegler, R. G., Hoover, R. N., Pike, M. C., Hildesheim, A., Nomura, A. M., West, D. W., et al. (1993). Migration patterns and breast cancer risk in Asian-American women. *Journal of the National Cancer Institute, 85*, 1819–1827.

Zoorob, R., Anderson, R., Cefalu, C., & Sidani, M. (2001). Cancer screening guidelines. *American Family Physician, 63*, 1101–1112.

Chapter 12

Global Perspectives on Violence, Injury, and Occupational Health

Carol Holtz

Violence

The United Nations' *World Report on Violence and Health* defines violence as "the intentional use of physical force or power, threatened or actual, against oneself, another person, or against a group or community, that either results in or has a high likelihood of resulting in injury, death, psychological harm, maldevelopment, or deprivation" (United Nations, 2005, p.1).

Violence is a world health issue that includes child abuse and neglect by caregivers, violence by youth (ages 10 to 29 years), intimate partner violence, sexual violence, elder abuse, self-inflicted violence, and collective violence, such as war or terrorism. Worldwide, an average of 4500 people die a violent death every day. In 2000, 1.2 million violent deaths occurred and half of them were from suicide, one third were from homicide, and one fifth were from war-related injuries (World Health Organization [WHO], 2002). The World Bank and the Inter-American Development Bank consider violence and insecurity to be major health obstacles. In the Americas, (United States, Canada, Mexico, Central and South America) 14.2% of the gross national product (GNP) or the equivalent of US $168 billion is lost or transferred because of violence. The human capital loss in GNP is 1.9%. Intentional violence is the first cause of death in many countries, and there are approximately 120,000 homicides worldwide a year. The majority of the victims are those in poverty and young males. Thirty to sixty percent of all hospital emergency visits are the result of violence of some kind. Of all violent acts, such as murder, child abuse, family abuse, assaults, or felonies, most are associated with alcohol consumption. Research indicates that children exposed to family violence have a higher risk of performing violent behavior in their adolescent years. In the United States violence was declared a public health emergency in 1992 by then Surgeon General, C. Everett Koop. In Latin American countries, the ministers of public health made the prevention of violence a public health priority in 1993. Later in 1996, the Pan American Health Organization and the World Health Assembly also made a similar resolution (Guerro, 2002; Mercy, Krugberg, Dahlberg, & Zwi, 2003).

The United States has high rates of homicide and deaths related to firearms as compared to other developed countries, but when considering all countries of the world, the United States has lower rates than many other countries, including developing countries. Homicide rates for Africa, Central America, and South America were three times the US rate. The US suicide rate of 10.6 per 100,000 in 2000 was lower than the global rate of 14.5 per 100,000. Suicide rates for Europe and the Western Pacific regions were twice the rate of the United States. Suicide was considered the 13th leading cause of death in the world for 2000, and homicide was considered the 22nd leading cause of death. In the United States, suicide was the 11th leading cause of death and homicide the 14th leading cause of death for 2000 (Guerro, 2002; Mercy, Krugberg, Dahlberg, & Zwi, 2003).

Domestic violence reduces the health of millions of women throughout the world. The American Psychiatric Association reports that 4 million American women experience a serious assault by an intimate partner each year. In the United States one study revealed that 22.1% of women reported physical assault by an intimate partner. Sexual assault by an intimate partner in the United States has been reported to be approximately 7.7%. Parental abuse has a severe impact on child health worldwide. Some research studies reveal a 50% rate of children who have been hit, kicked, or beaten by their parents. About 20% of women and 5% of men reported being sexually abused during their childhoods. In addition, 4–6% of elderly have experienced some form of abuse. Exposure to violence during childhood may result in later life consequences such as mental illness, depression, smoking, obesity, high-risk sexual behaviors, unintended pregnancies, alcohol, and drug use (Guerro, 2002; Mercy, Krugberg, Dahlberg, & Zwi, 2003).

Violence related to war may result in increased health services costs, reduction in productivity, and decreased property values. Violence may cross international borders especially when it is associated with illegal drug trade, small arms trade, sexual slavery, or terrorism.

Sometimes violence is contained within cultural practices, such as violence against women and female genital mutilation. A unique preventative method for curtailing domestic violence exists in some communities in India. A dharna is a public shaming and protest done in front of the home or workplace of abusive men. In countries where there are huge differences in the incomes of people who are wealthy in comparison to people living in extreme poverty, there are much higher rates of violence. Today, there are violence prevention programs promoted by the US Centers for Disease Control and Prevention (CDC), and in the many US state and city health departments (Guerro, 2002; Mercy, Krugberg, Dahlberg, & Zwi, 2003). See Figure 12-1.

The US public health approach recommends the following four steps to prevent violence:

1. Define the violence problem through systematic data collection.
2. Conduct research to find out why it occurs and who it affects.
3. Find out what works to prevent violence by designing, implementing, and evaluating interventions.

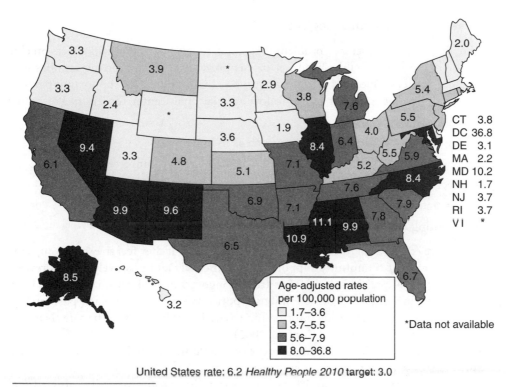

Figure 12-1 Homicide rates per state, 1999.

Source: National Vital Statistics System, National Center for Health Statistics, CDC.

4. Promote effective and promising interventions in a wide range of settings and evaluate their impact and cost effectiveness.

How people are raised in childhood affects the vulnerability and likelihood for becoming a victim or a perpetrator. Some examples include alcohol abuse, being a victim of child maltreatment, or a psychological or personality disorder. Close relationships with others also influence the possibility of becoming a victim or perpetrator such as when the following occur (UN, 2005):

- Poor parenting practices
- Marital discord and having friends who engage in violence
- Social, economic, and gender inequalities
- Weak economic safety nets
- Poor law enforcement
- Cultural norms about violence also determine violent situations.

Child Maltreatment and Neglect

Child maltreatment is a serious problem that can have long-term harmful effects on children. The main goal of public health efforts is prevention by supporting families with skills and resources. One method of prevention is by teaching and supporting parental nurturing skills. These consist of the following (National Center for Injury Prevention and Control, 2005b):

- Giving physical signs of affection such as in hugging
- Fostering self-esteem in children such as with positive reinforcement
- Recognizing and understanding children's feelings
- Engaging in effective communication with children
- Learning alternative methods to shaking, hitting, and spanking

Parents are encouraged to take a break from a situation if they feel they are losing control. The benefits of community support can significantly and positively affect previous parental behavioral practices. Volunteers from nongovernmental organizations and corporations can further help provide family support services. Through such partnerships parents and teachers can provide information to teach children how to be safe (National Center for Injury Prevention and Control, 2005).

A 2002 CDC child maltreatment report of 906,000 maltreated children, stated that within this study, 61% of the children experienced neglect, 19% were physically abused, 10% were sexually abused, and 5% were emotionally (psychologically) abused (see Figure 12-2). Moreover, shaken baby syndrome is a form of child abuse that affects 1200 to 1600 children per year, which may result in serious permanent damage or death. Twenty-five to thirty percent of shaken babies die from their injuries. Effects of child maltreatment may result in brain maldevelopment, sleep disturbances, panic disorder, and attention deficit/hyperactivity disorder. Consequences of child maltreatment may also result in problematic behavior as adults, including smoking, alcoholism, drug abuse, eating disorders, severe obesity, depression, suicide, and sexual promiscuity. Victims of child maltreatment are twice as likely to be physically assaulted as adults. Up to one third of parents who were maltreated as children are likely to maltreat their own children. Children most likely to suffer severe injury or death are those under age 4.

A report conducted in the Netherlands identified child abuse and neglect as important causes of child morbidity and death. Infants aged 6 months who were crying had been smothered, slapped, or shaken at least once. Results of the study indicate that clinicians should be aware of babies who cry a lot, and target interventions to parents to help them cope with the crying (Reijneveld, Brugman, Sing, & Verloove-Vanhorick, 2004).

Sexual Violence

According to the World Health Organization (2005), sexual violence occurs in all cultures and in every part of the world. Up to 20% of all women experienced an attempted or

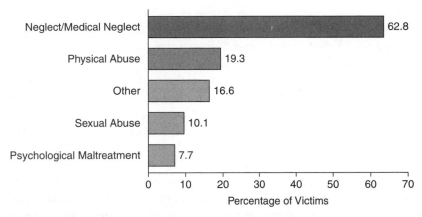

Figure 12-2 Percentage of child abuse and neglect victims by type of maltreatment, 2000.

Source: US Department of Health and Human Resources.

TABLE 12-1   Risk Factors That Can Contribute to the Need for Protective Factors for the Child

Risk Factors	Protective Factors Needed for the Child
Disabilities or mental retardation, increasing caregiver burden	Supportive family environment
	Nurturing parental skills
Social isolation of families	Stable family relationships
Parents' lack of knowledge of child development and needs	Household rules and monitoring of the child
	Parental employment
Poverty and unemployment	Adequate housing
Family disorganization and/or violence	Access to health care and social services
Substance abuse in family members	Caring adults outside the family who serve as role models or mentors
Young and single parents	
Poor parent–child relationships	Communities that support parents and attempt to prevent child abuse
Parental thoughts and emotions that support child maltreatment	
Parental stress and/or mental health issues	
Community violence	

Source: National Center for Injury Prevention and Control, 2005.

completed rape by an intimate partner during their lifetime. Up to one third of women have experienced rape as their first sexual experience. More that 50% of all rapes occur in women before age 18, and 22% of this group occur before age 12. In 80% of all rape cases, the victim knew the perpetrator. Although the majority of victims are women, men and children of both sexes also experience sexual violence. Sexual violence has a significant effect on the health of the population with consequences such as depression, unwanted pregnancy, sexually transmitted diseases, HIV/AIDS, and risk of development of high-risk sexual behaviors through sexual promiscuity. One longitudinal study estimated that in the United States over 32,000 pregnancies resulted from rape of women age 12 to 45 years. Of the rape victims, 4–30% contract HIV or STDs. Post-traumatic stress disorders (PTSD) are usually found 3 months after the rape, and victims can experience one or more of the chronic symptoms of anxiety, guilt, nervousness, phobias, substance abuse, sleep disturbances, depression, and sexual dysfunction. Rape victims are more likely than the general population to commit suicide.

Intimate Partner Violence

Domestic or intimate partner violence is the range of sexually, psychologically, and physically coercive acts used against adult and adolescent women by current or former male intimate partners. The CDC report on intimate partner violence indicated that 5.3 million intimate partners are victims of violence each year (National Center for Injury Prevention and Control, 2004a). This results in greater than 2 million injuries and 1300 deaths per year. Intimate partner violence occurs in all populations regardless of culture, socioeconomic status, or geographic location. Young women and those living in federal poverty are disproportionately more likely to be victims. As many as 324,000 women each year in the United States experience intimate partner violence during their pregnancy. Forty-four percent of women murdered by their intimate partners had visited an emergency room within the last 2 years of the homicide, and 93% had at least one injury visit. Firearms were the most common type of weapon used. In the United States approximately 40–70% of female murder victims were killed by their husbands or boyfriends and had a history of an abusive relationship.

The consequences of intimate partner violence include a 60% higher rate of health problems among these women as compared to women with no history of abuse. Some examples include chronic pain, gastrointestinal disorders, and irritable bowel syndrome. Reproductive health problems include unwanted pregnancy, premature labor and birth, sexually transmitted diseases, and HIV/AIDS. In addition, women often experience mental health problems such as anxiety and low self-esteem. They are more likely to abuse alcohol and make suicide attempts. These women are more likely to be unemployed and be recipients of public assistance. Both men and women experience intimate partner violence, but women are 2–3 times more likely to report their situations. Hispanic women and women of American Indian/Native Alaskan descent had a lower rate of reporting victimizations than non-Hispanic white women. Characteristics of perpetrators of intimate partner violence include the following:

- Young age
- Low self-esteem
- Low academic achievement
- Alcohol or drug use
- Witnessing violence as a child

The relationships of the perpetrators and the victims often consisted of the following (National Center for Injury Prevention and Control, 2004a):

- Marital conflict
- Marital instability
- Male dominance in the family
- Poor family functioning
- Emotional dependence and insecurity
- Belief in strict gender roles
- Desire for power and control of a relationship, and exhibiting anger and hostility toward the partner

Within the African-American community in the United States, high rates of domestic violence exist. Low socioeconomic status and poverty are often linked to the causes of violence. Although domestic violence cuts across race, socioeconomic status, education, and income, African-Americans experience a disproportionate amount of domestic violence compared with non-Hispanic white Americans. The National Black Women's Health Project identified domestic violence as the health issue of highest priority for African-American women. African-American women are at a greater risk than non- Hispanic white women for contracting HIV as a result of domestic violence. The number of deaths and serious injuries is greater in African-American communities. African-American women are more likely to kill a partner and are also twice as likely to be killed because of domestic violence than white women. Possible explanations are that African-American women do not always see themselves in danger and are less likely to seek assistance for violence. Other reasons are that African-Americans are more likely to be in poverty and have less access to transportation to geographically convenient shelters. In addition, lack of culturally competent healthcare providers has also resulted in hesitancy of African-American women to seek counseling and assistance for domestic violence (Bent-Goodley, 2004).

In a study of domestic violence in the Rakai District of Uganda, 30% of women had experienced physical threats or physical abuse from their current partner. Of those who had experienced domestic violence, greater than 50% reported injuries. The perpetrators' main characteristics include alcohol consumption and HIV-positive status.

Unfortunately, most of the study's participants (70% of men and 90% of females) reported that beating a wife or female partner was justifiable in some circumstances, which creates a challenge for prevention in some settings. One explanation for the relationship to HIV status is that women who believe that their partner is at high risk or is diagnosed with HIV may not want to have sexual relations with that partner. The resistance is met by physical violence (Koenig et al., 2003).

Watts and Mayhew (2004) relate that in sub-Saharan Africa, 13–49% of women have been hit or otherwise physically assaulted by an intimate male partner, with only 5–29% reporting their experience of physical violence. In Zimbabwe and in Ethiopia, 26% and 59% respectively, have been forced to have sex with their intimate partners. For women who experience violence, the abuse is continued and often intensified during pregnancy.

A study conducted in Finland using open-ended questions with battered women found that women who had been maltreated in their parental home, also experienced violence from their spouses. The study concluded that intimate partner violence was associated with childhood experience of maltreatment, their partners' weak identities, and conflicts between individualism and familism. Results indicated that nurses and other healthcare providers need to be more aware of symptoms of violence and have skills needed to discuss intimate moral and spiritual issues (Flinck, Paavilainen, & Astedt-Kurki, 2005).

In 2004, 67 women in Spain were murdered by their current husbands or boyfriends. Spain's medical community has long ignored the problems of domestic violence. With the passage of new laws, the minister of health has developed a program to help doctors and other healthcare professionals recognize signs of domestic violence, such as eating disorders or depression, and develop special training programs for counseling abused women (Loewenberg, 2005).

A study in Fuzhou, China, of 600 women at a gynecological clinic, revealed that 43% experienced intimate partner violence. Intimate partner violence is highly prevalent in China, with a strong association with male patriarchal values. Efforts to reduce this problem should be given a high priority in healthcare settings where woman can be seen (Xu, Zhu, O'Campo, Koenig, Mock, & Campbell, 2005). Notwithstanding developed and developing nations, intimate partner violence shares consistent patterns and characteristics of perpetrators and of those who are abused.

Intimate Partner Violence and Pregnancy

Domestic violence against women who are pregnant is a special case of intimate partner violence. The true incidence of physical abuse in pregnancy is not known, but it ranges from .9% to 26% in developing countries. Most victims are reluctant to report abuse. The effects on violence during pregnancy may result in a blow to the abdomen causing adverse outcomes such as preterm labor and delivery, chorioamnionitis (infection of the amniotic fluid), premature rupture of membranes, low birth weight babies, intrauterine growth retardation, hemorrhage, fetal injury, and also death of the mother and fetus. Indirectly, psychological stress and lack of access to prenatal care can also cause poor outcomes.

Related responses to domestic violence include polysubstance (alcohol, drugs, and tobacco) abuse.

In a study of 522 Nigerian pregnant women, 47.1% reported abuse from their intimate partner relationship. Of those abused, 11.7% experienced it for the first time during pregnancy. The majority of women (99%) refused to report the abuse to the police. The conclusion of the study indicated that healthcare workers need to be alert to the clues of abuse in order to protect the women from further abuse (Ezechi, Kalu, Ezechi, Ndububa, Nworkoro, & Okeke, 2004). In another study of 991 pregnant women in northern India, violence was higher when the husband/partner was less educated and when the man consumed opium, tobacco, and/or alcohol. The perpetrators were the intimate partner, the husband's mother, and the husband's brother (Khosla, Dua, Devi, & Sud, 2005).

School Violence

Violence is taking an increasing toll on American society. School violence is now a major problem that inhibits learning and causes physical and psychological harm to students. Homicide and suicide cause 25% of deaths of people ages 10 to 24 years in the United States. The potential for being threatened or injured by a weapon on school property has increased in recent years (Brener, Lowry, & Barrios, (2005). Children are bullied at home and also in their school environments. Victimized children often experience symptoms of withdrawal, anxiety, or depression, and many remain unhappy within their school environment. Prevention and intervention programs have been proven to reduce mental health problems during childhood.

Violence and War

Today many are faced with violence as a result of war and terrorism. These situations affect large groups of civilians who are confronted with civil strife, food shortages, and population displacements. Worldwide there is about 1 death per day per 10,000 people. Some countries with greater violence, such as the Democratic People's Republic of the Congo, have a mortality rate of 3.5 deaths per 1000 people per month (Waldman, 2005). Efforts to address the high rates of violent deaths need to continue to promote human security by taking the following measures (A new vision for human security, 2003):

- Protect people in violent conflict.
- Protect people from the proliferation of arms.
- Support migrants, refugees, and internally displaced persons.
- Establish funds for postconflict situations.
- Encourage fair trade to benefit the poor.
- Provide minimum living standards everywhere.
- Give high priority to universal access to basic health care.

- Develop an equitable global system for patient rights.
- Provide basic education.

Within nations, however, violence reduction can also be directed toward religious and political leaders who can work towards developing systems of openness and opportunity for their own constituents.

Bioterrorism also relates to war and is another major threat to world health. Safeguarding the public's health, safety, and security became a high priority after the attacks on the World Trade Center on September 11, 2001. On October 4, 2001, a Florida man was diagnosed with inhalation anthrax. An anthrax agent was dispersed throughout the US postal system in New York, Washington, DC, and other locations. This resulted in five deaths, thousands more tested, and many hundreds treated for this illness. As a result the Model State Emergency Health Powers Act, or Model Act, was developed. The Model Act provides states with power to detect and contain bioterrorism or a naturally occurring disease outbreak. Included are the following elements (Gostin et al., 2002):

- Preparedness—Preparing for a public health emergency
- Surveillance—Measures to detect and track public health emergencies
- Management of property—Ensuring adequate availability of vaccines, pharmaceuticals, and hospitals
- Protection of persons—Powers to compel vaccination, testing, treatment, isolation, and quarantine when clearly necessary
- Communication—Providing clear and authoritative information to the public

Injury

Injuries cause about 10% of all deaths worldwide with traffic accidents, self-inflicted injuries, violence, and war being the most common of traumatic deaths. There is a predicted increase in all types of injuries by the year 2020. Historically, global health-related problems tended to be from infectious disease, pollution, and malnutrition; but, at present, injury is gaining more attention as a major global health problem. A study comparing mortality from serious blunt trauma showed that the rates decreased as income increased. Examples included low income, Ghana; middle income, Mexico; and high income, United States. The higher rates of death were due to increased time necessary to transport patients to a hospital emergency room setting and care given in transit to the hospital (Leppaniemi, 2004; Mock, Quansah, Krishnan, Arreola-Risa, & Rivara, 2004; Mock, Joshipura, & Goosen, 2004).

The World Bank and the World Health Organization report that almost 12 million people die of traffic accidents each year, and the number could increase by 65% in the next 20 years. Most of the increase will be from deaths in developing countries. In the United States the estimated cost of serious trauma care for each person is far greater than care for cancer and cardiovascular diseases. Reduction of deaths and injuries from trauma could have a major worldwide positive economic impact. Significant advances in prehospital care with advanced life support (ALS), and basic life support (BLS) have improved mortality rates for serious injuries. Advances in technology in hospital emergency rooms and operative care, as well as intensive care unit (ICU) hospital care, have also significantly improved chances of survival for patients. Unfortunately many seriously injured patients living in developing countries may not have the benefit of such care, lack of technology, lack of funds, or transportation to healthcare facilities (Leppaniemi, 2004; Mock, Quansah, Krishnan, Arreola-Risa, & Rivara, 2004; Mock, Joshipura, & Goosen, 2004).

Injuries have traditionally been considered to be random and unavoidable accidents, yet today intentional and unintentional injuries are considered to be preventable events. Injuries are among the world's leading causes of death, disability, or disease and affect people of all races, ages, and socioeconomic status. Worldwide, road traffic accidents and self-inflicted injuries are the leading causes of injury deaths.

Worldwide, falls are the leading health injury problems in children 5–14 years. For those ages 15–29 years, road traffic accidents, self-inflicted injuries, interpersonal violence, war injuries, drowning, poisonings, and fire exposures are the leading causes of deaths. China is the only region that has drowning as one of the 15 leading causes of death and burden of disease. Low- and middle-income countries in Europe have poisonings as the leading cause of death for injuries (WHO, 2005; Silcock, 2003; Hyder, 2004).

There is a significant gap in the burden of trauma and injury in low- and middle-income countries of the world as compared to high-income countries. Fifteen percent of the world's population resides in high-income countries, with 60% of this high-income population having life spans of above 70 years. In contrast, the remaining 85% of the world's population lives in middle- and low-income countries, with only 25% of its population living past 70 years. The newly independent countries of Eastern Europe, which are in the category of middle-income countries, have the highest overall injury mortality rates. Countries in North America, Western Europe, Australia, and New Zealand, have the lowest world injury rates. The main reasons for higher rates of trauma and injury in low- and middle-income countries are inadequate systems of hospital and community-based emergency care. Roads used to transport trauma patients to hospitals are often unpaved and have few safety regulations. In addition there is often little recognition for road safety and public education in middle- and low-income countries. In response to this significant gap it is essential that trauma care services, research in trauma and injury, and comprehensive training programs for preventing injuries and violence that are unique to the specific demographic and environmental influences be developed (Hofman, Primack, Keusch, & Hryndow , 2005; Zhang, Norton, Tang, Lo, Zhuo, & Wenkui, 2004).

Injuries and violence are also a great problem for US older adults. To protect older Americans many programs are being developed that address the following (National Center for Injury Prevention and Control, 2003):

- Elder abuse and maltreatment
- Falls

- Traffic accidents with injuries
- Residential fire injuries
- Sexual abuse
- Suicide
- Traumatic brain injury

The CDC in partnership with the US National Highway Traffic Safety Administration is also working to reduce deaths caused by alcohol-related road traffic injuries (CDC, 2004b).

Road Traffic Injuries

A road traffic injury is a fatal or nonfatal injury that occurred as a result of a road traffic crash. A road traffic crash is a collision or incident that may or may not lead to injury, which occurs on a public road and involves at least one moving vehicle (WHO, 2004). In 1990 road accidents were the ninth leading cause of death in the world, and by 2020 they will be the third leading cause of death if nothing is done to stop the trend. Every year over 1.2 million people around the world are killed in traffic accidents. Ninety percent of deaths occur in poorer countries. In addition 20–50 times that number of people are seriously injured. In 2004, 3300 deaths and 66,000 serious injuries occurred daily. If this current trend continues, the numbers of those killed or seriously injured from road accidents will continue to increase by greater than 60% from 2000 to 2020. The majority of these deaths and injuries will occur in developing countries where more people are using cars, trucks, motorcycles, and mopeds, and more pedestrians are also vulnerable to injury and death from motor vehicles.

Since 1990, for example, traffic fatalities increased 237.1% in Colombia. China and Botswana had increases of 243% and 383.8% respectively. At present nothing appears to be impeding the trend. Since 1990 China has quadrupled its rate of motor vehicles usage to 55 million. In developing countries crashes are more likely to result in death than in developed countries. Crashes in developing countries often involve pedestrians or people in unprotected mopeds or motorcycles. The good news is that most of these injuries and mortalities are preventable (Silcock, 2003; Vehicle manslaughter, 2004; WHO, 2004).

In Mexico, the road traffic injuries and pedestrian injuries are a major public health problem. During 2000, 17,500 deaths occurred from traffic accidents. Pedestrians have the largest rates of deaths from traffic accidents in Mexico City. Baja California Sur has a death rate from traffic injuries of 28.7 per 100,000 people, the highest in Mexico, as compared to Chiapas, with a rate of 7.9 per 100,000 (Hijar, Vazquez-Vela, & Arreola-Risa, 2002)

Since its implementation of economic reform policies, China has made great progress in development of the road infrastructures. In the United States teen drivers are especially vulnerable to traffic deaths. Forty percent of all deaths of teens are from motor vehicle accidents. Teens age 16–19 were four times more likely than older drivers to have traffic accidents. Teenagers represent 10% of the population and 14% of all motor vehicle accidents. Also the presence of other teen passengers increases the risk of accidents for teen drivers. Male teens have double the number of deaths from car accidents as female teens. These accidents are particularly high during the first years that teenagers are eligible to drive. Teens are more likely than older drivers to do the following:

- Underestimate the dangers in hazardous situations
- Have less experience coping with difficult driving situations
- Speed
- Run red light
- Make illegal turns
- Ride with an intoxicated driver
- Drive while using alcohol and drugs
- Not using a seat belt

Male teens are less likely to use a seat belt than female teens (National Center for Injury Prevention and Control, 2004c).

US drivers over age 65 have higher rates of traffic accidents than all other drivers except teen drivers. In 2002 the majority of fatal traffic accidents of older drivers occurred during daytime (81%) and on weekdays (72%). Although older drivers were more likely than younger drivers to use a seat belt, drivers 65 and older are more likely to die from injuries than younger drivers. Injury rates are twice as high for older men than women. Factors related to injury and deaths for older drivers are caused by problems with vision, hearing, cognitive functions, and physical impairments (National Center for Injury Prevention and Control, 2004b,c).

Other Injuries (Poisons, Alcohol, Burns, and Drowning)

Poison

In 2000 US poison control centers reported that 2.2 million poison exposures occurred. Greater than 90% of the exposures happened in the home, and 52.7% occurred in children under age 6 years. The most common exposures of children were ingestion of household products such as cosmetics and personal care products, cleaning substances, pain relievers, foreign objects, and plants. For adults, the most common exposures are pain relievers, sedatives, cleaning substances, antidepressants, and bites or stings. Lead poisoning in children is a very preventable problem, though millions of children have this exposure. Elevated levels of lead in the blood cause problems in child cognitive growth and development (National Center for Injury Prevention and Control. 2002).

Alcohol

In the United States excessive alcohol consumption causes greater than 10,000 deaths per year, and between 20–30% of the patients seen in all emergency rooms have alcohol-related problems. Half of all alcohol-related deaths are the result of injuries from motor vehicle accidents, falls, fires, drowning, homicides, and suicides. Thirty percent of Americans will at some stage in their lives be involved in an alcohol-related crash (CDC, 2004b).

Preventable actions and programs can be developed, such as the following (CDC, 2004b):

- Suspend drivers licenses of those who drive intoxicated.
- Lower the blood alcohol level concentration for US adults to .08% in all states.
- Establish zero tolerance for drivers under 21 who consume alcohol. Establish sobriety check points and have community education about drinking and driving.
- Raise state and federal alcohol excise taxes.
- Have compulsory blood alcohol testing for all traffic accidents with injuries.

Burns

Burns are injuries of the skin and sometimes of the underlying tissue, muscle, nerves and organs. They can be caused by hot liquids, flames, hot surfaces, sunlight or radiation, electricity, or chemicals. Primary prevention is the most effective means of combating burns. Fire-related burns were responsible for 322,000 deaths worldwide in 2002. The majority were in developing countries. Greater than half of all the worldwide deaths were in Southeast Asia, in which 66% were females. Prevention of injurious fires can be achieved by taking the following measures (WHO, 2003):

- Enclose open fires, and limit the height of fires in homes, especially in developing countries.
- Promote use of safe stoves and fuels.
- Have housing fire safety regulations and inspections.
- Educate the public.
- Establish and comply with industrial safety regulations.
- Promote the use of smoke detectors, fire alarms, and escape systems for fires.
- Avoid smoking in bed.
- Promote the use of nonflammable children's pajamas.
- Lower the temperature of hot water taps in homes.

In the United States in 2002, four of every five fires occurred in the home, with cooking as the main cause of residential fires and smoking the second leading cause of fires. Most deaths are from smoke or toxic gas inhalation. Those at greatest risk for fires are children under 5 years of age, adults over 65 years, African-Americans and Native Americans, those living in poverty, those living in rural areas, and those living in substandard housing.

Fires occur more in the winter season, and more deaths occur to those without home smoke detectors (National Center for Injury Prevention and Control, 2003).

However, those in developing nations do not tend to have smoke detectors and more often cook by fire within their homes.

Drowning

Drowning is the process of experiencing respiratory impairment from the submersion or immersion in liquid resulting in death or morbidity. One third of all world drownings occur in the western Pacific region of the world, yet Africa has the highest world rate for a specific continent. In 2000, China reported 129,000 drowning deaths, and India had 86,000 drowning deaths. Both China and India have very high drowning death rates and together have 43% of the world's deaths by drowning. Drowning in younger children is generally a result of a lapse of supervision by parents or caregivers. Males drown twice as often as females. In 2000 approximately 409,272 people drowned worldwide. Drowning is the second leading cause of unintentional injury deaths, second only to traffic accidents. Ninety percent of drownings occur in low- and middle-income countries. Large numbers of drowning deaths are associated with major floods, unsafe or overcrowded boats, alcohol use, and epilepsy. Prevention intervention strategies include the following (WHO, 2001):

- Drain unnecessary accumulations of water in baths, ponds, buckets, and so on.
- Build a fence around swimming pools, ponds, lakes, and rivers, if possible.
- Teach people to swim.
- Train people to perform CPR when needed.

Occupational Health

Work-related injuries and illnesses are events or exposures in the work environment that cause or contribute to a health condition or significantly aggravate a preexisting condition. These illnesses or injuries may result in death, loss of consciousness, time away from work, restricted work activity, or medical treatment beyond first aid. Significant work-related injuries or illnesses may be diagnosed by a physician or other healthcare professional.

Occupational illnesses may consist of any of the following (Bureau of Statistics, 2004):

- Skin diseases or disorders caused by exposure to chemicals, plants, or other substances. The worker may get problems such as contact dermatitis, eczema, rash, ulcers, chemical burns, or inflammations.
- Respiratory problems associated with breathing hazardous biological products, chemicals, dust, gases, vapors or fumes. Examples include pneumonitis, pharyngitis, rhinitis, tuberculosis (TB), occupational asthma, toxic inhalation injury, or chronic bronchitis.
- Poisoning can occur from exposure to lead, mercury, arsenic, carbon monoxide, or hydrogen sulfide or other gases.

- Other occupational illnesses may include heatstroke, sunstroke, heat exhaustion, freezing, frostbite, decompression sickness, anthrax, HIV, or hepatitis B.

Occupational injuries could include broken bones, cuts, or fractured eardrums. Injuries may result in sick days away from work, a transfer to another location or assignment, or permanent job loss (Bureau of Statistics, 2004).

Workplace injuries, illnesses, and fatalities continue to remain at very high levels worldwide, which contribute to the worldwide burden of health.

In 2000 there were 2 million work-related deaths, and only 10–15% of workers worldwide have basic standard occupational health services. The World Health Organization (WHO) is implementing a global strategy to provide evidence for policy legislation and support of decision makers to estimate the burden of occupational diseases and injuries. It also disseminates information to promote workers' health. WHO also assists countries to develop or upgrade their national occupational health plans and assists in implementing the plans (WHO, 2005).

The movement of capital and technology and changes in the organization of work has outpaced the system for protecting workers' health. Women in particular have been affected by these employment patterns. They have taken on more jobs and worked longer hours, due to the double workload of household work and employment in formal or informal sectors, and often have low-skilled, low-paid jobs where rates of union membership are low. The work is often strenuous, monotonous, and they have little control over the job pace or content. For both men and women who work in agriculture, manufacturing, and mining sectors, there are associated high rates of injury from mechanical, electrical, and physical hazards. In African countries the injury rates in forestry, electricity production, mining, and manufacturing are all greater than 30 injuries per 1000 workers. In addition to the traditional problems of traumatic injury, respiratory disease, occupational dermatitis, and musculoskeletal injuries, workers are now suffering from asthmatic disorders and psychological stress. Estimates of the burden of occupational health diseases in southern Africa are underestimated 50 fold (Loewenson, 2001).

In the United States in 2002, 14.6 million workers made visits to physicians' offices for worker's compensation, and in 2003, 40.1 million workers went to hospital emergency rooms for work-related problems (National Institute for Occupational Safety and Health [NIOSH], 2005d).

The US Occupational Safety and Health Administration (OSHA) calculates that in the United States 6000 employees die each year from injuries in the workplace, and another 50,000 die from illnesses caused by exposure to workplace hazards. This costs US businesses greater than $125 billion dollars yearly. Within the United States federal criteria (OSHA standards) used to address worker safety consists of the following requirements (OSHA, 2002):

- Provide well-maintained tools and equipment.
- Provide medical examinations.

- Provide training by OSHA standards.
- Report accidents or fatalities within 8 hours.
- Keep records of work-related accidents, injuries, or illnesses.
- Post prominently employee rights and responsibilities.
- Provide employee access to their medical and exposure records.
- Do not discriminate against employees who exercise their rights under the OSHA Act.
- Post citations and violations at or near the worksite.
- Respond to survey requests.

Acute trauma at work is a leading cause of death and disability among workers in the United States. Acute trauma can occur with a sudden application of force or violence that causes injury or death. In 2000 there were 5915 workplace deaths from acute traumatic injury. The National Institute for Occupational Safety and Health (NIOSH) is currently conducting research to identify and prioritize the problems with injury surveillance studies, quantify and prioritize risk factors with analytic injury research, identify existing or new strategies to prevent occupational injuries with prevention and control research, and implement the most effective injury control measures with communication and dissemination of recent information and technology (NIOSH, 2005d)

Occupational health is often neglected in developing countries because of competing social, economic, and political issues. The majority of developing countries lack the ability to establish new occupational health policies and regulations (Nuwayhid, 2004). Today many US manufacturing jobs have moved to developing countries where labor and taxes are much more economical. Thus manufacturing has made a dramatic shift in the last decade from well-regulated, high-wage, often unionized plants to low-wage, unregulated, nonunion plants in the developing world. Workers in developing countries have often been subjected to high noise and temperature levels, unguarded machinery, and other safety hazards. In countries such as in Indonesia and Guatemala, limited or no safety regulations exist within occupational settings. Other countries such as China or Mexico may have safety regulations, but they may not be fully enforced. One problem, such as in Mexico, is its level of international indebtedness to private banks, the World Bank, and International Monetary Fund. This results in a level of national dependency on foreign investment, which discourages the host country to push for occupational health policies (Nuwayhid, 2004).

In a study of the occupational health of workers in South Africa, results indicated that the most common work-related problems were musculoskeletal diseases and respiratory diseases. Of the 8–9 million employed South Africans approximately 792,000 consult healthcare services every year for conditions related to or aggravated by their work (Kielkowski, Rees, & Bradshaw, 2004).

Working children in Nigeria often have health-related problems. They tend to work in unregulated industries, especially in the informal sector, such as on the streets, in markets, and other public places. These working children can be exposed to environmental hazards that result in accidents and communicable diseases (Omokhodion & Omokhodion, 2004).

Safety of Healthcare Providers

Nurses have one of the highest job-related injury rates of any occupation worldwide. The injury rate is even greater than construction or agriculture jobs. In the United States as of 2000, there were 2.7 million registered nurses and 700,000 licensed practical/vocational nurses. Major safety hazards include biological and infectious risks, chemical risks, environmental and mechanical risks, physical risks, and psychological risks. Respiratory illnesses and other communicable diseases, such as severe acute respiratory syndrome (SARS) and TB are examples of some of the health risks that confront healthcare providers. Healthcare workers are also subjected to the risk of blood-borne infections such as hepatitis B, hepatitis C, and HIV. Disinfectants and cold sterilants used to disinfect instruments can cause reactive airway problems and skin problems. Chemotherapy agents also can cause problems for nurses who administer them. Latex gloves can produce allergies, causing dermatitis or even anaphylaxis. Lifting heavy patients or equipment can cause significant musculoskeletal injuries, especially in the lower back. Psychiatric patients can cause physical and psychological trauma as well (Foley, 2004).

In the United States needlestick injuries have decreased from one million exposures in 1996 to 385,000 in 2000. This decline has resulted from the formation of OSHA's blood-borne pathogens standard. Reasons for the success in decreasing needlesticks may be attributed to the elimination of needle recapping and the use of safer needle devices, sharps collection boxes, gloves and personal protective gear, and universal precautions. Increased risk for HIV from needlesticks can result from deep injury, visible blood on the device, high viral titer status of the patient (especially a newly infected patient), or a patient in the terminal state, and the device being used to access an artery or vein. The US surveillance for healthcare workers identified devices most responsible for needlestick injuries, which consist of the following:

- Hypodermic needles (32%)
- Suture needles (19%)
- Winged steel needles (butterflies) (12%)
- Scalpel blades (7%)
- IV and catheter needles (6%)
- Phlebotomy needles (3%)

The most common circumstances that cause injuries involve hollow bore needles, which can be filled with blood (Wilburn, 2004).

Job Stress

In the American workplace 25% of employees view their jobs as the number one stressor in their lives. Job stress can be defined as the harmful physical and emotional responses that happen when the requirements of the job do not match the capabilities or resources or needs of the worker, leading to poor health or injury (see Figure 12-3).

Job stress is not the same as job challenge, which often energizes workers. Possible causes of job stress include differences in the individual personality and coping styles as well as certain working conditions of the job itself. Certain jobs in particular may more likely lead to stress than other jobs. Factors that lead to stress on the job include:

- Heavy workloads
- Infrequent rest breaks
- Long working hours
- Shift work
- Routine tasks that have little inherent meaning
- Getting little or no participation in decision making
- Poor communication in the organization
- Insensitivity to family needs
- Conflicting or uncertain job expectations
- Too much responsibility
- Job insecurity
- Unpleasant or dangerous physical conditions such as crowding, noise, or air pollution

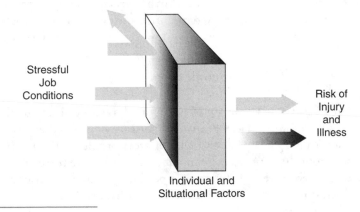

Stressful
Job
Conditions

Risk of
Injury
and
Illness

Individual and
Situational Factors

Figure 12-3 NIOSH model of job stress.

Source: NIOSH, 2004.

Healthcare expenses are 50% greater for workers who report high levels of job stress. An increase in job stress may result in an increase in risk for any or several of the following (NIOSH, 2004):

- Cardiovascular disease
- Musculoskeletal disorders
- Psychological disorders
- Workplace injuries
- Suicide
- Cancer
- Ulcers
- Impaired immune function

Some employers assume that stressful working conditions are expected and companies must constantly be increasing the pressure for workers in order to remain productive and profitable. However, stress in the workplace is often associated with greater absenteeism, tardiness, and job quitting. Low morale, health and job complaints, and employee turnover often are the first signs of job stress. Remedies for job stress include stress management and employee assistant programs to help employees cope with difficult work, personal stressors, and organizational change. Employers need to work with the employers to solve the problem early before it becomes too large, causing greater damage to workers or the company (NIOSH, 2004).

Reproductive Health

Job stress and workplace hazards can cause problems with reproductive health in employees. Reproductive disorders can include birth defects, developmental disorders, spontaneous abortion, low birth weight, preterm birth, and congenital anomalies. Other disorders include reduced fertility, infertility, impotence, and menstrual disorders (NIOSH, 2005c).

Occupational Lung Disease

Occupational lung disease is the most common work-related illness in the United States. Lung diseases at the workplace are usually caused by extended exposure to irritating toxic substances causing acute or chronic respiratory problems. Even a severe single exposure can cause chronic lung problems. Smoking can exacerbate the problems. In the United States in 2002, there were 294,500 newly reported cases of occupational illness in private industry, including 22,000 new respiratory conditions. Workers had a 2.5 per 10,000 rate of developing nonfatal respiratory conditions. These diseases are preventable but often not curable. Prevention measures include improving ventilation, wearing protective equipment, changing work procedures, and educating workers about prevention. Common work-related lung diseases worldwide include the following (American Lung Association, 2005):

- Occupational lung cancer—20–30% of males and 5–20% of females may have been exposed during their working years to agents that cause lung cancer.

- Occupational asthma—This is the most common form of occupational lung disease. In the United States 15–23% of new adult asthma cases are caused by occupational exposures. Exposures in the workplace can also exacerbate preexisting asthma.

- Asbestosis—This is a progressive disease that causes scarring on lung tissue due to exposure to asbestos. In the United States 1.3 million employees in construction and industry have had exposures on the job, and in 2002 there were 6343 deaths from asbestosis.

- Black lung disease (pneumoconiosis)—A chronic occupational lung disease contracted by the prolonged breathing of coal mine dust caused by the silica and carbon in the coal dust. About one of every 20 miners studied in the United States has X-ray evidence of black lung disease, and for some miners, the disease becomes more severe, called progressive massive fibrosis. Black lung disease is not reversible, and there is no specific treatment,

- Brown lung disease (byssinosis)—This is a chronic obstruction of the small airways in the lungs, causing impaired lung function. This is caused by dust from hemp, flax, and cotton processing. In the United States greater than 30,000 textile workers were affected by this problem.

- Silicosis—This is a disease resulting from exposure to free crystalline silica in mines, blasting operations, and in stone, clay, and glass manufacturing, which causes scar tissue in the lungs and increases the risk of TB.

- Hypersensitivity pneumonitis—This is caused by exposure to fungus spores from moldy hay, bird droppings, or other organic dust, causing the lung sacs to be inflamed, causing scar tissue, and decreased lung functioning.

Occupational Cancer

In Asian countries such as China and India, there is a continuous use of asbestos though there is substantial evidence of a link, even at low level exposure, to the development of pulmonary fibrosis and lung cancer in humans. This is due to poor occupational health and safety systems. The International Labour Organisation (ILO) reports that greater than 100,000 deaths a year occur from asbestos-related disease. The number of cases are expected to increase and then peak at about 2020, with about 1 million deaths occurring in this time period. Other studies have reported that there continues to be sufficient evidence to infer a causal relationship between particulate air pollution and respiratory deaths in infants up to one month of age (Joshi & Gupta, 2005; Radim, Binkova, Dejmek, & Bobak, 2005).

In Canada, fetal exposure to chemical agents via maternal exposure at work has shown to have a direct effect on the production of acute lymphoblastic leukemia in children. Exposures of industrial solvents (alkalines and mononuclear aromatic hydrocarbons) ranged from 2 years prior to pregnancy up to the time of birth (Infante-Rivard, Siemiatycki, Lakhani, & Nadon, 2005). In the United States about 20,000 cancer deaths and 40,000 new cases occur each year due to occupational exposures. When a known or suspected cancer-causing agent is present and types of cancer have been linked with exposure, especially for a group of people working in the same place, it is possible that the particular job or workplace may have carcinogens. The time of exposure to the carcinogens to the time of diagnosis of cancer may vary. Diagnosis of cancer may occur anytime from less than 1 year up to 15–20 years after exposure (NIOSH, 2005a).

Highway Work Zones

Globally, highway workers continue to be at high risk for injuries. Workers in highway construction work zones are exposed to the risk for injury from construction vehicles, vehicles and equipment within the work zones, and also from passing motor vehicles. Highway workers often work in conditions where there is low lighting, low visibility, inclement weather, and congested areas with exposure to high traffic. Within the United States from 1980 to 1995 at least 17,000 construction workers died from injuries on the job (NIOSH, 2005e).

Here are some tips drivers should follow to reduce injuries in highway work zones (US Federal Highway Administration, 2000):

- Dedicate full attention to the roadway.
- Disengage from distracting activities, such as changing radio stations and using mobile phones.
- Pay close attention to merge signs, flaggers, and do not change lanes within the work zone.
- Watch out—not only for workers in the zone, but also their equipment.
- Turn on vehicle headlights to become more conspicuous to workers and other motorists.

Agricultural Safety

Agriculture is among the world's most hazardous industries. Farmers are at high risk for fatal and nonfatal injuries. Leading causes of agricultural machinery injuries include entanglements, being pinned or stuck by machinery, falls, and runovers. Nonmachinery injuries include falls from heights, animal-related trauma, and being stuck against objects. Frequent injuries include limb fractures, open wounds, intracranial (head) injuries, and spinal cord injuries, as reported in a Canadian study of hospitalized farm injuries (Pickett et al., 2001). Workers in agriculture have double the mortality rates because of inadequate training and safety systems. In the US, agriculture workers make up only 3% of the workforce, but account for almost 8% of all work-related accidents. In Italy 9% of the workforce are farm workers, but they account for 28.9% of work-related injuries. The greatest dangers are with cutting tools and machinery such as tractors and harvesters, and exposure to pesticides and other chemicals (International Labour Organisation, 1997).

There were approximately 1,859,000 full-time workers in agriculture in the United States in 2003. In addition approximately 1.08 million children and adolescents under 20 years of age resided on the farms, and 593,000 were performing work on the farm. About 103 children are killed annually on farms, and 40% of these deaths are work related. In 2001, 22,600 children were injured on farms and 8400 were caused by farm work. Each year 110 farm workers are crushed to death by tractor rollovers. Every day about 228 farm workers have work-related injuries, and 5% of these injuries are permanent. In 1990, the US Congress developed extensive agricultural safety and health programs to address the high risk for injuries and preventable deaths. These programs conduct research and make recommendations for prevention of injuries and death from pesticide exposure, lung disease, musculoskeletal disorders, hearing loss, and stress (Frank, McKnight, Kirkhorn, & Gunderson, 2004).

References

A new vision for human security. (2003). *Lancet, 361*(9370), 1665.

American Lung Association. (2005). *Occupational lung disease fact sheet*. Retrieved October 24, 2005, from http://www.lungusa.org/site/pp.as[?c=dv:IL9O0E&b=35334

Bent-Goodley, T. (2004). Perceptions of domestic violence: A dialogue with African American women. *Health and Social Work, 29*(4), 307–316.

Brener, N., Lowry, R., & Barrios, L. (2005). Violence-related behaviors among high school students—United States, 1991-2003. *Journal of School Health, 75*(3), 81–85.

Bureau of Statistics. (2004). *Occupational safety and health definitions*. Retrieved October 24, 2005, from http://www.bls.gov/iif/oshdef.htm

Centers for Disease Control and Prevention (CDC). (2004a). *Preventing motor vehicle accidents*. Retrieved June 21, 2005, from http://www.cdc.gov/program

CDC. (2004b). *Preventing alcohol-related injuries*. Retrieved June 21, 2005, from http://www.cdc.gov/program

Ezechi, O. C., Kalu, B., Ezechi, L. O., Nwokoro, C., Ndububa, V., & Okeke, G. C. E. (2004). Prevalence and pattern of domestic violence against pregnant Nigerian women. *Journal of Obstetrics and Gynecology, 24*(6), 652–656.

Flinck, A., Paavilainen, E., & Astedt-Kurki, P. (2005). Survival of intimate partner violence as experienced by women. *Journal of Clinical Nursing, 14*, 383–393.

Foley, M. (2004). Caring for those who care: A tribute to nurses and their safety. *Online Journal of Issues in Nursing, 9*(3), 91–101.

Frank, A., McKnight, R., Kirkhorn, S., & Gunderson, P. (2004). Issues of agricultural safety and health. *Annual Review of Public Health, 25*, 225–245.

Gostin, L,, Sapssin, J., Teret, S., Burris, S., Mair, J., Hodge, J., et al. (2002). The model state emergency health powers act. Planning for and response to bioterrorism and naturally occurring infectious diseases. *Journal of the American Medical Association, 288*(5), 622–628.

Guerro, R. (2002). Violence is a health issue. *Bulletin of the World Health Organization, 80*(10), 767.

Hijar, M., Vazquez-Vela, E., and Arreola-Risa, C. (2002). Pedestrian traffic injuries in Mexico: A country update. *Injury Control and Safety Promotion, 10*(1–2), 37–43.

Hindin, M. (2003). Understanding women's attitudes towards wife beating in Zimbabwe. *Bulletin of the World Health Organization, 81*(7), 501–508.

Hofman, K., Primack, A., Keusch, G., & Hrynkow, S.(2005). Addressing the growing burden of trauma and injury in low- and middle-income countries. *American Journal of Public Health, 95*(1), 13–17.

Hyder, A. (2004). Road safety is no accident: a call for global action. *Bulletin of the World Health Organization, 82*(4), 240–240A.

International Labour Organisation. (1997). *ILO warns on farm safety.* Retrieved June 25, 2006, from http://ilo.org/public/English/bureau/inf/pr/1997/23.htm

Infante-Rivard, C., Siemiatycki, J., Lakhani, R., & Nadon, L. (2005). Maternal exposure to occupational solvents and childhood leukemia. *Environmental Health Perspectives, 113*(6), 787–792.

Joshi, T., & Gupta, R. (2005). Asbestos in developing countries: Magnitude of risk and its practical implications. *Human and Ecological Risk Assessment, 11*, 239–247.

Kalichman, S. C., and Simbayi, L. C. (2004). Sexual assault history and risks for sexually transmitted infection among women in an African township in Cape Town, South Africa. *AIDS Care, 16*(6), 681–689.

Khosla, A., Dua, D., Devi, L., & Sud, S. (2005). Domestic violence in pregnancy in North Indian women. *Indian Journal of Medical Science, 59*(5), 195–199.

Kielkowski, D., Rees, D., & Bradshaw, D. (2004). Burden of occupational morbidity in South Africa: Two large field surveys of self-reported work-related and work-aggravated disease. *South African Journal of Science, 100*, 399–402.

Koenig, M., Lutalo, T., Zhao, F., Nalugoda, F., Wab-Wire-Mangen, F., Kiwanuka, N., et al. (2003). Domestic violence in rural Uganda: Evidence from a community-based study. *Bulletin of the World Health Organization, 81*, 53–60.

Krugberg, E., Mercy, J., Dahlberg, L., & Zwi, A. (2002). The world report on violence and health. *Lancet, 360*, 1083–1088.

Lee, J. (2003). Science and the health of the poor. *Bulletin of the World Health Organization, 81*(7), 473.

Leppaniemi, A. K. (2004). Global trends in trauma. *Trauma, 6*, 193–203.

Loewenberg, S. (2005). Domestic violence in Spain. *Lancet, 365*, 464.

Loewenson, R. (2001). Globalization and occupational health: A perspective from southern Africa. *Bulletin of the World Health Organization, 79*(9), 863–868.

Maclean, R. (2004). Partner violence elevates the risk of HIV infection for South African women. *International Family Planning Perspectives, 30*, 148–149.

Mercy, J., Krugberg, E. G., Dahlberg, L., & Zwi, A. (2003). Violence and health: The United States in a global perspective. *American Journal of Public Health, 92*(12), 256–261.

Mock, C., Joshipura, M., & Goosen, J. (2004). Global strengthening of care for the injured. *Bulletin of the World Health Organization, 82*(4), 241.

Mock, C., Quansah, R., Krishnan, R., Arreola-Risa, C., & Rivara, F. (2004). Strengthening the prevention and care of injuries worldwide. *Lancet, 363*, 2172–2179.

National Center for Injury Prevention and Control. (2002). *Poisonings: Fact Sheet.* Retrieved June 5, 2005, from http://www.cdc.gov/ncipc/factsheets/poisoning.htm

National Center for Injury Prevention and Control. (2003). *Fires deaths and injuries: Fact sheet.* Retrieved June 5, 2005, from http://www.cdc.gov/ncipc/factsheets/fire.htm

National Center for Injury Prevention and Control. (2004a). *Intimate partner violence: Fact sheet.* Retrieved June 5, 2005, from http://www.cdc.gov/ncipc/factsheets/ipvfacts.htm

National Center for Injury Prevention and Control. (2004b). *Older adult drivers: Fact sheet.* Retrieved June 5, 2004, from http://www.cdc.gov/ncipc/factsheets/older.htm

National Center for Injury Prevention and Control. (2004c). *Teen drivers: Fact sheet.* Retrieved June 5. 2004, from http://www.cdc.gov/ncipc/factsheets/teenmvh.htm

National Center for Injury Prevention and Control. (2005a). *Sexual violence: Fact sheet.* Retrieved June 5, 2005, from http://www.cdc.gov/ncipc/factsheets/svfacts.htm

National Center for Injury Prevention and Control .(2005b). *Child maltreatment: Fact sheet.* Retrieved June 5, 2005, from http://www.cdc.gov/ncipc/factsheets/cmfacts.htm

National Institute for Occupational Safety and Health (NIOSH). (2003). *Traumatic occupational injuries.* Retrieved July 9, 2005, from http://www/cdc.gov/niosh/ injury/traumaviolence.html

NIOSH. (2004). *Stress at work.* Retrieved July 9, 2005, from http://www.cdc.gov/niosh/stresswk.html

NIOSH. (2005a). *Occupational cancer.* Retrieved October 24, 2005, from http://www.cdc.gov/niosh/topics/cancer

NIOSH. (2005b). *Occupational. Health care workers.* Retrieved October 24, 2005, from http://www.cdc.gov/niosh/topics/healthcare

NIOSH. (2005c).*Reproductive health.* Retrieved October 24, 2005, from http://www.cdc.gov/niosh/topics/repro

NIOSH. (2005d). *Occupational. Traumatic occupational injuries.* Retrieved October 24, 2005, from http://www.cdc.gov/niosh/injury

NIOSH. (2005e). *Occupational. Highway work zones.* Retrieved October 24, 2005, from http://www.cdc.gov/niosh/injury/traumazone.html

Nuwayhid, I. (2004). Occupational health research in developing countries. A partner for social justice. *American Journal of Public Health, 94*(11), 1916–1921.

Occupational Safety and Health Administration (OSHA). (2002). *OSHA fact sheet.* Retrieved October 1, 2005, from http://www.osha.gov

Occupational Safety and Health Administration. (2005). *OSHA's mission.* Retrieved 6/15/2005, from http://www.osha-slc.gov/oshinfo/mission.html

Omokhodion, F., & Omokhodion, S. (2004). Health status of working and nonworking school children in Ibadan, Nigeria. *Annals of Tropical Paediatrics, 24,* 175–178.

Peden, M., & McGee, K. (2003). The epidemiology of drowning worldwide. *Injury Control and Safety Promotion, 10*(4), 195–199.

Pickett, W., Hartling, L., Dimich-Ward, H., Guernsey, J. R., Hagel, L., Voaklander, D. C., et al. (2001). Surveillance of hospitalized farm injuries in Canada. *Injury Prevention, 7,* 123–128.

Radim, R., Binkova, B., Dejmek, J., & Bobak, M. (2005). Ambient air pollution and pregnancy outcomes: A review of the literature. *Environmental Health Perspectives, 113*(4), 375–382.

Reijneveld, S., Brugman, E., Sing, R., & Verloove-Vanhorick, S. (2004). Infant crying and abuse. *Lancet, 364,* 1340–1342.

Silcock, D. (2003). Preventing death and injury on the world's roads. *Transport Reviews, 23*(3), 263–273.

United Nations (UN). (2005). *Global campaign for violence prevention.* New York: UN.

US Federal Highway Administration. (2000). *National work zone safety awareness.* Retrieved August 8, 2007, from http://safety.fhwa.dot.gov/wz/index.htm

Vehicular manslaughter: The global epidemic of traffic deaths. (2004). *Environmental Health Perspectives, 112*(11), 629–631.

Waldman, R. (2005). Public health in war. *Harvard International Review, Spring,* 2005. 1283–1284.

Watts, C., & Mayhew, S. (2004). Reproductive health services and intimate partner violence: Shaping a pragmatic response in sub-Saharan Africa. *International Family Planning, 30*(4), 207–213.

World Health Organization (WHO). (2001). *Injuries and violence prevention. Facts about drowning.* Retrieved August 8, 2007, from http://www.who.int/entity/violence_injury_prevention/ publications/other_injury/en/drowning_factsheet.pdf

WHO. (2002). *Global burden of disease estimates—2002 rev.* Retrieved August 8, 2007, from http://www.who.int/healthinfo/bodestimates/en/index.html

WHO. (2003). *Injuries and violence prevention. Facts about burns.* Retrieved August 8, 2007, from http://www.who.int/entity/violence_injury_prevention/publications/other_injury/en/ burns_factsheet.pdf

WHO. (2004). *Road safety: A public health issue.* Retrieved June 15, 2005, from http://www.who.int/ features/2004/road_safety/en

WHO. (2005). *The injury chartbook: A graphical overview of the global burden of injuries.* Retrieved June 15, 2005, from http://www.who.int/violence_injury_prevention/publications/other_injury/ chartb/en

Wilburn, S. (2004). Needlestick and sharps injury prevention. *Online Journal of Issues of Nursing, 9*(3). Retrieved October 1, 2005, from http://web16.epnet.com/citation.asp?tb=1&_ug=sid+5/ co5B185%2D3FD4%2D4CIA%2D

Xu, X., Zhu, F., O'Campo, P., Koenig, M., Mock, V., & Campbell, J. (2005). Prevalence and risk factors of intimate partner violence in China. *American Journal of Public Health, 95*(1), 78–85.

Zhang, J., Norton, R., Tang, K. C., Lo, S., Zhuo, J., & Wenkui, G. (2004). Motorcycle ownership and injury in China. *Injury Control and Safety Promotion, 11*(3), 159–163.

Chapter 13

Global Perspectives on Nutrition

Carol Holtz, Kathy Plitnick, and Marvin Friedman

Introduction

Good nutrition is the basis for health and infant and children's growth and development. In addition, it is correlated to a more effective immune system and reduction of the number of diseases. Traditionally the World Health Organization's (WHO) goal was focused around the issue of malnutrition caused by nutritional deficiencies, particularly with regard to malnutrition induced by disease. Now included in the agenda for both developing and developed countries is the improvement of global nutrition related to malnutrition also caused by overnutrition and obesity. Worldwide, obesity and malnutrition are leading causes of such chronic diseases as cardiovascular disease, cancer, and diabetes. Deficiency diseases include scurvy (vitamin C deficiency), blindness, vitamin A deficiency, kwashiorkor (protein deficiency), goiter (iodine deficiency), pellagra (niacin deficiency), anemia (iron or folic acid deficiency), and many more. Significant morbidity, mortality, and economic costs are associated with nutritional imbalances (WHO, 2006a).

Malnutrition is considered to be the world's leading threat to life and health today. It is difficult to imagine living on less than US$1 per day yet 1.2 billion people in the world live on this amount. With this limited amount of income it is very difficult to maintain a healthy and adequate diet. Every day 24,000 people worldwide die from hunger and malnutrition, the majority of whom are young children. Nearly 33% of the world suffers from micronutrient malnutrition, which results in the following:

- Decreased mental and physical development
- Poor pregnancy outcomes
- Decreased work capacity for adults
- Increased illness
- Premature death
- Diseases
- Deficiencies in zinc, leading to immune deficiency, growth retardation, and diarrhea

- Bone loss
- Blindness

Not only are there problems from lack of quantity and quality of food, but there are also worldwide issues with overnutrition (obesity) as well. Two thirds of all people from developing nations are either overweight or obese, and increasing numbers of individuals from emerging or transition economy nations are also having similar health challenges. Overweight and obesity from both developed and developing nations are creating chronic health problems and costing hundreds of millions of dollars (CDC, 2003; WHO, 2006a). This is an even more extreme problem amongst individuals migrating from global areas, where food is not available, to developed countries where overeating is easy. WHO estimates that malnutrition is a contributing factor in at least 49% of the death burden of the world. Half of all malnourished children and a large proportion of malnourished adult women are in Bangladesh, India, and Pakistan, and in many other countries in Africa and middle Asia (Underwood, 2002).

The WHO's Nutrition for Health Development Department established major goals at the World Summit for Children in 1990 and the International Conference on Nutrition in 1992, which with some modification in 2003, are current and still relevant for 2006. They include the *elimination* of the following:

- Famine and related deaths
- Starvation and nutritional deficiency diseases caused by natural and man-made disasters
- Iodine and vitamin A deficiency

and *reduction* of the following:

- Starvation and widespread hunger
- Undernutrition especially in women, children, and the aged
- Other micronutrient deficiencies such as iron
- Diet-related communicable and noncommunicable diseases
- Barriers to breast-feeding
- Poor sanitation, hygiene, and unclean drinking water

Strategies for implementing these goals include (WHO, 2006a):

- Developing new nutritional health policies and programs
- Improving household food security
- Improving food quality and safety
- Preventing and treating infectious diseases

- Promoting breast-feeding
- Promoting diets with micronutrient supplements
- Assessing and monitoring nutritional programs

By the year 2015 worldwide nutritional issues will be mainly problems with food distribution, access, and availability. Some of the key future trends are the following (CDC, 2003):

- There will be a 20% increase in malnutrition in sub-Saharan Africa.
- The total number of people who are hungry worldwide increased in the 1990s (except for China), and will continue to grow.
- Iron deficiency and anemia will affect 3.5 billion people in the developing world.
- Food donations will decrease by one third.
- Famine will continue due to repressive governments, internal conflicts, or natural disasters.

Stunting and underweight problems are due to persistent undernutrition. In 2002 there were 180 million stunted children and 150 million underweight children. Ninety million of the underweight children live in Asia. During the past two decades progress has been made in Asia, yet not in sub-Saharan Africa (Merck Manual, 2002).

Types of Nutritional Challenges

Micronutrient Deficiencies

Micronutrient deficiencies include iron, iodine, and vitamin A as well as zinc, folate, and other B vitamins. In many settings more than one micronutrient deficiency exists, which necessitates interventions that address multiple micronutrient deficiencies. Areas of prevalence are especially greatest in Southeast Asia and sub-Saharan Africa. These deficiencies are mainly caused by inadequate food intake, poor quality of foods, poor bioavailability because of inhibitors, types of preparation, and presence of infections, especially as a result of poor water quality (Ramakrishnan, 2002).

Iron Deficiency Anemia

Iron deficiency is the most widespread nutrient deficiency in the world affecting greater than 2 billion people. It is best known in causing anemia, a condition in which there is an inadequate amount of red blood cells. Although iron deficiency is the main cause of anemia, other causes may be related to nutrient deficiencies such as vitamin B_{12} and folic acid, as well as nonnutritional causes such as malaria, genetic abnormalities (thalassemia), and chronic disease. Iron deficiency develops over time. Populations especially vulnerable to iron deficiency anemia are young children and women of child-bearing age. It is diagnosed as low hemoglobin or hematocrit levels. When there are decreased numbers of red blood cells, which normally carry oxygen throughout the body, the person then has a decreased oxygen level and has symptoms of weakness and fatigue. This problem has profound effects on infants and children by limiting learning capacity and impairing the immune system. Within the region of Southeast Asia, millions of people are affected by this problem, mainly adolescent girls, and childbearing age women (due to menstruation) and young children. Pregnant women with iron deficiency anemia are more likely to die in childbirth, as a result of postpartal hemorrhage, or have their fetus or newborn die as a result of decreased oxygen levels in the tissues. Research indicates that children who have this problem have a 5–7 point reduction in IQ score (Gleason, 2002). The main contributing factors include inadequate intake of iron, poor iron availability from cereal-based diets, and high intestinal worm infections. According to the WHO, iron deficiency anemia is second only to tuberculosis as the world's most prevalent and costly health problem. In India and parts of Africa greater than 80% of the population has this condition (Ramakrishnan, 2002; Ulrich, 2005; WHO, 2004).

The presence of overweight among children and adolescents has been increasing at a rapid rate in the United States and throughout the world. In the United States greater than 1 in 7 children is overweight. Results from a Centers for Disease Control and Prevention (CDC) research study of 9698 US children (2–16 years of age), conducted from 1988 to 1994, demonstrated that iron deficiency anemia has been linked to overweight and obesity in children. Results concluded that children and adolescents who were overweight or at risk for overweight were almost twice as likely to be iron deficient than normal weight children (Nead, Halterman, Kaczorowski, Auinger, & Weitzman, 2004). It is important to recognize that body weight alone is not a good index of nutritional status, as water retention from poor kidney function can result in misleading body weights.

The 2000 Global Burden of Disease Project, a study funded by the WHO and the World Bank, ranked iron deficiency ninth among the risk factors that contribute to human death and disability. This deficiency affects about one fifth of the world's population, or 1.4 billion people. In the United States since the 1940s it has been common to find iron-fortified foods, most notably bread (WHO, 2004).

Adding micronutrients to such products as table salt has been practiced for many years to replenish deficient levels of iodine, but a form of table salt with iron fortification has been manufactured to help combat iron-related anemia. Researchers working in North Africa have demonstrated that iron added to salt causes the color to change to a yellow brown, and may also sometimes have a rusty taste. Working in northern Morocco, researchers gave this new product to 75 children for 10 months. Results indicate that the children receiving the fortified salt had a reduction in anemia rates from 5–30% (Harder, 2004).

Iron is found primarily in meats, with liver being the best source of iron.

Niacin Deficiency (Pellagra)

Pellagra, also known as "black tongue," is found amongst populations that consume corn as the main staple of their diet, often seen in Mexico, Northern Italy, and South America. Because corn is deficient in the amino acid tryptophan, and since tryptophan is required for biosynthesis of niacin, these populations are particularly sensitive. Signs of niacin deficiency include photosensitivity, red skin lesions, dementia, and can lead to mortality. This condition is easily treated with niacin supplements. Genetically engineered maize is available that has a high tryptophan content and does not cause pellagra. A Nobel Prize was awarded for this development.

Folic Acid Deficiency

Folic acid is readily available from green leafy vegetables. Many diets are marginally deficient in these components. Folic acid is necessary for nucleic acid (i.e., DNA and RNA synthesis). A population marginally deficient in folic acid will appear normal at first glance. However, this deficiency results in birth defects, particularly cleft lip and palate and spina bifida. Because most populations are marginally deficient in this vitamin, it is logical that folic acid supplements should be taken during pregnancy. This may be a problem as most developmental anomalies are induced in the first 3 months of pregnancy, and for at least half of that time, most women do not know they are pregnant.

Vitamin A Deficiency

Vitamin A deficiency occurs when inadequate storage of vitamin A exits, which is caused by either inadequate intake of food rich in vitamin A or severe and repeated illnesses have taken place. Approximately 2 billion people in the world are at risk for vitamin A deficiency, along with iodine or iron deficiencies. The problem is especially high in Southeast Asia and sub-Saharan Africa. Pregnant women and young children are at greatest risk. In many of these areas more than one micronutrient deficiency exists, and therefore interventions must approach multiple micronutrient deficiencies. Severe vitamin A deficiency is usually exhibited by signs of night blindness and decreased levels of vitamin A (@ 0.35/dL). Serum retinol is the biochemical indicator of vitamin A status (Ramaskrishnan, 2002). Vitamin A is available from raw colored foods such as carrots or tomatoes.

Vitamin D Deficiency

This nutritional deficiency is unique amongst vitamin deficiencies. Vitamin D is required for the absorption of calcium and translocation to bones and teeth. Vitamin D deficiency in children results in rickets, which is failure of the long bones to mature. In adults it causes osteoporosis (fragile bones), and osteomalacia (bone thinning). Chronic vitamin D deficiency eventually also causes dermal lesions. What makes this vitamin unique is that the body easily produces a large amount of vitamin D from the reaction of sunlight and sterol (a cholesterol derivative). In the absence of sunlight the body cannot get enough vitamin D from diet. This disease was first seen amongst nuns in Europe who were always completely covered by their habits and generally worked inside. Now, vitamin D is added to milk, which is the major source of dietary calcium.

Iodine Deficiency Disorder

Iodine deficiency is the leading cause of preventable brain damage in childhood. Iodine deficiency is found in populations with no access to salt water fish (as sea water is high in iodine) or as a result of consuming vegetables such as broccoli that binds with iodine and makes iodine unavailable for absorption. During the last decade worldwide improvement has been related to low-cost prevention measures such as the iodization of salt. Under normal conditions the body has small amounts of iodine, housed mainly in the thyroid gland, utilized for the synthesis of thyroid hormones. Iodine deficiency causes hypothyroidism, (goiter) which can cause a syndrome called iodine deficiency disorders. In developed countries, iodine intake correlates with obesity and basal metabolic rate as the hormone requiring iodine, thyroxin, regulates basal metabolism rate. Symptoms are listed in Table 13-1.

TABLE 13-1   **Iodine Deficiency Disorders at Various Stages of Development**

Developmental Stage	Disorders
Fetus	Abortion
	Stillbirth
	Congenital abnormalities
	Increased perinatal mortality
Neonate	Neonatal goiter
	Neonatal hypothyroidism
	Mental retardation
Child and adolescent	Goiter
	Hypothyroidism
	Decreased mental function
	Impaired physical development
Adult	Goiter and complications
	Hypothyroidism
	Impaired mental function
	Spontaneous hyperthyroidism in the elderly
	Iodine-induced hyperthyroidism

Source: Adapted from Andersson, Takkouche, Egli, & de Benoist, 2003.

Data on urinary iodine and goiter are monitored at the WHO's Global Database on Iodine Deficiency Disorders. Disorders are deficiencies resulting from decreased intake of the element iodine, which is essential in minute amounts for normal growth and development. It is necessary that the iodine content be monitored during manufacturing to ensure that the prescribed levels are maintained. Thyroid failure causing irreversible brain damage can occur if the iodine deficiency occurs from fetal life up to 3 months of age. Iodine deficiency causes a decreased mean IQ loss of 13.5 points in children. During the past century, iodine fortification has been implemented into foods such as bread, milk, water, and salt. Salt has been the most common product because it is widely used and available. The WHO recommends 20–40 mg of iodine per kg of salt to meet daily iodine requirements, assuming that the average consumption is 10 g per day. Iodine fortification is safe, but excessive intake may produce hyperthyroidism (Andersson, Takkouche, Egli, & de Benoist, 2003).

In Southeast Asia 172 million people have goiter, and 599 million people are at risk. Problems caused by iodine deficiency include goiter, psychomotor defects, impaired mental function, and slow cognitive development. The universal iodization of salt has been very successful in bringing the prevalence down in many countries (Center for Global Development, 2006; WHO, 2003).

Nuclear events, such as occurred in Chernobyl, cause the production of I^{131}, the radioactive form of iodine. Consumption of this isotope results in thyroid cancer. Similarly, irradiation of the head and neck, as was common in acne therapy in the 1950s, also caused conversion of iodine to I^{131} and a consequent epidemic of thyroid cancer.

Protein–Energy Malnutrition

Protein–energy malnutrition (kwashiorkor) is a global health problem and is potentially fatal, causing death in children, mainly in developing countries where there is unsafe water, reductions in macronutrients, and deficiencies in many micronutrients. Kwashiorkor is an example of various levels of inadequate protein and/or energy intake. Although it mainly occurs in infants and children, it can be found in persons of any age in the lifecycle. In the United States secondary protein–energy malnutrition is seen in elderly people who live in nursing homes and in children in poverty. Protein–energy malnutrition may result from AIDS, cancer, kidney failure, inflammatory bowel disease, and other disorders. It usually appears in people who have chronic disease or chronic semi-starvation, and has three forms:

- Dry (thin, desiccated)—*Marasmus* results from near starvation with a deficiency of protein and calories. The marasmic child consumes little food, usually because the mother is unable to breast-feed, and appears very thin as a result of loss of body muscle and fat. This is the predominant form in most developing countries. It occurs when energy intake is insufficient for the body's requirements and the body uses up its own reserves. Marasmic infants have hunger, weight loss, growth retardation, and wasting of fat and muscle. The chronic phase of this disease is made acute when an incident of diarrhea takes place. This diarrhea usually takes on fatal consequences.

- Wet (edematous, swollen)—*Kwashiorkor* is an African word meaning first child–second child. This refers to the fact that the first child develops protein–energy malnutrition when the second child is born and replaces the first child at the breast. The weaned child is fed a thin gruel of poor nutritional quality and has organic failure to thrive. Edema results because the protein deficiency is greater than the energy deficiency. Increased carbohydrate intake is accompanied with decreased protein intake. A decrease in albumin causes the edema. Those affected get thinning and discoloration of the hair and have an increased vulnerability to infections. The body weight increases due to edema.

- Combined form (between the two extremes)—Called *marasmic kwashiorkor,* children have some edema and more body fat than marasmus.

Treatment of either of these two conditions includes the following:

- Correcting fluid and electrolyte imbalances
- Treating infections (causing diarrhea) with antibiotics
- Supplying macronutrients (primarily milk-based formulas) by diet therapy

Mortality is anywhere from 5–49% (Merck Manual, 2002).

Obesity

The WHO estimates that within the next few years, noncommunicable diseases may become the main cause of mortality and morbidity worldwide. Elimination of childhood fatality, particularly as a result of poor water quality, is key to this estimate. The world population has shifted towards highly refined foods of animal origin and towards meat and dairy products containing high levels of saturated fats. With reduced energy expenditure and more available food stuffs as a result of better food preservation, there has been a rise in obesity and noncommunicable diseases. The prevalence of obesity is growing worldwide, not only in most developed countries, but also in developing countries, mainly from the influx of modern technology and economic growth. These factors provide more inactivity and greater availability of food. Despite the use of diets and exercise plans for combating obesity, this problem continues to increase. One third of the world's population age 15 or older is overweight or obese.

Overweight and obesity are ranges of weight greater than what is considered healthy for a specific height. In addition, the conditions identify specific likelihoods of chronic diseases and health problems. Overweight is a body mass index (BMI) of 25–29.9 and obese is 30 and above. The BMI correlates the amount of body fat with height, but does not directly measure body fat. Other modes of measurement of body fat include skinfold thickness and waist circumference, calculation of waist-to-hip circumference ratios, and other diagnostic measurements such as ultrasound, computed tomography (CT), and magnetic resonance imaging (MRI). For children and adolescents, the BMI ranges are defined taking into account normal male and female variations of body fat for specific ages (CDC, 2006b).

US government surveys show that the average adult man age 20–74 weighs 191 pounds, and the average adult woman of the same age weighs 164 pounds. Approximately three quarters of all Americans age 15 years and older were overweight or obese in 2005. The average US adult currently weighs 24 pounds more than an adult in the early 1960s. The United States is the world leader in percentage of the population who are obese. The US population consists of 60% who are overweight and 21% who are obese. China, with 19% of the total population being overweight or obese, leads the world in numbers of people. In China the urbanization process has been linked to changes in diet, increase in television in homes, and reduced physical activity. The majority of the population is thin, but there are millions who are overweight, though generally not obese (Chopra, Galbraith, & Darnton-Hill, 2002; Johnson, 2006).

The function of fat is to provide a cushion, insulation, and energy storage, but excess fat causes numerous problems. When persons become obese, they are more likely to have problems such as the following:

- Diabetes
- Gall bladder disease
- Hypertension
- Dyslipidemia
- Breathlessness
- Apnea
- Heart disease
- Osteoarthritis
- Gout
- Increased risk for some cancers
- Reproductive hormone abnormalities
- Impaired fertility
- Low back pain
- Fetal defects

The BMI can be calculated as weight (kg) ÷ height (m)^2. A BMI ranging from 18.5 to 24.9 is a healthy weight range (USDA, 2005b).

Within the United States obesity problems contribute to 12% or $100 billion of US healthcare costs. The rate of obesity is rising at about 5% yearly (Marvin & Medd, 2005).

Obesity and overweight are chronic conditions that are caused from energy imbalance, created from eating too many calories and not getting enough physical activity. The body weight is the sum of genetic makeup, metabolism, behavior, environment, culture, and socioeconomic status. Genetics and environment may influence overweight and obesity, but personal choices of eating and physical activity can be modified. The United States has had changes in food options within grocery stores and restaurants. A large percentage of the packaged foods and fast foods are very high in salt, fat, sugar, and calories. In addition, portion size today is much larger compared to 20 years ago. Physical activity is beneficial for overall health. It helps to decrease the risk of colon cancer, diabetes, and hypertension; helps in weight control; contributes to healthy bones, muscles, and joints; reduces falls in the elderly; and helps relieve the pain of arthritis. It is particularly important to menopausal women to combat osteoporosis. Moderate activity of 30 minutes a day for five or more times a week will enhance overall fitness and help combat overweight and obesity (CDC, 2006b).

The economic cost of overweight and obesity in the United States and throughout the world is quite significant. Medical costs include preventive, diagnostic, and treatment services. In addition, decreased productivity, restricted activity, and absenteeism further increase costs. Loss of future income due to premature death is also a cost of overweight and obesity (CDC, 2006a).

Within developing nations there is also a growing trend towards overweight and obesity, especially among the high socioeconomic status individuals of the populations. Obesity is now increasing worldwide and is increasingly found in larger numbers within the lower socioeconomic status populations of developing countries as well (Monteiro, Moura, Conde, & Popkin, 2004).

Childhood obesity is also now considered a global epidemic problem even in developing nations. About 10% of the world's children, ages 5–17 years, are now considered overweight, and 2–3% of the same aged children are obese. This corresponds to 155 million overweight children and 30–45 million children who are obese, worldwide (Stettler, 2004).

Why are children becoming obese? One reason is that children who consume high-fat and carbohydrate-rich foods produce high levels of circulating insulin, enabling the body to store extra calories as fat. On the South Pacific island of Nauru, children as well as adults have access to cheap and easily accessible high-density, high-caloric foods and have become diabetes prone. In China, the one-child-per-family policy has produced millions of spoiled and overnourished children (little emperor's syndrome), leading to a rise in childhood obesity and also type 2 diabetes in children (Nash, 2003). Dramatic shifts in food consumption and physical activity patterns are occurring. In the last 10 years the traditional low-fat diet now seems to be more of a reflection of poverty than of concern for good nutrition and health (Monteiro, Moura, Conde, & Popkin, 2004).

Food Safety and Security

Food prevents illness and maintains normal growth and development. Food security may be defined as steady access to sufficient nutritious foods for an active healthy life. Those who have food security have access to clean, safe, and nutritious food at all times. They are able to acquire necessary foods without having to scavenge or steal. Food insecurity exits when there is a limited or uncertain availability of safe and nutritious food. Food may not be easily acquired in safe and socially acceptable ways. The long-term effects of food insecurity are ill health, reduction in physical and cognitive growth and development, disease vulnerability, and if untreated, eventually death (Hall & Brown, 2005).

Food insecurity in the United States occurred in 11.7% of married couple households in 2003, and was present in 32.3% of families with a female head of the household and no spouse. Today in the United States women are more likely to live in poverty than men, which greatly increases their risk of having food insecurity. In households with food insecurity often the first foods to be eliminated are fruits and vegetables, causing the family members to lack essential vitamins and minerals. This population is more likely to become overweight or obese from energy-dense foods that are often low in fruits and vegetables and contain more refined grain, sugars, and fats, which cost less per calorie. The women and children are ultimately at greater risk for chronic illnesses, including cancers and cardiovascular diseases (Olson, 2005). National survey data indicate that more than 50% of all Americans are overweight based on BMI, and 22% of adults are classified as obese. Surveys also indicate those people most likely to be overweight or obese have less formal education, lower family income, are African-American or Latino, and are female (Stallings, Wolman, & Goodner, 2001).

In addition to the previous concerns about food safety and security, food security now has a new meaning that may differ in comparison to previous years. Food now has also become a weapon of bioterrorism. Besides having concerns related to disease threats such as anthrax and smallpox, the world population now has major concerns relating to food and water supplies, which could be a source of intentional spread of illness. Toxic substances might be put into the food and water supply that could include radioactive particles, microorganisms (*E. coli* 0517:H7), salmonella, shigella, or botulism toxin (a very deadly substance) (Hall & Brown, 2005).

National policies and programs can promote food safety and improve the capacity for monitoring, assessing, and controlling food quality. Training is also needed for foodborne disease surveillance and control, as well as assessing for food contamination. Public education about food safety issues is essential. In the United States the food supply is considered reasonably safe, yet each year 76 million Americans get sick, 300,000 are hospitalized, and 5000 people die from food contamination. Contamination sources may be biological or chemical. The role of the US Food and Drug Administration (FDA) is to protect and inspect the food supply. The Department of Agriculture protects the meat supply as well as fish and unusual species, such as snakes, alligators, and ostriches as food stuffs. The CDC may investigate a disease outbreak or a cluster if it is not in the FDA or Department of Agriculture area of responsibility (CDC, 2003).

INFOSAN (International Food Safety Authorities Network) was developed by the WHO in cooperation with the Food and Agriculture Organization of the United Nations (FAO) to promote the exchange of food safety information and to improve collaboration among international food authorities. Its goal is preventing the international spread of contaminated food. The organization has 143 members representing most countries of the world (WHO, 2005a). One example of global concern is bird flu. This disease infects chickens in Southeast Asia as a result of failure to segregate these animals from wild birds. The chickens then enter commerce and may transmit the disease. While by 2006 there have been no unambiguously identified cases of this disease in humans caused by chickens, there is substantial evidence of this occurring.

Following natural disasters, food in affected areas may become contaminated and be at risk for outbreaks of food-borne diseases such as diarrhea, dysentery, cholera, and typhoid fever. Poor sanitation and lack of clean drinking water have caused massive food-borne diseases. Contaminated water may be considered as an unclean food and should be boiled or given additives (biocides) to be made safe before it is consumed or added to foods. Some examples of food and water issues after a major flood include the following (WHO, 2005b):

- Agriculture harvested from an area which has been flooded may be contaminated with microorganisms from raw sewage or microorganisms and chemicals in the flood water.

- Produce that was stored in the affected areas may be contaminated by flood waters.

- Foods that have not been contaminated need to be protected against sources of contamination.

- All foods distributed with mass feeding programs should be fit for human consumption and be nutritionally and culturally appropriate.

- Consumers need education in food preparation in more primitive conditions to promote food safety.

Nutrition and Poverty

The significance of poverty lies not only in low income. Perhaps more significant components of poverty include limited or no access to health services, safe water, literacy, and education. There is a two-way association between poverty and health. Poverty is one of the main factors related to poor health, and also poor health can lead to poverty. Poverty causes people to be exposed to environmental risks such as poor sanitation, unhealthy food, violence, and natural disasters. Those in poverty are less prepared to cope with their problems, making them at greater risk for illness and disability. Nutritional status depends on both food and nonfood factors. The nonfood factors include education and hygiene. As of 2002, 1.5 billion people of the world are exposed to poverty, particularly in the developing world. Those who live in extreme poverty are five times more likely to die before the age of 5 years, and two and half times more likely to die between the ages of 15 and 59 years than those in higher income levels (Pena & Bacallao, 2002).

Poverty affects nutrition throughout the life span, causing both infectious and noncommunicable diseases and a reduced learning capacity. Beginning in pregnancy the fetus, compromised with malnutrition, has slower intrauterine growth and as a result is small for gestation age. These children do not respond to environmental stresses as well as their larger counterparts. Lifetime challenges from malnutrition affect the normal cognitive, psychomotor, and affective behavior in children, and later as they become adults, they have less resistance to infection (a weaker immune system) throughout the life span. Pregnant teens in poverty are more likely to have malnutrition and again expose the fetus and newborn to even greater risks. Low height for age (stunting) is the most frequently seen manifestation of malnutrition worldwide. Greater than 30% of the world's children have stunting. Poor quality and quantity of milk during the first 2 years of life results in shorter and more disease-prone individuals. Adults in poverty often use their money to buy more high-energy (calories) foods of low nutritional quality, which may not resolve nutritional deficiencies in vitamins or protein, but contribute to overweight and obesity. Older adults affected by poverty often suffer a long history of poor nutrition and frequent illnesses (both infectious and noncommunicable). Many have to continue working to help with the adult children and grandchildren (Pena & Bacallao, 2002).

The most common scenario in developing countries is children, ages 2–5 getting bacterial infections from unsafe drinking water. This results in diarrhea which, without antibiotics, is virtually impossible to cure. The child goes into an electrolyte imbalance and a protein and calorie deficit. These children are not equipped with any reserve to fight this infection, and the consequences of this diarrhea are more often fatal. Antibiotic treatment along with oral rehydration therapy (ORT) early in the disease will save numerous lives on a global basis.

Nutrition Emergencies

The WHO assists with worldwide nutritional emergencies with numerous projects developed to provide assistance as needed. Some of their projects include the development of the following (WHO, 2006b):

- A manual that provides an explanation or how-to guide for managing nutritional needs of a community in an emergency, including the estimation of energy, protein, and nutrient requirements for a specific population
- A field guide to determine nutritional requirements, current nutritional status, and methods for prevention and treatment of protein–energy malnutrition and micronutrient deficiency diseases

- Specific guides for prevention and control of scurvy, pellagra, and thiamine deficiency
- Guides for feeding infants and young children
- Training modules for humanitarian aid workers
- Guides for caring for the nutritionally vulnerable people of a population
- Training modules for management of severe malnutrition

Burundi, a sub-Saharan African nation, has a significant problem with acute malnutrition in the general population, especially acute in children under 5 years. This is a consequence of the armed conflicts resulting in displacement of people, the inability of people to work their land, and the changes in weather patterns that has caused severe agricultural problems. To combat this situation, the International Medical Corp (IMC), an emergency nongovernmental organization (NGO), has implemented a comprehensive program for treatment and prevention of malnutrition in three Burundian provinces (Muyinga, Rutana, and Kirundo) since 1998. The program consists of three therapeutic feeding centers, one in each province, and 38 supplementary feeding centers, 12–14 in each province. The TFC centers provide inpatient, high-intensity treatment to the severely malnourished, and the supplementary feeding centers provide rations and treatment in an ambulatory (outpatient) center. UNICEF, USAID and other NGOs have partnered with the IMC to make a more dramatic impact in combating the acute malnutrition (Mach, n.d.).

Nutritional Support Programs

Programs to assist in improving nutritional health of developing nations are urgently needed to provide opportunities for health promotion by education, and diet changes reflecting specific local community cultural and health needs. In response to this need, the United States is presently supplying monetary funds via USAID to support nutritional programs. Recently, additional vitamins and minerals (food fortification) were added to common foods such as wheat flour, sugar, and cooking oil in Bangladesh, Central America, Eritrea, Ghana, Mali, Morocco, the Philippines, Uganda, Zambia, Bolivia, the Dominican Republic, Pakistan, and Uzbekistan. Increased vitamin A, for example, can reduce infant mortality by 30% (International Nutrition Foundation, n.d.; USAID, 2005).

GAIN (Global Alliance for Improved Nutrition) in September 2006 signed an agreement with UNICEF (United Nations International Children's Emergency Fund) to support flour fortification in Central and Eastern Europe in order to improve maternal, infant, and child health. GAIN is an organization created to fight vitamin and mineral deficiency. This type of malnutrition affects greater than 2 billion people globally, and produces major health problems such as limited cognitive, psychomotor function, blindness, and death (GAIN, 2006).

The International Micronutrient Malnutrition Prevention and Control Program (IMMpaCT) was established by the CDC in 2000 to eliminate vitamin and mineral deficiencies—the "hidden hunger." The CDC provides funding and technical assistance directly through cooperative agencies such as UNICEF, WHO, GAIN, USAID, and the Micronutrient Initiative (Geverding, 2006).

Within the United States the Women, Infants and Children (WIC) program was established in 1974 to safeguard low-income women, infants, and children up to age 5 who are at nutritional risk. This program provides nutritious foods to supplement diets, nutrition counseling, and healthcare referrals to low-income pregnant, breast-feeding, and nonbreast-feeding postpartum women, and to infants and children who are at nutritional risk. It is administered by the Food and Nutrition Service of the US Department of Agriculture. The majority of states provide vouchers that participants use at authorized food stores. Women who participate in the WIC program during their pregnancies have been shown to have fewer Medicaid costs, longer gestational periods, higher birth weights, and lower infant mortality for their babies and lower mortality for themselves than those who do not participate (USDA, 2005a).

Nutritional Challenges in Vulnerable Populations

Infants and Children

The vast majority of children who die today of hunger will not die in a high profile emergency, but rather pass unnoticed by anyone other than their families and neighbors. There are approximately 400 million hungry children in the world with an estimated 146 million under age 5 years. These children will most likely die or have long-term disabilities unless the following occurs (Gerberding, 2006):

- The children are identified and support from local organizations can reach them in their local communities.
- Local organizations are able to initiate interventions.
- Water purification and transport systems are established.
- Antibiotics can be made available.
- Complementary interventions such as childhood immunizations, education, and food security are also given.

Each year undernutrition contributes to the deaths of about 5.6 million children less than 5 years of age. In the least developed countries of the world 42% of the children are stunted in growth and 36% are underweight. Insufficient folic acid among childbearing-aged women contributes to 200,000 babies born with birth defects worldwide. Iron deficiency contributes 60,000 deaths among women in pregnancy and childbirth and decreases cognitive development in 40–60% of the children of the developing world. Food fortification, supplementation, and dietary improvements have been successful in eliminating most of these problems in the developed world and could result in similar improvements in the developing world (Gerberding, 2006).

As stated above, children under 5 years of age are generally much more vulnerable to higher rates of mortality during major emergencies such as earthquakes or tidal waves because of increased rates of communicable diseases and diarrhea as well as very high rates of undernutrition. During major emergencies donations of infant formula and other powdered milk products actually cause more harm than good. Infants and small children do better if they are breast-fed only. Mothers and infants need to be kept together and mothers should continue breast-feeding. In addition, maternal nutrition cannot be ignored and must also be addressed. Any breast milk substitutes for feeding infants and young children should be given only by carefully assessed needs under strict medical supervision and hygienic conditions. There should be no general distribution. Children older than 6 months should also be given fortified foods or micronutrient supplements under supervised programs (Labbock, Clark, & Goldman, 2004; Morris, 2006; UNICEF, 2005).

Safe water is also essential for nutrition. In settings with poor access to safe water and hygiene, children experience diarrhea and malnutrition. The diarrheal infections kill almost 2 million children under age 5 annually, and cause short- and long-term morbidity among millions more. Children with diarrhea frequently lose their appetites and do not absorb food, leading to nutritional deficiencies. In addition, malnourished children are at higher risk for diarrheal diseases. These children commonly have poor height and weight gains. Foods prepared with unsafe water or unclean hands expose children to diarrhea, causing illnesses and further promoting malnutrition (Gerberding, 2006). A significant percentage of infants anywhere from 4 to 6 months can be given complementary feedings, which are usually cereals or gruels (WHO, 2004).

The Progress for Children Report states that in the developing world there are 146 million children under 5 years who are underweight. Undernutrition is the cause of 5.6 million deaths per year. In countries such as India, Bangladesh, and Pakistan children also have iron deficiency anemia and iodine deficiency as well. From 1990 to 2002, China reduced the number of underweight children from 19% to 8%. (Global childhood malnutrition, 2006). Low birth weight (LBW) correlates with nutrition-related early childhood mortality. Thirty million newborns per year in developing countries (24% of the 126 million births per year) suffer from intrauterine growth retardation (IUGR). The world prevalence for of IUGR/LBW is 11% of all newborns in developing countries (13.7 million babies annually). Incidence in Asia (excluding Japan) is highest in the world with 28.3% (accounting for 80% of all newborns worldwide) and next is middle and Western Africa with 14.9% and 11.4% respectively. Almost 30% of South Asian women are moderately or severely underweight and do not gain a sufficient amount of weight during pregnancy to allow for fetal growth (Underwood, 2002). In rural areas of Southeast Asia breast-feeding is common for infants and young children, but this practice is decreasing in urban areas. There is a very interesting social structure where the poor and the wealthy perform breast-feeding, while the middle class, due to problems with the mothers having to work, use bottle feeding.

In Pakistan, for example, protein and calorie malnutrition is a significant health problem and contributes greatly to the morbidity and mortality in children. This area has been identified as a region with sex bias and female discrimination, including violence towards women. Boys are sent to school and given more nutrients when food is scarce. Preschool children, particularly girls, receive fewer calories than male children. In a study of 1878 children less than 3 years old, protein–energy malnutrition remained an important cause of death among preschool children in Pakistan. Female illiteracy, poverty, and overcrowding were found to be important risks for stunting (Shah, Selwyn, Luby, Merchant, & Bano, 2003).

Childbearing Women

Maternal malnutrition is disproportionately high in Asia and Africa and contributes to 87% of the 585,000 approximate maternal mortalities per year. The ratio is highest in Africa with 1 woman per 100 dying during births followed by a rate of .56 per 100 live births in Central Asia. Progress to reduce the maternal mortality has been targeted to improvements in nutrition as well as other nonnutritional causes. Among the causes of deaths, iron deficiency anemia is responsible for 15–20% of all maternal deaths (Underwood, 2002).

Older Adults

National estimates reveal that there are over 36 million older adults in the United States, 58% of which are females. Of this group food insecurity in Americans ranges from 6 to 16%. Good nutrition is particularly important for older adults because inadequate diets may contribute to or exacerbate diseases or delay recovery from illnesses. This group consistently has lower intakes of nutrients such as protein, iron, zinc, vitamin B_6 and B_{12}, riboflavin, and niacin. Of particular note is the incidence of scurvy in elderly men. These individuals eat primarily canned food and heat processing destroys ascorbic acid (vitamin C.) Poor nutrient intake increases the risk of chronic illnesses and greater vulnerability for the need for hospitalization. Poverty in older adults frequently causes them to do the following:

- Consume less than 3 meals per day.
- Have a lower intake of energy, vitamin C, iron, zinc, and calcium.
- Have iron deficiency anemia.
- Have reduced bone density or osteoporosis.
- Have oral health problems (tooth decay and gum disease).

Strategies to assist the older US adult to enhance food security needs include an increase in dieticians and health professionals and federal nutrition programs for elders such as Older Americans Act Nutrition Program (meals-on-wheels program) and the Food Stamp Program (Hall & Brown, 2005).

Aging adults often get anorexia of aging, a physiological process in which there is a decrease in appetite and food intake resulting in undesirable weight loss. In addition, the sense of smell and taste decline with age and can result in the consumption of a less varied and more monotonous diet leading to micronutrient deficiencies that decrease nutritional status and immune function. Research involving subjects in a study indicates that older adult males and females losing 10 pounds or more within a 10-year period of time had a higher adjusted mortality rate as compared to those with stable weight or weight gain. In addition hospitalized older adults with a BMI less than 18.5 have increased mortality rates. Undernutrition in the older adult has been shown to increase respiratory and cardiac complications, infections, and pressure ulcers. Nutritional supplemental liquids have been shown to reduce hospitalization, complications, and mortality. Specific micro (vitamins and trace metals) or macro (protein or cholesterol) supplementation may be quite useful. There is also evidence that vitamin supplementation increases cognitive functioning and ulcer healing. Research also indicates that in some situations the consumption of some alcohol with meals may increase food intake. For frail older adults delivery of food such as with the meals-on-wheels program may also help increase food intake (Visvanathan, 2003).

Nutrition Case Studies

Case Study: Micronutrient: Iodine Deficiency

Prior to the initiation of a nationwide program in China to eliminate iodine deficiency in 1995, over 20% of children between the ages of 8 and 10 years were found to have enlarged thyroid glands. In addition, there were approximately 400 million people living in China at risk for developing a disorder associated with iodine deficiency.

The National Iodine Deficiency Disorders Elimination Program was introduced by the Chinese government in an effort to combat this national health problem. The focus of the program was to produce, package, and distribute iodized salt nationwide. One challenge that had to be overcome for the program to be successful was that many people lived in salt-producing areas and on salt hills and consumed only raw salt and therefore were reluctant to pay for commercially produced salt.

The efforts of the program were primarily supported by the World Bank, UNICEF, and WHO. At its beginning, a nationwide health campaign was underway to inform the public of the ill effects of iodine deficiency and how essential it was to purchase only the fortified salt. Ensuring that the people across the nation would have access to the iodized salt, salt-producing factories were targeted to improve and increase their technology for production. New centers were also built for iodation and packaging. Licensing regulations, including quality control, were put into place by the government in an attempt to ban the sale of noniodized salt (Center for Global Development, 2006).

Five years after the initiation of the program, 94% of the country was receiving iodized salt as compared to only 80% at the start of the program. The quality of the product had also dramatically improved. The health of schoolchildren has shown a significant improvement. Total goiter rates have lowered to 6.5% in 2002 (Center for Global Development, 2006).

An Essential Micronutrient: Iodine

Iodine is a trace element that participates in the synthesis of thyroxine, a hormone secreted by the thyroid gland. Thyroxine stimulates cell oxidation and regulates the basal metabolic rate. It also helps regulate protein synthesis in the brain and other organs. The majority of iodine found in the body is contained in the thyroid gland. The recommended daily intake of iodine is 90 micrograms (mcg) for preschool children; 120 mcg for school children; 150 mcg for adults; and 200 mcg for pregnant and lactating women. Iodine is naturally found in seafood and in soil and water around the world. Iodine deficiency results when intake falls below the recommended levels. The principal disorder associated with deficient levels is enlargement of the thyroid gland, or goiter. Gland enlargement occurs as a result of continuous secretion of thyroid-stimulating hormone (TSH) despite low blood levels of thyroid hormone and the increase in the amount of thyroglobulin that accumulates in thyroid follicles. The gland thus increases in size and can weigh up to 700 grams or more. Iodine deficiency can also cause profound damage to the developing brain in utero and during the growing years of infancy and childhood. Stillbirths and miscarriages can result during pregnancy (Williams & Schlenker, 2003).

Case Study: Micronutrient: Vitamin A

To reduce vitamin A deficiency in sub-Saharan Africa, the International Potato Center supported by the Department for International Development has developed a sweet potato variety that is enhanced with the provitamin A form, beta-carotene. This orange-fleshed sweet potato is being promoted to alleviate vitamin A deficiency among children and pregnant and lactating women. A project led by South African scientists, school children between the ages of 5 and 10 years old were given a portion of boiled, mashed orange-fleshed sweet potato, weighing 125 grams, each day over 53 school days. A similar group of children received the same portion of white-fleshed sweet potato. Blood tests showed that the orange-fleshed sweet potato provided 2.5 times the recommended dietary allowance of vitamin A for that age group. The vitamin A stored in the liver in this group of children increased by 10% as compared to a 5% decline in vitamin A liver stores in those children consuming the white variety of sweet potatoes (South African Medical Research Council, 2004).

An Essential Nutrient: Vitamin A

Vitamin A is a fat-soluble vitamin that has many physiological functions:

- It helps with visual adaptation to light and darkness and prevention of night blindness.
- It is essential for optimal growth of soft tissues and bones.

- It maintains integrity of epithelial cells such as the mucous membranes.
- It maintains normal skin.
- It supports the immune system in the formation of T lymphocytes.

The recommended daily allowance for vitamin A is 300 mcg for children 1 to 3 years of age, 400 mcg for children 4 to 8 years of age, 600 mcg for children 9 to 13 years of age, 700 mcg for women and 900 mcg for men ages 14 and over. Two dietary sources of vitamin A exist. Retinol, or preformed vitamin A, is the natural form that can be found in animal food sources and is associated with fats. Beta-carotene is the provitamin A form and is found in orange-yellow and dark green leafy vegetables. The clinical signs of vitamin A deficiency results in conditions such as xerophthalmia, an abnormally dry and thickened surface of the cornea and conjunctiva, night blindness, and keratinization where epithelial cells become dry, flat, and hard (National Institutes of Health, Office of Dietary Supplements, 2006a).

Research Study: Micronutrient: Iron

Iron deficiency anemia has been a major health problem for over four decades in Sri Lanka. Women of childbearing age and those who are pregnant are at highest risk, as are preschool children and children in primary school. Anemia is especially high among groups of low socioeconomic status living in crowded environmental conditions and those prone to recurrent infections. A national survey found that 58% of children in primary school were identified as anemic (International Nutrition Foundation, n.d.).

A research study was conducted in Colombo, Sri Lanka, using 453 school children between the ages of 5 and 10 years, who presented with and without infection. The study examined the effects of iron supplementation on both iron status and morbidity and was designed as a longitudinal, randomized, controlled, double-blind supplementation trial. Baseline information was collected on each child that consisted of a detailed medical history, height and weight, venous blood sample, socioeconomic status, and morbidity from respiratory and gastrointestinal illness (deSilva, Atukorala, Weerasinghe & Ahluwalia, 2003).

The intervention consisted of iron supplementation for 8 weeks. The children were given 60 mg of elemental iron (ferrous sulfate) every day. The control group received placebo capsules of lactose. Field investigators followed-up with each of the children at their homes every 2 weeks to ensure high compliance. After supplementation was completed, all children were reassessed according to the preintervention parameters (deSilva, Atukorala, Weerasinghe & Ahluwalia, 2003).

Of the 363 children who completed the 8-week iron supplementation, 52.6% of the children had anemia. After the children took iron supplements, there was a significant improvement in iron status as indicated by the serum hemoglobin and ferritin concentrations in both groups of children with and without infections. In addition, those children who received the iron had a lower number of upper respiratory tract infections and total number of sick days (deSilva, Atukorala, Weerasinghe & Ahluwalia, 2003).

An Essential Nutrient: Iron

Iron is found in the body bound to protein and present in blood as the heme portion of hemoglobin and in muscle as myoglobin, bound to a transport protein as transferrin, and stored as a protein–iron compound as ferritin. It has many functions such as the following:

- Participates in the transportation of oxygen from the lungs to the tissues as a component of hemoglobin
- Acts as a catalyst of oxidative enzyme systems for energy production
- Converts beta-carotene to vitamin A
- Synthesizes collagen
- Removes lipids from the blood stream
- Detoxifies drugs in the liver
- Helps in the production of antibodies

The recommended daily allowance for iron for the following age groups is:

- 7 to 12 months—11 mg per day
- Children 4 to 8 years—10 mg per day
- Children 9 to 13 years—8 mg per day
- Children 14 to 18 years—11 mg per day for males; 15 mg per day for females
- Women aged 19 to 50 years—18 mg per day
- Men aged 19 to 50 years—8 mg per day
- Women aged 51+—8 mg per day
- Men aged 51+—8 mg per day

Iron can be found in organ meats such as liver, dark green vegetables, and grains. The principal deficiency associated with iron is anemia. Anemia can lead to various symptoms such as fatigue, pale skin, difficulty maintaining body temperature, glossitis, slow cognitive and social development, and decreased immune function. Common causes of iron deficiency anemia are increased iron losses, inadequate dietary intake, and inadequate absorption of iron usually secondary to diarrhea (National Institutes of Health, Office of Dietary Supplements, 2006b).

Case Study: Protein–Energy Malnutrition

Mr. Williams, a 70-year-old man with long-standing insulin-dependent diabetes mellitus, renal insufficiency, and heart failure is admitted to the hospital with fatigue, weakness, and weight loss. The nursing staff discovered a 4-inch diameter decubitus ulcer located over the sacrum. His caretaker gives a detailed history of his eating patterns over the previous 3 months indicating a progressive decline in his food intake. He is 5 feet 11 inches tall (180 cm) and his present weight is 125 pounds (56 kg). His calculated body mass index (BMI) is 17.2.

Causes of Unintentional Weight Loss in the Elderly

Unintentional weight loss can often occur in the elderly. There are many causes and situations that can signal and alert one to malnutrition, especially in the elderly population. Many chronic disorders of the cardiovascular, endocrine, gastrointestinal, and neurological systems can play a role in weight loss along with infections and malignancy. Psychiatric and eating disorders such as anorexia nervosa and bulimia also predispose an individual to weight loss. As one ages, grief and depression can result from separation from family or loss of a spouse, leaving a person living and eating alone. The side effects of many medications can also cause one to be anorexic and interfere with the utilization of food nutrients. Variables that actually interfere with the ability to eat include ill-fitting dentures, loss of teeth, problems with swallowing, and decreased sensation of taste and smell. All play a role in nutritional intake. Economic problems place the elderly at risk for malnutrition and include low socioeconomic status, insufficient income to purchase food, and inadequate living conditions such as the lack of heating or cooling and the lack of appliances to prepare meals (Jensen, Friedmann, Coleman, & Smiciklas-Wright, 2001; Williams & Schlenker, 2003).

Physical features of protein–energy malnutrition include the following:

- Reduction in body weight
- Muscle wasting with loss of strength
- Reduction in cardiac and respiratory muscular capacity
- Thinning of skin
- Decreased basal metabolic rate
- Hypothermia
- Edema
- Immunodeficiency
- Apathy

Treatment of Protein–Energy Malnutrition

Nutritional therapy for Mr. Williams is aimed at improving tissue integrity, muscle function, and immune function by providing enhanced amounts of protein and energy intake. Optimal dietary protein should be supplemented to the patient to ensure that an adequate supply of necessary amino acids is obtained for tissue synthesis. Calories need to be provided in amounts that will meet his energy output demands (Akner & Cederholm,

2001). Mr. Williams will also benefit from enhanced oral supplements to aid in healing of his pressure sore (European Pressure Ulcer Advisory Panel, n.d.). In addition, supplementation of arginine, vitamin C, vitamin A, and zinc has also been shown to be beneficial for the treatment of pressure sores (Langer, Schloemer, Knerr, Kuss, & Behrens, 2003; Schmidt, n.d.).

Essential Nutrition: Protein

Proteins are made up of amino acids that are necessary for the body to function properly, for growth, and for maintenance of body tissue. Proteins are the principal source of nitrogen and are essential for many body functions. These functions include the following:

- Building new and repairing old body tissues
- Supplying amino acids for making enzymes and hormones
- Regulating fluid and acid–base balance
- Providing resistance from disease
- Providing transport mechanisms
- Providing energy

Protein requirements are influenced by the rate of growth, body size, rate of protein synthesis, the quality of the protein, and the level of dietary fats and carbohydrates. The recommended dietary allowance (RDA) for both men and women is 0.80 grams per kilogram of body weight per day (Institute of Medicine, 2005). Additional protein is needed during illness and disease, trauma, prolonged immobilization, pregnancy, and lactation. Protein needs of infants and children vary according to their age and patterns of growth.

Sources of proteins can be described as either a complete protein or incomplete protein. A food that supplies a sufficient amount of the nine indispensable (essential) amino acids is called a complete protein. All proteins from animal sources are considered to be complete proteins. Foods from this group include chicken, beef, pork, fish, shellfish, eggs, and the milk food groups. Incomplete proteins are foods that lack one or more essential amino acids. This includes foods such as some fruits, grains, and vegetables (National Library of Medicine, 2006).

The following are the nine indispensable (essential) amino acids (Institute of Medicine, 2005):

- Histidine
- Isoleucine
- Leucine
- Lysine
- Methionine
- Phenylalanine

- Threonine
- Tyrptophan
- Valine

Case Study: Obesity

Dorothy is a 36 year-old female who has been diagnosed with hypertension by her family doctor. Her other significant medical history includes insulin-dependent diabetes mellitus. She reports that she has always had a sedentary job and lifestyle. Dorothy's weight is 204 pounds, height 66 inches, and she has a waist circumference of 38 inches. Her blood pressure is 170/95 mmHg and a heart rate of 86. She has acknowledged that she has been taking her blood pressure at home and it has been at least 156/95 on several occasions.

According to the USDA Dietary Guidelines for Americans (2005b), Dorothy's BMI is 33 indicating that she is in the category of obesity (see Figure 13-1). Another index that can be useful to identify obesity is the measurement of waist and waist/hips circumference.

BMI	19	20	21	22	23	24	25	26	27	28	29	30	31	32	33	34	35
Height							Weight in Pounds										
4'10"	91	96	100	105	110	115	119	124	129	134	138	143	148	153	158	162	167
4'11"	94	99	104	109	114	119	124	128	133	138	143	148	153	158	163	168	173
5'	97	102	107	112	118	123	128	133	138	143	148	153	158	163	158	174	179
5'1"	100	106	111	116	122	127	132	137	143	148	153	158	164	169	174	180	185
5'2"	104	109	115	120	126	131	136	142	147	153	158	164	169	175	180	186	191
5'3"	107	113	118	124	130	135	141	146	152	158	163	169	175	180	186	191	197
5'4"	110	116	122	128	134	140	145	151	157	163	169	174	180	186	192	197	204
5'5"	114	120	126	132	138	144	150	156	162	168	174	180	186	192	198	204	210
5'6"	118	124	130	136	142	148	155	161	167	173	179	186	192	198	204	210	216
5'7"	121	127	134	140	146	153	159	166	172	178	185	191	198	204	211	217	223
5'8"	125	131	138	144	151	158	164	171	177	184	190	197	203	210	216	223	230
5'9"	128	135	142	149	155	162	169	176	182	189	196	203	209	216	223	230	236
5'10"	132	139	146	153	160	167	174	181	188	195	202	209	216	222	229	236	243
5'11"	136	143	150	157	165	172	179	186	193	200	208	215	222	229	236	243	250
6'	140	147	154	162	169	177	184	191	199	206	213	221	228	235	242	250	258
6'1"	144	151	159	166	174	182	189	197	204	212	219	227	235	242	250	257	265
6'2"	148	155	163	171	179	186	194	202	210	218	225	233	241	249	256	264	272
6'3"	152	160	168	176	184	192	200	208	216	224	232	240	248	256	264	272	279
	Healthy Weight						Overweight					Obese					

Locate the height of interest in the leftmost column and read across the row for that height to the weight of interest. Follow the column of the weight up to the top row that lists the BMI. BMI of 19 to 24 is the healthy weight range, BMI of 25 to 29 is the overweight range, and BMI of 30 and above is in the obese range. Due to rounding, these ranges vary slightly from the NHLBI values.

Figure 13-1 Adult BMI chart.

Source: US Department of Agriculture, 2005.

There are two recommendations for overweight and obesity; calorie reduction and exercise promotion.

The best choice that is indicated for weight loss is to undergo a change in diet and physical activity patterns. Recommendations include a reduction in total calories initially by 500 or more per day while maintaining appropriate proportions of protein, carbohydrates, and fats in the diet, typically resulting in a loss of approximately 1 to 2 pounds per week, a common goal of most weight-loss programs (USDA, 2005b). Increasing energy expenditure is also very important in the reduction of weight. Exercise has many beneficial effects on nearly every system in the body. Regular physical activity helps reduce the risk of dying of heart disease and decreases the risk for developing diabetes, hypertension, stroke, and colon cancer. Physical activity contributes to weight loss; assists in controlling weight; maintains healthy bones, muscles, and joints; reduces the incidence of falls among the elderly; assists in relieving pain associated with arthritis; and reduces the symptoms related to anxiety and depression (American Heart Association, 2006). Recommendations from the Centers for Disease Control and Prevention and the American College of Sports Medicine state that adults should engage in *moderate-intensity* physical activities for at least 30 minutes on 5 or more days of the week" (CDC, 2006b).

Obesity risk factors include the following (Williams & Schlenker, 2003):

- Cardiovascular disease
- Hyperlipidemia
- Hypertension
- Stroke
- Diabetes mellitus
- Cancer
- Surgical complications
- Pregnancy complications

References

Akner, G., & Cederholm, T. (2001). Treatment of protein-energy malnutrition in chronic nonmalignant disorders [Electronic version]. *American Journal of Clinical Nutrition, 74*, 6–24.

American Heart Association (2006). *Physical activity.* Retrieved November 8, 2006, from http://americanheart.org

Andersson, M., Takkouche, B., Egli, I., & de Benoist, B. (2003). The WHO global database on iodine deficiency disorders: The importance of monitoring iodine nutrition. *Scandinavian Journal of Nutrition, 47*(4), 162–166.

CDC. (2003). *Food safety and nutrition.* Retrieved October 5, 2006, from http://www.cdc.gov/nceh/globalhealth/priorities/foodnutrition.htm

CDC. (2006a). *Overweight and obesity: Economic consequences.* Retrieved October 17, 2006, from http://www.cdc.gov/needphp/obesity/economic_consequences.htm

CDC. (2006b). *Overweight and obesity: Contributing factors.* Retrieved October 17, 2006, from http://www.cdc.gov/needphp/obesity/contributing_factors.htm

Center for Global Development. (2006). *Case 14: Preventing iodine deficiency disease in China.* Retrieved October 21, 2006, from http://www.cgdev.org

Chopra, M., Galbraith, S., & Darnton-Hill, I. (2002). A global response to a global problem: The epidemic of overnutrition. *Bulletin of the World Health Organization, 80*(12), 952–958.

deSilva, A., Atukorala, S., Weerasinghe, I., & Ahluwalia, N. (2003). Iron supplementation improves iron status and reduces morbidity in children with or without upper respiratory tract infections: A randomized controlled study in Colombo, Sri Lanka [Electronic version]. *American Journal of Clinical Nutrition, 77,* 234–241.

European Pressure Ulcer Advisory Panel. (n.d.). *Nutritional guidelines for pressure ulcer prevention and treatment.* Retrieved November 6, 2006, from http://www.epuap.org

GAIN. (2006). *GAIN signs grant agreement with UNICEF to support flour fortification in the CEE/CIS region.* Retrieved October 5, 2006, from http://www.gainhealth/ch/FN/index.cfm?contentid=fp5C67729.1143.F7CC.3

Gerberding, J. (2006). *Initiative to combat child hunger.* FDCH Congressional Testimony: 9/26/2006. Committee name: Senate Foreign Relations. Accession number: 32Y1742177555. Retrieved October 17, 2006, from http://wf2la7.webfeat.org/ WSvZG1118/ url=http://web.ebscohost.com/ ehost/delivery?vid

Gleason, G. (2002). Iron deficiency anemia finally reaches the global stage of public health. *Nutrition in Clinical Care, 5*(5), 217–219.

Global childhood nutrition. (2006). *Lancet, 367,* 1459.

Hall, B. & Brown, L. (2005).Food security among older adults in the United States. *Topics in Clinical Nutrition, 20*(4), 329–338.

Harder, B. (2004). Double credit. *Science News, 166*(18), 276–277.

Institute of Medicine. (2005). Protein and amino acids. In *Dietary reference intakes for energy, carbohydrates, fiber, fat, fatty acids, cholesterol, protein, and amino acids (macronutrients).*Retrieved November 8, 2006, from http://www.nap.edu/catalog/10490.html

International Nutrition Foundation. (n.d.). *Case studies on successful micronutrient programs: The Sri Lankan experience.* Retrieved October 25, 2006, from http://www.inffoundation.org

Jensen, G. L., Friedmann, J. M., Coleman, C. D., & Smiciklas-Wright, H. (2001). Screening for hospitalization and nutritional risks among community-dwelling older persons [Electronic version]. *American Journal of Clinical Nutrition, 74,* 201–205.

Johnson, B. (2006). The not-so-skinny: U.S. population weighs in as the world's most obese. *Advertising Age, 77*(20), 43.

Labbok, M., Clark, D. & Goldman, A. (2004). Breast-feeding: Maintaining an irreplaceable immunological resource. *Nature Reviews, 4,* 565–572.

Langer, G., Schloemer, G., Knerr, A., Kuss, O., & Behrens, J. (2003). Nutritional interventions for preventing and treating pressure ulcers. *Cochrane Database of Systematic Reviews, 4,* No. CD003216.

Mach, O. (n.d.). *Improving nutrition in Burundi.* Global Health Council, International Medical Corp. Retrieved October 17, 2006, from http://www.globalhealth.org/reports/printview-report.php3?id=53

Marvin, S. & Medd,W. (2004). Fat city. *World Watch, 18*(5), 10–14.

Merck Manual. (2002). *Protein-energy malnutrition.* Retrieved October 8, 2006, from http://www.merck.com/mrkshared/mmanual/section1/chapter2/2c.jsp

Monteiro, C., Moura, E., Conde, W., & Popkin, B. (2004). Socioeconomic status and obesity in adult populations of developing countries: A review. *Bulletin of the World Health Organization, 82*(12), 940–946.

Morris, J. (2006). World Food Programme. Statement by James T. Morris, Executive Director World Food Program to the United States Senate, Foreign Relations Committee. Hearing: *Ending Child Hunger and Undernutritional Initiative.* September 26, 2006.

Nash, M. (2003). Obesity goes global. *Time, 162*(8), 53–54.

National Institutes of Health. (2006b). *Dietary supplement fact sheet: Iron.* Retrieved October 25, 2006, from http://ods.od.nih.gov

National Institutes of Health. (2006a). *Dietary supplement fact sheet: Vitamin A and carotenoids.* Retrieved October 25, 2006, from http://ods.od.nih.gov

National Library of Medicine. (2006). Medline Plus. *Medical encyclopedia: Protein in diet.* Retrieved November 12, 2006, from http://www.nlm.nih.gov

Nead, K., Halterman, J., Kaczorowski, Auinger, P. & Weitzman, M. (2004). Overweight children and adolescents: A risk for iron deficiency. *Pediatrics, 114*(1), 104–108.

Olson, C. (2005). Food insecurity in women. *Topics in Clinical Nutrition, 20*(4), 321–328.

Pena, M. & Bacallao, J. (2002). Malnutrition and poverty. *Annual Reviews of Nutrition, 22,* 241–253.

Ramakrishnan, U. (2002). Prevalence of micronutrient malnutrition. *Nutrition Reviews, 60*(5), S46–S52.

Schmidt, T. R. (n.d.). *What's new in nutrition: Wound care in long-term care.* Retrieved November 7, 2006, from http://www.novartisnutrition.com

Shah, S., Selwyn, B., Luby, S., Merchant, A. & Bano, R. (2003). Prevalence and correlates of stunting among children in rural Pakistan. *Pediatrics International, 45,* 49–53.

South African Medical Research Council. (2004). *Not an ordinary sweet potato.* Retrieved October 21, 2006, from http://www.mrc.ac.za/mrcnews/ sep2004/sweetpotato.htm

Stallings, S., Wolman, P., & Goodner, C. (2001). Contribution of food intake patterns and number of daily food encounters to obesity in low-income women. *Topics in Clinical Nutrition, 16*(4), 51–60.

Stettler, N. (2004). Comment: The global epidemic of childhood obesity: Is there a role for the paediatrician? *Obesity Reviews, 5*(Suppl. 1), 1–3.

Ulrich, C. (2005). Iron plays a major role in nutrition. *Human Ecology, 32*(3), 7–11.

Underwood, B. (2002). Health and nutrition in women, infants, and children: Overview of the global situation and the Asia enigma. *Nutrition Reviews, 60*(5), S7–S13.

USAID. (2005). *USAID announces contribution to global nutrition.* Retrieved October 5, 2006, from http://www.usaid.gov/our_work/global_health/home/ News/nutrition_program.html

USDA. (2005a). *About WIC.* Retrieved October 5, 2006, from http://www.fns.usda.gov/wic/ aboutwic/mission.htm

USDA, (2005b). Dietary guidelines for Americans. *Weight management* (Ch. 3). Retrieved November 6, 2006, from http://www.health.gov/dietaryguidelines/dga2005/document/html/chapter3.htm

Visvanathan, R. (2003). Under-nutrition in older people: A serious and growing global problem! *Journal of Postgraduate Medicine, 49,* 352–360.

WHO. (2003). *Goals: Nutrition for health development.* Retrieved October 5, 2006, from http://w3.whosea.org/nhd/goal.htm

WHO. (2004). *Challenges for the 21st century. Nutrition in Southeast Asia.* 74–80.

WHO. (2005a). INFOSAN. *Building a food safety network to prevent foodborne disease.* Retrieved June 19, 2007, from http://www.who.int/foodsafety/fs_management/flyer_info_eng.pdf

WHO. (2005b). *Ensuring food safety in the aftermath of natural disasters.* Retrieved October 17, 2006, from http://www.who.int/foodsafety/ foodborne_disease/emergency/en/print.html

WHO. (2006a). *Challenges.* Retrieved October 6, 2006, from http://who.int/nutrition/ challenges/en/print.html

WHO. (2006b). *Nutrition in emergencies*. Retrieved October 5, 2006, from http://who.int/nutrition/topics/emergencies_collaboration/en/print.html

WHO and UNICEF. (2005). WHO, UNICEF, the International Red Cross and Red Crescent societies call for support for appropriate infant and young child feeding in the current Asian emergency, and caution about unnecessary use of milk products. Retrieved June 10, 2007, from http://www.who.int/topics/nutrition/tsunami-statement/en

Williams, S. R., & Schlenker, E. D. (2003). *Essentials of nutrition & diet therapy* (8th ed.). St. Louis: Mosby.

Chapter 14

Global Perspectives on Mental Health

Mary Ann Camann

Overview

Few would argue that mental health is a valued component of health, but worldwide, the effect of mental illness on overall health is poorly understood. This becomes an important factor when healthcare dollars are allocated. In 2003, the World Health Organization (WHO) issued the report *Investing in Mental Health* and reinforced the concept that "For all individuals, mental, physical and social health are vital and interwoven strands of life . . . mental health is crucial to the overall well-being of individuals, societies, and countries" (World Health Organization [WHO], 2003a). Further, in describing the extent of the effect of mental health on general health, mental health was defined as "a state of well-being in which the individual realized his or her own abilities, can cope with the natural stresses of life, can work productively and fruitfully, and is able to make a contribution to his or her community" (WHO, 2003a, p. 4). This broad definition of mental health puts mental health issues firmly in the arena of global health and population-focused health policy.

In this chapter an historical overview of the global understanding of mental health will be presented in a policy-making and policy implementation context. The extent of the effects of mental illness on health worldwide will be explored, including an overview of the prevalence of mental illness and the concept of disease burden. Issues related to mental health and illness, such as cultural variations on understanding and stigma, will also be discussed as well as a review of mental health issues and programs in various parts of the world. Finally, the most recent findings on mental illness as compiled in the WHO Mental Health Atlas will be presented as they point toward issues that will continue to need attention in the future.

Global Perspective—The Results of Research and Technology

The first annual World Mental Health Day, as initiated by the World Federation for Mental Health, was held on October 10, 1992, to call attention to the lives of persons who experience mental illnesses. This marked a growing awareness of the effects of mental health and illness on overall health and productivity worldwide. However, it would take much work over nearly a decade to increase awareness of mental health issues before the landmark publication of the *World Health Report 2001: New Understanding, New Hope*, which included an extensive section dedicated to mental health and was viewed as giving mental health the place it deserves on the world health agenda (Levav & Rutz, 2002). On World Health Day, 2001, the WHO Director General Dr. Gro Harlen Brudtland proclaimed: "We focus on mental health in recognition of the burden that mental and brain disorders pose on people and families. An estimated 400 million people suffer from mental or neurological disorders and psychosocial problems and those related to alcohol and drug abuse. The simple truth is that we have the means to treat many disorders. We have the means and scientific knowledge to help people with their suffering" (WFMH, World Mental Health Day, 2004).

Not coincidentally this time span also marked the culmination of the "Decade of the Brain" declared by the National Institute of Mental Health (NIMH), in the United States. President George Bush issued a proclamation designating 1990–1999 as a decade to continue study of the brain, to expand the burgeoning knowledge of the workings of the brain, and acknowledge the needs of millions of Americans affected each year by disorders of the brain ranging for neurogenetic diseases to degenerative disorders such as Alzheimer's, stroke, schizophrenia, autism, and impairments of speech language and hearing. This event marked the recognition of the increase in knowledge about the brain that was encouraged by the mapping of the brain's biochemical circuitry; study of how the brain's cells and chemicals develop, interact, and communicate with the rest of the body; and breakthroughs in molecular genetics and understanding of the connection between the body's nervous and immune system (White House, 1990).

Although the proclamation of the Decade of the Brain was significant in itself, it also heralded the scientific advances that changed the way many had viewed the mind and brain. Philosophical and religious leaders as well as the general public had to address the changes based on the visualization of brain activity through advanced imaging such as PET scans, and begin to reconcile this biological view with long-held beliefs about human identity and understanding of the self (Boyle, 2001). This struggle would have implications for the acceptance of developing neuroscience around the world and subsequent development of health policy and programs in the future.

The work that was done during the Decade of the Brain brought together many public and private entities in the United States and abroad for discussion about the science of brain function as well as the economic implications of health and diseases. During this time the World Health Organization, the World Bank, and Harvard University also worked on development of a single measure of disease burden to capture the effects of various illnesses on daily life through the disability-adjusted life-year (DALY), which expresses years of life lost to premature death and years lived with a disability. This work was reported in the *World Health Report*, 1996. The DALY measure "provided a comparative tool to analyze and prioritize health challenges worldwide, regionally, and nationally" (Magee, 2000). "The results of the WHO study confirmed what many health workers in mental health promotion and injury prevention had suspected for some time: that neuropsychiatric disorders and injuries were major causes of lost years of healthy life" (Lopez, 2005, p. 1186).

In 1999, the *Surgeon General's Report on Mental Illness in the United States* was issued; it was the first such report in the nation's history. It heralded an "understanding of the importance of mental health in the overall health and well-being and to the strength of a nation and its people" (U.S. Department of Health and Human Services [USDHHS], 1999). Donna Shalala, Secretary of Health and Human Services, noted in the introduction to the surgeon general's report that "We are coming to realize . . . that mental health is absolutely essential to achieving prosperity . . . [and there is] an opportunity to dispel the myths and stigma surrounding mental illness" (USDHHS, 1999, p. I). The implications of the surgeon general's report on mental health care in the United States will be discussed in detail later, but it clearly marked the beginning of a more inclusive, population-based mental health policy. The report also focused on the disparities in the availability of, and access to, services in the mental health field, and the stigma and hopelessness that often surrounds the issue. It set the tone for national policy and echoed the themes of the WHO *World Health Report* (1999).

Closely following the surgeon general's report, the *World Health Report 2001, Mental Health: New Understanding, New Hope* was issued and firmly placed mental health in the arena of global health. The director general stated clearly that "WHO is making a simple statement: mental health—neglected for far too long—is crucial to the overall well-being of individuals, societies, and countries and must be universally regarded in a new light" (WHO, 2001c, p. ix). The report marked the continuation of a collaborative effort to develop a global campaign on depression management, suicide prevention, schizophrenia, and epilepsy (WHO, 2001c). In keeping with the emphasis on disease burden, it was acknowledged that most illnesses, mental and physical, are influenced by a combination of biological, psychological, and social factors, setting the stage for advocacy for the cause of mental health and treatment of mental illness all over the world.

Legal and Ethical Issues

Global Burden of Disease

The 1996 Global Burden of Disease study was created to measure the burden of disease and injury in a manner that could also be used to assess the cost-effectiveness of interventions, in terms of the cost per unit of disease burden prevented. Disease burden represents the gap between a population's actual health status and a reference point—expected years of healthy life. The measure of disease burden takes into consideration egalitarian principles of how long a person should live regardless of socioeconomic status, race, or level of education. Disease burden also addresses the time lived with disability as well as lost healthy time due to death. Most people can agree that some disabilities are more serious than others and produce variations in the effects of the illness on the healthy days of individuals (Murray & Lopez, 1996).

The Global Burden of Disease findings demonstrated that disability plays an important role in determination of the overall health status of a population and so placed disability on the public health agenda, in addition to morbidity and mortality. In doing so the study illustrated the long-underestimated burden of psychiatric conditions. "Of the 10 leading causes of disability worldwide in 1990, measured in years lived with a disability, 5 were psychiatric conditions: unipolar depression, alcohol use, bipolar affective disorder, schizophrenia, and obsessive-compulsive disorder. Altogether, psychiatric and neurological conditions accounted for 28% of all years living with disability" (Murray & Lopez, 1996, p. 300).

The Global Burden of Disease study was instrumental in focusing on mental illness in terms of disease burden that cut across world regions and economic status. Combined with increased knowledge of the physiology of brain workings, it set the stage for worldwide health officials to address mental health as an important and economically significant public health issue. By the time of the publication of the *World Health Report 2001*, the concept of the burden of mental illness was understandable to the world at large, and it had been established that mental illness cut across all cultures and nations and was not a respecter of social or economic status.

Demographics of Mental Illness

The picture of mental health and illness globally is not pleasant. At the time of the *World Health Report 2001* it was reported that one in four people in the world are or will be affected by mental or neurological disorders at some point in their life. About 450 million people currently suffer from mental illness, placing mental disorders among the leading causes of illness and disability globally.

Where treatments were available, nearly two thirds of people with a known mental disorder never sought help from health professionals. Lack of understanding, stigma, discrimination, and neglect block individuals and population groups from benefiting from known effective treatment (WHO, 2001b). Lack of resources and the direction of resources toward mental health care is also a significant factor in dealing with mental disorders.

> Mental disorders are not the exclusive preserve of any special group: they are truly universal . . . and can be found in people of all regions, all countries, and all societies. Mental and behavioral disorders are common among persons seeking care in primary healthcare settings, constituting about 24% of individuals. The most common diagnoses in primary care settings are depression, anxiety, and substance abuse disorder. These disorders are present either alone or in addition to one or more physical disorders. There are not consistent differences in prevalence between developed and developing countries (WHO, 2001c, chap. 2, p. 1).

The prevalence numbers took on additional significance when it was estimated that one in four families has at least one member currently suffering from a mental or behavioral disorder, and they are often required to provide physical and emotional support and bear the impact of stigma and discrimination present worldwide and also, in many cases, the expense of treatment (WHO, 2001c). The economic costs also affect the population in proportionally different manners. It is estimated that mental and behavioral disorders cause considerable disruption in the lives of those who are affected and their families, which in turn increases the overall cost of health care and contributes to a loss of productivity and quality of life.

Additionally, conflicts such as "war and civil strife and disasters affect a large number of people and result in mental health problems. In 2000, it was estimated that about 50 million people were refugees or internally displaced. . . . Millions are also affected by natural disasters that take a heavy toll on the mental health of the people involved, many of whom live in developing countries, where capacity to take care of these problems is limited" (WHO, 2001c, chap. 2, p. 19).

Development of Mental Health Policy

Health policy is always developed in the larger social and political environment. Health policy is a work in progress that acknowledges the current state of health, invites discussion, focuses attention on specific issues, and at its best creates a sense of priority and encourages development of services and evaluation of effectiveness of the impact of services on human life. The *World Health Report 2001* made available new knowledge about the understanding of mental and behavioral disorders. It also offered possible solutions and policy options to governments and policy makers that could influence strategic decision making and point toward positive changes in the acceptance and treatment of mental disorders (WHO, 2001b). It is beyond the scope of this chapter to explore all policy issues and the ramification of policy directions, but suffice to say that policy development is a slow process and affected by many internal and external issues, as well as, available resources and public understanding and will.

In the *World Health Report 2001*, 10 broadly conceived recommendations for action were made. These recommendations will be visited later in the chapter as regional programs are presented, but an abbreviated list is presented as follows:

- Provide treatment in primary care, as it enables the largest number of people to get easier and faster access to services. It implies that general health personnel be trained in the essential skills of mental health care and has implications for education and training.

- Make psychotropic drugs available. Include essential psychotropic drugs in every country's essential drug list as they can ameliorate symptoms, reduce disability, shorten the course of many disorders, and prevent relapse.

- Give care in the community, as community care has a better effect on quality of life of individuals with chronic mental disorders that does institutional treatment. Such care is also cost-effective, respects human rights, and can lead to early interventions and limit the stigma of seeking treatment.

- Educate the public. Educational and awareness campaigns on mental health should be launched in all countries to reduce barriers to treatment and care by increasing awareness of the frequency of mental disorders, their treatability, the recovery process, and the human rights of people with mental disorders.

- Involve communities, families, and consumers in the development and decision making regarding policies, programs, and services taking into account age, sex, culture, and social conditions.

- Establish national policies, programs and legislation for sustained action based on current knowledge and human rights considerations. Mental health reforms, including budgetary allocations, should be part of the larger health system reforms.

- Develop human resources, especially in developing countries to increase and improve the training of mental health professionals, who will provide specialized care as well as support the primary healthcare programs. Specialist mental healthcare teams ideally should include medical and nonmedical professionals, such as psychiatrists, clinical psychologists, psychiatric nurses, psychiatric social workers, and occupational therapists, who can work together toward the total care of individuals in the community.

- Link with other sectors. Sectors such as education, labor, welfare, and law and nongovernmental organizations should be involved in improving the mental health of communities.

- Monitor community mental health through the inclusion of mental health indicators in health information and reporting systems to determine trends, detect mental health changes resulting from external events such as disasters, and assess the effectiveness of mental health prevention and treatment programs, all the while building the case for the provision of resources.

- Support more research. Increase research on a wide international basis to understand variations across communities and to identify factors that influence the cause, course, and outcomes of mental disorders, and to increase understanding of the biological and psychosocial aspects of mental health as a method of understanding mental disorders and the development of more effective interventions.

These recommendations have provided the foundation for further work in global mental health policy and programs and are revisited in WHO's *Project Atlas, Atlas Mental Health*, which reports on progress made in each area on a regular basis (WHO, 2001a). In the year 2001, of the 185 countries studied, which cover 99.3% of the world's population, 41% had no mental health policy, 25% had no legislation on mental health, 28% had no separate budget for mental health, 41% do not have treatment facilities for severe mental health disorders in primary health care, 37% had no community care facilities, and about 65% of the beds for mental health care are in mental institutions (WHO, 2001a). These statistics illustrate the deficits in mental health care and point out the need for increased attention to mental health needs globally. To better focus on regional issues a review is presented that includes analysis of scope, effectiveness, and cultural and economic issues as indicated.

Regional Mental Health Issues and Outcomes

There are no worldwide subdivisions or sets that can address all cultural and ideological issues in mental health care. The thrust of the World Health Organization's efforts is to focus on scientific research and good practices, while acknowledging that many cultures base local policies and programs on religious or ideological beliefs. The WHO efforts also focused on the role of stigma and exclusion that presents barriers to care on an individual and population basis. The action plans also acknowledge the fear factor and stigma that promotes care in institutions rather than communities. The plans also offer examples of programs that have been successful when community care is developed (Levav, & Rutz, 2002). In this section regional mental health policies, programs, and outcomes will be examined. Exemplar programs will be presented when available, and examples will be used to illustrate problems and successes.

North America

United States of America

In a combined statement issued with the *Report of the Surgeon General on Mental Health in the United States*, the directors of the Substance Abuse and Mental Health Services Administration (SAMHSA), Nelba Chavez, the National Institute of Mental Health (NIMH), Steven Hyman, and the Center for Mental Health Services, Bernard Arons, called the report a challenge to the nation, and to U.S. communities, and health and social services, policy makers, employers, and citizens to take action and collaborate on generation of needed knowledge about the brain and behavior and to translate the knowledge to the service systems and citizens. The surgeon general at that time, Dr. David Satcher, called for a social resolve to make the needed investment to change attitudes about mental health and usher in a healthy era of mind and body for the nation (USDHHS, 1999). The fact that this 1999 report was the first surgeon general's report ever issued on the topic of mental health and mental illness was significant and followed on the heals of the efforts embodied in the Decade of the Brain. The report emphasized two main findings:

1. The efficacy of mental health treatments is well documented, and a range of treatment exists for most mental disorders. This provided a basis for a call for understanding of mental health and mental illness as a public health issue and one which contributes to significant disability.

2. The report also viewed mental health and mental illness as points on a continuum pointing toward needed efforts along the entire continuum, while acknowledging the complex and multifaceted mental health system in the U.S. that does not always function in a coordinated manner.

The surgeon general's report (DHHS, 1999) heralded the inclusion of mental health care in the overall healthcare schema, and created a vision for the future that encouraged good access to a range of mental health treatment programs, and that continued to build on the scientific bases of neuroscience, molecular genetics, and pharmacotherapies. The report urged the reduction of stigma by the dispelling of myths with accurate knowledge, while improving public awareness of effective treatment. Further, the supply of mental health services and providers was called for in different venues that could ensure that state-of-the-art treatment would be delivered in a manner that was adjusted to age, gender, race, and culture by facilitating entry into treatment and by reduction of financial barriers to treatment. The report was greeted with enthusiasm by consumers and mental health advocates. Indeed, it did mark a major emphasis on the essential inclusion of mental health care in healthcare discussions, but few direct programs resulted from the report.

Consequently in 2001, President George W. Bush created the New Freedom Commission on Mental Health in order to conduct a comprehensive study of the United States mental health service delivery system and issue advice on methods to improve the system and fill the gaps in the mental health system. By 2003 the commission had issued its report confirming "that recovery from mental illness is now a real possibility. . . yet for too many Americans with mental illness, the mental health services and supports they need remain fragmented and disconnected—often frustrating the opportunity for recovery. Today's mental healthcare system is a patchwork relic—the result of disjointed reforms and policies" (USDHHS, 2003, p. 4). The report incorporated the views of consumers, families, and professionals. Six goals were formulated to direct the focus on recovery and transformation of the mental healthcare system.

The recovery movement has become a significant motivator of reform. Many important and innovative programs carry on this work, addressing the goals within the often disconnected mental healthcare system. The National Alliance for the Mentally Ill noted 12 such programs.

TABLE 14-1   Goals: In a Transformed Mental Health System . . .

Goal 1 Americans understand that mental health is essential to overall health.

Goal 2 Mental health care is consumer and family driven.

Goal 3 Disparities in mental health services are eliminated.

Goal 4 Early mental health screening, assessment, and referral to services are common practice.

Goal 5 Excellent mental health care is delivered and research is accelerated.

Goal 6 Technology is used to access mental health care and information.

Source: USDHHS, 2003.

One such program, the Network of Care for Behavioral Health, is a Web-based and text-based community that addresses the need for information and access and was developed to be a single point of entry in providing critical information, communication, and advocacy tools with ways to access emergency services. It is linked with state and county services and offers up-to-date information on important findings in the mental health field (Network of care, 2006). Currently there are only 13 states that have links to the site.

The Nurse-Home Visiting Program is another innovative program focused on prevention of mental illness and was developed by David Olds and lately supported by the Robert Wood Johnson Foundation. Based on work over a 15-year period by David Olds, the program focuses on prevention of mental illness by providing nurse home visits to targeted new mothers. Some of the outcomes of the first project have been repeated in subsequent versions. "For mothers: 80% reduction in abuse of their children, 25% reduction in maternal substance abuse, and 83% increase in employment. For children (15 years later): 54% to 69% reduction in arrests and convictions, less risky behavior, and fewer school suspensions and destructive behaviors. This is the only prevention program trial in the field with a randomized, controlled design and 15 years of follow-up" (NAMI, 2005; Nurse Family Partnership, 2006).

The program began in rural New York 20 years ago, and its benefits have been replicated in Denver, Colorado, and in minority populations in Memphis, Tennessee. When compared with paraprofessional visits in similar programs nurse-visited mothers were more likely to enter the workforce and had fewer pregnancies before the first child's second birthday. Nurse-visited children born to mothers who were more psychologically vulnerable had better language development and ability to control their behavior at ages 2 and 4. The visited mothers interacted better with their children and showed some reported reduction in psychological distress. To date the program is operating in 270 communities in 23 states (Nurse Family Partnership, 2006).

Another group of programs is centered at Boston University, Center for Psychosocial Rehabilitation, and is affiliated with Sargent College of Health and Rehabilitation Sciences and the Rehabilitation Counseling Program. Their many programs are centered around rehabilitation and recovery programs, including their Hope and Health program, their Training for the Future program, individual services in recovery and research, and evaluation projects. The work is focused on "increasing knowledge in the field of psychiatric rehabilitation and applying the knowledge to train treatment personnel, to develop effective rehabilitation programs, and to assist in organizing both personnel and programs into efficient and coordinated service delivery systems" (Center for Psychiatric Rehabilitation, 2006).

Obviously, there are many outstanding programs devoted to the needs of the mentally ill. However, the National Alliance for the Mentally Ill recently completed a comprehensive survey and grading on 39 criteria of state adult public mental healthcare systems that service people with serious mental illnesses. They reported that "nationally, the system is in trouble, and its grade is not better that a D. Only five states received a B and eight failed altogether," confirming what the New Freedom Commission on Mental Health called a fragmented system in shambles (NAMI, 2006). To encourage development of more effective programs, NAMI also published a list of state innovations and best practices so that programs could learn from each other.

Canada

Canada also established a Canadian Mental Health Commission "to provide leadership to make mental health a long-term priority of governments: facilitating the exchange of research and best practices, reducing fragmentation of mental health and illness policies and programs, and developing a strategy to increase awareness and reduce stigma around mental illness" (Canadian Collaborative Mental Health Initiative, 2005a). The Canadian Collaborative Mental Health Initiative was funded for 2 years by Health Canada's Primary Health Care Transition Fund. The Canadian healthcare system is focused on the primary care model (CPA/CFPC, 2003). When reviewing patterns of use it was found that one in every five Canadians experience a mental illness during their lifetime. The collaborative also addressed the complex interplay between physical and mental illnesses. The collaborative sought to maximize the shared care focus in mental health care through evaluation of various initiatives. The collaborative involved a consortium of 12 national organizations representing mental health consumers, families, and caregivers, community providers, dietitians, family physicians, nurses, occupational therapists, pharmacists, psychologists, psychiatrists, and social workers. One of the first activities of the initiative was to survey regarding "buy in" of the various groups, resulting in an engaged community of interest that provides ongoing advice. The initiative produced 10 research papers and 12 toolkits to ensure dissemination of the information (Canadian Collaborative Mental Health Initiative, 2006).

Several initiatives developed out of the collaborative focused on integration of mental health services within primary care as a method of delivering mental health care as the traditional models that expected persons to come to mental health services were not working (Kates, Crave, Crustola, Nikolaou, & Allen, 1997). A collaborative process was developed where mental health professionals were paired as consultants, either on-site or in shared space. The details of how to make it work varied. One example focused on knowledge exchange at a family medicine clinic in Nova Scotia, which provides an academic teaching environment for family medicine residents and clinical staff, including family physicians, nurses, social workers, and psychiatrists. This program focused on knowledge transfer via use of electronic patient records, weekly rounds, monthly case discussions, and three shared care retreats held annually (Kates, Crustolo, Farrar, & Nikolaou, 2001).

Another initiative developed a geriatric psychiatry outreach team, bringing together psychiatrists, registered nurses, social workers, and a neuropsychologist to provide consultation to two family practice clinics and one community health center as well as home-based assessment when appropriate. The collaborative also sponsors a shared care conference annually.

All activities were based on a shared belief that Canadians are entitled to a health system with the capacity to help them meet both their physical and mental health needs—

whether those needs are illness prevention, early detection, treatment, rehabilitation, or recovery. The consortium produced a general toolkit for providers and policy makers on planning and implementing collaboration between mental health and primary care services; additionally, the consortium produced a two-volume report on emerging trends in mental health care, including descriptions of over 90 Canadian initiatives (Canadian Collaborative Mental Health Initiative, 2005b, p. 25). In all, 61% (55 programs) of long-term mental health initiatives were started during the years of the collaboration (2000–2004) (Canadian Collaborative Mental Health Initiative, 2005b, p. 28).

There is considerable agreement in North America on the scope of mental health problems, but very different approaches to collaborative and coordinated mental health prevention and care. Although outstanding examples exist, the system's main focus is on keeping the system working with the consumer as the focus and streamlining access to care. Much work remains to be done.

Latin America

The Latin American region includes many different cultural groups. In geopolitical terms, there are 13 countries in South America, 5 in Central America, plus Mexico and 13 other countries in the Caribbean basin (Pan American Health Organization, 2005). The Pan American Health Organization (PAHO) began a process in 2001 to consider new priorities for mental health care. In November 2005 a regional conference was held in Brazil convening governmental mental health officers, organizations of the civil society, and consumers and family members to the Regional Conference on Mental Health Services Reform 15 years after the Caracas Declaration (1990). The conference focused on the state of mental health care in the Americas and on improvement of mental health care through replacement of the service model based on the psychiatric hospital with community alternative care and through actions to safeguard the human rights and the social inclusion of persons affected by mental disorders. The main thrust of the discussion considered the use of the primary health care strategy adopted by PAHO. Jointly, the conference participants declared the importance of preserving human rights and linking psychiatric care to primary health care. They also declared that the training of mental healthcare workers should be based on a community-based service model that included psychiatric inpatient care, when necessary, in community hospitals.

Studies conducted by the PAHO/WHO found that "around 30% of the total population of Latin America and the Caribbean was partially or totally excluded from access to health goods and services" (Acuna & Bolis, 2005, p. 3). Exclusion from health care was a particular issue to persons with mental illness and made them vulnerable related to stigmatization. Stigmatization could be viewed as a social variable or self-exclusion based on a belief that there is no effective treatment (Acuna & Bolis, 2005) The number of people with mental disorders in the region of the Americas is forecasted to increase from 114 million in 1990 to 176 million in 2010. Policies that focus on access to services and community-based care are necessary to meet the demand (Pan American Health

Organization, 2005). However, 64.5% of Latin American countries have specific mental health policies and 80.6% have plans and programs, which is higher than many other regions (Alarcon, 2003). Consequently, actions geared toward dissemination of knowledge about mental health and the effective treatment of mental illness, as well as protection of human rights, will be important to the success of any policy or program.

One such program is an 8-year training program based on the delegation of responsibilities among various levels of workers including recovered patients, mid-level professionals, religious leaders, and mental health specialists including psychologists and psychiatric nurses. The evaluation of the program in Santiago, Chile, and Cordoba, Argentina, noted its low cost-benefit ratio that was achieved by using the natural resources of the community (Marconi, 1996).

Another training program involved primary care nurses in Panama who were trained to recognize depression and provide notification to primary physicians and provision of supportive interventions. This program had its greatest impact on the detection of moderate cases of depressive disorders and indicated that more education may be necessary (Moreno, Saravanan, Levav, Kohn, & Miranda, 2003).

One other program addressed understanding of mental illness by addressing attitudes toward mental illness in Dominica. In this program, case vignettes depicting persons experiencing psychosis, alcoholism, depression, and childhood hyperactivity were viewed by community leaders, nurses, teachers, police officers, and community members. The person in the psychosis vignette was identified by 84% of the leaders and by 71% of the community members, but fewer than 30% identified the other situations as involving mental illness, but would refer someone with mental health problems to a medical practitioner if it was identified (Kohn, Sharma, Camilleri, & Lavav, 2000).

Another program expanded on the recommendation of primary care interventions through a program that enrolled women in three primary care clinics in Santiago, Chile. The women were randomly assigned to a stepped-care program or usual care. The stepped care improvement program consisted of a stepped-care approach that involved structured psychoeducational systematic monitoring of clinical progress and a pharmacotherapy program that was delivered for 7 weeks with a booster session at weeks 9 and 12. This study demonstrated far greater improvement among those randomized to stepped care, with 70% recovered at 6 months compared with 30% among those given standard care (Araya, Rojas, Fritsch, Gaete, Rojas, & Simon, 2003). This program provided a cost-effective intervention that was suitable for low-socioeconomic population groups.

Based on the broad policy recommendations and the demonstration programs, it would seem that mental health programs would most likely be effective if they addressed understanding of mental health issues and treatment and if they could be provided along with mental health care delivered as part of the primary care system.

Europe

Countries in the WHO European Region face challenges with mental health problems, with over 100 million people suffering from anxiety and depression, 21 million suffering from alcohol use disorders, 7 million from Alzheimer's disorders and other dementias, 4 million from schizophrenia, 4 million from bipolar affective disorder, and 4 million from panic disorders—accounting for 19.5% of all disability-adjusted life-years (WHO, 2005a). Individual governments increasingly recognize the importance of mental well-being for all citizens as a fundamental part of quality of life (WHO, 2005a). Services across the region are varied. Community care has been shown to offer a better quality of life and greater satisfaction to consumers and family caregivers. Across the region the number of institutional beds is decreasing. A quarter of European countries have no services available in the community, and more than 50% of all patients are still treated in large mental hospitals. Other issues involve funding, and in some countries 85% of the money devoted to mental health is spent on maintaining large institutions. Many do not have care available from primary healthcare professionals, and many do not have a therapeutic drug policy or an essential drug list. There are also great variations in the availability of mental health professionals. There is a wide gap in services needed versus services available. In a survey published by the European Union in 2003, 90% of individuals saying that they had mental health problems reported that they received no care or treatment in the previous year. Even in Western Europe about 45% of people suffering from depression got no treatment (WHO, 2005a).

In recognition of the state of mental health care in the European Union, the members assembled and set out an action plan for mental health solutions. The basic plan included the following:

- Develop comprehensive national mental health legislation and policies.
- Address health allocations in budgets to reflect priorities and needs.
- Evaluate parity and coverage in social and private insurance-based systems.
- Develop primary care services with the capacity to detect and treat mental health problems by expanding the numbers and skills of primary care staff.
- Plan and implement specialty community-based services available 24 hours a day, with multidisciplinary staff for persons with severe mental illness.
- Provide access to psychotropic medications and simple psychotherapeutic interventions in the primary care setting, especially for individuals with long-term and stable mental disorders who live in the community.
- Guarantee access to necessary and affordable medicines for people with mental problems to achieve appropriate prescription and use of these medicines.
- Ensure equitable distribution of mental health workers across the population by creating incentives.
- Inclusions of children, adolescents, and the elderly as priority groups and at-risk groups such a migrant families.
- Develop mental health services sensitive to the needs of young and elderly people, operated in close collaboration with families, schools, day care centers, and community agencies.

- Support the implementation of community development programs in high-risk areas (WHO, 2005b, chap 5).

Many projects are being piloted at this time and partnerships are being fostered to increase understanding and improve treatment. One such project is the Cooperation with General Practitioners Project sponsored by the European Alliance Against Depression (EAAD).

One of the reasons for the underdiagnosis and undertreatment of depression can be seen in deficits at the primary care level (e.g., lack of knowledge concerning diagnosis and treatment of depression, underestimation of the severity of the disorder). In the framework of EAAD, these deficits are being tackled by establishing a close cooperation with general practitioners (GPs) and other primary care doctors.

To improve ability and knowledge concerning the processes of detection, diagnosis, and treatment of depressive disorders, advanced training courses for GPs are being conducted in EAAD intervention regions using highly interactive training packages including role playing and group discussions. Furthermore, information material and decision aids (e.g., video tapes for GPs and patients, patient files, screening tools) are being distributed among primary care doctors to support the decision making concerning individual cases of depressive patients in their practice. Currently there are 18 European countries participating in training and information dissemination projects (Mental Health Europe, 2005).

The Mental Health Europe project is carrying out the project Good Practices for Combating Social Exclusion of People with Mental Health Problems and working on assessment of which practices are transferable to other European countries, taking into account the major existing socioeconomic and cultural differences. The project addresses coordination and cooperation around the issues of health and social services in communities, employment, education, housing, transport, leisure, and civil and human rights (Mental Health Europe, 2005).

A major report was recently issued by the European Commission titled *Included in Society*, which focuses on the placement of mentally disabled people in large residential institutions, which in itself constitutes a major human rights violation. The report exposes the institutional excesses, while showcasing successful programs such as supported living in Bucharest. This program provides accommodation for 12 people with mental health problems, as well as support and counseling in order to develop their coping skills and ability to deal with daily domestic activities, in four ordinary flats in different areas of Bucharest (European Commission, 2003, p. 17).

Another highlighted program involves a parents school aimed at parents of children with mental health problems. The aim of the project is to assist parents to develop their own solutions, to make informed decisions, and to reduce the intensity of the burden of care. In the program the parents get support and information on improving relationships and creating effective methods of communication, as well as assistance in creating independent self-help groups (European Commission, 2003).

In Europe there are islands of hope in a region that has much institutional history and stigma to overcome. But Europe has serious plans for its future. The gap is wide between policy and practice and among various countries. The move toward greater community focus and away from institutional care is an economic issue as well as a social and political issue. Innovations and demonstrations provide a pathway to future success.

Africa

Africa is a vast land that encompasses many diverse peoples and has been the site of much strife and war. "Most of its countries also are characterized by low incomes, high prevalence of communicable diseases and malnutrition, low life expectancy, and poorly staffed services" (Gureje & Alem, 2000). Mental health is most often low on the list of policy priorities. In 1988 and 1990 the African Region of the World Health Organization adopted two resolutions to improve mental health services, and each state was expected to formulate mental health policies, programs, and action plans. When progress was addressed 2 years later some modest achievements had been made, but the progress was not satisfactory. The current goals are directed toward changing the negative perception of mental disorders by the public and reducing the incidence and prevalence of mental disorders while providing adequate care for persons with mental illness (Gureje & Alem, 2000).

A conference in 2003 focused on the crisis situation in Africa caused by wars, civil strife, and natural disasters. At the time of the meeting 23 of the 46 countries of the WHO African Region were experiencing some kind of emergency—creating greater than nine million refugees and more than 35 million internally displaced persons in Africa and many types of healthcare crises including mental illness (WHO, 2003b).

In most parts of Africa attitudes toward mental illness are influenced by traditional beliefs in supernatural causes and remedies, which often leads to stigmatization of mentally ill persons and to reluctance or delay in seeking care. Citizens and policy makers often believe that mental illness is largely incurable or unresponsive to orthodox medical practice. In one survey in South Africa where 25% of patients who see general practitioners experience mental illness and nearly 20% of high school students per year have contemplated suicide, it was reported that they would rather die than admit they suffer from some sort of mental illness (Science in Africa, 2002). Additionally, there is a HIV pandemic in some African communities, and the mental health consequences of AIDS contribute to overall psychiatric morbidity in the region, as well as the consequences of hunger, displacement, and lack of material resources. Compounding the fear of mental illness is the lack of mental health workers in most countries and having only a limited drug formulary in most countries. Nearly half of the countries in Africa have just one hospital for the mentally ill. Further, because many families do not understand the manifestation of mental illness in their family members, they may chain or tie them up and administer beatings (Kaplan, 2006).

Clearly there are many challenges to providing mental health care in Africa that cannot be overcome by policy statement and goal setting. Several programs however provide beacons of hope for the future. In one project, traditional mental health practitioners (TMHPs) in Nigeria were included in a program to foster working relationships between orthodox mental health practitioners and traditional mental health practitioners. The project involved pre- and post-training evaluations and training on the types of mental illness, treatment of mental illness, including follow-up, after care, relapse prevention, and other primary prevention measures. The post-training evaluation showed there was a higher percentage of TMHPs that could recognize all the symptoms of mental illness listed. The post-intervention evaluation also noted a change in the attitude of the TMHPs toward persons with mental illness including the belief that persons should not be sent out of the community and how they should be treated. Beating of the mentally ill had been a long-time practice where caning was seen as an effective treatment for the mentally ill. After the intervention, beating was less likely to occur. Another outcome was that traditional mental health professionals were more likely to refer patients to orthodox mental health providers (Adelekan, Makanjuola, & Ncom, 2001).

In another program conducted in Uganda, a site of war and rebellion for nearly two decades, local people were recruited to implement a program to treat depression in adults. Dr. Paul Bolton led the program where 250 persons from 30 villages were assessed as suffering from major depression and assigned to one of 30 groups. Fifteen of the groups received psychotherapy sessions for 16 weeks, and the other half received none. At the end of the period, those who received the therapy were significantly less depressed than the control group. Additionally, 14 of the 15 therapy groups were still meeting 6 months later, having transformed themselves into economic support groups so that members could help each other by lending money and helping each other develop small businesses (McNeil, 2005). A similar program was implemented with Ugandan teenagers in refugee camps that had similar results. In all of the programs, Bolton begins by asking the people open-ended questions about how they view mental health, and then goes on to develop a sustainable program utilizing a relatively inexpensive and simple intervention. Also in Uganda, Bolton utilized a system and function assessment of depression to increase the likelihood that understanding of the impairment of depression would build justification for the allocation of scarce resources to mental health issues (Bolton, Wilk, & Ndogoni, 2004).

Where poverty is endemic, low-cost public mental health programs are vital, as well as programs that train and involve community workers. Culturally sensitive programs that include significant local involvement are important to change attitudes and offer hope to persons with mental illness.

Asia and the Western Pacific

In 2003 in Beijing, Dr. Henk Bekedam spoke at the Second International Mental Health Development Conference, and noted that "While many aspects of physical health have improved in the region of the past 50 years, mental health has worsened" (Bekedam, 2003). He also acknowledged that the burden of mental health goes hand-in-hand with rapid urbanization and social changes such as poverty and physical illness. To address these difficult realities, the region adopted three basic goals:

1. Reduce the human, social, and economic burden produced by mental and neurological disorders, including intellectual disability and substance abuse and dependence.

2. Promote mental health.

3. Give appropriate attention to psychosocial aspects of health care and the improvement of quality of life.

Bekedam further called for the integration of mental health into health care and primary care (Bekedam, 2003).

As in Europe, mental health activities in the countries of the South East Asia Region had been concentrated on hospital-based psychiatry. In the report on the work of WHO in the South East Asia Region they called for mental health services that could be integrated into the primary healthcare system, and the development of innovative community-based programs. As in Africa, considerable attention has been paid to crisis situations such as tsunami relief efforts and provision of basic health care and the demands of bird flu outbreaks. Additionally, areas in Asia have also been marked by war and insurgent activities that contribute to human suffering and mental illness.

One study that examined factors that influence Asian communities' access to mental health care noted that both health professionals and the general public have considerable knowledge deficits regarding mental illness and mental health. Shame and stigma were commonly reported. The sense of shame was significant, and it was noted that the shame connected with mental illness for Chinese people meant that "you can't go out and face other people" (Wynade, Chapman, Org, McGowan, Zeeman, & Yeak, 2005, p. 90). Another commonly reported barrier to seeking care was the level of knowledge about mental illness, which was related to the level of education and country of origin, and religion. Karma, the law of cause and effect in Eastern spirituality and beliefs about reincarnation, are important concepts in many Eastern religions. Consequently, having a child with mental illness results in the parents feeling that they were being punished for conduct in their past lives. Others might believe that a mentally ill person was possessed by evil spirits, or that bad blood was passed down from the child from the mother. Even if a general practitioner would ask about mental illness, concern about family reputation and shame would prohibit discussion of the illness. These beliefs often result in a mental illness being hidden from the community, and family members not doing anything about the illness, or hope that it would go away. Seeking help for mental illness was seen as a last resort (Wynaden et al., 2005).

As in other regions, the World Health Organization has focused on training and education as important first steps in developing mental health services. The World Health Organization has supported a variety of activities such as training nurses in Fiji to detect symptoms of mental illness in primary care and provide treatment. In China, workshops to train trainers were conducted to increase recognition and management of common mental disorders in general practice. In the Republic of Korea, a workshop was held on the development of a model for community-based mental health services. In Vietnam and Mongolia, projects were developed to produce a community-based mental healthcare text and to use an ICD-10 coding system to diagnose and manage common mental health disorders at the primary healthcare level (WHO, 2004).

Efforts have been expended to change understanding and reduce reliance on institutional care in other countries as well, but much still needs to be accomplished. In Jakarta, the Lawang mental hospital has been reduced to 700 patients from over 4,200 patients, and the atmosphere has been changed to reflect changes in therapy and nonchemical approaches, but police continue to get calls to remove mentally ill people from the highways where they have been put out by their relatives because they are too ashamed to seek help (*Jakarta Post*, 2006). One project is attempting to provide basic needs by encouraging effective community-based care including treatment and support by also addressing the issues of poverty and stigma through creating partnerships with governments and community groups to create sustainable programs. The program links medical model mental health treatment with community development approaches such as programs on how to earn a living and creation of small-scale horticultural projects that provide a family livelihood and reduce stigma (Kaplan, 2006).

There are some promising approaches in process. When a mood disorders center was opened in Hong Kong, the center's phone lines were heavily used with people asking for help. The hotline bypassed the long-held taboo against talking about depression and other mood problems, and provided a point of contact regarding reports of chronic fatigue, headaches, and poor memory, that are often correlates of depression. In this way bad moods can be blamed on physical health, bypassing the associated stigma. The mood disorders center, developed by the Chinese University of Hong Kong, also trains family doctors to better recognize and treat anxiety disorders and depression as a face-saving way for people to seek treatment (Saywell & McManus, 2001).

Summary

It is clear that considerable attention to mental health and mental illness issues needs to continue and involve more government entities as well as community agencies. There is increased evidence of the biopsychosocial nature of both mental illness and mental health and evidence that mental illness has profound impact on the lives of persons affected, their families, and communities. This public evidence has increased the global profile of international mental health, but sustained and sustainable action remains limited. Especially in developing countries, each new public health challenge moves mental health into the background. Mental disorders have clear economic cost. Persons experiencing mental illness often experience reduced productivity at home and in the workplace. "Mental disorders also have a range of consequences on the course and outcomes of comorbid chronic conditions, such as cancer, heart disease, diabetes, and HIV/AIDS, and persons with untreated mental disorders are at heightened risk for poor health behaviors, noncompliance with prescribed medical regimens, diminished immune functioning, and unfavorable disease outcomes" (WHO, 2002, p. 3).

Understanding of the importance of mental health and the treatment of mental illness does not necessarily produce resources and programs. The WHO Mental Health Atlas, a compendium of global data from 192 countries, was updated in 2005 "shows no substantial change in global mental health resources since 2001. There continues to be marked and growing differences in availability between high- and low-income countries. Only 62% of all regions have mental health policies with the Western Pacific 48%, South-East Asia 54.5%, and Africa 50%, falling behind in planning and implementation of mental health services (WHO, 2005a, p. 15). As discussed earlier, competing priorities for serious health problems, natural disasters, and war push mental health issues to a low priority despite increased understanding of the effects of mental illness on the population.

Community care continues to be a high priority, but is available in only 68.1% of the countries covering 83.3% of the world's population. In the Americas and Europe more than 75% have community care programs with considerable variations in geographic access. Community care is also highly correlated to income level with only 51.7% of low-income countries having it versus 97.4% in high-income countries (WHO, 2005a, p. 19).

On a more positive note, 89.3% of countries have a therapeutic drug policy and essential list of drugs. The drug list is made up of basic and traditional psychotropic drugs that can be produced in generic formulations. This coverage is most likely related to the increase in mental health care in primary care, which has been an important health policy direction. Eighty-seven percent of the world reports having mental health in primary care, but only 61% have treatment facilities for severe mental disorders in primary care. There are only 19.8% of psychiatric beds in general hospitals worldwide. Consequently there is a reliance on large mental hospitals in 68% of the world, and this often also results in issues related to human rights in many countries (WHO, 2005a).

When available personnel and training of primary care workers are considered, the deficits become obvious. Worldwide there are only 1.2 psychiatrists per 100,000 population and only 2 psychiatric nurses per 100,000 population. The state of mental health care is most evident in the decrease of 2.8% of the number of countries stating that they had a specific budget line for mental health in their health budgets (WHO, 2005a). "One fifth of the countries reported spending less than 1% of their health budget on mental health, in contrast to the estimate that 13% of all disease burden is caused by neuropsychiatric disorders" (Patel, Saraceno, & Kleinman, 2005, p. 1313).

There is much work to be done in educating healthcare providers and the population about mental illness and its effective treatment. The major policy directions of including mental health care in primary care and the community setting will come about only when governments and individuals demand such care and see the benefit of the outcomes for individuals and populations. Opportunities are present for developing countries to apply current knowledge and the lessons of exemplar programs to their developing healthcare policies and programs. In countries where there are few mental health services, and mentally ill persons already live in the community with family as caregivers, it is relatively easy to find support for community care programs and mental health care delivered as part of the primary care system. Training efforts directed at primary care workers are likely to be most effective in those countries. Community-based programs could increase support for inclusion of mental health care in healthcare budgets (Thornicroft & Maingay, 2002).

Development of culturally congruent programs illustrate that major mental disorders can be treated in an efficient and cost-effective manner with low-cost and technically simple treatment. Community and primary care treatment programs need the support of philanthropic organizations as well as government entities to increase understanding of the effectiveness of such programs. The issue of drug availability can be increased if mental illness is included as an exemption category in the trade-related intellectual property rights international agreement; this would make it possible for developing countries to produce generic versions of drugs patented after 2005 (Patel, Saraceno, & Kleinman, 2005). In keeping with the spirit of the first Global Mental Health Day, mental health needs to have its place on the world health agenda. The case needs to continue to be made that good mental health care enhances overall health and the prosperity of the population.

References

Acuna, C., & Bolis, M. (2005). *Stigmatization and access to health care in Latin America: Challenges and perspectives.* Washington, DC: Pan American Health Organization.

Adelekan, M. I., Makanjuola, A. B., & Ncom, R. J. E. (2001). Traditional mental health practitioners in Kwara State, Nigeria. *East African Medical Journal, 78*(4), 190–196.

Alarcon, R. (2003). Mental health and mental health in Latin America. *World Psychiatry, 2*(1), 54–56.

Araya, R., Rojas, G., Fritsch, R., Gaete, J., Rojas, M., & Simon, G. (2003). Treating depression in primary care among low-income women in Santiago, Chile: A randomised controlled trial. *Lancet, 361,* 995–1000.

Bekedam, H., (2003). *Speeches: WHO representative in China on the occasion of the second international mental health development conference.* China: WHO.

Bolton, P., Wilk, C., & Ndogoni, L. (2004). Assessment of depression prevalence in rural Uganda using symptom and function criteria. *Social Psychiatry and Psychiatric Epidemiology, 39,* 442–447.

Boyle, P. (2001). Bulletin: Religion and the brain: The decade of the brain. *Park Ride Center, 19,* 1–6.

Canadian Collaborative Mental Health Initiative. (2005a). Canadian collaborative mental health initiative applauds the establishment of landmark commission. *Canada NewsWire Ltd,* Nov. 28.

Canadian Collaborative Mental Health Initiative. (2005b). *A review of Canadian initiatives, Vol I, Analysis of Initiatives.* Canadian Collaborative Mental Health Initiative.

Canadian Collaborative Mental Health Initiative. (2006). *Health Canada primary care transition fund, 2006 Canadian Collaborative Mental Health Initiative, final report.* Retrieved May 1, 2006, from http://www.ccmhi.ca

Caracas Declaration. (1990). Regional conference for the restructuring of psychiatric care in Latin America. Caracas, Venezuela, November 11–14, 1990.

Center for Psychiatric Rehabilitation. (2006). *About the center for psychiatric rehabilitation.* Retrieved August 9, 2007, from http://www.bu.edu/cpr/about/index/html

CPA/CFPC. (2003). *Shared mental health care: Strengthening the relationship between mental health and primary care providers: A document from the CPA/CFPC Working Group—April 2003.* Retrieved August 9, 2007, from http://www.shared-care.ca/cpacfpc.shtml

European Commission. (2003). *Included in society: results and recommendations of the European research initiative on community-based residential alternatives for disabled people.* Retrieved August 9, 2007, from http://www.community-living.info/contentpics/226/Included_in_Society.pdf

Gureje, O & Alem, A, (2000). Mental health policy development in Africa. *Bulletin of the World Health Organization, 78*(4), 475–481.

Kaplan, A. (2006). Basic needs: Helping the mentally ill live productively. *Psychiatric Times, 23*(7), 51.

Kates, N., Crustolo, A., Farrar, S., & Nikolaou, L. (2001). Integrating mental health services into primary care: lessons learnt. *Family Systems & Health, 19*(1), 5–12.

Kates, N., Crave, M., Crustolo, A., Nikolaou, L & Allen, C. (1997). Integrating mental health services within primary care: A Canadian program. *General Hospital Psychiatry, 19*(5), 324–332.

Kohn, R., Sharma, D, Camilleri, CP. & Lavav I. (2000). Attitudes towards mental illness in the Commonwealth of Dominica, *Pan American Journal of Public Health, 7*(3), 148–154.

Jakarta Post. (2006). *Mental illness is not divine retribution,* April 19. p. 17.

Levav, I. & Rutz, W. (2002). The WHO World Health Report 2001—New understanding, new hope. *Israel Journal of Psychiatry Related Science, 39*(1), 50–56.

Lopez, AD. (2005). The evolution of the Global burden of disease framework for disease, injury and risk factor quantification: developing the evidence based for national, regional and global public health action. *Globalization and Health, 1*(5), 1144–1186.

Magee, M. (2000). The global burden of disease. Health politics. Pfizer Medical Humanities Initiative. Retrieved from http://www.healthpolitics.org/archives.asp?previous=prog_01

Marconi, I. J. (1996). Teaching of mental health in Latin America. *Acta Psiquiátrica y Psicológica de América Latina, 22*(4), 277–281.

McNeil, T. (2005). An offer of hope: A pioneering BU effort bring mental health programs to the developing world. *The Bostonian,* Winter 2005–2006.

Mental Health Europe. (2005). EU Project: Good practices for combating social exclusion of people with mental health problems. Sante Mentale Europe, Brussels.

Moreno, P., Saravanan,Y., Levav, I., Kohn, R., Miranda, CT. (2003). Evaluation of the PAHO/WHO training program on the detection and treatment of depression for primary care nurses in Panama. *Acta Psychiatrica Scandinavica. 108,* 61–65.

Murray, C. J. L., & Lopez, A. D. (Eds.). (1996). *The global burden of disease: A comprehensive assessment of mortality and disability from diseases, injuries and risk facts in 1990 and projected to 2020.* Cambridge, MA: Harvard University Press on behalf of the World Health Organization and the World Bank.

NAMI. (2006). *Grading the states report, 2006.* Retrieved August 9, 2007, from http://www.nami.org/content/navigationmenu/grading_the_states/project_overview/overview.htm

NAMI. (2005). Model program: Intervening early to prevent mental health problems. Retrieved August 9, 2007, from http://www.nami.org

Network of Care, (2006). A reference guide to your network of care web-site for behavioral health. Retrieved August 9, 2007, from http://missouri.networkofcare.org/common/MOBrochure.pdf

Nurse Family Partnership. (2006). The nurse family partnership, helping first time parents succeed. Retrieved August 9, 2007, from http://www.nursefamilypartnership.org

Pan American Health Organization. (2005). Mental disorders in Latin America and the Caribbean Forecast to Increase. *Press release.* Retrieved August 9, 2007, from http://www.paho.org/English/ DD/PIN/pr051209.htm

Patel, V., Saraceno, B., Kleinman, A. (2005). Beyond evidence: The moral case for international mental health. *American Journal of Psychiatry, 163,* 1312–1315.

Saywell, T., & McManus, J. (2001). Behind the smile: Silent suffering. *Far Eastern Economic Review, 9,* 26–31.

Science in Africa. (2002). *The mental health information centre—Brain awareness week information.* Retrieved August 9, 2007, from http://www.scienceinafrica.co.za/2002/march/mhic.htm

Thornicroft, G., & Maingay, S. (2002). The global response to mental illness, *British Medical Journal, 325,* 608–609.

White House. (1990). Presidential Proclamation 615, *Decade of the Brain: 1990–1999, by the President of the United States of America.* Retrieved August 9, 2007, from http://www.loc.gov/loc/brain/ proclaim.html

USDHHS. (2003). President's new freedom commission on mental health, 2001. DHHS Publication No. SMA-03-3832.

US Department of Health and Human Services (USDHHS). (1999). *Mental health: A report of the surgeon general. Executive summary.* Retrieved August 9, 2007, from http://www.surgeongeneral.gov/ library/mentalhealth/home.html

World Federation for Mental Health (WFMH). (2004) World mental health day: The relationship between physical and mental health. Retrieved August 9, 2007, from http://www.wfmh.org/ wmhday/about.html

World Health Organization (WHO). (1999). *The World Health Report 1999—Making a difference.* Geneva, Switzerland: Author.

WHO. (2001a). *Fact Sheet: Project atlas: Mapping mental health resources around the world.* Retrieved August 9, 2007, from http://www.who.int/entity/whr/2001/media_centre/en/ whr01_fact_sheet3_en.pdf

WHO. (2001b). Mental disorders affect one in four people—Press release. Geneva, Switzerland: Author.

WHO. (2001c). Burden of mental and behavioural disorders. In *The World Health Report 2001: Mental Health: New Understanding, New Hope.* Geneva, Switzerland: Author.

WHO. (2002). *Mental health global action programme.* Retrieved August 9, 2007, from http://www.who.int/mental_health/actionprogramme/en/index.html

WHO. (2003a). *Investing in mental health.* Retrieved August 9, 2007, from http://www.who.int/ entity/mental_health/media/investing_mnh.pdf

WHO. (2003b). *Press Release: Emergencies cited as major threat to human health in Africa, as wars cost region $15 billion per year.* Retrieved August 9, 2007, from http://www.afro.who.int/press/ 2003/pr20030313.html

WHO. (2004). *The work of WHO in the south-east asia region, 2004.* Retrieved August 9, 2007, from http://www.searo.who.int/EN/Section898/Section1447.htm

WHO. (2005a). Mental Health Atlas 2005. Geneva, Switzerland: Author.

WHO. (2005b). Mental health: Facing the challenges, building solutions. Geneva, Switzerland: Author.

Wynaden, D., Chapman, R., Org, A., McGowan, S., Zeeman, Z., & Yeak, S. (2005). Factors that influence Asian Communities' access to mental health care, *International Journal of Mental Health Nursing, 14*(2), 88–92.

Chapter 15

Global Perspectives
on Environmental Health

Marvin Friedman

Environmentally induced diseases can result from lack of knowledge about the adverse effects from electromagnetic, ionizing, and nonionizing radiation and environmental chemicals or from intentional or ethical decisions that weigh the pros and cons of competing alternatives resulting in population exposure to toxic chemicals. In this chapter we give examples of how epidemics have resulted from a failure to know and understand environmental risk both from man-made stimuli and natural contaminants as well as those which resulted from societal, economic, or ethical decisions. We briefly provide a framework on how these decisions can be evaluated and made. We also present a regulatory framework under which many governments implement these decisions. At the end, the reader will have a broader and deeper understanding of how man interacts with his environment.

Global Issues—Lessons in Environmental Health

Much has been written and speculated on the issue of global health and sustainable development. Speculation about problems for which there is not hard data is difficult and unreliable. However, environmental problems can be solved through application of diligent scientific procedures.

What Happened to the Mink?

In the early 1980s, reproductive complications were observed in mink (Aulerich & Ringer, 1977). Several dietary components were evaluated to determine whether they were the cause of this failure for mink to reproduce. Neither the Coho salmon, which made up the major component of their diet, nor other species of Great Lakes fish appeared to cause this response in experimental mink. Diets and carcasses were evaluated for mercury and chlorinated pesticides, and there was no correlation. Analysis of the pathological signs suggested that PCBs (polychlorinated biphenyls) might be the causative agent. However, no other species was presenting these signs. Feeding of groups of mink on 30 ppm PCB diets or salmon from the Great Lakes, the signs were identical to those of wild mink. It turned out that mink are extremely sensitive to the reproductive effects of PCBs and that there were enough PCBs in Great Lakes Coho salmon to induce the reproductive effects.

The next issue became to determine where the PCBs came from. It was determined that the major use of PCBs was as a heat transfer agent in electrical transformers (IARC, 1978). At first glance, this use would not suggest the high levels of PCBs that were observed in the mink and Coho salmon. However, PCBs are not metabolized to any large extent and therefore were stable in the environment. Because they were fat soluble and only marginally water soluble, the PCBs accumulated in the fat of the fish, which then accumulated in the fat of the mink. During the winter, as the mink lost their fat, blood levels of PCBs would increase sharply. The PCBs caused increased drug metabolism that was reflected in alteration of circulating sex hormone levels that then adversely affected reproduction.

The science did not end here. It turned out that PCBs were contaminated with another chlorinated, environmentally stable hydrocarbon, TCDD (tetrachlorodibenzodioxin or dioxin), which was three orders of magnitude more toxic than PCBs (Mandal, 2005). This substance was even more widely distributed and was found not only associated with PCBs but also in landfills associated with paper mills that chlorinated their waste at elevated temperatures. This lead to a change in the process in which chlorine dioxide and not chlorine is used. Chlorine replacement due to environmental contamination will be a continuing theme in this chapter. This is costly and does not necessarily translate to developing countries.

Parenthetically, the PCB toxic response was replicated in humans when a Japanese family used PCBs for cooking instead of cooking oil. The signs of toxicity were the same.

In this chapter we will evaluate what makes one species more sensitive than another, how we characterize the toxicity of materials, and how we can extrapolate risk to environmental exposures. Although there was no human reproductive toxicity observed in these studies, the studies did cause a careful evaluation by regulatory agencies of the safety of Great Lakes fish, particularly to the Canadian aboriginal population who consume large quantities of these animals.

What About the Cats in Japan?

In the 1950s, the domestic house cat population demonstrated a highly unusual central neurotoxicity characterized by staggered gait and other signs. This was referred to as Minimata disease (Takeuchi, D'Itri, Fischer, Annett, & Okabe, 1977). A chemical plant had initiated manufacture of acetaldehyde and dumped waste methyl mercury in the bay. Methyl mercury, being fat soluble and not metabolized by fish, accumulated in fish in the bay. The cats ate these fish exclusively in their diet. Subsequently, people living in Minimata showed the same neurological signs, which also included tunnel vision and learning deficits.

Methyl mercury is a well-known neurotoxin that causes neuropathies in experimental animals and has been studied as a pesticide. In the 1960s, grain was shipped to Iraq for planting that was treated with methyl mercury as a pesticide (Rustam & Handi, 1994). This pesticide was purple in color, and it was not expected that people would eat the grain; rather, they were instructed to plant it. They prepared it as bread, and there was a clear dose-response of bread consumption and tunnel vision, peripheral neuropathies, terata, and other forms of methyl mercury toxicity.

Methyl mercury is a component of sea water and accumulates in pelagic (oceangoing) fish. Considerable debate has taken place as to the safety of pelagic fish due to methyl mercury contamination. Island populations consuming diets almost exclusively of fish have been studied. To date these results are inconclusive (CLS, C.o.L.S, 2000).

When methyl mercury is used as an herbicide, such as on golf courses, where the water is not free flowing like the ocean, the concentration can become excessive and the fish a source of toxicity.

Why Do We Discuss Selenium?

The biological effects of selenium represent the best example of environmental health and toxicology. Selenium is a metal that is found in abundance in many parts of the world and concentrates in some plants. Most selenium is consumed as the sulfur amino acids methionine and cysteine, as the selenium can replace the sulfur. There is a nutritional requirement for selenium in several biochemical pathways. In New Zealand, China, and Finland, for example, selenium deficiency was a major public health problem. Selenium intake is less than 50 mcg/day. Selenium deficiency is characterized as a cardiomyopathy and muscle pain (Dodig & Cepelak, 2004; Reuterswiff, Krol, & Lecure, 2006). In contrast there are other areas of the world where selenium is present in excess (Dodig & Cepelak, 2004). In these areas a characteristic neurotoxicity is observed. These levels are in excess of 250 mcg/day. Consideration of selenium deficiency or excess in the absence of knowledge of the other biological properties might lead to other toxic effects.

Vitamin A

Vitamin A, α-tocopherol, is a necessary component of diet. Vitamin A is needed for vision, and its absence results in night blindness, among other effects. It is a fat-soluble vitamin concentrated in the liver (Fishman, 2002; Russell, 1967). It, like selenium, also has toxic properties when consumed in excess. This toxicity has been documented among arctic explorers and Eskimos who consume polar bear. Polar bears live on a diet rich in fish, which are rich in vitamin A. When arctic explorers consumed polar bear liver, their dose of vitamin A was enormous. So a nutrient that receives little attention in the Western diet can be a serious toxin in other conditions. A deficiency of vitamin A is characterized by night blindness followed by connective tissue disorders. Chronic toxicity affects the skin, the mucous membranes, and the musculoskeletal and neurological systems. Vitamin A toxicity is not necessarily restricted to polar bear consumption as megadose vitamins are becoming popular.

Lessons to Be Learned

All materials have toxicity at high enough doses. In the case of methyl mercury and PCBs, those animals with the highest consumption were harbingers of human exposure. With selenium and vitamin A, there are toxicities from both deficiencies and excesses. Just because a material is required does not mean it has no toxicity.

Principles of Environmental Health

Definitions

For the purposes of this chapter, infectious agents will be excluded to the extent possible. Very frequently there is a trade-off between infectious agents and chemicals: examples include food preservatives and water purification not to mention antibiotics and other pharmaceuticals and antiseptics. Due to the ability of microorganisms to reproduce, infectious disease almost always represents a greater public health concern than chemical contamination.

Assessment of environmental health is accompanied by technical terms that have clear definitions. Sometimes these definitions have connotations that public health professionals must ignore. For example, workplace exposure to toxic substances is different from environmental exposure. However, contamination of the rivers with pharmaceutical agents is an environmental event. The use of estrogens as birth controls agents in women would not be considered environmental. However, these hormones were excreted in urine and ended up in river water (Shore, Gurevitz, & Semesh, 1993). This resulted in developmental and reproductive problems in striped bass that almost killed the species. Prior to delineating the impact of environmental chemicals on public health, it is important to clarify these terms.

Environment

The environment is defined as the air we breathe, the water we drink, and the food we eat. None of these environmental components is pure in the chemical sense. That is, there is no chemical definition of air, water, or food as each of these are mixtures and have both major and minor components contributed by natural sources. For example, the air in the forest contains chemical substances (e.g., terpenes) that volatilize from trees in the forest. Although these substances are natural components of the forest air, they are intentional additives in cleaning products, and in some cases have pesticidal and biocidal activity. The same applies to food. Although a synthetic diet can be constructed from purified starches, proteins, and fatty acids, no one consumes this diet. Therefore, a qualifier is usually appropriate with an environmental component, such as "forest air," or "Great Lakes water."

Environmental Agent

This is the chemical or infectious agent or radiation source that is alleged to induce an environmental health incident. There are two critical characteristics of such an agent.

First, what is the quality of data linking the agent with the effect? Although Koch's postulates can be applied to infectious agents, it is more difficult to apply them directly to environmental health. Koch's postulates are as follows:

1. The pathogen must be present in all hosts diagnosed with the disease.
2. The pathogen must be isolatable from the diseased host.
3. The pathogen must be purifiable.
4. The purified pathogen must cause the specific disease.
5. The pathogen must be isolated from the host used in step 4.
6. The pathogen in step 5 must be shown to be the same pathogen purified in step 3.

To do this, one would have to demonstrate that the environmental agent was present in the affected population, that the agent could cause the environmental outcome, and that it was present in sufficient quantities to account for the effects. Secondly, there must exist an analytical technique for the agent in question. Of course, that requires a detailed definition of the environmental agent. For example, it is not appropriate to suggest that neurological behavior observed in the cats at Minimata Bay were caused by methyl mercury. The neurological signs must be demonstrated in experimental animals following methyl mercury treatment. Methyl mercury had to be isolated from the cats at doses which would cause the disease. The first step in any environmental evaluation is always the development of an analytical method.

Adverse Health Effect

Adverse health effect is usually defined in preclinical toxicology as any significant deviation from the norm. However, in the human environment, this is not always easy. The best example of such difficulty in defining adverse health effects lies in the manufacture of hypnotics. These substances are safe and effective in people even when used in large doses. Sleep induction is a therapeutic response. However, in the manufacturing environment, they cause the workers to fall asleep on the job; this is an adverse outcome. Therefore the definition of adverse health effect becomes subjective. It is the induction of an effect that the exposed population does not intend or want. This has already been demonstrated with environmental exposure to estrogens that can also inhibit reproduction in the environment.

Risk

Risk is the probability that an adverse outcome will occur. Individual risk is the probability that an individual will suffer from an adverse outcome. The opposite of individual risk is population risk. Population risk is the expected number or percentage of adversely effected individuals in a population that will suffer an adverse outcome. Exposure of three people to a material that will cause one adverse event in a million is different from exposing 300 million people to that risk.

Risk has three components: exposure, causation, and dose-response. The calculation and interpretation of risk will be dealt with in great detail later.

Ecology

Receptors for adverse events are not restricted to humans but are also present in wildlife, including fish. Due to the varied spectrum of species and their different physiologies, a substantial difference in sensitivity has been observed. Subtle questions can be asked with regard to protection of the environment. For example, are environmental evaluations performed by protecting most of the species exposed or the total population?

Toxicology

Toxicology is the study of the adverse effects of materials, chemicals, or radiation on living organisms. Although not explicit in the definition, what makes a toxicologist different from other scientists is that a toxicologist relates dose and response rather than just studying response. The terms *adverse effects* and *toxicological effects* are used interchangeably in this chapter.

Physiologically or Toxicologically Significant Adverse Health Effects

Although this issue seems apparent, it is very difficult to deal with. For example, an environmental substance that causes weight loss at a specific dose is considered to be inducing an adverse effect. However, when that same substance is evaluated as a pharmaceutical for that purpose, it is considered therapeutic. Looking at the same situation in reverse, one can look at a material that can be used safely and effectively as a hypnotic. The dose at which it manifests the hypnotic response is not a toxic dose but rather a pharmacologically beneficial event. However, when this material is manufactured in the workplace and exposure takes place at a level sufficient to induce a hypnotic dose, the workers fall asleep, and there are substantial problems thereafter.

As a perspective, one can consider how to evaluate additives for food that decrease calorie availability or promote weight loss. If one evaluates an inert ingredient such as a nonmetabolizable starch for use in breads, cookies and cakes, FDA requires at least a 100-fold safety margin be administered. Of course adding 100 times the amount to be used in breads, cakes, and cookies will result in body weight loss, as the test animals do not eat enough food to compensate. It then appears that there is a toxic response characterized by weight loss. These additives are food additives and not drugs so a margin of safety is required. The definition of *adverse effect* is not always obvious.

Similarly, with large sample sizes or sensitive assays, small effects that have no physiological significance can be detected while the response has no physiological significance. The terms *statistical significance* and *toxicological significance* relate to different findings. The former is dependent on characteristics of the assay and the sample size while the latter deals with hazards. It is important to evaluate whether effects observed in populations around the world are real adverse health effects or statistical anomalies caused by large sample sizes or sensitive assays.

Global Catastrophic Risk

There are a few risks whose consequences can be so significant that normal considerations of cost, benefit, weight of the evidence for data, and concentration dependency are not considered. The most obvious of these is global warming. This results from destruction of the ozone layer of the atmosphere and consequent warming of the surface of the earth by a few degrees centigrade. The postulate is that release of carbon dioxide or fully halogenated hydrocarbons (to be discussed later) into the atmosphere can decrease the density and effectiveness of the stratospheric filter for radiation. Although the data is poor and the effects immeasurable, if true, this would mean a global catastrophe. Therefore, the threat must be dealt with as if it were absolutely true. These mega-events are not common, but when present require an entirely different way of thinking about risk. Treatment of drinking water, safety of vaccines, and contamination of food stuffs all fit into this global catastrophic risk.

Principles of Toxicology

A detailed and comprehensive treatise on toxicology is beyond the scope of this chapter. However, there are some very critical concepts that can be covered here.

Intrinsic Activity

Intrinsic activity can be defined as the maximum response that can be induced by a material. It can be seen in Figure 15-1, which is an idealized schematic. Of the four curves, two have the same intrinsic activity and two have the same potency. For intrinsic activity, the maximum response is 40 at both high and low potency while the maximum at the low dose is 8. Intrinsic activity is a biological property of a substance. For example, the diuretic properties of a substance such as melamine or the porphyrin-modifying properties of lead and iron are intrinsic activities. These may be considered as a physical property of the substance. These are generally determined in animal experiments or in vitro studies, but sometimes these are determined in humans first as anecdotal observations, such as the observation that vinyl chloride was a human carcinogen. In the European Union intrinsic activity is categorized. Category 1 is an activity known to occur in man, category 2 is one that will probably occur in man, and category 3 is one that has been identified only in animals.

Intrinsic activity does have degrees of effectiveness associated with it. That is, the maximum effect of a substance can be different between two substances. For example, one substance may induce more chromosomal anomalies than another at the maximum dose tested.

One can compare the bladder cancer-inducing activity of chemicals as an example. Several materials such as melamine or cyclamate will precipitate in the bladder. This precipitate can irritate the walls of the bladder and cause tumors to be produced. Very seldom does the incidence of tumors produced by this mechanism exceed 15% even at doses like

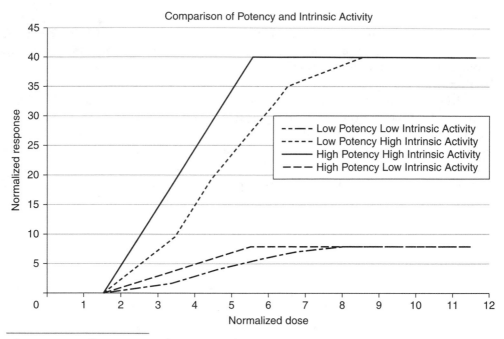

Figure 15-1 Comparison of potency and intrinsic activity.

6000 ppm in the diet (Melnick, Boorman, Haseman, Montali, & Huff, 1984; Heck & Tyl, 1985). In contrast, some aromatic amines cause bladder cancer in rats in 50% of the animals (Bioassay of 4,4′-Methylenebis-(N,N-dimethyl)benzeneamine, 1979).

Potency

Potency relates to the dose at which an effect is observed. The units of expression of potency are either expressions of doses where no responses occur or expressions at doses where a 50% response occurs. In the case of the doses with no response, the no observed adverse effect level (NOAEL) is used. This is dependent on the dose spacing and sensitivity of the assay to detect responses. The NOAEL is the experimental dose at which no adverse effect has been observed. This experimental point is highly dependent on the protocol, quality of data, experimental design, and sample size. The poorer the design, the lower the quality of the data or the smaller the sample size, the higher the NOAEL.

In the case of measuring 50% response, ED50 (effective dose in 50% of the population), LD50 (lethal dose to 50% of the population), or benchmark dose (BMD; a curve fitting exercise) is used (Bioassay of 4,4′-Methylenebis-(N,N-dimethyl)benzeneamine, 1979). These are the most reproducible experimental observations. Finally, a mathematical curve fitting can be used that will generate the best fitting curve. This takes into account all of the data points. This mathematical expression can then generate a theoretical 10% dose-response, which is the BMD. Since this is a mathematical curve fitting, virtually any dose can be used or the statistical bounds could also be used. In Figure 15-1, the ED50 is 4 while for the lower potency material it is 6.

The concepts of potency and intrinsic activity underscore the inability to compare the adverse effects of substances. Either potency or intrinsic activity can be a variable.

Legal and Ethical Issues

Laws and Regulations

Government in democratic nations is accomplished in two ways. Laws are passed by an elected legislature that provides direction for governance. Within these laws is the delegation of responsibility to or establishment of an executive agency for implementation and enforcement of these laws.

The executive agencies deal with the details of management of nations. As an example, the US Congress passed the Federal Insecticide, Pesticide and Rodenticide Act which gave the EPA control over the labeling of pesticides and the FDA responsibility for establishing limits (tolerances) for pesticides in food. This separation of authority between legislative and executive branches is not unique to the United States but is global in nature. Serious abuses in this system occur when there is no legislative branch to write the laws but when the executive branches write the laws, the regulations, and perform the enforcement. This system then leads to corruption and environmental deterioration.

Legal challenges to regulations, which make for interesting news, deal with whether the regulatory agency has the authority to perform a specific task as identified by legislation, or whether the regulatory agency has acted as described by law. Citizens may then challenge the regulatory enforcement on the basis that it was either not correctly carried out by law or that the law did not authorize the agency to act the way it did. Perhaps the best example of regulation and legislation is the failed attempts of the FDA to regulate cigarette smoking. Clearly, the FDA is responsible for a major component of public health, and clearly cigarette smoking is counter to public health. However, there was no authorization in the Food, Drug, and Cosmetic Act to allow the FDA to regulate smoking. Cigarette smoke was neither food nor food additive. Congress chose not to change the legislation that could have authorized FDA regulation. It also was not a drug as there were no claims being made for cigarette smoke. It was only recently that the FDA embarked on regulating cigarettes smoke by declaring cigarettes as a drug delivery system, delivering nicotine as a drug (CDC, 2007; FDA, 1995). This allegation brought cigarettes under the Food, Drug, and Cosmetics Act and FDA regulation. Otherwise, independent of the adverse health effects of cigarettes, the FDA was powerless to regulate tobacco smoke.

Regulation vs. Ethics

Ethics become an issue when there are no laws or regulations to be enforced. The critical issue associated with ethical decisions lie in values. Values have many varied definitions.

These include moral values, ethical values, family values, religious values, and so on. Based on the soft and personal nature of values, interpreting them for environmental decision making is virtually impossible. Ethical considerations must either be converted to some form of regulation or not be major decision criteria for environmental issues. An example of an ethical decision is Proposition 6 in California, a regulation to ban consumption of horse meat (CDC, 2007; Promotion of horse slaughter, 1998). There was no public health issue involved in this proposition and no laws under which to regulate horse meat. The state made a decision that it was unethical to slaughter horses for the purpose of human consumption.

What Is the Environment?

Simply stated, the environment consists of the air we breathe, the water we drink, and the food we eat. Public health concerns about each of these are very different.

Air Pollution

There are four major classes of air-polluting gases. These are irritating chemicals, asphyxiating chemicals, air toxics, and atmospheric reactants.

Irritants

Irritants damage the surface of the respiratory tract. Highly water-soluble irritants such as formaldehyde cause irritation of the upper respiratory tract, and less water-soluble irritants such as nitrogen oxides, cause lower respiratory tract irritation. Hydrogen chloride is very water soluble and is an upper respiratory tract irritant. This causes effects in the nose, for example. As a response to upper respiratory tract irritants, individuals will hold their breath or breath more shallowly. The major chronic effect of upper respiratory tract irritants is loss of sense of smell through toxicity to the olfactory epithelium. Sulfur dioxide is also an upper respiratory tract irritant. It is extremely import to differentiate irritants from foul-smelling materials. Odor is not necessarily a characteristic of toxic vapors. Foul smells are designed to elicit an avoidance response.

Oxides of nitrogen such as nitrogen dioxide are lower respiratory tract irritants. Exposure to these substances is accompanied by chest pains. The other major environmental irritant gases are ozone and chlorine. These gases oxidize the lower respiratory tract. In each case there is fibrotic/scarring lesion in the irritated portion of the lung with an accompanying loss of function. They can also cause emphysema and other typical pulmonary lesions.

Asphyxiants

Asphyxiants cause suffocation or lack of oxygen transport to the body. The major asphyxiant is carbon monoxide. The result of carbon monoxide overexposure is a chemical asphyxiation. Carbon dioxide induces a similar response but at marked higher concentrations.

Toxics

The third class of pollutant gases is toxics. Toxics are gases that are absorbed through the lungs and have adverse systemic effects. For example, hydrogen cyanide has direct effects on the blood and not on the lungs. There are a wide variety of other materials that when inhaled produce systemic toxicity. Anesthetic and neurotoxic gases, such as ether and toluene, are in this class. Virtually any material when inhaled can be absorbed into the lung to some extent.

High molecular-weight polymers and water-insoluble chemicals are not absorbed. These materials are deposited into the lungs and remain there. They may be removed by a system that moves them up the trachea for excretion or to be swallowed. The body defenses against these materials may have a side effect of irritating the adjacent lung tissue. Macrophages are designed to kill bacteria in the lungs by producing peroxide. An effect of some particulates is to kill the macrophages and thereby cause peroxide in the lungs which is toxic.

Finally, exercise can accentuate lung toxicity through increase in the respiratory rate. With increased respiration, the dosage increases.

Atmospheric Reactants

Chemical reaction of pollutants with atmospheric constituents can induce serious environmental degradation. The two major classes of these are smog and greenhouse gases.

Smog. Photochemical smog is a concern in most major urban centers. Smog is caused by a reaction between sunlight and emissions, mainly from human activity such as automobile exhaust and fireplaces. Photochemical smog is the chemical reaction of sunlight, nitrogen oxides (NO_x) and volatile organic compounds (VOCs) in the atmosphere, which leaves airborne particles (called particulate matter) and ground-level ozone. Nitrogen oxides are released in the exhaust of fossil fuel-burning engines in cars, trucks, coal power plants, and industrial manufacturing factories. VOCs are vapors released from gasoline, paints, solvents, pesticides, and other chemicals.

Greenhouse Gases. Some organic substances, the most notable and avoidable being fully halogenated substances such as chlorofluorocarbons, decrease the atmospheric filter for sunshine. The greenhouse gases may interact with ozone, which filters sunlight and provides a stable temperature on Earth. Perhaps the most significant of these gases is carbon dioxide which is produced by burning fossil fuels and by the setting of concrete. Methane comes from livestock farming and rice paddies. Sunlight and other radiation form free radicals from methane and carbon dioxide, which then interact with ozone.

Water Pollution

Water Treatment—Trihaloalkanes

Pollution of drinking water can take the form of chemical or microbial contamination. Microbial contamination is beyond the context of this chapter, except that it necessitates chemical treatment of water. In the absence of chemical treatment, epidemics of cholera and typhus can occur, as well as *E. coli* infection. On a global basis water contamination is a leading cause of death as an inducer of diarrhea.

Treatment of microbial contamination is not difficult, but it is costly. It generally involves killing the organisms with chlorine, chlorine dioxide, or ozone. The costly part is not only the treatment phase but also the transport of the water to the site of use. In developing countries without water purification plants, boiling water is effective. In general, chemical oxidants are added to the water to sterilize it. Historically the most popular of these is chlorine. Chlorine is an inexpensive and effective agent for this purpose. The downside of chlorine use is that it is difficult and risky to transport and that one of the results of the chemical reaction between chlorine and the biological agents in water is the production of chloroform and other trihalomethanes that are carcinogens at high doses in experimental animals. Chemical reaction rate constants show that the bromine analogues—bromoforms—are also produced. For this reason, newer treatment facilities are using either peroxide or chloramine. Peroxide is very effective at eliminating other chlorination byproducts such as TCDD, which is among the most toxic of all organic chemicals and highly persistent. Paper mills, which may have a very high organic content waste, will use the more costly peroxide process to avoid TCDD production. Chloramine is also not without its disadvantages, as it appears to increase the level of nitrosamines in the water. Nitrosamines are highly carcinogenic chemicals more commonly found in nitrite-preserved meats. Evaluation and trade-off of these treatment methods is closely analogous to the ethical decisions discussed previously. Possibly the worst alternative is microbiological contamination. Only peroxide is without a potentially toxic sequella. Yet the concentrations of halogenated contaminants is very low and the nitrosamine concentration is less than 0.5% of dietary intake. Regulatory risk assessment methods assume that there is no risk-free dose.

Persistent Organics
Water contamination results in pollution from two sources. First and most obvious is drinking the water itself. Secondly, and not as obvious, are the seafood harvested from the water. The ability of materials to accumulate and persist in wildlife is a measurable characteristic of organic and inorganic chemicals. Some of the most recognizable of these persistent chemicals are DDT, PCBs, and TCDD. The environmental concern is not that these are toxic at ambient concentrations, but rather they can accumulate in biota to reach toxic levels as discussed earlier with methyl mercury. On a global basis these persistent organic pollutants are being banned with the same aggressiveness that those that cause global warming are being banned.

Clearly, low cost chlorination will continue to predominate in countries where social costs cannot be born by the economy. In the Western world, one of other methods will be selected.

Toxics

In the same way that there are toxic substances in the air, there can also be toxic substances in water. Toxics are defined as materials in water that exert toxic effects through systemic absorption. Establishing an acceptable dose for materials in water is difficult. In addition estimating consumption of water toxics is complicated. In the United States, individuals move frequently and their exposure to any particular drinking water source will be limited to 10 years. They will have an average consumption of 3 liters of water per day.

Toxics in drinking water include pesticides, heavy metals, nitrosamines, halogenated materials from chlorination, and other pollutants, depending on the area, ground water, purification, and so on. There is currently no way to remove metals from drinking water, so these represent a special problem. Symptomatology in a population exposed to chemically contaminated drinking water will not be restricted to a single individual but rather large numbers in the overall population. For example, contamination of water with large amounts of iron salts will result in liver and blood problems in many people. If a single individual is found, the causative agent is not likely from drinking water.

A special subset of this population is people who have wells. Since the well can be contaminated in its construction, use, or the water supply it accesses, a family can have toxic symptoms separate from the overall population. For example, a family in Japan lined its well with an acrylamide polymer that had not sufficiently polymerized to remove the acrylamide (Igisu, Glote, Kawamura, Kato, & Izumi, 1975). The entire family then came down with acrylamide neurotoxicity while the rest of the population remained healthy.

Biological Oxygen Demand

When microorganisms in water metabolize pollutants to nontoxic carbon dioxide, they utilize oxygen in this process. As a side note, the degradability of an organic chemical is measured as the demand it presents on oxygen. However, this oxygen depletion can be disastrous to animals in the water that require oxygen, such as fish. Fish kills can be caused by adding to water various nutrients that microorganisms metabolize, thus depleting the available oxygen. Another way to stimulate growth of oxygen-depleting organisms is to add a cofactor to the water that had previously been growth limiting. Runoff of phosphate from agricultural and suburban land provides much needed phosphate to algae that then grow and deplete oxygen. This reaction is ruinous to many lakes and estuaries such as the Everglades. Globally this problem is more extensive as the equation for the value of conservation versus agricultural production favors agricultural production in the developing world.

Food

Inclusion of food in this chapter is not meant to imply that food is toxic. However, food can serve as a source of pharmacologically active substances that must be considered in disease causation. These substances can arise through storage, manufacture, cooking, or as an integral part of the food being consumed. For example Guam inhabitants chew on cycad nuts (The cycad story extended, 1970). As a result these individuals have a disease similar to amyotrophic lateral sclerosis (ALS, also Lou Gehrig's disease).

There are two ways of looking at food contamination. Historically, epidemiologists have been primarily concerned with low levels of very potent contaminants. However, there may be an even higher risk associated with high levels of low potency substances. For example, the presence of nitrosamines in nitrite-preserved foodstuffs has been the subject of extensive research. These substances cause cancer at low doses in virtually every species tested including humans. However, their presence in foodstuffs appears so low that they do represent a public health risk. They are generally the result of food preservation by nitrite or conversion of nitrate to nitrite in the stomachs of neonates and subsequent in vivo nitrosation. They are found in low levels in drinking water as a result of chloramine purification, also. In contrast, polyunsaturated fatty acids are another cancer risk with very little animal data in support. But these chemicals are present in very high levels with very significant doses and even being of low potency may represent a much greater risk than the potent nitrosamines. The argument approaches absurdity when nitrosamines are compared with the use of salt. Salt represents a real public health problem, even as a naturally occurring substance (Hussein & Brasel, 2001).

Storage

Contamination of food during storage can be a major source of toxic substances. Peanuts provide perfect example of this problem. Peanuts, being approximately 50% fat, are an excellent substrate for mold growth. The mold *Aspergillus flavus* has been particularly well studied (Hussein & Brasel, 2001). This mold produces a unique metabolite, aflatoxin, which is amongst the most carcinogenic substances known. In many areas of the world, such as central Africa, this mold growth results in a substantial increase in liver cancer. There are areas of China with the same increased cancer incidence from aflatoxin consumption. Peanuts are not the only aflatoxin substrate. *Aspergillus* can grow on corn, wheat, and so on. The FDA monitors aflatoxin contamination very closely. Foodstuffs are carefully assayed for aflatoxin content.

There are many storage molds that produce very potent toxins (Howlett, 1996). A laundry list will not be provided as this list grows continually with the discovery of new molds.

Manufacture

Contamination of food and beverages by chemicals during manufacture is a heavily regulated issue in the developed world. Many developing nations follow US FDA or EU regulations for their internal food manufacture industries. The United States and the European Union have different approaches (Hattan & Kahl, 2002; Evaluation of certain food contaminants, 2006). In the United States, industry must supply FDA not only with safety information that is coordinated with expected exposure, but also with efficacy data in the case of direct food additives. Chemicals are evaluated on a single use basis. That is, if a chemical is used in more than one process, each process is evaluated independently. It is also evaluated independent of the food stuff. For example the fortification of breakfast cereals does not consider the presence of these nutrients in the milk added to the cereal.

In contrast, the EU has a list of substances that are accepted for food use. In addition the EU also has a list of chemicals not allowed for use in foods. Efficacy is not an issue in the EU.

An example is the addition of calcium to breakfast cereal. The FDA would consider the nutrient properties of calcium and set a standard for addition of calcium in breakfast cereal. It would not consider the calcium level in milk added to the breakfast cereal arguing that cereal can be consumed without milk. In the EU, calcium salts would be approved for use in foodstuffs. It may be added to cereal or even milk.

Cooking

The most apparent cooking contaminants are associated with grilling food at high temperatures. The charred surfaces of meats and other grilled food stuffs are rich in polynucleated aromatic hydrocarbons (PAHs). These materials are carcinogenic, mutagenic, and induce reproductive disorders at elevated concentrations. This chemistry occurs at elevated temperatures from all organics. For example in fires or automobile exhaust there can be high levels of these materials. They were highly significant air pollutants and are now tightly regulated in the developed world.

In contrast, heating amino acids, the major component of proteins, causes the production of heterocyclic amines (HCA). The major source is muscle meat. Epidemiologists have linked this cooking process with cancer of the stomach. Frying, broiling, and barbequing cause much more HCA production than baking or microwaving as they induce higher temperatures in the foodstuff.

In the same fashion as HCAs are produced by heating muscle meat at high temperatures, acrylamide is produced by heating starchy foods in excess of 230(F[24]. Acrylamide had long been established as a human neurotoxin due to its mishandling in industry. It is an industrial intermediate used in the manufacture of polymers for water treating, mining, paper manufacture, and sludge dewatering. Excessive heating of the amino acid asparagine in the presence of reducing sugars also produces acrylamide. In the mid 1980 acrylamide was found to cause cancer in laboratory rats and to influence chromosomal segregation in male reproductive tissue. It is found in greatest quantities in those starchy foods cooked at the highest temperatures such as potato chips. It is only this elevated cooking process that must necessarily drive out the water so that the temperature can exceed the boiling point of water. For example, acrylamide has been found in the crust of bread but not in the middle.

Saturated fatty acids have been found in low levels in meats. However in order to increase shelf life, foodstuffs have been treated with antioxidants to keep the unsaturated fatty acids from going rancid. This elevates the saturated fatty acid content. Saturated fatty acids have been associated with many maladies including memory loss and cancer.

Intrinsic Pharmacologically Active Chemicals
There is no end of naturally occurring chemicals in food that have pharmacological activity. For example the puffer fish in Japan is rich in tetrodotoxin. This substance is an extremely toxic neurotoxin. Preparation of this puffer fish must be done by a licensed individual who can remove the poisonous gland. Some mushrooms contain (α-aminitin, which became the anticancer drug amantadine. The presence of these agents has spawned an effort by the pharmaceutical industry to seek biological substances that occur naturally. The presence of these substances in foodstuffs does not have a large impact on the Western world where diets are relatively standard. But in the developing world, it is a different story. Consumption of cycad nuts in the Philippines has resulted in amyotrophic lateral sclerosis.

In the Western world concern about foodstuffs focuses on the materials that are present in large amounts and have low potency such as cholesterol. In the developing world, the more potent contaminants become more important. That is not to say that there is not also toxicity from low potency chemicals. Iron toxicity is rampant in some areas of China and Africa as a result of cooking in rusty pots.

Food allergies are another area where intrinsic properties of food represent serious medical hazards. To some individuals, peanuts are extremely toxic. The incidence of this is low, perhaps 1 per million. However with 300 million inhabitants in America, it is questionable whether this can be economically regulated (Schoessler, 2005).

Sustainable Development

According to the United Nations, sustainable development is the process of developing land, cities, business, communities, and so on, so that it "meets the needs of the present without compromising the ability of future generations to meet their own needs" (The environment becomes a political issue, 1988). One of the factors that sustainable development must overcome is environmental degradation, but it must do so without forgoing the needs of economic development, social equality, and justice. To accomplish this, a balance must be struck between industrial development, pollution control with an absence of environmental degradation, and attention to the needs for the future. We have discussed air pollution with its toxics and oxidants, water pollution with its toxics and persistent organic chemicals, and protecting our food supply. An unsustainable situation occurs when natural capital (the sum total of nature's resources) is used up faster than it can be replenished. Sustainability requires that human activity, at a minimum, only uses nature's resources at a rate at which they can be replenished naturally. Implicit in this concept is that pollution prevention is as important or more important than pollution development.

References

Aulerich, R. J., & Ringer, R. K. (1977). Current status of PCB toxicity to mink, and effect on their reproduction. *Archives of Environmental Contamination and Toxicology, 6*(2-3), 279–292.

Bioassay of 4,4'-Methylenebis-(N,N-dimethyl)benzeneamine for possible carcinogenicity (CAS No. 101-61-1). (1979). *National Toxicology Program Technical Report Service, 186*, 1–11.

Centers for Disease Control and Prevention (CDC). (2007). *Selected actions of the U.S. government regarding the regulation of tobacco sales, marketing, and use.* Atlanta, GA: Author.

CLS, C.o.L.S. (2000). *Toxicological effects of methylmercury.* Washington, DC: National Academy of Sciences.

Dodig, S., & Cepelak, I. (2004). The facts and controversies about selenium. *Acta Pharmacopeia. 54*(4), 261–276.

Evaluation of certain food contaminants. (2006). *World Health Organization Technical Reporting Service,* 930.

FDA. (1995). Regulations restricting the sale and distribution of cigarettes and smokeless tobacco products to protect children and adolescents; proposed rule regarding FDA's jurisdiction over nicotine-containing cigarettes and smokeless tobacco products; notice. *Federal Register,* p. 41314–41787.

Fishman, R. A. (2002). Polar bear liver, vitamin A, aquaporins, and pseudotumor cerebri. *Annals of Neurology, 52*(5), 531–533.

Hattan, D. G., & Kahl, L. S. (2002). Current developments in food additive toxicology in the USA. *Toxicology, 181–182*, 417–420.

Heck, H. D., & Tyl, R. W. (1985). The induction of bladder stones by terephthalic acid, dimethyl terephthalate, and melamine (2,4,6-triamino-s-triazine) and its relevance to risk assessment. *Regulatory Toxicology and Pharmacology, 5*(3), 294–313.

Howlett, J. (1996). ILSI Europe Workshop on Food Additive Intake: Scientific assessment of the regulatory requirements in Europe, 1995. Brussels summary report. *Food Additives and Contaminants, 13*(4), 385–395.

Hussein, H. S., & Brasel, J. M. (2001). Toxicity, metabolism, and impact of mycotoxins on humans and animals. *Toxicology, 167*(2), 101–134.

IARC. (1978). IARC monographs on the evaluation of the carcinogenic risk of chemicals to humans. Polychlorinated biphenyls and polybrominated biphenyls. *IARC Monograph Programme on the Evaluation of the Carcinogenic Risk of Chemicals to Humans, 18*.

Igisu, H., et al. (1975). Acrylamide encephaloneuropathy due to well water pollution. *Journal of Neurology, Neurosurgery, and Psychiatry, 38*(6), 581–584.

Mandal, P. K. (2005). Dioxin: a review of its environmental effects and its aryl hydrocarbon receptor biology. *Journal of Comparative Physiology, 175*(4), 221–230.

Melnick, R. L., Boorman, G. A., Haseman, J. K., Montali, R. J., & Huff, J. (1984). Urolithiasis and bladder carcinogenicity of melamine in rodents. *Toxicology and Applied Pharmacology, 72*(2), 292–303.

Prohibition of Horse Slaughter and Sale of Horse Meat for Human Consumption Act of 1998. California Proposition 6. 1998.

Rederstorff, M., Krol, A., & Lescure, A. (2006). Understanding the importance of selenium and selenoproteins in muscle function. *Cellular and Molecular Life Sciences, 63*(1), 52–59.

Russell, F. E. (1967). Vitamin A content of polar bear liver. *Toxicon, 5*(1), 61–62.

Rustam, H., & Hamdi, T. (1994). Methyl mercury poisoning in Iraq. A neurological study. *Brain, 97*(3), 500–510.

Schoessler, S. Z. (2005). The perils of peanuts. School Nurse News, 22(4), 22–26.

Shore, L. S., Gurevitz, M., & Semesh, M. (1993). Estrogen as an environmental pollutant. *Bulletin of Environmental Contamination and Toxicology, 51*(3), 361–366.

Takeuchi, T., D'Itri, F. M., Fischer, P. V., Annett, C. S., & Okabe, M. (1977). The outbreak of Minamata disease (methyl mercury poisoning) in cats on Northwestern Ontario reserves. *Environmental Research, 13*(2), 215–228.

The cycad story extended. (1970). *Food, Cosmetics, and Toxicology, 8*(2), 217–218.

The environment becomes a political issue. (1988). Highlights of the Brundtland Commission Report. *UN Chronicles, 25*(1), 38–39.

Volpe, M. (2004). Hypertension therapy: mixing, matching, and meeting targets. *Advances in Therapy, 21*(2), 107–122.

Chapter 16

Global Health in Reproduction and Infants

Carol Holtz

Suzanne Grisdale

This chapter will address the international health issues related to male and female reproduction, which includes human rights and public policy, infertility, family planning (contraception), pregnancy, childbirth, and infant health. These issues will relate health beliefs, customs, practices, and issues in both developed and developing countries.

Background

According to the Alan Guttmacher Institute (2003), sustained and increased investment in reproductive health services increases benefits to women, families, and societies. In addition, it contributes to general economic growth of a nation, equality in gender, and democratic governance. Poor or inadequate sexual and reproductive health contributes to one third of the world's burden of disease for women of childbearing age and one fifth of the total world population. The greatest need is among the poorest people in the developing countries. Improved contraception in developing countries could prevent 52 million unintended pregnancies.

Alam and Ashraf, within the UN, plead for better reproductive health in poor nations. They reveal the reproductive health challenges of today in developing countries as where they state, "Today in developing countries, poor reproductive health is responsible for one fifth of the burden of disease and 40% in sub-Saharan Africa. Poverty, poor health, and fertility are still the highest in the least developed countries where the population has tripled since 1955 and will triple again in the next 50 years" (Alam & Ashraf, 2003, p. 1843).

The Global Burden of Disease Initiative, which was developed by the World Health Organization (WHO), the World Bank, and the Harvard School of Public Health, began the estimation of world health impact from major diseases and behaviors, including reproduction and sexual behavior. Other efforts focused on the economic costs and benefits of health interventions. Sexual and reproductive health issues represent 18% of the world's total burden of disease and 32% of the burden of women of childbearing age (15–44 years). Medical benefits of health interventions can be measured by *disability adjusted life years* (DALYs). This is a measure developed by the Global Burden of Disease project to evaluate potential health interventions. Maternal causes, such as hemorrhage or sepsis, problems with labor, or abortion cause 13% of all DALYs lost by childbearing-aged women. Perinatal causes, such as low birth weight or birth trauma are responsible for 7% of all DALYs lost. For example, the increased use of contraception from 0% to 20% in sub-Saharan Africa is highly cost-effective in preventing many maternal and infant health problems and deaths (Alan Guttmacher Institute, 2003).

Germain (2004, p. 65) states, "One of the greatest disparities between rich and poor countries is maternal mortality." The risk of dying from pregnancy in sub-Saharan Africa is 1 in 16. This compares to 1 in 4000 in many European countries. Seventy percent of the world's maternal mortality occurs in only 13 countries. Greater than 500,000 women of childbearing age die every year from causes related to pregnancy and childbirth. In addition, 3.9 million babies die within the first month of life. Countries with poor maternal and infant health generally have weak healthcare systems, are in a social crisis, or both. Sex discrimination and lack of healthcare services, lack of equal rights, and lack of power for women all contribute to this health problem. Violence against women, rape, and sexual coercion threaten women's human rights and reproduction (Germain, 2004).

Progress has been made in various areas of reproductive health. The global population growth rate has slowed to 77 million people per year, but while fertility rates have decreased in some countries, such as Mexico, they are still very high in other countries, such as Ethiopia. Contraceptive use has increased, but now an estimated 201 million women in developing countries have unmet needs for birth control, and 60 million unplanned pregnancies occur annually. About 19 million unsafe abortions occur each year. More people are aware of sexually transmitted diseases; yet about 340 million people worldwide still have great concerns about sexually transmitted diseases (STDs). Infant mortality rates have improved somewhat, yet at least 529,000 women die each year from pregnancy or childbirth complications. The highest rates are for those women living in sub-Saharan Africa, where 920 maternal deaths per 100,000 live births occur each year in contrast to the rate of 24 deaths per 100,000 live births in Europe (Feki, 2004).

Definition of Reproductive Health

At the 21st session of the United Nations General Assembly in 1999, an overall plan for reproductive health and rights, called the Programme of Action, was created. Governments were asked to work in cooperation with nongovernmental organizations (NGOs) and to increase investments to improve quality of reproductive health. According to the United Nations Conference on Population and Development, the following is a definition of reproductive health:

> Reproductive health is a state of complete physical, mental, and social well-being and not merely the absence of disease or infirmity, in all matters relating to the reproductive system and to its functions and processes. Reproductive health therefore implies that people are able to have a satisfying and safe sex life and that they

have the capability to reproduce and freedom to decide if, when, and how often to do so. Implicit in the last condition are the rights of men and women to be informed and to have access to safe, effective, affordable, and acceptable methods of family planning of their choice, as well as other methods of their choice for regulation of fertility that are not against the law, and the right of access to appropriate health-care services that will enable women to go safely through pregnancy and childbirth and provide couples with the best chance of having a healthy infant. In line with the above definition of reproductive health, reproductive health care is defined as the constellation of methods, techniques, and services that contribute to reproductive well-being by preventing and solving reproductive health problems. It also includes sexual health, the purpose of which is the enhancement of life and personal relations and not merely counseling and care related to reproduction and sexually transmitted diseases (United Nations, 2004).

Murphy (2003) suggests that gender inequality results in poor reproductive and mental health outcomes, including unwanted pregnancy, unsafe abortions, maternal mortality, STDs, and depression. In poor countries with strong male dominance, women usually have little control of their sex lives, are rarely able to choose with whom to marry, when to have sex, how many children to have, or whether to use contraception or protection against sexually transmitted diseases. Men are often permitted to have multiple sex partners, and women remain ignorant and passive about sexuality, thus increasing their risk of exposure to HIV and other sexually transmitted diseases. Women often internalize the local cultural norm that they are inferior to males. This may also reflect female feticide and infanticide in some countries. Women's greater rate of malnutrition contributes to maternal and infant mortality. Pregnant women who are also malnourished have low-birth-weight babies. During pregnancy the women may have anemia, making them vulnerable to postpartal hemorrhage, leading to shock and death.

Reproductive Rights

According to the United Nations' Programme of Action of the International Conference on Population and Development, 1995, para.7.3, as cited in *World Population Monitoring 2002* (United Nations, 2004):

> Reproductive rights embrace certain human rights that are already recognized in national laws, international human rights documents, and other consensus documents. These rights rest on the recognition of the basic right of all couples and individuals to decide freely and responsibly the number, spacing, and timing of their children and to have the information and means to do so, and the right to attain the highest standard of sexual and reproductive health. It also includes their right to make decisions concerning reproduction free of discrimination, coercion, and violence, as expressed in human rights documents. . . . The promotion of the

responsible exercise of these rights for all people should be the fundamental basis for government- and community-supported policies and programs in the area of reproductive health, including family planning. As part of their commitment, full attention should be given to the promotion of mutually respectful and equitable gender relations and particularly to meeting the educational and service needs of adolescents to enable them to deal in a positive and responsible way with their sexuality.

Reflecting upon the above UN document, the key issues of reproductive human rights consist of the following: (1) family planning, (2) adolescent issues, (3) reproductive rights, (4) HIV/AIDS, and (5) violence against women.

An example of lack of personal reproductive rights is reflected by the following law in China. On June 1, 1995, the Chinese government passed the Maternal and Infant Health Care Law to decrease the number of congenital anomalies (birth defects) in the country. This law requires that couples obtain a premarital exam for serious genetic diseases and "relevant medical disorders," as well as prenatal testing. If a serious disorder is found the law dictates that long-term contraception or sterilization must take place or the couple may not marry. People who have diseases or problems such as schizophrenia, psychoses, leprosy, HIV/AIDS, and sexually transmitted diseases are subject to this law. Within this law is also a mandated right for all pregnant women to have the right to prenatal care, which includes education about pregnancy and general health care, and health care for the newborn. Encouragement is given to the couple to electively abort a pregnancy in which a fetus is known to have a serious genetic disorder or a serious defect, or a pregnancy in which the life of the mother may be jeopardized from the pregnancy (Law of the People's Republic of China on Maternal and Infant Care, 1995).

Also in China women lack personal rights to bear more than one child without permission from the government. Rural women are allowed one or two children, and ethnic minority women have fewer restrictions. For women of the majority Han ethnicity, if a second child is permitted, it is usually to be spaced 4–5 years after the first child is born. In some rural communities, if the first child is a girl, permission is given for a second child. Pregnant women who do not have permission from the government for the birth of a child may go outside their residential area to give birth and hide this birth. These women do not get any prenatal care or have a skilled birth attendant. They expect to pay a fine, but they are able to avoid being forced to terminate the pregnancy against their wishes (Short & Zhang, 2004).

Adolescent Reproductive Health

Adolescents and young adults often face a transition into adulthood with insufficient knowledge and experience. It is important to educate them for effective health promotion and prevention of diseases and unwanted pregnancies. Menarche (the age at which reproduction is physically possible) varies greatly across societies. From a recent study of

67 countries, findings conclude that menarche is reached early in developed societies as compared to developing societies. It is associated with socioeconomic class, literacy rates, and nutrition. The onset of sexual activity today typically takes place during adolescence, a period of growth, experimentation, and identity search. Lack of access to health information may be due to social, cultural, and sometimes legal barriers. This results in adolescents who are often poorly informed and do not make responsible choices, which may lead to sexual and reproductive health problems (United Nations, 2004).

In the United States about one million adolescents, ages 11–19, become pregnant every year and 500,000 give birth. These pregnancies account for 13% of all births. Data show a decline in teen pregnancies and births in recent years. Yet, in the United States teen childbirth rates are at least five times greater than teens of other Western countries. Increases in rates of teen pregnancies contribute to the overall increased rates of premature labor, low-birth-weight babies, and perinatal mortality. African-American teens have the highest rates of pregnancy complications when compared to other racial groups. In addition, older African-American pregnant women (20–29) also had higher rates of prematurity, low birth weights, and infant mortality when compared to older Caucasian women (Gilbert, Jandial, Field, Bigelow, & Danielsen, 2004).

Sexual activity in the United States among younger teenage girls and boys has declined in recent years, and contraception use for teenagers has increased. According to a study by the US Department of Health and Human Services, sexual activity rates for females who have never married, ages 15–17, dropped from 38% in 1995 to 30% in 2002. More teenagers are avoiding or postponing sexual activity, which can lead to sexually transmitted diseases, unwanted pregnancy, or emotional experiences that they are not prepared to handle. Today sexually active teens are also more likely to use contraception, and this has led to decreases in teen pregnancy and birth rates (National Center for Health Statistics, 2004a).

The decline in the US teen birth rates has been attributed to delayed initial sexual activity, increased use of contraception, and education about the HIV virus and pregnancy prevention. Compared to nonpregnant teenagers, teenage mothers are less likely to graduate from high school, are more likely to score below average in language and reading skills, have lower self-esteem, and have more symptoms of depression. Children of adolescent mothers are at greater risk for prematurity, low birth weight, child abuse, neglect, and poverty. Seventy-five percent of teenage mothers receive public assistance within 5 years of delivering a baby. Costs for society to provide health care, food, housing, employment training, and foster care are $7 billion per year. Many prevention programs are initiated to reduce the number of pregnancies and STD rates among adolescents. They attempt to increase social skills, promote educational goals, and support open communication between parents and teens. Abstinence-only programs teach that abstinence is the only certain way to avoid unmarried pregnancy, STDs, and other health problems. However, most abstinence-only programs have failed to show significant improvement in rates of sexual intercourse or pregnancy (As-Sanie, Gantt, & Rosenthal, 2004).

Jones and Boonstra (2004) report the results of a study regarding confidential reproductive health services for minors. They concluded that recent legislative efforts to mandate parental involvement for minor adolescents seeking birth control may contribute to increase rates of teenage pregnancy. They state that, instead, voluntary parental involvement is needed.

An estimated 14 million young women worldwide, ages 15 to 19, gave birth each year from 1995 to 2000, and 12.8 million of those adolescent women were from developing countries. Adolescent women in developed countries give birth at a rate of 29 per 1000 women, while in developing countries the rate is 133 per 1,000 women, with adolescent women in Africa having the highest rates. In many countries in Asia, increases in age in marriage and low incidences of premarital childbearing resulted in low rates of adolescent pregnancies (United Nations, 2004).

In most developed countries of the world the majority of teenagers become sexually active, and at least 75% have had sexual intercourse by the time they are 20 years old. Teenagers in the United States are becoming sexually active and with more partners, as compared to teenagers of other developed countries such as Canada, Sweden, France, and the United Kingdom. Teenagers in the United States also have a high rate of pregnancy, childbearing, and abortion as compared to other developed countries. A major factor is that the US teenagers use fewer types of contraception than teens in other developed countries. This decrease in use is due to negative attitudes toward teen sexual activity and restriction of access to reproductive health services as well as lack of motivation to prevent pregnancy (Alan Guttmacher Institute, 2004).

Teenage pregnancy rates have declined during the last 25 years in developed countries due to high motivation to complete education and get employment experience before having a baby. Teens have greater sex education and access to contraception. Adolescent pregnancy rates vary greatly among countries, with an exceptionally high rate of 102 per 1000 (15 to 19 years old) in the Russian Federation and a lower rate of 12 per 1000 (15 to 19 years old) in the Netherlands. The United States, Belarus, Bulgaria, Romania, and the Russian Federation have a teen pregnancy rate of 70 or more per 1000 (15 to 19 years old). Childbearing (birthing) rates in developed countries vary from a low of 3.9 per 1000 in Japan, to a high of 54.4 in several countries including the United States (Alan Guttmacher Institute, 2004).

Abortion rates for teenagers in developed countries also vary greatly from a rate of 10–20 per 1000 (15 to 19 years old) in the Czech Republic, Denmark, England, Wales, Finland, Norway, and Sweden to a high rate of 56 per 1000 (15 to 19 year olds) in the Russian Federation. The youngest adolescents are more likely than older ones to have an abortion (Alan Guttmacher Institute, 2004).

Sexually transmitted diseases disproportionately affect teenagers as compared to older women of childbearing age. Syphilis, gonorrhea, and chlamydia are the most common STDs in teens. The United States has higher rates of STDs than other developed countries such as England, France, Canada, and Sweden. This is due to lower use of condoms and higher numbers of sexual partners by US teenagers (Alan Guttmacher Institute, 2004).

Cultural Influences

Muslim culture directly affects programs and policies involving adolescent reproductive health. Islamic law condemns prostitution, homosexuality, and premarital sex. The interpretation of the Koran presents challenges for the reproductive health programs for teenagers. Some religions in Morocco, a mostly Muslim country in northern Africa, oppose sex education and condom promotion for unmarried adolescent use, while others stress that the Hadith includes clear guidelines for sex education. In Iran in the late 1980s fatwas declared that family planning methods were allowed. In Egypt since the 1960s all major family planning and reproduction health programs have worked with religious leaders and supported family planning. Morocco and Tunisia tend to encourage nongovernment organizations (NGOs) to target the population's adolescent health issues and problems (Beamish & Abderrazik, 2003).

Fertility

Age of childbearing varies greatly among countries. In Africa ages of women who are bearing children are evenly distributed between younger and older women, but in most other major areas of the world the majority (two thirds) of childbearing takes place before age 30. In many developed countries today, the age at which women have their first child has increased. They are having children later in life and having fewer children than previous generations. This has resulted in a below-replacement fertility rate in many developed countries. Lower fertility rates in developed countries are caused by industrialization, urbanization, modernization of societies, improved access to education, improved survival of children, and increased use of contraception (United Nations, 2004).

Men are physiologically capable of reproducing longer than women and often marry later and become fathers at older ages than women. Women, who have children closely spaced in age and give birth at ages less than 18 years, or older than 34 years, have higher risks of morbidity and mortality for both themselves and their babies (United Nations, 2004).

Culture

In the Arab culture the bride's status in her husband's household is unstable until she gives birth to her first baby and proves that she is fertile, and then she is obligated to have a second child because of the fear that an only child may die and leave the parents childless. After the second child is born the pressure to continue having children exists if there are only female children. Women are expected to continue having children until at least one son is born. The need to have a male child is great, in order to preserve the family name. Muslims believe that their religion requires them "to be fruitful and multiply" (Kridli, 2002).

Infertility

Infertility is the biological failure to conceive by normal sexual activity without contraception or to carry a pregnancy to full term, affecting both men and women of reproductive age. This is in contrast to intentional childlessness that may be due to cultural, social, economic, or psychological factors. The infertility rates are especially high in sub-Saharan Africa where many have reproductive tract infections caused by STDs, particularly gonorrhea, and HIV infections. Unsafe abortions may also be responsible for infertility problems to those in countries with transition economies. In developed countries infertility is higher than expected in spite of available legal abortions and treatment of STDs. This infertility is mainly due to significant delays in childbearing. In many cultures infertility causes stress, social exclusion, and stigma. In some cultures, women who are infertile, may be divorced, neglected, abused, and given lower social status. Universally, infertility usually results in serious psychological stress for the couple. Approximately 8–12% of couples worldwide experience infertility problems of some type (United Nations, 2004).

In the United State about 6.1 million Americans or 10% of all people of reproductive age are affected by this problem. Testing for men begins with an analysis of the semen, looking at number, shape, and movement. Sometimes hormones are also tested. For women, checks for ovulation may be done. Depending on the test results, different types of treatments can be performed. Between 85% and 90% of infertile couples can be treated with drugs or surgery. Assisted reproductive therapy (ART) uses special methods to help infertile couples, involving the woman's eggs and the male sperm. These procedures are often very expensive and are not usually covered by health insurance. Donor eggs or frozen embryo are sometimes used (United Nations, 2004).

Cultural and Religious Issues

Religion and culture are often major influences on sexuality and reproduction. According to Jewish law an infertile couple should undergo diagnosis and treatment. Christianity states that marriage does not confer upon spouses the duty to have a child, but the right to have intercourse. Sterility can be an occasion for other important services to humanity such as adoption, educational work, assistance to families, and to disadvantaged children. Polygamy is practiced today in many Islamic societies, which creates more opportunities for fertility within a family structure. According to the Jewish culture and religion, most infertile couples will do almost anything to have a child, including the use of reproductive technology. Israel, a predominately Jewish country, is one of the leading countries of the world in the research and development of reproductive technology. Insemination of husband's sperm is permitted, and some groups of Jews permit insemination of another man's sperm if absolutely necessary. In vitro fertilization and embryo transfer are also permitted by most groups of Jewish people. The Roman Catholic church states that assisted reproduction, including artificial insemination, in vitro fertilization, and embryo transfer are not allowed. Most religious groups have more liberal attitudes toward infertility interventions and treatments. Islam allows all treatments for infertility as long as it only involves the husband and wife. Adoption is not permitted. Within Judaism, fetal reduction for multiple gestation pregnancies is allowed by most Jews. Catholics consider this an abortion, which is not permitted. In Islam fetal reduction is allowed if the other fetuses or the mother's life is in jeopardy (Schenker, 2005).

The moral status of the human embryo is quite controversial in the United States. Embryos created in the in vitro fertilization (IVF) clinics are not all used for pregnancy implantation. Clinics could put "extra" created embryos in cryopreservation, as donated for reproductive use for couples, research, or disposal. Disposal of excess embryos creates many moral and ethical issues, which are widely debated. Currently about 400,000 embryos are frozen in storage in the United States, and many others exist in other countries as well. Depending on the culture, religion, and geographic location, human embryos are considered to be anything from a cluster of cells to an actual human being (Gurmankin, Sisti, & Caplan, 2004).

Family Planning and Contraception

Family planning allows people to decide the number, spacing, and timing of the birth of their children. Research clearly links adequate spacing of the birth of children with decreased maternal and infant morbidity and mortality. At present, 60% of the world's individuals or couples use family planning as compared to 10% in the 1960s (Table 16-1). Contraception is the intentional prevention of a pregnancy by natural or artificial methods. Family planning and contraception use are closely correlated to women or couple's urbanization, education, socioeconomic status, and approval by culture.

TABLE 16-1 Worldwide Contraceptive Use

Country	Percentage of Population Using Contraceptives (%)
Africa	<10
Eastern Europe	35
Russian Federation	70–74
Western Europe	71–77
Latin America	73
United States	82
China	83

Source: United Nations, 2004.

From a survey of women 15–44 years of age in the United States, the most common forms of contraception are as follows:

- Oral contraceptive pill
- Female sterilization
- Male condom
- Male sterilization
- Injectable Depo-Provera

Nearly 98% of all women who have had sexual intercourse have used at least one type of contraception (National Center for Health Statistics, 2004a).

A recent study of five European countries, France, Germany, Italy, Spain, and the United Kingdom, was conducted to determine contraceptive use. Results indicated that oral contraceptives were the most frequently used method. Male and female sterilization were the most widely used methods of the 40 years and older age groups, while 23% of the subjects did not practice contraception at all (Skouby, 2004).

According to a United Nations report, in China premarital sex is no longer taboo, and norms and behaviors are changing. Most sexually active people do not want a pregnancy, yet many lack knowledge of contraception. Many unmarried women are embarrassed about obtaining contraception and do not want their sexual activity to be revealed. Many believe that family planning centers are for married women only, yet the government has made these services available to all (United Nations, 2004).

In Diandong County within the Yunnan province of China, the population is predominately Han Chinese, and 94% work in agriculture. The current population policy permits rural couples to have two children, with a spacing of 4–5 years between children. Couples who exceed the birth quota may be fined from US$374 to US$500. The majority of women believe that having a son is extremely important. Female infants were much more likely to die than male infants. Deaths of female infants were often unrelated to illness or disease. Women with "unapproved by government" births were found to be less likely to get adequate prenatal and postpartal care than women with "approved by government" births (Li, 2004).

According to a Muslim jurist, who uses the Quran, a fatwa (ruling) related to family planning in Islam, family planning is permitted. There is a wide variation in opinion of Muslim authorities regarding family planning. There are today some Muslims who do not believe in family planning and state that children are a great asset, and the larger the number of Muslims, the greater the power. Today, the higher court in Jordan believes that family planning is acceptable in Islam, yet decisions are left to the couple (Hasna, 2003).

Mogilevkina and Odlind (2003) report that historically in the Ukraine, as in other countries of the former Soviet Union (now known as the Commonwealth of Independent States), abortion was used as a method of birth control. This policy reflected negative attitudes towards contraception. Their data from 1999 showed that the abortion ratio was

121 per 100 deliveries, and the abortion rate was 36.7 per 1000 women of reproductive age. Today, contraception services are increasing, yet abortion remains common and 32.5% of women do not use any form of contraception.

Emergency Contraception

One example of a moral dilemma regarding emergency contraception, reported by Zwillich (2005), states that in the United States a small group of conservative pharmacists refuse to fill prescriptions for the emergency contraception medication called levonorgestrel sold by Barr Pharmaceuticals Inc., which prevents pregnancy when taken within 72 hours of unprotected sex. The drug works by inhibiting ovulation, interfering with fertilization, and blocking implantation in the wall of the uterus.

Abortion

Definition

Elective abortion is the voluntary termination of a pregnancy, which in most cases, is done prior to viability of the fetus. In 1973, the United States Supreme Court ruled that induced abortions must be legal in all states as long as the pregnancy is under 12 weeks. Individual states can regulate abortion in a second trimester pregnancy and prohibit abortion that is not life threatening. In the third trimester of pregnancy some states can also mandate additional regulations regarding the procedure, such as requiring a 24-hour waiting period for counseling or requiring parental approval for minors (Childbirth by Choice Trust, 1999).

History of Elective Abortion

According to the Childbirth by Choice Trust (1999) abortion has been practiced in almost all regions throughout the world since the earliest of time. Women have been faced with unwanted pregnancies and have chosen to abort a fetus regardless of religious or legal sanction and often risk their lives in the process. In primitive societies abortions were induced by poisons, herbs, sharp sticks, and pressure on the abdomen, causing vaginal bleeding. Ancient Chinese and Egyptians used surgical instruments, much like modern ones of today. Socrates, Plato, and Aristotle were known to suggest abortion, while Hippocrates recommended it on occasion. St. Augustine (354–430 A.D.) related that the animation and sensation occurred at 40 days after conception. Prior to the first 40 days, abortion was not considered homicide. Pope Innocent III wrote that quickening, the time of perception of fetal movement, was the moment that abortion became homicide. In 1869 Pope Pius IX, declared excommunication for those who had an abortion at any stage of fetal development. From the late 1800s until World War II, abortion was restricted almost everywhere in the world. Later, countries in Eastern and Central Europe relaxed some of the laws, followed by most of the developed countries during the 1960s and 1970s (Childbirth by Choice Trust, 1999).

World Perspectives

At present, two thirds of the world's population allows abortion upon request. Abortions are carried out in every country in the world regardless of the law. In places where it is prohibited (such as Muslim Asia, Latin America, and Africa) hidden abortions are a significant health problem to women. Maternal deaths occur as a result of hidden abortions that can cause hemorrhage, bleeding, infection, and damage to reproductive organs (Childbirth by Choice Trust, 1999).

Worldwide, nations have different ways of addressing the rules and regulations regarding abortion. In 1997 South Africa established a woman's right to an abortion upon request up to 12 weeks of gestation. It allows abortion through 20 weeks of pregnancy if the mother's physical or mental health is endangered. A program was established to train licensed registered midwives to perform them at primary care facilities (Dickson-Tetteh & Billings, (2002). In Mexico elective abortion is a well-publicized issue, and is punished by law, which dates back to 1931. Mexico has no clear law regarding abortion. Exception is made for saving a mother's life, or if the pregnancy was a result of rape. In some states if a fetus is severely malformed an abortion can be done legally. The state of Yucatan accepts economic reasons as valid for having a legal abortion. Currently the federal government labels those who have many children and are economically poor, as irresponsible. In spite of the public and government attitudes about elective abortion, as many as 850,000 induced abortions are performed each year, both legally and illegally (Castaneda, Billings, & Blanco, 2003; Erviti, Castro, & Collado, 2004).

The statistics regarding abortion are dependent upon the country's legal status on this issue. In many countries throughout the world including the United States, where abortion is legal, reporting of statistics is not always required, and therefore data collection and reporting may be very difficult (see Table 16-2).

About 15 million legal abortions are performed annually, with China, the Russian Federation, the United States, and Viet Nam performing 80% of the world's legal abortions (United Nations, 2004).

Greater numbers of women from North America, Western Europe, Australia, New Zealand, and Latin America (with the exception of Brazil) who have elective abortions are unmarried, as compared to women of Eastern Europe and the former Soviet Union, who are mostly married. In countries such as Germany, Hungary, Israel, Italy, and the Netherlands, about half are married and half are unmarried. In some societies, abortion is used as a method of family planning, especially among married women. In most countries women in their twenties have the highest pregnancy rates and also the highest rates of abortions. Abortion is legal in many areas of the world, yet the criteria varies. Some countries only permit abortions to save the woman's life. The laws are generally more restrictive in the developing world than in the developed nations. Unsafe abortion is the

TABLE 16-2   Abortion Rates of 14–44-Year-Olds, 1999

Countries	Abortion Rates (%)
Soviet Union (the Russian Federation, Belarus, and the Ukraine)	> 60
Estonia, Romania, Bulgaria, and Latvia	50–59
Republic of Moldova, Viet Nam, Hungary, and Kazakhstan	40–49
Lithuania, Slovenia, Czech Republic, Armenia, Georgia, China, Slovakia, Sweden, Croatia, Turkmenistan, and Canada	30–39
Macedonia, Singapore, Australia, United States, Japan, New Zealand, United Kingdom, Italy, Denmark, Norway, and France	20–29
Germany, Spain, Israel, Tajikistan, the Netherlands, Belgium, and Uzbekistan	10–19
Brazil, Chile	4.1
Chile	5
Columbia	3.6
Dominican Republic	4.7
Peru	5.6
Mexico	2.5

Source: United Nations, 2004.

termination of a pregnancy by a person lacking the necessary skills or in an environment lacking minimal medical standards. In countries where abortion is strictly illegal or very restrictive, unsafe abortions are performed against the law and can also cause unnecessary morbidities and mortalities. Globally, 1 in 8 maternal deaths are due to an unsafe abortion. The highest rates of deaths by unsafe abortions are in Africa with a rate of 7 deaths per 1000 of unsafe abortions, followed by Asia with 4 deaths per 1000 of unsafe abortions. The most frequent complications from unsafe abortions are sepsis, incomplete abortion, hemorrhage, and abdominal cavity injury (United Nations, 2004).

Fifty million abortions take place every year in the world, which end 25% of all pregnancies worldwide. Of these abortions, 20 million are unsafe, and 95% of those unsafe occur in developing countries. Unsafe abortions cause 80,000 maternal deaths per year, while others who survive may suffer blood loss, pain, infection, damage to internal organs, and infertility (Murphy, 2003).

According to a study conducted by Lofstedt, Shusheng, and Johansson (2004), in China high gender ratios of males at birth are due to abortion practices. Between 1984 and 1987 rates of abortions for female fetuses in Huaning County, Yunnan Province, in

China increased, creating a ratio of 107 males to 100 females, while between the period from 1988–2000 the ratio rose again to 110 males to 100 females.

Maternal Mortality and Morbidity

Maternal mortality is a major global problem that affects families and society as a whole. Obstetrical complications are the leading cause of death for women of reproductive age in developing countries today. Tragically, despite progress in some countries, an estimated 529,000 deaths occur each year. Ninety-nine percent of these deaths occur in developing countries and most could be prevented. Maternal health services and maternal mortality rates are very specific indicators of the general functioning of healthcare systems of a country. A maternal death is defined as the death of a woman while pregnant or within 42 days after the termination of a pregnancy. This is irrespective of the duration, site, cause, or management of the pregnancy. *Direct maternal deaths* are due to obstetrical complications during pregnancy, labor and delivery, or post partum. It may be related to interventions, omissions, incorrect treatment, or other events. Examples are sepsis, pregnancy induced hypertension, or delivery complications. *Indirect maternal deaths* are due to a previous existing disease or from a disease that developed during pregnancy, yet not directly due to obstetrical causes. It may be a disease that was exacerbated during pregnancy. Examples include malaria, HIV/AIDS, or cardiovascular disease (United Nations Population Fund [UNFPA], 2004).

A common indicator is the *maternal mortality rate*, which is the number of maternal deaths per 100,000 woman of reproductive age for a specific period of time, which is usually one year. There are numerous problems related to getting accurate data because many countries do not indicate on the death certificate that a woman was pregnant or recently pregnant. In addition, there is a significant amount of underreporting and misclassification of actual deaths. The causes of maternal mortality worldwide are ranked in this list:

1. Hemorrhage

2. Sepsis

3. Hypertensive disorders

4. Abortion complications

5. Obstructive labor

In addition to deaths, many women suffer complications that have long term effects. For example, a woman could get an amniotic fluid embolism or a cerebrovascular disorder causing a chronic disability; or a hemorrhage necessitating a hysterectomy, resulting in early loss of fertility. Family planning, good nutrition, and prenatal care have been shown to reduce maternal mortality (Horon, 2005; United Nations, 2004).

A close relationship exists between the maternal mortality ratios and proportion of births attended by skilled health personnel. A skilled health person can be a midwife, physician, or nurse who has skills needed to manage normal (uncomplicated) pregnancies, deliveries, and postpartal care. Worldwide 63.3% of all births are attended by a skilled healthcare worker. However, traditional birth attendants, whether trained or not, are not counted in this category of healthcare workers (WHO, 2005a).

According to Graham and Hussein (2004), women who die as a result of pregnancy or childbirth are often not counted in statistics. Approximately 500,000 women, worldwide, die each year due to maternal causes. Underreporting of these deaths ranges from 17% to 63% in developing countries, yet even in developed nations such as the United Kingdom, 19% of the maternal deaths did not report causes. In most developed countries, misclassification, rather than total omission, is the major problem.

One successful example of a significant drop in maternal mortality rate is in Egypt. A 52% decrease occurred from 1992 to 2000. In addition to their prenatal care education about birth, self-care during pregnancy, and danger signs, many of the women also received higher education during the same time period. This also allowed them to get better jobs, and receive better health benefits (Campbell et al., 2005).

Cambodia also has attempted to decrease its exceptionally high maternal mortality rate. Many mothers needlessly die from unsanitary water, poor sanitation, and lack of basic health care. Cambodia has a maternal mortality rate of 450 per 100,000 live births, one of the highest in the world. The infant mortality rate is also high at 166 per 1000 live births. Life expectancy at birth is 47.5 years. As of 2005, only 9% of pregnant women have more than four prenatal checkups, and 44% have only one. The majority (68%) of deliveries still take place without any birth attendants. A special program by the Reproductive and Child Health Alliance, a nongovernment organization, has worked to increase the skills of lay birth attendants and to encourage births at health centers (Chatterjee, 2005).

After 20 years of war and conflict, women in Afghanistan have tremendous needs. According to the 2000 estimates, the maternal mortality rate in Afghanistan is the second highest in the world, after Sierra Leone with 1900 per 100,000 live births. Afghanistan has a maternal mortality rate of 1600 deaths per 100,000 live births. Women in Afghanistan have limited access to quality health services, adequate food, shelter, and clean water. In addition the women have lack of choices for marriage partners, access to birth control, or rights to not be beaten by their husbands when disobeying them. Causes of this high rate of maternal mortality in Afghan women are due to early marriage and childbirth, frequent childbirth with lack of spacing between births, and lack of power to seek health care; however, women with more education had a higher rate of skilled birth attendants at delivery and better rates of survival (Egmond et al., 2004).

Accessing Reproductive Health Care

Prenatal care reduces maternal and newborn complications through regular checkups by a trained nurse midwife or physician. This care includes risk assessment, treatment for medical conditions or risk reduction, and education. In the United States, access to prenatal care has increased through the availability of Medicaid coverage for pregnancy-related services. An important element in reducing health risks for mothers and children is increasing the numbers of births with assistance by medically qualified people. Proper medical attention and hygienic conditions during delivery can reduce the risk of complications and infections that cause serious illness or death to either mother or baby. Women who do not receive prenatal care are more likely to deliver at home with no medically qualified birth attendant (CDC, 2004).

Two United Nations millennium development goals (MDGs) relate to drastically improving maternal and child health by the year 2015. Currently, public health expenditures in the 75 countries with the highest maternal and child health problems, account for approximately US$97 billion dollars per year (WHO calls for new approach, 2005).

The likelihood of mothers entering prenatal care increases with age and education, and decreases with numbers of children. The risk of poor birth outcomes is greatest in women ages 15 and under. Prenatal care needs to begin with the initial pregnancy and continue throughout pregnancy. The American College of Obstetricians and Gynecologists recommends at least 13 visits for a full-term low-risk pregnancy. More frequent visits are needed for a high-risk pregnancy (a pregnancy with complications such as diabetes or hypertension). In the United States over three fourths of women receive adequate prenatal care; however, this rate varies with race and ethnicity. In addition to the prenatal visits to a healthcare provider, women are encouraged to attend with their spouse/partner/friend a series of childbirth education classes. Classes include fetal development, physiology of labor and birth, exercises and self-help techniques for labor, role of support persons, care of the newborn, and opportunities for questions (CDC, 2004).

In a US study, women who receive no prenatal care often have more preterm births (less than or equal to 37 weeks gestation), and their babies have lower birth weights. The women in the study were also more likely to be uninsured, have more children, older, less educated, and more likely to use alcohol, tobacco, and drugs. Syphilis and HIV was also found in 5% of the women studied. Results indicated that intensive encouragement is needed to get women to use more prenatal care, in order to decrease many of the poor birth outcomes (Maupin et al., (2004).

China has more than 345 million women of reproductive age. Since the economic reforms which began in the late 1970s and early 1980s, the national government gradually shifted responsibility for health care to local units, such as counties, townships, and villages. This change has resulted in people in poor rural areas having to pay for at least half of their health care out of pocket. This has resulted in women having to pay for half of their prenatal care visits, with often no insurance coverage. In China, current birth control and family planning regulations require most women to seek permission to conceive and carry a child to term. Under the one-child-per family policy, regulations may vary for women living in rural areas (Short & Zhang, 2004).

Case Study

In the state of Oaxaca, Mexico, in the pueblo (village) of Zaachila, the majority of indigenous Indian women never have had any prenatal care, even though Mexico is reported to have universal health care as the right for every Mexican citizen. The problem is that within this village there is acute poverty and a shortage of local healthcare facilities. An 8-hour trip to receive health care is too long and costly for most of the pregnant women, especially with small children (Newman, 1996).

A Comparison of Customs and Practices of Pregnancy, Delivery, and Postpartum Care in Africa, China, and Mexico

Africa

Throughout most of Africa, birth is considered a natural event in a woman's life. Womanhood is often considered incomplete unless the woman gives birth to a child. Children are very important to African families and are viewed as the parents' social security in older age (Nyinah, 1997). Childbearing is an important time in a woman's life and has social, ritual, and morale significance in all African communities (Selepe & Thomas, 2000). Each country is diverse in its beliefs and practices pertaining to the childbearing period, and the following section will include information about South Africa, Zambia, Ethiopia, and Ghana.

Pregnancy

Africa is rich in traditional practices pertaining to the pregnancy period. Even though modern antenatal services are offered for free in South Africa, the majority of South African women prefer to visit traditional healers first before receiving modern health care (Mchunu & Bhengu, 2004). However, sometimes using a traditional healer is not a matter of preference when access to care is difficult. In rural areas, clinics often lack money needed to keep supplies in stock (Wintergreen, 2005). Villages are often miles or even days away from modern hospitals. Due to the lack of transportation and money, this prevents women from accessing needed care (Buor & Bream, 2004). Many women, instead, visit traditional birth attendants for prenatal care due to the accessibility and low cost. Traditional birth attendants often have little to no professional medical training, but learn through experience and by demonstrations from other birth attendants in the community. Many traditional birth attendants feel that they acquired their skills through God, and their job is to facilitate communication with supernatural powers that govern pregnancy and childbirth. They monitor for complications that may arise, and only then refer the woman to a modern clinic for further evaluation (Gaskin, 1999).

The traditional birth attendants watch over the pregnant woman to monitor social taboos, such as the diet of the pregnant woman. In Zambia, for example, traditional birth attendants tell women to avoid eggs because it is believed that eggs will cause the baby to be born without hair. Having a baby with no hair is considered an embarrassment to the woman and her family. Fish is also avoided because it believed to cause abnormalities in the infant. During pregnancy in many African communities, it is recommended that the woman eat liver, nuts, and vegetables, especially green leafy vegetables in order to "get more blood" (Gaskin, 1999; Maimbolwa, Yamba, Diwan, & Ranjo-Arvidson, 2003).

Many cultural practices are in place to prevent the fetus from becoming too large, thus reducing the chance of a difficult delivery. For example, in many African communities pregnant women are supposed to avoid sugar, fats, and oils in order to prevent having a large baby (Gaskin, 1999). Woman are also discouraged from sleeping a lot or reducing their workload, because it is thought that the mother's laziness will cause the baby to become lazy, which makes labor long and difficult (Selepe & Thomas, 2000; Gaskin, 1999). In Zimbabwe, women use a plant root that produces a soapy substance to prepare for the delivery. This substance is used to massage the perineal area until the woman's fist can fit inside her vagina, which is thought to prepare the birth canal for labor and make the delivery less difficult (Wintergreen, 2005).

Other important social taboos involve sexual restrictions. In South Africa, sex is allowed during the pregnancy up until the ninth lunar month. This is to prevent the fetus from becoming "dirty" with sperm (Selepe & Thomas, 2000). A similar practice is found in Zambia, except that women are not allowed to engage in sexual activities after the eighth month of pregnancy. It is believed that if a woman did not follow this prescription, then the baby would be born with "white stuff", or vernix. Vernix (a normal white cheesy substance) is considered dirty, and it is believed to destroy the infant's eyes (Maimbolwa et al., 2003). Birth attendants might also require a payment for delivery of an infant born dirty with vernix. In Zambia it is also taboo for women to partake in sexual relationships outside of their marriage during pregnancy. This is believed to cause problems with the mother and the baby, or could result in a miscarriage due to the fact the blood would be different from that of the father's blood (Maimbolwa et al., 2003).

Superstitions and folk beliefs also restrict women's activities during pregnancy. An example of a folk belief is the avoidance of plaiting the hair. This is believed to cause knots in the umbilical cord, thus killing the fetus. Crossing rivers is also avoided in order to prevent the spontaneous abortion of the fetus. A belief in spirits and other supernatural powers also plays a role in the pregnancy. To prevent spirits from harming the fetus, pregnant women often wear protective wristbands made from sacrificed animals (Selepe & Thomas, 2000).

Childbirth

The place in which births occur and the attendants that oversee the birthing process differ from country to country in Africa. However, most births in Africa are home births and are attended by traditional birth attendants. In Zambia, 53% of pregnant women deliver at home and they are assisted by birth attendants with no formal training, or *mbusas* (Maimbolwa et al., 2003). In Nigeria, 66% of all births are in traditional birth homes.

These birth homes are located slightly away from the rest of the community in order to ensure the privacy of the laboring woman (Izugbara & Ukwayi, 2003). Most of these birth homes are run by untrained birth attendants. In Ghana, 70% of births occur in the home, and the birth attendants are usually an elderly female relative (Nyinah, 1997).

As in pregnancy, many laboring women still entrust their care to traditional birth attendants for delivery in the home setting for many reasons. Some reasons include the fact that the traditional birth attendant speaks the local language; shares common cultural and health belief practices, including disposal of the placenta and freedom of birthing positions; provides emotional support; and generates trust, as compared to medical personnel in clinics and hospitals (Mchunu & Bhengu, 2004; Maimbolwa et al., 2003). There is also a common belief among many Africans that ancestral spirits are present in the grandmother's hut. Many believe that the ancestral spirits will protect the mother and the baby if the delivery takes place in this hut (Selepe & Thomas, 2000).

A common theme in most African communities is that childbirth is a woman's event. Men are excluded from participating in the birth, and do not provide support to the laboring woman. Most participants in the birthing process include female family members. In South Africa, labor support is provided by the woman's mother, mother-in-law, and grandmother. Newlywed women in the villages are also permitted to watch in order to prepare for what lies ahead of them (Selepe & Thomas, 2000). Zambia's birthing customs are similar to those of South Africa. For example, labor support is provided by female family members, but the mother-in-law is excluded. There also is a social taboo for the mother-in-law to see her daughter-in-law naked (Maimbolwa et al., 2003).

In Zambia, when a woman's labor begins, only her family is notified. It is believed that if others find out about her labor, they will bewitch her out of jealousy and cause complications in the delivery (Maimbolwa et al., 2003). Conversely, in Ethiopia, childbirth is a community event for all women and children, including boys under the age of seven. The women in the village gather outside the hut in which the woman is laboring, which is frequently the house of the woman's mother. They support the mother by singing songs and carrying heavy rocks on their shoulders in the belief that it will relieve the burden of the mother's pain and encourage her to continue her labor (Craig, 2005).

Women, who give birth using traditional birth attendants, labor in various positions. In Zambia and Ghana women deliver in a semisquatting or kneeling position (Maimbolwa et al., 2003; Nyinah, 1997). In Zambia, women support the laboring woman by holding her from behind while she is in a squatting position. The women will tie a piece of cloth around the mother's abdomen and pull from behind. This is to encourage her to push during the second stage of labor. The Zambian birth attendants will also insert a piece of cloth into the mother's anus, which is done to prevent fecal matter from contacting the fetus and thought to prevent the infant from being delivered through the rectal opening (Maimbolwa et al., 2003). Although women in Ghana are not restricted to certain laboring positions, they are expected to remain in control of their emotions and to refrain from screaming or shouting (Nyinah, 1997). In most African countries, the placenta is buried soon after the delivery in order to prevent it from being used in witch-craft to harm the infant or mother (Craig, 2005; Maimbolwa et al., 2003; Nyinah, 1997).

Traditional birth attendants intervene in the birthing process in various manners to hasten the delivery. In Zambia and Ghana, they administer traditional herbal medicines by inserting them into the vagina or through oral drink concoctions. These herbs have been identified as *Apaparitnus africanus*, which is shown to produce a response similar to oxytocin (Pitocin), a commonly used modern medication to stimulate or enhance the laboring process (Maimbolwa et al., 2003; Nyinah, 1997). Many traditional birth atten-dants also elicit the gag reflex as a method to accelerate labor. A common theme throughout many African countries is that a difficult labor is caused by the family's actions or not adhering to the cultural taboos. During difficult labors or deliveries, women are encouraged to confess their unfaithfulness or infidelity to their husbands. If the woman dies during childbirth, it is attributed to her hiding the truth and is consid-ered a shameful event for her entire family (Pearson & Shoo, 2005; Maimbolwa et al., 2003).

Postpartum and Infant Care

Soon after birth in Ghana and Zambia, the mother and infant are given cleansing baths. In Ghana, the infant is given a drink mixture of water, alcohol, and herbs in order to facil-itate the passing of meconium (black tarry initial feces) (Nyinah, 1997). Herbs are also applied to the umbilical cord to aid in healing in Ghana, while in other parts of Africa mashed leaves or cow dung is applied to the umbilical cord stump to prevent evil spirits from entering the child (Gaskin, 1999). The application of substances on the umbilical cord stump is thought to be a contributing factor to the high incidence of neonatal tetanus, a common cause of death of many African infants. Women in Ghana expel the colostrum (yellowish white premilk), because they believe it is unwholesome for the infant. Breastfeeding is not started until the mother's milk is fully established (usually by the third day), and in the meantime, the baby is fed sugary drinks (Nyinah, 1997).

In many countries in Africa, women are expected to rest for up to 40 days postpartum. In Ethiopia, new mothers are considered unclean and are not allowed to enter a church or cook food for others. Mothers in Ethiopia are not left alone with the infant for the first 10 days because the community believes that the new mothers are susceptible to crazy thoughts and are considered at high risk for harming themselves or their babies. Mothers eat a porridge made of roasted barley and clarified butter because it is believed to have healing properties. For this same reason, new mothers also apply clarified butter for one to two weeks on any perineal tears that occurred during childbirth (Craig, 2005). Postpartum practices in Ghana are initiated so that the new mother can rest and her body can heal. New mothers are relieved from all chores, are told to abstain from sex, and are not allowed to leave the home (Nyinah, 1997).

The women are fed nourishing herb mixtures that are thought to expel blood clots from the vagina and aid in lactation. They are not permitted to eat foods that contain sugar because it is thought to cause postpartum hemorrhage in the mother and colic and diarrhea in the infant (Nyinah, 1997). The postpartum rest period is much shorter in Zambia than in Ethiopia and Ghana. Mothers in Zambia are expected to refrain from cooking until the infant's umbilical cord falls off. This is believed to prevent the mother from becoming diseased. Zambian mothers are also supposed to refrain from having sex for 3 to 7 months after the birth of the infant, which is a longer time period than in most African countries (Maimbolwa et al., 2003).

China

In China many practices and beliefs pertaining to the childbearing period are not only influenced by the culture and family but also by politics. As previously discussed in this chapter, China in 1979 adopted a one-child policy that limits the number of children a family can have in order to curtail the socioeconomic consequences of the population growth. Although this policy varies at the local level, all pregnancies must be approved by the government in order to qualify for health benefits from the government and to avoid fines and penalties. The government in China also encourages people to marry later in life, thus waiting longer to have a child (Kartchner & Callister, 2003).

China's government policies have created many consequences, such as female infanticide due to the cultural preference of having a male child. Currently there are 118.5 boys to every 100 girls in China. In 1998, the government banned the use of ultrasounds to determine the sex of the fetus in order to close the gap between the number of males and females that was caused by the high abortion rate of females. Many women do not seek prenatal care if their pregnancy is not approved by the government in order to avoid the fines or simply because they cannot afford the care without government assistance, which often leads to a higher maternal and infant mortality rate when prenatal care is not obtained (Short & Zhang, 2004; Kartchner & Callister, 2003).

Pregnancy
Many Chinese believe that the emotional state of the pregnant woman can affect the fetus. Feelings of sadness or anger are thought to negatively affect the fetus, so pregnant women often try to remain in a positive mood throughout pregnancy (Kartchner & Callister, 2003).

Some Chinese women receive *shiatsu*, or a type of massage that uses the thumbs to apply pressure to specific points on the pregnant woman's body. This aids in relaxation and decreases anxiety, thus providing benefits to the mother as well as the fetus (Mancino, Melluso, Monti, & Onorati, 2005).

Many women adhere to dietary restrictions during pregnancy in order to protect the fetus and prevent spontaneous abortion. For example, foods such as watermelon, bananas, and bean sprouts are avoided to prevent early labor (Monti, 2000; Do, 2000). Some women avoid eating shellfish such as clams, shrimps, and crabs due to the belief that these foods can cause the baby to easily develop rashes after birth. There are no restrictions on sexual intercourse during pregnancy; however, some women refrain from intercourse during the first trimester due to the fear of a miscarriage. Women also avoid strenuous exercise and heavy lifting during this time (Do, 2000).

Childbirth

About 90% of all births in China occur in sterile conditions and are performed by an obstetrician or midwife (Paulanka & Purnell, 2003). However, while most urban women give birth attended by doctors or trained midwives in hospitals, almost 69% in rural areas still give birth at home (Short & Zhang, 2004). A traditional belief in many rural areas is that suffering will come to the family if the baby is not born at home (Feng, 2005). Childbirth is considered a "woman's business," and most obstetrical healthcare providers are female (Kartchner & Callister, 2003). For this same reason, men are usually not present in the delivery room. Female family members are present for the delivery and support the laboring woman instead of the husband (Kartchner & Callister, 2003; Ip, Chien, & Chan, 2003). Most women give birth without any medications, even in modern hospitals and are expected to remain stoic throughout the delivery (Kartchner & Callister, 2003). Crying out during labor is thought to deplete the body of energy stores needed to push the baby out in the second stage of labor. It is also thought to create a negative environment in which the infant is entering the world.

Postpartum and Infant Care

The postpartum period is an extremely important time for most Chinese women. It is a period that is rich in traditional beliefs and practices that were developed as early as the sixth century B.C. The postpartum period is referred to as *tso yueh-tzu*, or the sitting month (Chu, 2005).

The *yin-yang* theory is based on the belief that a balance must be maintained in the body of hot and cold in order to prevent illness and disease. After the birth of a child, the woman is considered to be in a state of *yin*, or a cold condition. In the *yin-yang* theory, blood is considered hot, so the loss of blood during childbirth causes a cold condition in the woman's body (Kim-Godwin, 2003; Kartchner & Callister, 2003). For this reason, she is to avoid allowing more *yin* from entering her body in an attempt to restore the needed balance of *yin* and *yang*. *Yin* foods that are avoided during this period include fruits and raw vegetables, cold water or refrigerated drinks, cabbage, mung beans, crab, and horseradish (Chu, 2005; Tien, 2004; Kartchner & Callister, 2003; Do, 2000). Instead, the postpartum diet should consist of foods and drinks that are hot in nature such as chicken, liver, yellow wine, ginger, dates, beef, eggs, and spicy foods (Holroyd, Twinn & Yim, 2004; Kartchner & Callister, 2003; Matthey, Panasetis & Barnett, 2002). These foods are thought to restore balance in the woman's body and help to ensure adequate milk production for breastfeeding (Holroyd et al., 2004).

Behavioral restrictions are initiated in the postpartum period for the woman's body to heal and to prevent future somatic ailments, such as arthritis. During this month, the woman should get as much rest as possible by staying in bed and abstaining from sexual intercourse. She is also to avoid drafts and chills by not going outside of the house and remaining fully clothed. Traditionally, bathing, hair washing, and teeth brushing are not permitted in order to prevent the new mother from becoming chilled. An older family member, usually the woman's mother or mother-in-law, stays with the family during this month to help with the household chores and to make sure the new mother adheres to the rituals (Tien, 2004). Even though most urban births take place in modern Westernized hospitals, these traditional postpartum rituals are still widely practiced. However, many Chinese women admit to not following the rituals as strictly as women have in the past, breaking traditions by showering and brushing their teeth (Kartchner & Callister, 2003).

Mexico

Many of the prevalent health beliefs in Mexico are a combination of European, or Spanish, beliefs and aboriginal beliefs. The fusion of the two health beliefs systems occurred after the Spanish conquest of Mexico in the 1500s (Lartigue, Lubin, Maldonado-Duran, & Munguia-Wellman, 2002). The culture is rich in folk beliefs that are still practiced and are thought to protect the mother and her infant from harm.

An important concept in the Mexican culture is familialism. Mexican families are more extended in nature. Families are extremely important in the Mexican culture and members of the family are highly interdependent on each other. Children are important to the entire family and are seen as a gift from God. Childbirth is considered an event for the entire family. Familialism also plays a central role in the tremendous support a new mother receives during the childbearing and postpartum period.

Pregnancy

Many traditional beliefs and practices in the Mexican culture relate to the humoral theory. This theory is based on the belief that the four conditions in the human body—hot, cold, moist, and dry—must remain in balance. A pregnant woman is considered to be in a hot state, and she must be careful not to expose herself to cold foods or environments that would not harmonize with the hot state of pregnancy. A dramatic shift in the hot and cold balance is thought to cause illness or miscarriage. The diet during pregnancy is also determined by this theory and should consist of foods that are considered hot in nature such as chicken, spicy foods, toasted tortillas, and beef. Cold foods that are avoided during pregnancy include fruits, beans, and cold beverages (Lartigue et al., 2002).

Throughout pregnancy, women will take special vapor baths called *tamazcal baths*. These baths are similar to a sauna in that water is poured over hot stones to fill the room with warm water vapors. The baths are taken in order to eliminate toxic products in the body through sweat. These baths are thought to be beneficial because they compliment the hot state of pregnancy. Women will also receive *ser sabadas* during pregnancy. These massages are performed by a traditional healer, or *curandera*. The massages not only help the mother to relax and release negative tension, but the abdomen is also manipulated in order to help the fetus assume the correct position for delivery (Lartigue et al., 2002).

Superstitions and folk beliefs play an important role during pregnancy. For example, exposure to an eclipse is thought to cause the death of the infant through a miscarriage or stillbirth and malformations such as a cleft lip or palate. The fear of eclipses originates from a belief of the Aztecs. The belief is that an eclipse occurs because the sun is running out of energy, thus causing many misfortunes to unborn babies. It is common for pregnant women to wear metallic objects wrapped with a red string around their waists in order to protect the baby from danger. *Susta* and *muinas*, or fright and anger, are also to be avoided at all costs during pregnancy. These emotions are thought to negatively affect the mother and fetus. It is believed that the sudden fright of a pregnant woman can cause the fetus to lose its soul. If this occurs, the *curandera* can perform a ritual, which includes administering herbal drinks to the pregnant woman, in order to return the soul to the baby (Lartigue et al., 2002).

Childbirth

Many Mexicans view pregnancy and childbirth as a normal bodily process that does not require medical interventions. For this reason, many women in Mexico prefer to receive care from traditional birth attendants, or *parteras*, even though the nationalized health-care system has made modern medical services readily available to almost all women. It is estimated that one in four women are cared for by someone other than a trained medical provider (Hunt, Glantz, & Halperin, 2002). In a recent study, women preferred *parteras* because of their attitudes concerning intervening in the birthing process, preference of laboring and birthing in the home environment, and sharing of authority and decision making (Hunt et al., 2002). Among many Mexican woman there is also a mistrust of the modern, Westernized medical establishments due to the high rates of caesarean sections (Bretlinger et al., 2005).

Most labor support is provided by the laboring woman's mother or mother-in-law. Although childbirth is considered a woman's affair, with most labor support provided by female family members, husbands will also provide support during the laboring process (Hunt et al., 2002). Childbirth is considered a family event, so many family members may come to support the woman. Women freely choose their positions during labor and are encouraged to walk frequently to hasten the labor. Most women prefer the squatting position during the second and third stage of labor. Mexican women freely express their emotions during childbirth. After the birth, the placenta is buried near the family's home, and the cord stump is later buried in the same place (Lartigue et al., 2002).

Postpartum and Infant Care

The 40-day recuperation period following childbirth is referred to as *la cuarentena*. Both the mother and infant are thought to be in a vulnerable stage during this time, so they must adhere to dietary and activity restrictions. After the birth of the infant, both the mother and baby are considered to be in a hot state and must remain protected from the cold. The newborn will often be wrapped in many blankets to keep the baby warm. To protect the mother from the cold elements, bathing and hair washing are restricted during this time, along with cold and acidic foods such as oranges, tomatoes, lemons, and grapefruits. The mother refrains from housework and sexual activities as well. The woman's mother, mother-in-law, or grandmother will often move in with the family during this time to assist them with the transition. During this period, the husband will often perform household duties, which are usually considered the woman's duties (Kim-Godwin, 2003).

Most Mexican's believe that the colostrum is harmful to infants because it is considered old milk (Skeel & Good, 1988). Women will often refrain from breastfeeding until the mature milk comes in. In traditional societies the babies are fed sugar water and herbs or chamomile tea with sugar, while in the modern cities, formula supplementation is used until the mature milk supply is established (Monti, 2000). Women will often drink chicken soup and *atole*, which is a mixture of sugar, milk, and oatmeal or cornmeal while breastfeeding because it is believed to increase their milk supply (Skeel & Good, 1988). Women also avoid drafts, cool breezes, walking barefoot on the floor, and looking at a red sunset while breastfeeding. These actions are thought to cause the breast milk to dry up. Women may choose to stop breastfeeding if they have become upset, scared, or angry. These emotions are thought to cause the breast milk to spoil(Lartigue et al., 2002; Skeel & Good, 1988).

Parents will often wrap a band of cloth, or *fajero*, around the newborn's abdomen and place an object over the umbilicus. This is done to prevent an umbilical hernia and *mal aire* from entering through the umbilicus. The concept of *mal aire* is from a belief of the Aztecs in which air entering through an orifice in which it is not supposed to enter can cause a disease or illness (Lartigue et al., 2002).

Infant Health

Infant mortality

The following is a list of terms useful for discussing infant mortality (Kochanek & Martin, 2005):

- Infant mortality rate—Deaths of infants aged less than 1 year per 1000 or 100,000 live births. It is the sum of the neonatal and postneonatal mortality rates.
- Neonatal mortality rate—Deaths of infants aged 0–27 days per 1000 live births
- Early neonatal mortality rate—Deaths of infants aged 0–6 days per 1000 live births
- Late neonatal mortality rate—Deaths of infants aged 7–27 days per 1000 live births

- Late fetal mortality rate—Fetal deaths of 28 or more weeks of gestation per 1000 live births

- Perinatal mortality rate—Late fetal deaths plus early neonatal deaths per 1000 live births plus fetal deaths

- Low-birth-weight rate—Births with weight at delivery of less than 2500 grams per 100 live births

- Moderately low-birth-weight rate—Births with weight at delivery of 1500 grams to 2499 grams per 100 live births

- Very low-birth-weight rate—Births with a rate at delivery of 1500 grams per 100 live births

- Term—Births at 37–41 weeks of gestation

- Preterm—Births at less than 37 completed weeks of gestation per 100 live births

Infant mortality worldwide differs greatly between and within developing and developed countries (Table 16-3). The highest rate areas are in sub-Saharan Africa. The fol-

TABLE 16-3 Developing Countries: World's Highest Infant Mortality Rates with Accompanying Life Expectancies, 2004

Country	Infant Mortality Rate (per 1000 live births)	Life Expectancy (years)
Afghanistan	161	42
Angola	192.5	36.8
Bangladesh	64.3	—
China	25.3	—
Egypt	33.9	—
Guatemala	36.9	—
India	57.9	—
Iran	42.9	—
Kenya	62.9	44.9
Mexico	21.7	—
Mozambique	137.1	37.1
Russian Federation	17	66.4
South Africa	62.2	44.2
Zimbabwe	67.1	37.8

Source: CIA, 2005.

lowing are some of the unusually high infant mortality rates worldwide, which are deaths per 100,000 live births.

In contrast, developed countries have much lower infant mortality rates and higher life expectancies (Table 16-4).

As can clearly be seen from the above worldwide statistics, the United States does not have the lowest infant mortality rate in the world, even though more money per capita is spent on health care in the United States than anywhere else in the world. Within the United States, the infant mortality rates also differ greatly depending on each state (see Table 16-5), which is influenced by education, income, cultures, geography, and politics (US Census Bureau, 2001).

As can be seen in Table 16-5, the northern states clearly have lower infant mortality rates than many of the southern states.

The US Department of Health and Human Services has a wide range of programs to prevent infant mortality. These programs include the improvement of access to prenatal and newborn care, which includes Healthy Start, Medicaid, and State Children's Health Insurance (SCHIP). It also supports educational programs teaching infant care and prevention of malnutrition, and research to prevent birth defects, premature births, and sudden infant death syndrome (CIA, 2005). Birth defects are the leading cause of infant mortality in the United States, which account for 20% of infant deaths each year. About 150,000 babies are born annually with congenital abnormalities. Many, who survive, have long-term morbidities and disabilities (United Nations, 2004).

Infant mortality rates differ greatly in the United States within the categories of race and ethnicity. Figure 16-1 compares various rates within selected groups.

TABLE 16-4   Developed Countries with Lower Rates of Infant Mortality and Higher Life Expectancies

Country	Infant Mortality Rate (per 1000 live births)	Life Expectancy (years)
Australia	4.8	80.3
Austria	4.7	—
Canada	4.8	—
Finland	3.6	—
Israel	7.2	79.2
Sweden	2.8	80.3
United States	6.6	77.4

Source: CIA, 2005.

TABLE 16-5   Selected US Infant Mortality Rates per State

State or District	Infant Mortality Rate (per 1000 live births)
Delaware	10.7
District of Columbia (Washington, DC)	10.6
Mississippi	10.5
Louisiana	9.8
Alabama	9.4
South Carolina	8.9
New Hampshire	3.8
Utah	4.8
Massachusetts	5
Minnesota	5.3

Source: US Census Bureau, 2001.

As stated in the *World Health Report 2005,* hundreds of millions of women and children have no access to health care, and mortality rates could substantially be reduced by increasing access to prenatal and child care. Worldwide, approximately 530,000 babies die each year, greater than 1 million are stillborn, and more that four million newborns die within the first days or weeks of life. In addition, 10.6 million children die before their fifth birthday. About 90% of the children that die under age 5 deaths die from preterm births, birth asphyxia, and infections, such as lower respiratory, diarrhea, malaria, measles, and HIV/AIDS (WHO, 2005; WHO calls for new approach, 2005).

The majority of neonatal deaths are within low-income and middle-income countries, and about half occur at home. In many poor countries infants die unnamed and unrecorded. "The availability of good medical care tends to vary inversely with the need for it in the population served" (Lawn, Cousens, & Zupan, 2005, p. 891). Challenges include HIV/AIDS, pneumonia, diarrhea, malaria, and vaccine preventable infections, as well as increasing poverty.

In the period from 1996–2005, there was an increase in neonatal deaths in sub-Saharan Africa (5%), and elsewhere decreases in rates such as the Americas especially Latin America (Lawn, Cousens, & Zupan, 2005):

- Latin American countries (–40%)
- Eastern Mediterranean countries (–9%)
- European countries (–18%)

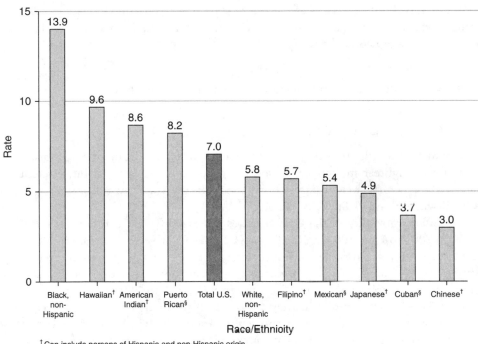

Figure 16-1 Infant mortality rates,* by selected racial and ethnic populations, United States, 2002.

*Per 1,000 live births.

Source: National Center for Health Statistics, 2005.

- Southwest Asian countries (–21%)
- Western Pacific (–39%)
- Overall world decrease of –16%.

Mortality is greatest in the first 24 hours after birth (25–45%). About 75% of all neonatal deaths worldwide occur during the first week of life. Up to 70% of deaths could be prevented if good neonatal care were implemented. Ideally a woman could choose to have a skilled birth attendant present during a delivery, and if a complication should occur, she and the newborn could have a much greater opportunity for better care. Women in Asia and sub-Saharan Africa most often do not have this opportunity. Rates for caesarian section deliveries are low in the countries with the highest mortality, such as much of Africa. Within the poorest countries, the richest women have 2–3 times greater rates of antepartal care and about 6 times the rate of skilled birth attendants as compared to the poorest women (Knippenberg et al., (2005).

In developed nations that keep accurate statistics, less than 3% of neonatal deaths occur whereas, in many developing countries the vital statistics may come from verbal reports. Causes of neonatal deaths include the following:

- Preterm births (low birth weight)
- Severe infections (sepsis, pneumonia, tetanus, and diarrhea)
- Asphyxia
- Congenital abnormalities

In many developing countries babies are not weighed at birth and often gestational age in unknown. Eighteen million babies worldwide are estimated to be low birth weight, with half of the low-birth-weight babies born in Southeast Asia (Lawn, Cousens, & Zupan, 2005; Lawn, Shibuya, & Stein, 2005).

The infant mortality in the United States increased from 6.8 infants per 1000 live births in 2001 to 7 per 1000 live births in 2002. This was the first increase in infant mortality rate in 40 years. Included in this increased rate were low birth weight, preterm, and "very preterm" infants. The main increase in infant mortality from 2001 to 2002 was related to the increase in infants born weighing less than 759 grams (1 pound, 10.5 ounces). These deaths were exclusively due to newborns dying in the first 4 weeks of life. The majority of these very low-birth-weight infants die within the first year of life. Multiple gestation (twins, triplets, etc.) births, more than half of which are born preterm or low birth weight, have contributed greatly to the recent increases in preterm and low birth weights. The preterm rate for singleton births (one baby per pregnancy) alone increased 7 percent during this 2001–2002 time period (MacDorman, Martin, Mathews, Hoyert, & Ventura, (2005).

Infant mortality for African-American babies is still a poorly understood and unresolved problem in the United States. Although progress has been made to lower infant mortality for all ethnic and racial groups, a significant disparity remains between African-American and European American infant mortality rates. Regardless of maternal age, education, income, or marital status, the African-American infant is twice as likely to die as the Caucasian infant. This disparity is often associated with high rates of preterm delivery, as well as low- and very low-birth-weight neonates. Despite many efforts, preterm deliveries still remains high at 18.4% in African-American births as compared to 9.1% of European American births. Some interventions such as treatment of urinary tract infections, cerclage, and treatment of bacterial vaginosis reflect improvements in rates, but overall the rates are still double in African-American women. The risk of infant mortality increases greatly as birth weight decreases (Professional Education, 2000).

Infant Abandonment in China

New research on the abandonment of children in China reveals that some of the population policies may lead to abandonment of "excess" daughters so that couples may have a son. Among 237 families who abandoned their daughters, most did so because of the gender of their child; 90% of the children were girls and 86% were healthy. Sixty percent of the abandoned boys were disabled or severely ill. Other couples who were infertile emerged spontaneously to adopt these abandoned girls. Those who already had a son were also willing to adopt an abandoned girl (Johnson, Huang, & Wang, 1998).

Diarrhea in Children in Developing Countries
Diarrheal diseases remain an important cause of infant and childhood morbidity and mortality in developing countries. These deaths have significantly declined in recent years due to oral rehydration therapy (fluids and electrolytes). Most of the diarrheal problems in children in developing countries are infectious in origin stemming from contaminated water supplies from various municipal and open water sources (rivers, streams, creeks, and wells). Normally most episodes of diarrhea resolve within a week. Infectious diarrhea lasts more than 14 days. Significantly high mortality rates are associated with diarrhea that lasts more than 2 weeks. Persistent diarrhea is often associated with poor nutritional status resulting in a significant risk for death. Breastfeeding should be continued and even encouraged during episodes of diarrhea. Special diets and vitamins are recommended for nutritional management. Antimicrobial agents are not usually prescribed with the exception of specific infections such as *Shigella*, *Salmonella*, and *Vibrio* species (Alam & Ashraf, 2003).

Sexually Transmitted Diseases (STDs)

The highest rates of sexually transmitted diseases are within the urban populations among men and women between 15 to 35 years age range. Women generally become infected earlier than men. Of particular concern are adolescents who may have unplanned sexual relations without adequate information about the diseases, treatment, and prevention. Sexual intercourse prior to menarche, such as in the cases of child brides, causes even greater vulnerability. Rape and incest victims are especially vulnerable to STDs. Those who are most vulnerable are of childbearing age, in poverty, abuse drugs, and are uneducated, institutionalized, or living within an unstable social environment. Most of the 20 or more pathogens transmitted by sexual intercourse can be treated with antibiotics yet still remain a large problem in developing as well as developed countries (United Nations, 2004).

Table 16-6 gives examples of classic worldwide STDs.

Prevention and Treatment Care

Prevention helps stop the spread of sexually transmitted diseases by interrupting the transmission, reducing the infection duration, and preventing complications. Primary prevention begins with sex education about the diseases and prevention methods for safe sex behavior such as abstinence and condom use. Treatment care involves access to health-care practitioners, making an accurate diagnosis based on laboratory tests, and giving the

TABLE 16-6 Classic Worldwide STDs, Bacterial and Viral

Disease—Classification	Pathogen	Signs and Symptoms
Syphilis (bacterial)	*Treponema pallidum*	Anogenital ulcers, swelling, skin rash
Gonorrhea (bacterial)	*Neisseria gonorrhoea*	Urethral discharge, cervicitis, lower abdominal pain in women, newborn conjunctivitis, may be asymptomatic
Chlamydia (bacterial)	*Chlamydia trachomatis*	Urethral discharge, cervicitis, lower abdominal pain in women, neonatal conjunctivitis, may be asymptomatic
HIV/AIDS (viral)	Human immunodeficiency virus	Lymph node swelling, fever, weight loss, skin rash, may be asymptomatic
Herpes genitalis (genital herpes) (viral)	Herpes simplex virus type 2 (HSV-2)	Anogenital vesicular lesions and lacerations
Genital warts (viral)	Human papilloma virus (HPV)	Anogenital warts, cervical warts, cervical cancer
Viral hepatitis (viral)	Hepatitis B virus (HBV)	Nausea, malaise, fever, enlarged liver, jaundice, liver cancer, cirrhosis

Source: United Nations, 2004.

appropriate medication and education. Lack of treatment can cause mortality and morbidity (United Nations, 2004).

HIV Infection and Reproduction

About 700,000 children under 15 years of age are infected with HIV every year in the world, and greater than 90% of them are in sub-Saharan Africa. Adding HIV to pregnancy causes an increase in numerous risk factors, which in turn can cause an increase in maternal mortality rates. HIV-infected pregnant women are at an increased risk of having HIV positive children, stillbirth, low birth weight, and preterm babies. Children of HIV-positive mothers (irrespective of the child's HIV status) also have a higher mortality due to maternal ill health or death. Options for contraception are limited in many developing countries. HIV-infected women should use male or female latex condoms to protect their partners from sexually transmitted diseases. In addition to condoms, contraception can be oral, injectable, or implantable. One problem is that oral contraception may interfere with antiretroviral medications, and special consideration must be made for these situations (Duerr, Hurst, Kourtis, Rutenberg, & Jamieson, 2005).

There are an increasing number of men and women in the United States and elsewhere in the world who are faced with the fact that they are HIV positive and wish to have children. As many as 28% of HIV-infected people in the United States wish to have children and many in sub-Saharan Africa and Europe also have a desire to reproduce. Pregnancy seems to have little effect on HIV disease progression if women are receiving antiretroviral therapy. Male and female condoms are suggested for protection against unwanted pregnancy and STDs. In countries, such as those in sub-Saharan Africa, the social stigma of not having children may be equal to or greater than the stigma of the HIV disease itself. Concerns about having an HIV-infected child and the stigma of HIV and pregnancy are also problematic. Artificial insemination is often used as a means of conception without fear of transfer of the disease to the partner or spouse (WHO, 2000a).

The World Health Organization recommends exclusive breastfeeding from birth to 6 months of age. In the general population exclusive breastfeeding for the first 6 months of life protects against infant morbidity and mortality from gastrointestinal and respiratory infections. Breastfeeding causes more transmission of the HIV virus from mother to child, and avoidance of breastfeeding has been recommended in *developed* countries. Yet in *developing* countries infants who are breast fed and have the HIV virus are better off with breastfeeding alone than mixed feedings. In 1999 there were 620,000 children who were HIV positive, living mainly in sub-Saharan Africa. Antiretroviral medications have clearly reduced the mother-to-child transmission of the virus. In developing countries children cannot be assured safe, feasible, affordable, and sustained breast milk substitutes (Bland, Rollins, Coutsoudis, & Coovadia, 2002; Papathakis & Rollins, 2003).

Violence Against Women

According to the United Nations Declaration on the Elimination of Violence Against Women of 1993, as cited in *World Population Monitoring,* "Violence against women is any act of gender-based violence that results in, or is likely to result in physical, sexual, or psychological harm or suffering to women, including threats of such acts, coercion or arbitrary deprivation of liberty, whether occurring in public or private life" (UN, 2004, p. 123). Problems begin in societies that give a higher recognition or value to males. Preferential treatment to males may affect the health and education of children. In societies where the husband is recognized as the dominant person with the most power in the relationship, women may be married without their consent and may be subject to domestic violence. Women are often vulnerable because of their economic dependence on men in many cultures. Violence against women also includes sexual exploitation of women refugees, rape as a weapon of war, and trafficking of women in prostitution. Violence against women needs to be considered a legal crime, and women need to get support and/or assistance in helping to protect themselves and their children (United Nations, 2004).

Women are subjected to worldwide violence from intimate partners and sexual violence from strangers. Men who were abused or who witnessed marital violence in their homes are more likely to abuse their wives or partners and their children. Each year in the United States 1.5 million women are physically abused or raped by an intimate partner. Rape and other acts of violence are common in refugee camps and by enemies in war. In many cultures, women who have been raped, or even in the company of a nonrelative male, are killed by family member males, in order to preserve the "honor" of the family. These killings are known as "honor killings" (Murphy, 2003).

Female Genital Mutilation

Female genital mutilation (also called female circumcision) is experienced by girls and sometimes young women prior to marriage, and this occurs outside the medical system. It involves the partial or complete removal of the external female genitalia or other injury to female genital organs. The majority of these procedures also include the removal of the clitoris and labia minora. The following are different types of female mutilation:

- Type I—Excision of the prepuce, with or without excision of part or the entire clitoris

- Type II—Excision of the clitoris with partial or total excision of the labia minora

- Type III—Excision of part or all of the external genitalia and stitching/narrowing of the opening (infibulation)

- Type IV—Pricking, piercing, or incision of the clitoris and/or labia; stretching of the clitoris and labia; cauterization by burning of the clitoris and surrounding tissue; scraping of tissue surrounding the vaginal orifice or cutting of the vaginal cuts; introduction of corrosive substances or herbs into the vagina causing it to bleed, or tightening or narrowing the vaginal cavity.

The most common type of female genital mutilation is excision of the clitoris and the labia minora (80% of all cases); and the most extreme form is infibulation (15% of all cases). The health consequences of these procedures vary according to the type and severity of the procedure. Long-term consequences include cysts, abscesses, keloid scars, damage to the urethra causing urinary incontinence, dyspareunia (painful sexual intercourse), sexual dysfunction, and painful childbirth. In addition women may suffer anxiety and depression. The estimated number of girls and women who had this procedure is 100–140 million. Each year 2 million girls are subjected to this procedure. Reasons for these procedures are the following (WHO, 2000b):

- Reduction or elimination of sexual desire in the female

- Maintain chastity or virginity before marriage and fidelity during marriage

- Increase male sexual pleasure
- Promote female hygiene and external sexual appeal

Approximately 30 countries in Africa, some in Asia, and also immigrants to Europe, North America, Australia, and New Zealand report this issue within their own countries. Within these countries, cultural norms dictate that women undergo this procedure so that they can be pure for marriage. Often women who had this procedure done to them support having the procedure done to their daughters because of community pressure within the culture (United Nations, 2004). Amnesty International and the World Health Organization consider this procedure to be an infringement of human rights. In the United States these procedures became a crime in 1997, with the enactment of the Female Genital Mutilation Act of 1996 (Ellwood, 2005).

Male Reproductive Health

The Alan Guttmacher Institute addresses global perspectives of male reproductive health needs and issues (Alan Guttmacher Institute, 2002). Most men in the world wish for intimate and sexual relationships and a stable family. The reproductive health needs of men have historically received little attention. Unplanned pregnancies, infertility, STDs, including HIV, can have a major impact on men's lives. The male traditional role can be gloomy due to poverty and lack of job perspectives, which can make many men fatalistic about their futures. Presently, men in sub-Saharan Africa have a significant reduction in life span, which may also decrease the motivation for adhering to preventive health measures. Less than half of these men age, 15–24, use any form of contraception, compared to 63–93% of the developed countries. Urbanization may weaken support systems and also decrease the desire for large numbers of children. Many men are increasing their education, yet job opportunities are often not available. This leaves poor urban men with great frustrations. Men between the ages of 15 and 24 become more independent and begin to initiate sexual relationships. In most countries of the world, men had their first sexual encounter by age 20. Few men in their teens marry and/or have children. Men usually marry and become fathers in their late 20s and 30s and begin to settle down. The more educated a man is, the more likely he will consider and use a method of family planning with his spouse or partner. Fifty percent of men in the world become fathers in their mid to late 20s. Men in their 40s and 50s usually have had all the children they wish. Male and female sterilization is common in males and females in developed countries, and also in China. STDs are highest in men in sub-Saharan Africa, Latin America, and the Caribbean areas. HIV/AIDS rates are the highest in the world in sub-Saharan African men and women. In many regions of the world men migrate to other areas to find work, living at times for several years before returning to their families. During this time away from home, they may have sexual relations with other women, contract STDs and subsequently bring these diseases back to their sexual partners back in their home communities.

Conclusion

This chapter has given a worldwide perspective of male and female reproductive health issues, and cultural beliefs and practices emphasizing pregnancy, childbirth, postpartal health, and infant health. Disparities in statistics demonstrate much of the perpetual inequality of health status, access to health care, available resources, research data collection, and reporting worldwide. These health disparities exist not only between developing and developed nations, but also within both developed and developing nations, especially among those countries with populations that are heterogeneous in income, race, ethnicity, and socioeconomic status.

References

Alam, N., and Ashaf, H. (2003). Treatment of infectious diarrhea in children. *Therapy in Practice, 5*(3), 151–165.

Alan Guttmacher Institute. (2003). In their own right. Addressing the sexual and reproductive health needs of men worldwide. Retrieved June 25, 2005, from http://www.guttmacher.org

As-Sanie, S., Gantt, A., & Rosenthal, M. (2004). Pregnancy prevention in adolescents. *American Family Physician, 70*(8), 1517–1524.

Beamish, J., & Abderrazik (January 2003). Adolescent and youth reproductive health in Morocco. *Policy Project*, 1–30.

Bland, R., Rollins, N., Coutsoudis, A., & Coovadia, H. (2002). Breastfeeding practices in an area of high HIV prevalence in rural South Africa. *Acta Paediatrics, 91*, 704–711.

Bretlinger, P., Sanchez-Perez, H., Cedeno, M., Morales, G., Hernan, M., Micek, M., et al. (2005). Pregnancy outcomes, site of delivery, and community schisms in regions affected by the armed conflict in Chiapas, Mexico. *Social Science and Medicine, 64*(5), 1001–1014.

Buor, D., & Bream, K. (2004). An analysis of the determinants of maternal mortality in Sub-Saharan Africa. *Journal of Women's Health, 13*(8), 926–937.

Campbell, O., Gipson, R., Issa, A., Matta, N., El Deeb, B., El Mohandes, et al. (2005). National maternal mortality ratio in Egypt halved between 1992–1993 and 2000. *Bulletin of the World Health Organization, 83*(6), 462–471.

Castaneda, X., Billings, D. & Blanco, J. (2003). Abortion beliefs and practices among midwives (Parteras) in a rural Mexican township. *Women and Health, 37*(2), 73–87.

CDC. (2004). *Healthy People 2010*. Maternal, infant, and child health. Retrieved June 3, 2005, from http://www.healthypeople.gov/Document/HTML/Volume2/16MICH.htm

Chatterjee, P. (2005). Cambodia tackles high maternal mortality. *Lancet, 366*, 281–282.

Childbirth by Choice Trust. (1999). Abortion in law, history and religion. Retrieved June 6, 2005, from http://www.cbctrust.com/abortion.html

China's law on maternal and infant health care. (n.d.). Retrieved June 12, 2005 from http://acad.swarthmore.edu/bio5/tong/International%20Laws/china's_law_on_maternal_and_infant_health_care

Chu, C. (2005). Postnatal experience and health needs of Chinese migrant women in Brisbane, Australia. *Ethnicity and Health, 10*(1), 33–56.

CIA. (2005). World Factbook: United States infant mortality rate. Retrieved June 2, 2005, from http://www.indexmundi.com/united_states/infant_mortality_rate.html

Craig, D. (2005). Women's secrets: Childbirth in rural Ethiopia. *Midwifery Today, 75*, 30–31.

Dickson-Tetteh, K., & Billings, D. (2002). Abortion care services provided by registered midwives in South Africa. *International Family Planning Perspectives, 28*(3), 144–150.

Do, H. (2000). *Chinese: Cultural profile.* University of Washington, Harborview Medical Center Web site. Retrieved July 7, 2005, from http://ethnomed.org/ethnomed/cultures/chinese/chinese_cp.html

Duerr, A., Hurst, S., Kourtis, A., Rutenburg, N., & Jamieson, D. (2005). Integrating family planning and prevention of mother-to-child HIV transmission in resource-limited settings. *Lancet, 366,* 261–263.

Egmond, K., Naeem, A., Verstraelen, H., Bosmans, M., Claeys, P., & Temmerman, M. (2004). Reproductive health in Afghanistan: Results of a knowledge, attitudes and practices survey among Afghan women in Kabul. *Disasters, 28*(3), 269–282.

Ellwood, A. (2005). Female genital cutting, "circumcision" and mutilation: Physical, psychological and cultural perspectives. *Contemporary Sexuality, 39*(1).

Erviti, J., Castro, R., & Collando, A. (2004). Strategies used by low-income Mexican women to deal with miscarriage and spontaneous abortion. *Qualitative Health Research, 14*(8), 1058–1068.

Feki, S. (2004). The birth of reproductive health: A difficult delivery. *PLOS Medicine, 1*(1), 10–13.

Feng, J. (2005). Reducing infant mortality. *Beijing Review, 48*(26), 30–31.

Gaskin, I. (1999). Indigenous customs in childbirth and child care. *Birth Gazette, 15*(1), 22–25.

Germain, A. (2004). Reproductive health and human rights. *Lancet, 363,* 65–66.

Gilbert, W., Jandial, D., Field, N., Bigelow, P. & Danielsen, B. (2004). Birth outcomes in teenage pregnancies. *Journal of Maternal-Fetal and Neonatal Medicine, 16,* 265–270.

Graham, W., & Hussein, J. (2004). The right to count. *Lancet, 363,* 67–68.

Gurmankin, A., & Caplan, A. (2004). Embryo disposal practices in IVF clinics in the United States. *Politics and the Life Sciences, 22*(2), 4–8.

Hasna, F. (2003). Islam, social traditions and family planning. *Social Policy & Administrative Issues, 37*(2), 181–197.

Holroyd, E., Twinn, S., & Yim, I. (2004). Exploring Chinese women's cultural beliefs and behaviours regarding the practice of "doing the month." *Women and Health, 40*(3), 109–123.

Horon, I. (2005). Underreporting of maternal deaths on death certificates and the magnitude of the problem of maternal mortality. *American Journal of Public Health, 95*(3), 478–482.

Hunt, L., Glantz, N., & Halperin, D. (2002). Childbirth care-seeking behavior in Chiapas. *Health Care for Women International, 25,* 98–118.

Ip, W., Chien, W., & Chan, C. (2003). Childbirth expectations of Chinese first-time pregnant women. *Journal of Advanced Nursing, 42*(2), 151–158.

Izugbara, C., & Ukwayi, J. (2003). The clientele of traditional birth homes in rural southeastern Nigeria. *Health Care for Women International, 24*(3), 177–192.

Johnson, K., Huang, B., & Wang, L. (1998). Infant adoption and abandonment in China. *Population and Development Review, 24*(3), 469–510.

Jones, R., & Boonstra, H. (2004). Confidential reproductive health services for minors: The potential impact of mandated parental involvement for contraception. *Perspectives on Sexual and Reproductive Health, 36*(5), 182–191.

Kartchner, R., & Callister, L. (2003). Giving birth: Voices of Chinese women. *Journal of Holistic Nursing, 21*(2), 100–114.

Kim-Godwin, Y. (2003). Postpartum beliefs and practices among non-Western cultures. *American Journal of Maternal/Child Nursing, 28*(2), 74–78.

Kochanek, K., & Martin, J. (2005). Supplemental analyses of recent trends in infant mortality. *International Journal of Health Services, 35*(1), 101–115.

Knippenberg, R. Lawn, J., Darmstadt, G., Begkoyian, G., Fogstad, H., Walelign, N., et al. (2005). Neonatal survival. Systematic scaling up of the neonatal care in countries. Retrieved June 29, 2005, from http://the lancet.com

Kridli, S. (2002). Health beliefs and practices among Arab women. *Maternal and Child Nursing, 27*(3), 178–182.

Lartigue, T., Lubin, S., Maldonado-Duran, M., & Munguia-Wellman, M. (2002). Latino families in the perinatal period: Cultural issues dealing with the healthcare system. *Great Plains Research, 12*(1), 75–100.

Law of the People's Republic of China on Maternal and Infant Care. (1995). Population and Family Planning. Law on maternal and infant health care. Retrieved June 12, 2005, from http://www.unescap.org/esid/psis/population/database/poplaws/law_china/ch_record006.htm

Lawn, J., Shibuya, K., & Stein, C. (2005). No cry at birth: Global estimates of intrapartum stillbirths and intrapartum-related neonatal deaths. *Bulletin of the World Health Organization, 83*(6), 409–417.

Lawn, J., Cousens, S., & Zupan, J. (2005). 4 million neonatal deaths: When? Where? Why? *Lancet, 365*(9462), 89–900.

Li, J. (2004). Gender inequality, family planning, and maternal and child care in rural Chinese county. *Social Science and Medicine, 59*, 695–708.

Lofstedt, P., Shusheng, L., & Johansson, A. (2004). Abortion patterns and reported sex ratios at birth in rural Yunnan, China. *Reproductive Health Matters, 12*(24), 86–96.

MacDorman, M., Martin, J., Mathews, M., Hoyert, D., & Ventura, S. (2005). Supplemental analysis of recent trends in infant mortality. Explaining the 2001-02 infant mortality increase: data from the linked birth/infant data set. *National Vital Statistics Report, 53*(12).

Maimbolwa, M., Yamba, B., Diwan, V., & Ransjo-Arvidson, A. (2003). Cultural childbirth practices and beliefs in Zambia. *Journal of Advanced Nursing, 43*(3), 263–274.

Mancino, P., Melluso, J., Monti, M., & Onorati, E. (2005). Preparation for childbirth in different cultures. *Clinical and Experimental Obstetrics and Gynecology, 32*(2), 89–91.

Matthey, S., Panasetis, P., & Barnett, B. (2002). Adherence to cultural practices following childbirth in migrant Chinese women and relation to postpartum mood. *Health Care for Women International, 23*, 567–575.

Maupin, R., Lyman, R., Fatsis, J., Prystowiski, E., Nguyen, A., Wright, C., et al. (2004). Characteristics of women who deliver with no prenatal care. *Journal of Maternal-Fetal and Neonatal Medicine, 16*, 45–50.

Mchunu, G., & Bhengu, B. (2004). The knowledge and attitudes of traditional birth attendants towards HIV/AIDS and their beliefs related to perinatal care: A study conducted in KwaZulu Natal. *Curationis: South African Journal of Nursing, 27*(1), 41–51.

Mogilevkina, I., & Odlind, V. (2003). Contraceptive practices and intentions of Ukrainian women. *European Journal of Contraception and Reproductive Health Care, 8*, 185–196.

Monti, D. (2000). Food customs and their role in pregnancy and infant feeding. *International Journal of Childbirth Education, 15*(4), 18.

Murphy, E. (2003). Being born female is dangerous to your health. *American Psychologist, 58*(3), 205–210.

National Center for Health Statistics. (2004a). Teens delay sexual activity: Using contraception more effectively. Retrieved June 1, 2005, from http://www.cdc.gov/nchs/pressroom/04news/teens.htm

National Center for Health Statistics. (2005). Supplemental analysis of recent trends in infant mortality. Retrieved July 9, 2005, from http://www.cdc.gov/nchs/ products/pubs/pubd/hestats/infantmort/infantmort.htm

Newman, L. [CNN World News Correspondent]. (1996). Poor access to health care endangers pregnant Mexican women. Retrieved June 30, 2005, from http://www.cnn.com/WORLD/9607/25/mexico.healthcare/index.html

Nyinah, S. (1997). Cultural practices in Ghana. *World Health, 50*(2), 22–24.

Papathakis, P., & Rollins, N. (2003). Are WHO/UNAIDS/UNICEF-recommended replacement milks for infants of HIV-infected mothers appropriate in the South African context? *Bulletin of the World Health Organization, 82*(3), 164–171.

Pattinson, R. (2004). Maternal Health Chapter 7. Health Systems Trust. *South African Health Review.* Retrieved June 12, 2005, from http://www.hst.org.za/publications/248

Paulanka, B., & Purnell, L. (2003). *Transcultural health care: A culturally competent approach* (2nd ed.). Philadelphia, PA: F.A. Davis Company.

Pearson, L., & Shoo, R. (2005). Availability and use of emergency obstetric services: Kenya, Rwanda, Southern Sudan, and Uganda. *International Journal of Gynecology and Obstetrics, 88*(2), 208–215.

Professional Education. (2000). Black infant mortality problem still unsolved. Retrieved June 1, 2005, from http://www.state.nj.us/health/bibs/education/1unsolved.html

Schenker, J. (2005). Assisted reproductive practice: Religious perspectives. *Reproductive BioMedicine Online.* Retrieved June 21, 2005, from http://www.rmonline.com

Selepe, H., & Thomas, D. (2000). The beliefs and practices of traditional birth attendants in the Manxili Area of KwaZulu, South Africa: A qualitative study. *Journal of Transcultural Nursing, 11*(2), 96–101.

Short, S., & Zhang, F. (2004). Use of maternal health services in rural China. *Population Studies, 58*(1), 3–19.

Simkin, P. (2003). Emotional support for the woman with an epidural. *International Journal of Childbirth Education, 18*(3), 5–7.

Skeel, L., & Good, M. (1988). Mexican cultural beliefs and breastfeeding: A model for assessment and intervention. *Journal of Human Lactation, 4*(4), 160–163.

Skouby, S. (2004). Contraceptive use and behavior in the 21st century: A comprehensive study across five European countries. *European Journal of Contraception and Reproductive Health Care, 9,* 57–68.

Tien, S. (2004). Nurses' knowledge of traditional Chinese postpartum customs. *Western Journal of Nursing Research, 26*(7), 822–832.

United Nations (UN). (2004). *World population monitoring 2002. Reproductive rights and reproductive health.* New York: UN.

US Census Bureau. (2001). State rankings—statistical abstract of the United States. Infant mortality rate—-2001. Retrieved June 2, 2005, from http://www.census.gov.statab/ ranks/rank17.html

WHO. (2000a). Pregnancy and HIV/AIDS. (2000). Retrieved June 18, 2005, from http://wholint/mediacentre/factsheets/fs250/en/index.html

WHO. (2000b). Female genital mutilation. Retrieved June 27, 2005, from http://www.who.int/ mediacentre/factsheets/fs241/en/index.html

WHO. (2005a). Reproductive health and research. Skilled attendant at birth. 2005 estimates. Retrieved June 11, 2005, from http://www.who.int/reproductive-health/global_monitoring/ skilled_attendant.html

WHO. (2005b). *World health report 2005.* Retrieved August 10, 2007, from http://www.who.int/whr/ 2005/en/index.html

WHO calls for new approach to save lives of children. (2005). *Indian Journal of Medical Science, 59*(4), 173–174.

Wintergreen. (2005). Birth without borders: The clash of modern and traditional. *Midwifery Today, 75,* 17–19.

Zwillich, T. (2005). US pharmacies vow to withhold emergency contraception. *Lancet, 365,* 1677–1688.

Chapter 17

Global Health of Children

Kathie Aduddell

Introduction

This chapter describes children's health in our world today as well as strategies to alleviate specific health concerns for children. The chapter begins with an introduction that identifies the number of children in the world today and the undue burden these children face in living on earth. In 2006, as the Global Health Council (GHC) indicated, 20 children die every minute of every day (2006). The chapter then reviews the historical perspective to children's health and how organizations such as the United Nations (UN) and the World Health Organization (WHO) began to call attention to children's health. Further description and explanation in this chapter provides the measurements of health currently being utilized to identify the problems that children face in the world as well as the criteria to evaluate the effectiveness of programs and projects to assist children. Continued exploration of the leading causes of death in children provides an in-depth analysis of the current situation for children in the world and the global ramifications of children's health problems. The final part of the chapter reviews the documented approaches and international strategies to alleviate these health concerns for children and addresses future challenges.

Current United Nations Children's Fund (UNICEF) data indicates there are 71 million children younger than 18 years old living in the United States while there are 2.1 billion children younger than 18 years old in other parts of the world (UNICEF 2006). According to various national and international organizations, children and adolescents represent approximately 30–40% of the world's population (WHO, 2003; US Census Bureau, 2004; UNICEF, 2006). The mortality rate of children 5 years and younger is 8 deaths per 1000 children in the United States and 86 deaths per 1000 children for the overall child population of the world (US Census Bureau, 2004). The Global Health Council (2006) translates these facts into approximately 1000 infants dying each hour; 970 of these deaths occur in developing countries. Another way to state this sobering fact is that every minute of every day, 20 children die somewhere in the world. They not only bear an undue share of the global disease but also the conditions that lead to disease and death. In particular, 30,000 children die each day because they are poor.

Although considerable progress has been made in many nations and countries, children are still vulnerable to the many health threats in today's world—poverty, political instability, environmental degradation, gender discrimination, economic crises, poor public infrastructures, inadequate health systems, and growing health issues such as HIV/AIDS (WHO, 2003; Kotch, 2005). Ninety percent of children are born in developing countries or low- and middle-income countries where many of these health issues are even greater (Torjesen & Olness, 2004; Kotch, 2005; Lopez, Mathers, Ezzati, Jamison, & Murray, 2006). Unfortunately, population projections show a continual rapid growth in the developing countries of Africa, south central Asia, Southeast Asia, west Asia, and South and Central America with modest or slowing growth rates in the more industrial nations such as east Asia, North America and Europe (WHO, 2003; Torjesen & Olness, 2004; WHO, 2005). In addition, children from these developing countries and nations are also moving into Europe and North America as refugees, immigrants, or international adoptees (Jenista, 2001).

Children continue to be exposed to various policies and practices that put them at risk for death, unhealthy conditions, and failure to develop properly. Children are often the most vulnerable members of society, thus their health serves as a marker for the well-being of a society and its future potential. Children not only require the basic survival needs of food, water, adequate shelter, and appropriate hygienic requirements, they also require basic social interactions and safe, supportive environments that allow for nurturing, healthy play, and optimal growth and development. Foundations of health as well as healthy habits are established during childhood. These health habits or lack thereof become part of an adult's methods to survive and flourish leading to a healthy society and world. It thus becomes vital to acknowledge and understand the background and historical perspective of global children's health as well as current health concerns for children and future challenges.

Background and Historical Perspective

According to Kotch (2005), the understanding and concern for the health of the world's children is closely linked to the world's political history, wars, colonialism, and trade. For example, during the colonial period, schools of tropical medicine were established in western Europe to understand and examine the nature, origin, and transmission of diseases from the colonies that were dangerous to Europeans; they did not necessarily examine the introduction of European diseases (e.g., measles and smallpox) to the colonies or the native population. Over time these schools grew in importance. In 1913, the Rockefeller Foundation established the International Health Commission, which focused on the control or elimination of specific diseases that affected trade and the productivity of workers. Kotch (2005) further explains that the growth in world trade led to concerns about transmission of diseases such as cholera or the plague between countries by way of trading vessels, which could lead to ships being quarantined. These concerns eventually led to the adoption of a common sanitary code to improve the sanitation in ports and establish fair and consistent quarantine measures. This was the initial development of the Pan-American Sanitary Code. The United Nations (UN) was created after World War II as a vehicle for peace and conflict resolution among nations; specialized agencies of the UN were developed to focus on promotion and protection of health (Kotch, 2005). Two such agencies are the United Nations International Children's Emergency Fund (UNICEF), which was developed to assist the thousands of orphans and abandoned children that resulted from the war; and, the World Health Organization (WHO), which began in 1948 as an intergovernmental institution to promote and protect global health.

Over the years WHO has called attention to the plight of children through such efforts as the World Summit of Children held in1990 (WHO, 2003). Major gains have been made in reducing child mortality; however, there has been a stagnation or even reversal of trends since the World Summit. For example, between 1970 and 1990, the under-5 mortality rate dropped by 20% every decade, but between 1990 and 2000 it dropped by only 12% (WHO, 2005). Just six countries account for 50% of the global childhood deaths (WHO, 2005). Today's ever-increasing globalization comes with profound health implications, such as increased disease transfer and mobility risks, an increased exchange of goods and information between countries in response to health problems, and the changing roles of national governments and international organizations in the health field (Kotch, 2005). The emergence and global spread of the bird flu or severe acute respiratory syndrome (SARS) in 2003, the reemergence of tuberculosis (TB) as an increasing public health threat in the developed world, and the pandemic concern of HIV/AIDS illustrate the truly global nature of today's health threats (Kotch, 2005). Although many of these threats affect the adult population of the world, attention needs to be drawn to the children who are also affected, by directly acquiring these diseases or by having family members or parents acquire and sometimes die from such health problems.

As a result of ever-increasing globalization and its profound implications for the health of the world, 189 member nations of the UN unanimously adopted the *Millennium Declaration* in 2000 (United Nations, 2000). This international document provides an overall mission, a set of guiding principles, and a list of specific objectives. These objectives target specific world issues, concerns, and problems related to the health and development of the world's population, and have completion dates in the twenty-first century. Included in this document are specific development goals, including three that specifically target the health of children. These goals are listed in Table 17-1 (United Nations, 2004). Although all eight goals affect children in various ways, these three bring attention specifically to children's health. In addition, other documents have followed, such as the UN's *Special Session for Children* published in 2002, which recognized the growing need for a new social agenda for children and their families (United Nations, 2002). In 2003, WHO's document, *Strategic Directions for Improving the Health and Development of Children and Adolescents,* summarized seven priority areas for action and defined specific principles to guide their implementation. The purpose of these documents and summits is to emphasize the importance of investing in children's and adolescents' health and

TABLE 17-1   United Nations Millennium Health Goals

Goal	Target Deadline
Four: Reduce child mortality	By 2015 reduce the mortality rate by two thirds among children
Five: Improve maternal health	By 2015 reduce the ratio of women dying in childbirth by three quarters
Six: Combat HIV/AIDS, malaria, and other diseases	By 2015 halt and begin to reverse the spread of HIV/AIDS and lower incidences of malaria and other major diseases

Source: United Nations, 2004

development as a cost-effective strategy to secure future prosperity for countries and nations.

Childhood Mortality and Morbidity Statistics: Measuring Health in Children

Health problems of children vary widely among countries and nations of the world. Torjesen and Olness attribute this variation to numerous factors ranging from climate and geography to gene frequencies (2004). In general, an acceptable measure of the health of children is mortality rates. Some authors identify it as the ultimate indicator of poor child health outcomes (Kotch, 2005). Mortality rates are calculated as the number of deaths occurring in an age range divided by the number of children entering that particular age range in a given period of time.

As mentioned earlier in the chapter, the mortality rate of children 5 years and younger is 8 deaths per 1000 children in the United States but 86 deaths per 1000 children for the overall child population of the world (US Census Bureau, 2004). The under-5 mortality rate captures the entire high-risk period in high-mortality settings and so is the most widely used and critical indicator to summarize child health from an international perspective (Kotch, 2005; UNICEF, 2003). This information is obtained through samples from vital registration systems in some countries, and in others, from population-based surveys such as the Demographic and Health Surveys (DHS) and UNICEF Multiple Indicator Cluster Surveys (Kotch, 2005).

The estimated global under-5 mortality rate declined from 197 deaths per 1000 live births in 1960 to 82 deaths per 1000 live births in 2000 (UNICEF, 2004a). Spectacular reductions in childhood mortality were achieved during the 1980s, reducing childhood mortality by one third. The 1990 World Summit for Children set a goal of reducing childhood mortality by an additional third by the year 2000 (Global Health Council, 2006). Although the decline in child mortality rate showed considerable progress over several decades, this progress was not uniform, specifically with certain areas of the world showing much less improvement (Global Health Council, 2006). There is some evidence that the rate of decline of child mortality has actually slowed or even increased in some areas, which causes great concern (Ahmad, Lopez, & Inoue, 2000; WHO, 2005). Approximately 90% of child deaths occur in 42 countries (Kotch, 2005; Global Health Council, 2006). The largest number of child deaths occur in India, Nigeria, China, and Pakistan, but the highest mortality rates occur in Sierra Leone, Niger, Angola and Afghanistan. This means 25% of all children die before their fifth birthday (Ahmad et al., 2000; Black, Morris, & Bryce, 2003; WHO, 2005). In comparison, less than 1% of children die before their fifth birthday in the United States.

What Are the Health Problems for Children?

According to WHO (2005), 99% of deaths in children younger than 5 years of age are due to malnutrition, perinatal and neonatal conditions, pneumonia, diarrhea, measles, malaria, and HIV/AIDS. WHO (2005) identifies the three major causes of deaths in children in countries with relatively high levels of child mortality to be diarrhea, pneumonia, and neonatal causes. According to WHO (2005), specific diseases, however, cause more deaths in specific regions, such as malaria being the significant cause of death in sub-Saharan Africa and AIDS being the cause in east and southern Africa. As the mortality rate declines in specific regions, the cause of death shifts from diarrhea, pneumonia, and vaccine-preventable diseases such as measles to neonatal causes such as birth asphyxia and low birth weight (Kotch, 2005; Byrce, Boschi-Pinto, Shibuya, & Black, 2005). In regions with low child mortality rates, the cause of death is due to neonatal conditions such as congenital anomalies and injuries. An indication of this is the infant mortality rates and the cause of infant deaths in the United States (Kotch, 2005).

Neonatal Deaths

The Global Health Council (2006) indicates approximately 37% of all child deaths occur during the neonatal period, or during the first 28 days of life. The leading causes of death for these nearly 4 million neonates include severe infection, birth asphyxia, complications of prematurity including low birth weight, and tetanus (Global Health Council, 2006; Lopez et al., 2006). Because there is evidence of incomplete records or underreporting in various regions of the world, these deaths may be much higher. Tetanus, alone, causes 200,000 newborns to die each year under circumstances such as cutting the umbilical cord with an unsterile instrument (Global Health Council, 2006).

WHO indicates that malnutrition is the single largest contributor to premature death in children. One in every 4 children, or about 150 million children, are malnourished (UNICEF, 2004b). When infants are born weighing less than 2500 grams they are at a greater risk of death and disease than infants at normal and above normal birth weights. Many times malnutrition results from the mother having poor nutrition and being deficient of essential minerals and vitamins such as vitamin A or zinc, which lead to increase risk of the child dying from diarrhea, pneumonia, measles, or malaria (WHO, 2003; Global Health Council, 2006). In addition, children born to unhealthy mothers are at risk for being underweight, which can lead to difficulty combating illness. These infants face a world that is less able to provide a safe and nurturing environment necessary for healthy growth and development (WHO, 2003).

Pneumonia

Approximately 19% of children's deaths can be attributed to pneumonia or other acute respiratory infections (Global Health Council, 2006). Many of these deaths result because the child is already weakened by malnutrition or other diseases when pneumonia is acquired. This occurrence is also associated with indoor pollution resulting from the use of certain types of fuel combined with poor ventilation (Global Health Council, 2006). Pneumonia, although serious, can be effectively treated with the appropriate health care and availability of antibiotics, especially since most fatal childhood pneumonia is of bacterial origin (Global Health Council, 2006). This fact raises a serious health dilemma about the availability of health resources in developing countries or nations.

Diarrheal Disease

Diarrheal diseases such as cholera, shigellosis, and rotavirus kill over 1.8 million children each year (Global Health Council, 2006). Because children are more vulnerable to dehydration and electrolyte imbalances, diarrheal conditions may lead to death in children more quickly than in adults. Death can occur even more easily in children with vitamin deficiencies or nondiarrheal infections. When poor sanitation conditions exist, such as unsafe drinking water or lack of proper food storage, food- and waterborne diarrheal infections develop easily making prevention extremely difficult.

Death from diarrheal diseases is mostly preventable and can be avoided with the use of inexpensive oral rehydration solutions while the child has diarrhea. WHO and UNICEF have advocated zinc supplement tablets during diarrhea episodes to help prevent recurrences. Diarrhea can also be prevented through better nutritional practices in early childhood, particularly exclusive breast feeding until the age of 6 months and the appropriate introduction of complementary foods during the weaning period (Global Health Council, 2006). Just by using these two practices, child mortality can be reduced by 20%. Other interventions outside the health sector, such as the provision of safe drinking water and clean sanitation facilities also play a major role in stopping needless diarrhea-related deaths in children.

Malaria and Measles

According to the Global Health Council (2006), over 800,000 children under 5 years of age die each year from malaria. This accounts for 8% of childhood deaths. In addition, 4% of children under the age of 5 die from measles, which can be prevented by ensuring children are vaccinated (Global Health Council 2006). Malaria is the leading cause of hospitalization, mortality, and morbidity in children living in areas such as sub-Saharan Africa. These deaths can be prevented by using insecticide-treated bed netting and spraying with insecticides to decrease the infestation of mosquitoes. According to the Global Health Council (2006), both this intervention as well as the successful treatment of malaria with artemisinin derivatives are gaining attention. Unfortunately, the cost of these new drugs and their lack of availability are presenting some barriers in eradicating this deadly disease.

HIV/AIDS

Unfortunately the HIV/AIDS pandemic has spread to over 2.2 million children under the age of 15 with over 90% of these children residing in sub-Saharan Africa (Global Health Council, 2006). Most of the children under 5 years of age became infected through their mothers during childbirth or through breastfeeding. As WHO (2003) indicates, the HIV pandemic poses a particular threat to children, as evidenced by the estimated 800,000 infants infected in 2001 mainly through mother–child transmission. In addition, over 15 million children, most living in sub-Saharan Africa, have lost one or both parents to AIDS; there are many ways children are affected by this deadly spread of infection. At present, approximately 1800 children become infected with HIV every day (Global Health Council, 2006). In addition, investigations of HIV prevalence rates reveal that most countries in sub-Saharan Africa with high HIV prevalence rates also experience increased under-5 mortality rates (Adetunji, 2000). Other regions identified for the potential of emerging epidemics include the Caribbean, China, India, central Asia, and eastern Europe (Kotch, 2005).

Kotch (2005) indicates that the political and financial commitments to dealing with HIV/AIDS have increased over the past decade through various initiatives of the UN, WHO, and the US President's Emergency Plan for AIDS Relief. Most of these initiatives focus on four main strategies: primary prevention of HIV in young women; avoidance of unintended pregnancies among HIV-infected women; provision of antiretroviral drugs (ARVs) targeted at preventing HIV transmission from HIV-infected women to their infants, safe delivery, counseling, and support for safer infant feeding practices; and providing care and support for mothers and their families. The treatment of children with AIDS also presents barriers because of the lack of availability and accessibility of pediatric formulations for these drugs. Also the cost of these drugs are slightly higher for children, and the administration is more complicated to regulate because children must have their medications adjusted as they grow (Global Health Council, 2006; Dawson, 2006). Thus few children with HIV/AIDS in sub-Saharan Africa get antiretroviral therapy because it is easier and cheaper to give to adults (Dawson, 2006). Another concern is the heavy emphasis on one single disease within severely resource-limited areas of the world, which could draw resources away from other health issues and concerns (Claeson, Gillespie, Mshinda, Troedsson, & Victora, 2003; Walker, Schwartlander, & Bryce, 2002).

Injuries

About 300,000 children under the age of 5 die each year from injuries caused by traffic accidents, fires, drowning, falls, and poisoning (Global Health Council, 2006). Over a 10 year period from 1999 to 2000, more than 20 million children were displaced by disasters (Torjesen & Olness, 2004). WHO attributes over 1 million deaths of children and adolescents to injuries and violence. With many of these deaths occurring in low-income countries, injuries are also among the leading causes of mortality and life-long disability for those who survive in higher-income countries.

Other Causes of Death in Children

About 10% of all child deaths under 5 years of age are due to other causes such as additional infectious diseases, childhood cluster diseases like pertussis and tetanus, and other nutritional deficiencies (Global Health Council, 2006). Additional factors lead to disease, disability or chronic poor health. For example, malnutrition among pregnant women leads to stunted growth and impaired learning in children. Over 50 million children in the world are malnourished, and 1 in every 3 children under age 5 from low-income countries shows evidence of being stunted (WHO, 2003). Good nutrition is the foundation for healthy development and prevention of illness. Children who are not breast fed are six times more likely to die by the age of 1 month than children who receive at least some breast milk. Children are also at a particularly vulnerable period from the end of 6 months onwards when breast feeding is no longer sufficient to meet all nutritional requirements (WHO, 2003). In addition, children around the world are losing one or both parents to AIDS, which leads to more homeless children and children in poverty, a condition that has many health problems associated with it. Globalization has created an abundance of opportunities for many, but it has also resulted in a deepening of socioeconomic disparities in all regions of the world.

Larger Ramifications of Children's Health Problems

The major determinants of childhood mortality can be traced to specific global issues such as poverty, a lack of essential public health resources such as safe water and appropriate sanitation, an absence of prenatal care, inadequate diet, exposure to insect vectors of disease, and a lack of basic health and preventive services (Global Health Council,

2006). These conditions and situations put children at a higher risk of death from numerous other conditions and diseases. For example, as already discussed, malnutrition from lack of an inadequate diet underlies and contributes to approximately 53% of all child deaths (Global Health Council, 2006). There are also larger ramifications of these conditions leading to unrealized human potential and negative effects on individuals, families, communities, and countries in terms of productivity, economics, and politics (Torjesen & Olness, 2004).

Impaired Learning and Other Disabilities

The effects of poor nutrition continue throughout a child's life by contributing to poor school performance, reduced productivity, and other measures of impaired intellectual and social development (WHO, 2003). Galler and Barrett (2001) have documented that a few months of malnutrition in the first year of life is linked to learning disabilities, attention problems, and reduced school performance in 65–70% of children. These children may also drop out of school and have difficulty finding employment if they lack access to special education and training. Over a million children who survive birth asphyxia each year develop problems such as learning difficulties, cerebral palsy, and other disabilities (WHO, 2005). Disabilities affect 1 in 10 children in developing countries with the major causes of these disabilities being premature birth, malnutrition, infections, injuries, child neglect and understimulation, which are all preventable (WHO, 2003). These conditions can be prevented through early identification, early interventions and rehabilitation for children at risk of developing disabilities, or who already have them.

Disasters and Child Trafficking

Between 1999 and 2000, over 20 million malnourished children were displaced by disasters (Torjesen & Olness, 2004). It is also vital to pay special attention to the rising numbers of orphans who have lost parents due to HIV infection, disasters, or violence. In 2000, more than 10 million children younger than 15 years old had lost one or both parents to AIDS (Torjesen & Olness, 2004). Whether it is natural events such as the 2005 tsunami, industrial accidents such as the 1984 chemical disasters in Bhopal, or the many wars including the Middle East conflict, children are greatly affected. Many of these children live on the streets or are lost to institutionalization. If they have not lost their parents and other family members, they are still at risk for infectious diseases, malnutrition, and psychological trauma with the potential for lifelong damages. Children displaced from wars in Southeast Asia, central Africa, and Bosnia, have shown a high prevalence of mental health problems continuing years after resettlement (Torjesen & Olness, 2004).

Other issues include trafficking, smuggling, physical and sexual exploitation, and economic exploitation, which are realities for children in all regions of the world (WHO, 2003). It is estimated that 1.2 million children fall victim annually to child trafficking (UNICEF, 2003). This occurs when children are exploited in agricultural and domestic service as documented in sub-Saharan Africa, or forced into prostitution as seen in Southeast Asia, the Republic of Modlova, Romania, and Ukraine. In addition, WHO (2003) estimates that 300,000 children in Africa have been coerced into military service as soldiers, porters, messengers, and other positions.

Health Issues Later in Life

Many of these health conditions and issues become lifelong problems for children. For example, children may survive injuries but live with a long-term disability. Victims of interpersonal violence, such as children who were subjected to sexual abuse, are twice as likely to become depressed and four times as likely to attempt suicide (WHO, 2003). Once affected, a child's health and development is permanently altered.

Adolescents

Unfortunately, adolescents are often thought to be healthy simply because they survived any early childhood health issues. This premise has lead to a lack of attention to adolescents' health and social needs. This neglect led approximately half of all new HIV infections to occur in this age group in 2000 (WHO, 2003). Further, the estimated mortality in ages 10 to 19 years is over 1.4 million young men and women annually. These deaths are caused by injuries from unintentional causes, suicide, violence, pregnancy-related complications and illnesses, all which can be treated and prevented (WHO, 2003). This age group also has such health problems as the highest rates of new sexually transmitted infections, which occur in youth 15 to 24 years of age; use of psychoactive substances such as amphetamines, opioids, and cocaine; undernutrition and micronutrient deficiencies in girls, which lead to adverse pregnancy outcomes; and unhealthy diets and lack of physical activity leading to unprecedented increases in obesity and risk for chronic diseases such as diabetes, hypertension, and cardiovascular disease (WHO, 2003). Again, the choices and habits established during this period of life will greatly influence the future health status of these up-and-coming adults.

Mental Health

Approximately 10–20% of children have one or more mental or behavioral problems (WHO, 2003). In addition, over 90,000 adolescents commit suicide globally each year (WHO, 2003). Conflict, poverty, forced migration, and nutritional deficiencies affect the intellectual and social development of children. This presents challenges and barriers leading to consequences for the children's well-being and productivity as it relates to mental health.

Marginalized Groups

Overt or implicit discrimination results in marginalized groups of children and adolescents, which leads to vulnerability (WHO, 2003). Examples include children who are permanently disabled or seriously injured by armed conflict, children displaced as refugees, street children, children suffering from natural and man-made disasters, children of migrant workers and other socially disadvantaged groups, and children who are victims of racial discrimination, xenophobia, and intolerance. Other groups include the orphans of the world and the children that have been exploited economically, sexually, or physically.

One example of this marginalization involves the refugees of ongoing military conflict such as in Sudan. The Nations Health Report (2004) provides some staggering statistics and facts about the excess of one million people who were refugees from the military conflict in Sudan. Malnutrition rates were up to 39% with 58% of children 6 months to 5 years having diarrhea and measles outbreaks. As many as 200 children were dying every month from violent acts, starvation, and disease. Many of these children worked the streets and would return home but not to a protective, nurturing family. In every country, children who live or spend most of their lives on the street are more at risk for malnutrition, HIV infection, drug abuse, and violence (UNICEF, 2003).

Approaches to Child Health Around the World

Two thirds of children's deaths can be successfully averted by existing preventive and therapeutic strategies (Global Health Council, 2006). Many of these proven prevention and treatment interventions used to improve child survival, such as exclusive breast feeding, immunizations, micronutrient supplementation, (particularly vitamin A and zinc), complimentary feeding, antibiotics for pneumonia, dysentery, sepsis, oral rehydration therapy for diarrhea, antimalarial drugs, and insecticide-treated bed netting, can be implemented even in resource-poor environments.(Kotch, 2005; Lopez et al., 2006). These strategies could prevent 63% of the 10 million child deaths that occur each year (Jones, Steketee, Black, Bhutta, & Morris. 2003). The WHO Expanded Program on Immunizations as well as the Diarrheal Disease Control Program are examples of effective programs with measurable impacts on child health (Bryce et al., 2003; Claeson et al., 2003). Launched in 1974, these programs focused on immunizing children against six major infectious diseases (diphtheria, pertussis, tetanus, tuberculosis, polio, and measles) before their first birthday. Great success was documented in various countries, but specific regions still lagged behind (Bryce et al., 2003).

Broader approaches, such as the WHO Integrated Management of Childhood Illnesses (IMCI), were launched in the 1990s to improve case management skills of health staff, make improvements in the health systems to support effective management skills, and enhance family and community practices (Kotch, 2005). The IMCI was a positive step towards providing higher-quality, comprehensive care for children in developing countries. The program used healthcare algorithms written at or slightly above the level of a village healthcare worker and targeted children younger than 5 years old, the age group with the highest death rate from common childhood diseases (Torjesen & Olness, 2004). Complex analyses indicate that mortality from diarrheal diseases fell from 2.4 million deaths in 1990 to about 1.6 million deaths in 2001 as a result of efforts in diarrhea case management, including the use of oral rehydration therapy (Lopez et al., 2006).

WHO (2003) called for priority areas of action in their report, *Strategic Directions for Improving the Health and Development of Children and Adolescents*. These priority areas, as identified in Table 17-2, require focused attention because they affect the physical well-being as well as the psychosocial development of children and adolescents. In addition, the report includes three specific guiding principles in order to implement the strategic actions. These include: (1) address inequities and facilitate the respect, protection, and fulfillment of human rights as outlined in the *Convention on the Rights of the Child*; (2) take a life-course approach that recognizes the continuum from birth through childhood, adolescence and adulthood; and (3) implement a public health approach by focusing on major health issues and applying a systematic development model to ensure the availability and accessibility of effective, relevant interventions.

Another way to examine the approaches to global health for children is to review the global maternal-child health (MCH) program strategies. These strategies can be split into two categories: disease-specific interventions and broad community-based strategies often identified as primary healthcare initiatives (Claeson & Waldman, 2000). Claeson and Waldman (2000) provide examples of disease-specific programs including attempts to eradicate malaria in the 1950s, 1960s, and 1970s as well as campaigns to eradicate smallpox and polio. These highly focused initiatives each aimed to have a dramatic impact on a single disease. They found some success such as the eradication of smallpox but also experienced failures such as the attempts to eradicate malaria. Due to these mixed results, there was a shift toward a broader community-based primary healthcare strategy in the late 1970s which focused on universal MCH services, family planning, improved sanitation and clean water supplies achieved through equitable distribution of resources, community participation, emphasis on preventive rather that curative services, and a multisectoral approach (Claeson & Waldman, 2000; Kotch, 2005). Another improvement made in the primary healthcare strategy is the emergence of selective care that prioritizes health problems that have higher mortality or morbidity. The strategy also includes cost-effective interventions that will aid the largest possible number of people such as growth monitoring, oral rehydration, breast feeding, and immunization (Kotch, 2005).

The obstacles of implementing general health strategies are similar to the obstacles of child-survival strategies. These obstacles include high staff turnover, poor management and supervision, and inadequate funding, all which continue to cause problems over and above the difficulty of acquiring adequate services in specific areas and regions (Kotch, 2005). The loss of children due to avoidable or treatable conditions is needless. The drastic decline in childhood mortality rates in the 1980s verifies that interventions are successful, especially if the global health community, political leaders, governments, foundations, and private citizens make commitments and provide needed resources (Global Health Council, 2006). Four major obstacles identified by the Global Health Council (2006) are displayed in Table 17-3. The current response to the death of children and the

TABLE 17-2   Priority Areas for Actions Identified by WHO

Priority Area	Specified Action
Maternal and Newborn Health	Reduce neonatal mortality, provide skilled birth attendants with adequate facility support, promote prenatal care, and tackle the mother–child transmission challenge.
Nutrition	Provide adequate nutrition to mothers and their children, promote breast feeding, and implement the *Global Strategy for Infant and Young Child Feeding*.
Communicable Diseases	Avert over 50% of childhood deaths by preventing communicable disease, specifically pneumonia, diarrhea, malaria, measles, and HIV infection. Also prevent other diseases that pose a greater risk to children than adults, which include syphilis, tuberculosis, meningitis, dengue, Japanese encephalitis, leishmaniasis, and trypanosomiasis. Move beyond addressing single diseases and towards integrated approaches for prevention and management of common diseases.
Injury and Violence	Draw attention to the prevention of injury and violence, which lead to death or lifelong disability in more than 1 million children and adolescents. Modify environments, change designs or structures, apply and reinforce regulatory measures, provide parent training and social support to families, and change unsafe behaviors through education. For the greatest success, combine the three strategies of regulatory measures, environmental changes, and education.
Physical Environment	Use interventions to improve water supply, sanitation, and hygiene, which can reduce child mortality by 65%. Also implement other interventions to improve indoor air pollution, prevent injuries and minimize other environmental risk factors. Focus on the WHO's six priority issues—household water security, hygiene and sanitation, air pollution, disease vectors, chemical hazards, and injuries and accidents.
Adolescent Health	Focus attention on support for mental, sexual, and reproductive health; the rights of adolescents to information, skills, services, and protection from exploitative relationships; and support to develop responsible behavior.
Psychosocial Development and Mental Health	Long-term consequences for well-being must be examined to prevent these concerns. Implement early interventions in areas of feeding, play and communication as appropriate.

Source: Adapted from WHO, 2003.

TABLE 17-3	Obstacles to Implementing Child Survival Strategies
First	The highest rates of under-5 mortality occur in a limited number of the poorest countries.
Second	Many of these countries have been involved in war or civil conflict.
Third	The government is unwilling to or incapable of providing health services effectively.
Fourth	The poor are marginalized and most difficult to reach.

implementation of strategies to prevent these deaths is fragmented and uncoordinated; therefore the Global Health Council proposes four major actions: effective leadership, strengthened health systems, evidence-based health delivery system guidelines, and evaluation systems to monitor progress towards improved survival.

Another important focus for eliminating health problems and issues for children and adolescents is to establish a developmental approach. WHO (2003) outlined five developmental phases with possible health outcomes and examples of interventions. Implementing this approach within a public health strategy that already targets the aforementioned obstacles could achieve the highest possible levels of health and well-being.

Future Challenges

So how can professional healthcare providers help children around the world? What type of skills and systems are needed by these individuals and institutions? Millions of children die each year from preventable causes. If they only had appropriate and timely access to five basic and inexpensive health prevention and therapeutic inventions, these children would survive (Rx for Child Survival, 2005).

The Global Health Council (2006) adds to the list by advocating these additional methods: (1) the continuance of breast feeding through a child's first year, (2) sanitation including clean water and waste disposal, (3) prevention of mother–child transmission of HIV in countries with a high prevalence of HIV through the use of antiretrovial drugs, and (4) the use of zinc therapy for diarrhea. These types of inventions are not expensive and could eliminate much unnecessary childhood death. If these interventions were available, there would be major decreases in child death for a fairly low cost (Global Health Council, 2006).

Research and Technology

The United States has done an extraordinary job of documenting events surrounding perinatal health using the vital records system. This is not the case for the health of children, on a population basis (Kotch, 2005). From a research population database perspective, the United States knows very little about early childhood health with the exception of mortality and immunization status (Kotch, 2005). Some states monitor blood lead levels, hospitalizations, and injuries, as well as school physical examinations, but these efforts are not uniform across the country (Kotch, 2005). We need this data to effectively monitor and explore trends and issues that effect children's health in order to advocate for policy, initiatives, and programs to promote and maintain children's health care. More efforts are needed to move toward population-wide surveys and surveillance of child health parameters. Some authors suggest one third of the births in the developing world are not registered (Torjesen & Olness, 2004). WHO (2003) recommends a public health model with strong research and technical implementation. Priority should be given to research and development activities relevant to the needs of children and adolescents that would inform policy, lead to new technologies, and improve delivery strategies.

Various Influences Such as Politics, Economics, and Culture

Not only do health problems differ in various areas of the world, but also communities, countries, and nations set priorities and deal with children's health differently due to the local concerns, resources, and needs. So many factors influence children's health from political instability and violence in a country or nation to the economic conditions and family resources that determine the healthcare decisions and resources provided for the children within a family. Children must depend on their parents, advocates, and policy makers to articulate appropriate child healthcare policies and implement relevant programs (Akukwe, 2000). More than 30% of children or approximately 600 million live in developing countries where they live on less than one US dollar a day (UNICEF, 2004a). Even in the world's richest countries, 1 in every 6 children still live below the national poverty level (UNICEF, 2004a). WHO (2005) estimates that poverty is directly responsible for the death of 12 million children annually under the age of 5. For example, in sub-Saharan Africa, most of the countries with stagnant or reversing child mortality rates also have the highest incidence of extreme poverty (WHO, 2005).

Many of the world's children are diverse in ethnic and cultural backgrounds and will need to be understood by healthcare providers. Cultural and religious practices may limit or counteract the effectiveness of medical and health practices (Torjesen & Olness, 2004). For example, the survival of an infant relies on more than its health at birth, but is also dependent on the race and ethnic status of the mother, the socioeconomic status of the parents, the residence of the parents, the preconception health status of the mother, and the level of maternal education (Akukwe, 2000). In the United States, women with fewer than 12 years of education have higher rates of delayed prenatal care, infants with low birth weight, and neonatal deaths compared to the women with higher educational levels (Akukwe, 2000).

TABLE 17-4 Three Major Factors Related to Inequality in Health Outcomes

Factor	Associated Conditions
Lower Socioeconomic Status	Less use of antenatal and delivery care
	Exposure to poor sanitation, crowding, and undernutrition
	Less preventive health or appropriate and timely treatment for illness
Gender	Low status for women in various global areas leads to greater exposure of health risks such as gender-based violence and exposure to HIV (Blanc, 2001; Shiffman, 2000; WHO, 2003; Dunkle et al., 2004).
	Stronger preference for sons leads to infanticide and neglect of female children in areas of the world such as northern India, China, and parts of east Asia (Victora et al., 2003; WHO, 2003).
Education	Educated women and their children are less likely to die than their less educated counterparts (Kotch, 2005).
	An increase in education leads to improved domestic health care and hygiene and increased use of health services.

A recurrent theme that develops in examining the health of children of the world is the inequality in health outcomes within and among countries worldwide. Although unfortunate health outcomes are seen in the poorer regions of the world, examination of data from the wealthiest countries also shows inequality within specific countries (Macinko, Shi, & Starfield, 2004). Various authors, national, and international documents identify three major factors that draw particular focus to this inequality: socioeconomic status, gender, and education (Kotch, 2005; Black et al., 2003; Victoria et al., 2003; WHO, 2003). Table 17-4 provides some of the conditions associated with each of these factors. Education of women and their children, higher socioeconomic status, and greater value and respect of women lead to more favorable health outcomes for children in countries and regions throughout the world (Kotch, 2005; Black et al., 2003; Victoria et al., 2003). Poverty and health are inextricably linked. Thus, the world must work towards eliminating poverty in order to improve health.

The United Nations Children's Fund (2004a) advocates four major goals to benefit children throughout the world. Accomplishing these goals would result in individual well-being and productivity for all children and adolescents with the overall result of healthy global communities. Today, fostering healthy families is a necessary global imperative. To continue to move beyond simple survival to ensure health, growth, and full development for all children, adolescents, and their families requires strong commitments from political leaders, clear identification of children's health as a priority, and strategic investments from nations' budgets followed by investments in comprehensive and integrated efforts that have proven cost-effective and have outcomes leading to improved child and adolescent health (WHO, 2003; Kotch, 2005).

The majority of the childhood death that occurs can be prevented worldwide if children receive appropriate and timely access to health care and interventions (Global Health Council, 2006; Bryce et al., 2003; Jones et al., 2003; Shiffman, 2000). These children die because of stagnant progress, missed opportunities, and growing inequities in the provision of basic services. This is a worldwide public health disaster (Venis, 2003). The international millennium development goals provide a clear strategy. Specific international organizations provide further guidance and strategic direction. The world needs to continue to seek creative and effective approaches in order to cross political, socioeconomic and cultural barriers so that all children will be adequately served, supported and protected. Hopefully, the value of the world's children will be understood and there will be an increased effort to guide and protect the world's future.

References

Adetunji, J. (2000). Trends in under-5 mortality rates and the HIV/AIDS epidemic. *Bulletin of the World Health Organization, 78*(8), 1200–1206.

Ahmad, O. B., Lopez, A. D., & Inoue, M. (2000). The decline in child mortality: A reappraisal. *Bulletin of the World Health Organization. 78,* 1175–1191.

Akukwe, C. (2000). Maternal and child health services in the twenty-first century: Critical issues, challenges, and opportunities. *Health Care for Women International, 21,* 641–653.

Black, R. E., Morris, S. S., & Bryce, J. (2003). Where and why are 10 million children dying every year? *Lancet, 361,* 2226–2234.

Blanc, A. K. (2001). The effect of power in sexual relationships on sexual and reproductive health: An examination of the evidence. *Studies in Family Planning, 32,* 189–213.

Bryce, J., el Arifeen, S., Pariyo, G., Lanata, C., Gwatkin, D., & Habicht, J. (2003). Reducing child mortality: Can public health deliver? *Lancet, 362,* 159–164.

Byrce, J., Boschi-Pinto, C., Shibuya, K., & Black, R. E. (2005). WHO estimates of the causes of death in children. *Lancet, 365,*1147–1152.

Claeson, M., Gillespie, D., Mshinda, H., Troedsson, H., & Victora, C. (2003). Knowledge into action for child survival. *Lancet, 362,* 323–327.

Claeson, M., & Waldman, R. J. (2000). The evolution of child health programmes in developing countries: From targeting diseases to targeting people. *Bulletin of the World Health Organization, 78,* 1234–1245.

Dawson, D. (2006). *New hope for children with HIV/AIDS. AIDMatters.* Retrieved August 2, 2006, from http://www.talcuk.org/aidmatters

Dunkle, K. L., Jewkes, R. K., Brown, H. C., Gray, G. E., McIntyre, J. A., & Harlow, S. D. (2004). Gender-based violence, relationship power, and risk of HIV infection in women attending antenatal clinics in South Africa. *Lancet, 363,* 1415–1421.

Galler, J. F. & Barrett, L. R. (2001). Children and famine: Long-term impact on development. *Ambulatory Child Health, 7,* 85–95.

Global Health Council. (2006). *Child health.* Retrieved March 30, 2006, from http://www.globalhealth.org/view_top.php3?id=226

Jenista, J. A. (2001). The immigrant, refugee or internationally adopted child. *Pediatric Review. 22*(12), 419–429.

Jones, G., Steketee, R. W., Black, R. E., Bhutta, Z. A., & Morris, S. S. (2003). How many child deaths can we prevent this year? *Lancet, 363*, 65–71.

Kotch, J. B. (2005). *Maternal and child health: Programs, problems, and policy in public health* (2nd ed.). Boston: Jones and Bartlett Publishers.

Lopez, A. D., Mathers, C. D., Ezzati, M. Jamison, D. T., Murray, C. J. L. (2006). Global and regional burden of diseases and risk factors, 2001: Systematic analysis of population health data. *Lancet, 367*, 1747–1757.

Macinko, J. A., Shi, L. Y., & Starfield, B. (2004). Wage inequality, the health system, and infant mortality in wealthy industrialized countries, 1970–1996. *Social Science and Medicine, 58*, 279–292.

Murray, C. J. L., Salomon, J. A., Mathers, C. D., & Lopez, A. D., (Eds.). (2002). *Summary measures of population health: Concepts, ethics, measurement and applications*. Geneva, Switzerland: World Health Organization.

Rx for Child Survival. (2005). *Rx for child survival campaign–A global health challenge*. Retrieved March 30, 2006, from http://www.pbs.org/wgbh/rxfosurvival/campaign/about.html

Shiffman, J. (2000). Can poor countries surmount high maternal mortality? *Studies in Family Planning, 31*, 274–289.

Singer, P. A., Salamanc-Buentello, F., & Daar, A. S. (2005). Harnessing nanotechnology to improve global equity. *Issues in Science and Technology*. Summer 2005, 57–64.

The Nation's Health. (2004). *Malnutrition, violence threaten Sudanese refugees*. October 2004.

Torjesen, K. & Olness, K. (2004) Child health in the developing world. In Behrman, R. E., Kliegman, R. M., and Jenson, H. B. *Nelson Textbook of Pediatrics* (17th ed., pp. 12–14). Philadelphia: Saunders.

UNICEF. (2003). *State of the world's children*. Geneva, Switzerland: United Nations.

UNICEF. (2004a). *End of the decade databases*. Retrieved March 6, 2004, from http://www.childinfo.org/index2.htm

UNICEF. (2004b) *UNICEF At A Glance*. New York. Retrieved on January 2004, from http://www.unicef.org

UNICEF. (2006). *State of the world's children, 2006*. Geneva, Switzerland: Author. Retrieved March 30, 2006, from http://www.unicef.org

United Nations. (2000). *The millennium declaration*. Retrieved September 2000 from http://www.un.org/documents/ga/res/55/a55r002.pdf - A/RES/55/2

United Nations. (2002). *Special session for children*. Retrieved May 16, 2004, from http://www.un.org/documents

United Nations. (2004). *Millennium development goals*. Retrieved May 16, 2004, from http://www.un.org/millenniumdevelopmentgoals

US Census Bureau. (2004). *Global population profile 2002*. Retrieved June 6, 2004, from http://www.census.gov/prod/2004pubs/wp-02.pdf

Venis, S. (2003). Commentary. *Lancet, 361*, 2172.

Victora, C. G., Wagstaff, A., Schellenberg, J. A., Gwatkin, D., Claeson, M., & Habicht, J. P. (2003). Applying an equity lens to child health and mortality: More of the same is not enough. *Lancet, 362*, 233–241.

Walker, N., Schwartlander, B., & Bryce, J. (2002). Meeting international goals in child survival and HIV/AIDS. *Lancet, 360*, 284–289.

WHO. (2003). *Strategic directions for improving the health and development of children and adolescents*. Geneva, Switzerland: World Health Organization. Retrieved March 30, 2006, from http://www.who.int/child-adolescent-health/publications/OVERVIEW/CAH_Strategy.htm

WHO. (2005). *The World Health Report, 2005-Make every mother and child count*. Geneva, Switzerland: World Health Organization.

Chapter 18

Global Health of the Older Adult

David B. Mitchell

Introduction

Grow old along with me!
The best is yet to be,
The last of life, for which the first was made:
Our times are in His hand . . .

—Robert Browning (from "Rabbi Ben Ezra," 1864)

Who is the *older adult*? Is it a person who is *elderly*? When does one become *old* or—to put it another way—when does *aging* begin? Under normal circumstances, a newborn baby begins its life with the same biological and psychological apparatus regardless of where in the world it is born. However, older individuals are clearly not all equally equipped. Although it is often said that all generalizations are false, including this one, a major hallmark of aging is that there are a variety of life span developmental trajectories (Nesselroade, 2001). A key concept to understanding the older adult is an appreciation of individual differences in patterns of aging, because there is no prototypical older adult. For example, one 79-year-old may be frail, suffering from osteoporosis, and experiencing significant deficits in strength and hearing. Another older person—of the same chronological age—might be in peak physical and mental condition (see Figure 18-1). How do aging and the experiences of elderly individuals vary around the world, as a function of different environments, cultures, religions, and political landscapes? We will attempt to answer some of these questions in this chapter.

Gerontology (from *geron*, the Greek word for "old man") is most commonly defined as the scientific study of aging. The term was introduced by Élie Metchnikoff in 1903. A broader definition of gerontology also includes: studies of the processes associated with aging; studies of mature and aged adults; studies of aging scholarship from the perspective of art, philosophy, history and literature; and applications for the *benefit* of older adults (Kastenbaum, 2001). Not to be confused, geriatrics is a subfield of gerontology concerned specifically with the *medical* aspects of aging. The American Geriatrics Society was established in 1942 (Butler, 2001b).

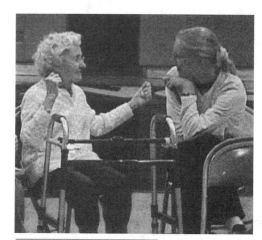
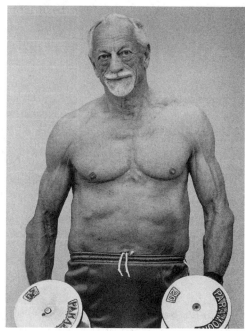

Figure 18-1 Two individuals of the same chronological age (79) with significantly different aging experiences. The image on the left is from the SPARHKS program at Kennesaw State University, courtesy of Dr. Angela Baldwin Lanier. The image on the right is a photo of Dr. John Turner by Etta Clark (1995).

Source: Clark, 1995.

In the field of gerontology, studies of older populations typically use the index of chronological age, starting at age 65. However, the passage of time per se does not cause the biological changes associated with age (Arking, 2006, p. 4). Because most biologists believe that aging begins at conception (Hayflick, 1996), the age of 65 is arbitrary and certainly not biologically precise. Furthermore, even though there are normative ages to define specific stages of maturation, including adolescence and menopause, there is no such thing as a normative age at which a person "turns old." The historical reason for the particular age of 65 is based on a story about German chancellor Otto von Bismarck who lived from 1815 to 1898. Bismarck noted that his major political rivals were federal employees over the age of 65. He succeeded in pushing through legislation that required retirement at age 65, and then "ascended to power with ease" when he was 56 years old (Hayflick, 1996, p. 108). Ironically, he held his position as chancellor until age 75. The 65+ criterion has long been the standard in most American (He, Sengupta, Velkoff, & DeBarros, 2005) and European aging research, and is still the cut point used in current

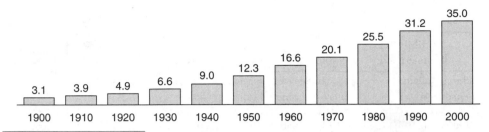

Figure 18-2 Number of older adults in the United States in the twentieth century (in millions).

Source: He Sengupta, Velkoff, & DeBarros, 2005.

studies of global aging (Kinsella & Phillips, 2005). However, this particular chronological milestone may not serve as well for research conducted in third and fourth world countries, because, as we will see in the next section, a relatively smaller proportion of people in less developed countries survive past 65 years old.[1] Nevertheless, with the exception of the United Nations Programme on Ageing (2001), which prefers to use age 60, the 65+ criterion is the most commonly used index for defining those in the *older adult* category.

Chronological age is still the best marker available for making global comparisons of aging phenomena. We will start with data from the US Census Bureau to describe the increase in the older portion of the population over the past century. Then we will examine the same phenomenon across the globe. It is clear from Figure 18-2 that the number of older people in the United States increased greatly during the past century. The population as a whole also grew substantially (from 76 million in 1900 to 281 million in the 2000 census[2]), so a simple count—even in millions—could be misleading. Perhaps the growth in the number of older people simply parallels the overall growth of the country as whole. However, this is not the case. A more informative perspective is provided in Figure 18-3 where the number of older adults in America is plotted as a *percentage* of the total population. It is clear from this graph that the size of the older population has

---

[1]Various terms are used to differentiate national developments. In the United Nations usage, more developed, developed, and industrialized refer to countries in Europe and North America, and to Australia, New Zealand, and Japan. All other countries are referred to as less developed, developing, and nonindustrialized (Kinsella & Phillips, 2005). The terms less developed and more developed will be used in this chapter.

[2]The US Census Bureau estimated that the US population reached 300 million on October 17, 2006. As explained on their Web site, the current birthrate still exceeds the death rate: "The estimate is based on the expectation that the United States will register one birth every 7 seconds and one death every 13 seconds.... while net international migration is expected to add one person every 31 seconds. The result is an increase in the total population of one person every 11 seconds" (US Census Bureau, 2006).

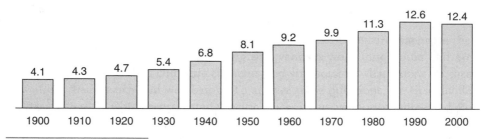

Figure 18-3 Older adults as a percentage of total US population in the twentieth century.

Source: He et al., 2005.

grown disproportionately, increasing at a much faster rate than the entire population. In other words, while the entire population increased almost fourfold, the older adult population increased more than tenfold. This phenomenon is called *population aging,* defined as "the process by which older individuals come to form a proportionately larger share of the total population" and "is one of the most distinctive demographic events in the world today" (Chakraborti, 2004, p. 33).

The aforementioned demographic facts have led to an increased interest in the field of gerontology. Prior to 1974, the United States did not have a national health institute dedicated to aging, and now—just over 30 years later—the National Institute on Aging has a budget of over 1 billion dollars and sponsors a number of important research projects aimed at increasing our understanding of aging and improving the lives of older Americans. The increased interest in gerontology is apparent on a global basis as well, as evidenced by the convening of the Second World Assembly on Aging, which took place in Madrid 20 years after the United Nations (UN) convened the First World Assembly on Aging in Vienna in 1982 (National Research Council, 2001). In Figure 18-4, it is clear that although the percentage of older adults worldwide increased only slightly (2%) from 1950 to 2000, it is projected to increase dramatically during the first half of the twenty-first century (United Nations, 2002).

Mortality and Morbidity Statistics

> *Old age is the most unexpected of all the things that happen to a man.*
>
> —Leon Trotsky (*Diary in Exile,* entry for May 8, 1935)

Before we consider life expectancy and mortality rates around the world, it is crucial to understand the distinction between two widely used measures: *life expectancy* and *maximum life span* (Hayflick, 1996). Life expectancy involves taking a statistical snapshot of a population during a particular year and calculating an arithmetic mean based on their age

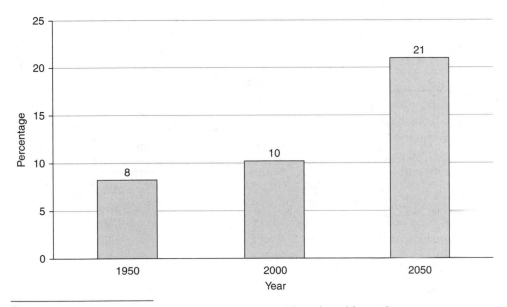

Figure 18-4 Older adults (60+) as a percentage of total world population.

Source: Adapted from United Nations, 2002.

at death. Although it is most commonly calculated from the time of birth, life expectancy can be calculated from any age. Maximum life span, on the other hand, is simply the longest life span (or longevity) recorded. The human record is currently 122 years.

As before, we will start with data from the US Census to describe how life expectancy has changed in the United States over the past century, and then we will examine the same phenomenon across the globe. Figure 18-5 reveals the astonishing fact that the average life expectancy from birth has increased dramatically in the United States, from only 47 years in 1900, to 77 years in 2000. However, this increase in life expectancy is often misinterpreted. For example, one headline proclaimed, "People in U.S. Living Longer" ("People in U.S.," 2005). Journalists such as *New York Times* columnist William Safire also make this mistake, saying "When you look back over the last 50 or 75 years...you see these enormous advances in science where you are actually extending the life of a human being from 47 in 1900 to 77 today" (Morgan, 2006, p. 24). Although far less sensational, a more accurate headline stated: "U.S. Life Expectancy up to 77.6" ("U.S. Life Expectancy," 2005). In other words, individuals are not setting new longevity records, but more people are surviving into the stage of old age, as defined as older than 65 years.

Unlike life expectancy, the most compelling fact about the maximum life span is that *it has not changed.* That is, since these data have been recorded over the last few thousand years of human history, there have always been a few people that live to be older than 100 years, close to the maximum of about 120 years of age. One prominent biologist goes

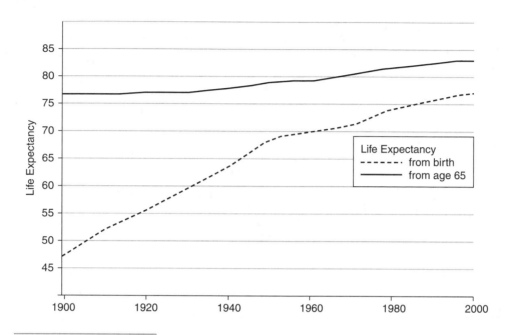

Figure 18-5   Changes in mean life expectancy, United States, 1900–2000. Note the dramatic change in life expectancy from birth, contrasted with much less change in remaining life expectancy for those who reached age 65.

Source: He et al., 2005; Hayflick, 1996.

so far as to say that "there is no evidence that the maximum human life span has changed from what it was about a hundred thousand years ago" (Hayflick, 1996, p. 66). According to more recent history, the prophet Moses lived to exactly 120 years old, dying on his birthday in 1273 B.C.E. Over 1600 years ago (according to Athanasius, patriarch of Alexandria), Saint Anthony died in 356 C.E. at the age of 105 (Perls & Silver, 1999). In 1899, Mr. Geert Boomgaard of the Netherlands died at the age of 110. In England, Ann Pouder died in 1917 at the age of 110, and in the United States, Louisa Thiers lived to be 111 years old, passing away in 1926.[3] In 1906, the biologist Metchnikoff (1912) interviewed a certain Mme. Robineau who was age 106, and included her photograph in his book. Most recently, Jeanne Calment (Figure 186) died in 1997 at the age of 122 (Allard, Lèbre, & Robine, 1998). Although this may set a new record, a 2-year increase over the past

---

[3]The Gerontological Research Group, which includes Dr. Thomas Perls, Director of the New England Centenarian Study (Perls, 2004), maintains a carefully validated list of supercentenarians, defined as anyone who has lived to be 110 years old or older. Boomgaard, Pouder, and Thiers top this list, which includes supercentenarians born in 29 different countries.

Figure 18-6　Madame Jeanne Calment (Arles, France), photographed in 1995 at the age of 120. She died in 1997 at the age of 122.

Source: Courtesy of the Gerontology Research Group, www.grg.org, 2006.

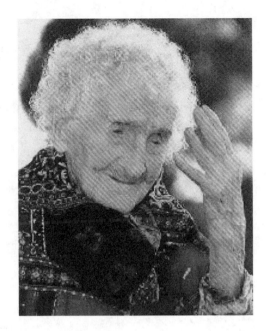

3279 years of recorded human history is not nearly as impressive as the changes we have seen in average life expectancy.

In addition, if life expectancy is calculated from ages beyond birth, very little change has occurred. As far back as 1693, Edmund Halley (famous for the comet bearing his name) reported that although life expectancy was only 33 years as calculated from birth (in the city of Breslau), for those who made it to 80 years old, they could expect to live an average of 6 more years (Hayflick, 1996). In the United States, life expectancy at age 65 increased only 6 years from 1900 to 2000 (from 11.9 to 17.9 years beyond 65, for a total of 76.9 to 82.9 years; see top line in Figure 18-5). In the same time period, life expectancy only increased 1.7 years at age 85.

Yet another way to understand the changes in life expectancy is to plot the percentage of people surviving to a given age, according to calendar years. For example, in the United States in 1900, only 88% of newborn babies reached their first birthday; by 2000, the number was up to 99% (He et al., 2005). These changes are plotted in Figure 18-5. As more people survive into older age ranges, the survival curve starts to approximate the shape of a rectangle. If all of us survived to the maximum life span, the survival curve would become *rectangularized*. As seen in Figure 18-7, the US population is moving in that direction. The same phenomenon is happening globally, but at a much lower rate and slower pace.

Another type of rectangularization can be seen in the *population pyramids* in Figure 18-8. In 1900, these data did have a pyramidal shape, but by the year 2000, this demographic structure had grown fatter in the middle, so that it had what is called a midriff bulge, and

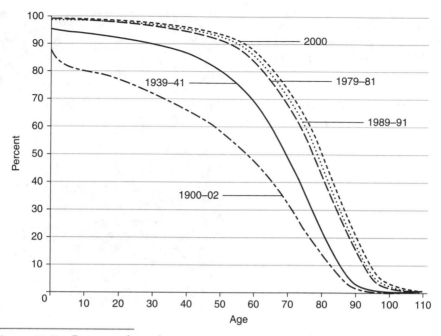

Figure 18-7 Percent of people surviving to certain ages for selected years in the United States.

Source: He et al., 2005.

now the upper tip is also widening. (The pyramid metaphor may have to be dropped in the near future.)

It is estimated that there were 461 million people worldwide over the age of 65 in 2004 (Kinsella & Phillips, 2005), which represents 7% of the world's population. Paradoxically, because industrialized countries tend to have more elderly than nonindustrialized countries, 59% of these older adults live in developing countries (He et al., 2005). These figures reveal a lopsided proportion of older adults in Africa, Asia, Central America, the Caribbean, and Oceania. As for the shape of the worldwide population structure, developing countries are still much more pyramidal, but in due course, the statistical prediction is that their population pyramids will also become rectangularized. This phenomenon is shown graphically in Figure 18-9, comparing more developed countries with less developed countries, with data from 1950 and 1990, and projections for 2030. The percentages of people 65 years of age and older are shown for different regions of the world in Figure 18-10. Note that sub-Saharan Africa is expected to experience the smallest increase over the next 30 years, due in large part to the HIV/AIDS epidemic. Of the 18.8 million people who died of AIDS by 2001, 79% were in Africa (Kinsella & Phillips, 2005). Countries with the highest percentages of older adults are plotted in Figure 18-11. Based on 2001 and 2004 census data, the populations with the longest life expectancies are

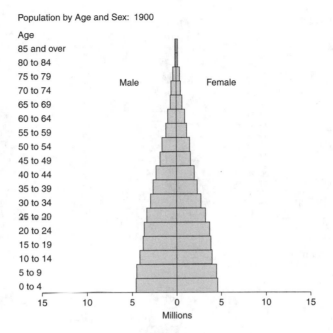

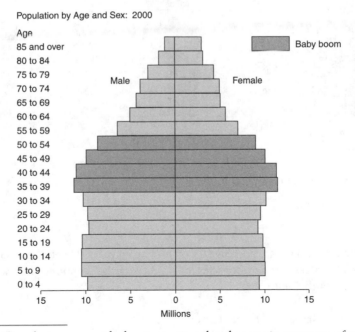

Figure 18-8 Population pyramids demonstrating the changes in structure of age groups in the United States.

Source: He et al., 2005.

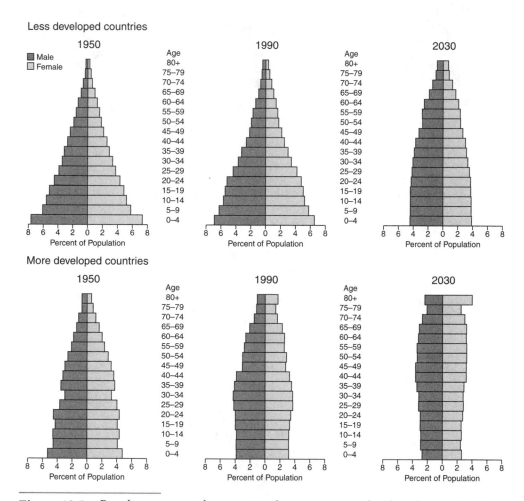

Figure 18-9   Population pyramids comparing less versus more developed countries (data from 1950 and 1990 with projections for 2030).

Source: Kinsella & Phillips, 2005.

Japanese females at 86 years and Swedish males at 78 years (He et al., 2005). The populations with the shortest life expectancies, only 33 years, are females in Botswana and males in Swaziland (Haub, 2006).

Disability Adjusted Life Expectancy

Beyond basic life expectancy, the World Health Organization uses a concept known as the *disability-adjusted life expectancy* (DALE), meaning the expected number of years to be lived

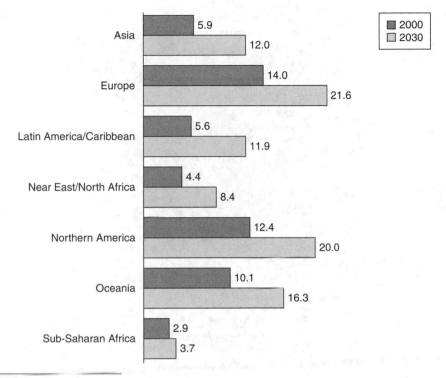

Figure 18-10 Percent of the population aged 65 and older in various regions (2000, projected for the year 2030).

Source: He et al., 2005.

in full health (cf. Chakraborti, 2004). Japan has the highest DALE of 74.5 years, while the country of Sierra Leone has the lowest DALE of less than 26 years.

Oldest-Old, Centenarians, and Supercentenarians

Among those older than 65 years, further distinctions are now recognized: *young-old, oldest-old* (more than 85 years old), and centenarians (100 years and older) (He et al., 2005). Centenarians are the fastest growing segment of the oldest-old. Surprisingly—given the age-related functional decline of people in their sixth, seventh, eighth, and ninth decade of life—about 25% of centenarians are in very good health (Perls, 2004). There are two centenarian research centers located in the United States, one in Massachusetts and the other in Georgia. The New England Centenarian Project is directed by Dr. Thomas Perls, and the Georgia Centenarian Study is directed by Dr. Leonard Poon. Although little information is available on the prevalence of centenarians around the world, Vaupel and Jeune

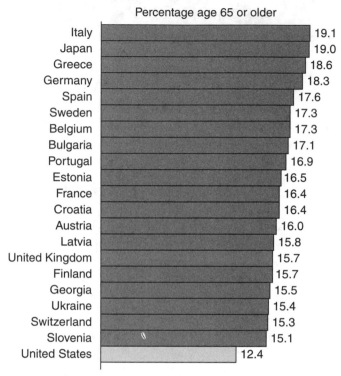

Percentage age 65 or older

Country	Percentage
Italy	19.1
Japan	19.0
Greece	18.6
Germany	18.3
Spain	17.6
Sweden	17.3
Belgium	17.3
Bulgaria	17.1
Portugal	16.9
Estonia	16.5
France	16.4
Croatia	16.4
Austria	16.0
Latvia	15.8
United Kingdom	15.7
Finland	15.7
Georgia	15.5
Ukraine	15.4
Switzerland	15.3
Slovenia	15.1
United States	12.4

Note: United States ranks 38th.

Figure 18-11 Countries with the greatest percent of older population.

Source: Kinsella & Phillips, 2005.

(1995) estimated that in 1990 there were approximately 8800 people age 100 and older in Japan and the western European countries combined.

Supercentenarians (age 110 and older) are a much smaller and even more elite group. According to the Gerontological Research Group, there are 76 validated supercentenarians alive in the world today (as of October 2006), only 10 of whom are men. This gender gap is discussed in the next section.

Gender Differences

Although males outnumber females at birth, by midlife the gender ratio is reversed. The relative proportion of females to males continues to expand as age increases. This dramatic life span change is depicted graphically in Figure 18-12. The *gender differential* in life expectancy shown in Figure 18-12 is especially true in more developed countries, where the average gender gap is about 7 years. Gender differences are typically smaller in less

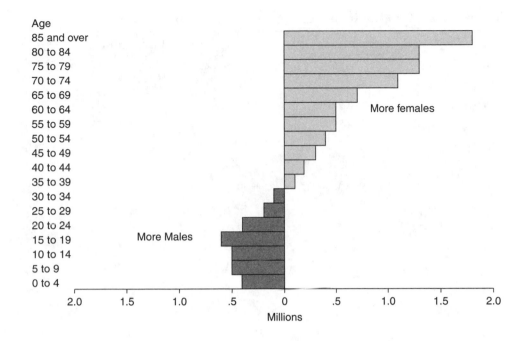

Figure 18-12   Different numbers of males and females as a function of age.

Source: He et al., 2005.

developed countries, and are even reversed in some south Asian and Middle Eastern countries. In some of these cultures, women have a lower social status, which, combined with a preference for male children, has a negative impact on female life expectancy. A sample of gender ratios in 20 countries is presented in Table 18-1. Some researchers have labeled this phenomenon as the "feminization of the elderly" (Chakraborti, 2004, p. 58). As mentioned earlier, the percentage of females increases with age, but gender ratios are less favorable for women living in developing countries. For example, among those 80 and older, women comprise 71% in Europe versus 59% in Africa.

Research and Technology

In speaking of modern gerontology research, "it is more beneficial to opt for a healthy and vigorous, albeit finite, life than to search in vain for the elixir of immortality" (Arking, 2006, p. 5). As some gerontologists have suggested, we need to focus more on adding life to years, and less on adding years to life (Maddox, 1994). In both theory and practice, most current gerontological research and policy is committed to the goal of *successful aging*

TABLE 18-1   Gender Ratios Among People Aged 65 and Older

More Developed Countries		Less Developed Countries	
Australia	79	Bangladesh	117
Bulgaria	72	Brazil	70
France	69	Ethiopia	84
Germany	68	Fiji	85
Italy	71	Ghana	89
Poland	62	Honduras	90
Russia	46	India	103
Ukraine	51	Iran	98
United Kingdom	74	Mexico	84
United States	71	Zambia	79

Note: Ratios are number of men per 100 women.
Source: Kinsella & Phillips, 2005

(Rowe & Kahn, 1998). Biologists have emphasized that "gerontology is committed not to a search for immortality but to the elimination of premature disability and death" (Arking, 2006, p. 5). Nowhere is this truer than in the arena of global aging, because life spans for the majority of people, at least in developing nations, fall far below what can and should be expected.

The advances in communication and computer technologies "offer a promising future for older adults" (Mundorf & Brownell, 2001, p. 224). More and more older adults are logging on to the Internet to use such sites as www.SeniorNet.org, which celebrated its 20th anniversary in 2006, and to use the worldwide web for e-mail, purchases, and medical information. Data from the US Census Bureau in 2005 revealed that 35% of older adults had a computer, and 29% had internet access (Greenberg, 2005). New technologies are also playing a key role in new employment opportunities for older workers, at least in the United States (Riggs, 2004). Although no data are available, it is likely this trend is occurring in other developed countries (e.g., Japan and Europe).

A significant portion of the research effort is to develop strategies and technology to help older adults *age in place* (Rogers & Fisk, 2006). Although some of these initiatives involve providing good old-fashioned low-tech social support; "birthday cards are one option being explored to keep health providers in contact with older clients" at the University of Auckland in New Zealand ("Helping elderly stay at home", 2006), other countries, such as Korea, have more ambitious plans involving robot maids for their elderly (Tae-gyu, 2006).

Work by Dr. Wendy Rogers and her colleagues (an interdisciplinary team of psychologists, engineers, and computer programmers at the Georgia Institute of Technology) has resulted in the creation of an *aware house*, in which communication and control systems (involving cameras, sensors, and computers) maximize the independence of older adults living alone by monitoring many of their daily activities, ranging from recipe reminders during cooking to more complex tasks such as measuring insulin accurately (Rogers & Fisk, 2006). The advantage of such a home is that the older person can function without requiring around-the-clock help from a nurse or other live-in assistant. Of course, expense is a serious obstacle, making this concept entirely impractical in developing countries at this time.

Another related innovation is *telemedicine*, illustrated in the following vignette:

> Ruth, a functionally independent older adult, awakes and sits down at her computer. She helps manage her husband's chronic illness. Today, he has an appointment with a specialist. At 09:00, they have a live conversation with the specialist by videoconference, and the physician recommends a change in her husband's medications. After the appointment, Ruth checks her e-mail and receives a message from her online caregiver support group to schedule a chat later that afternoon. Ruth quickly responds that she is available and switches off the computer to begin her day. (Stronge, Rogers, & Fisk, 2007, p. 1)

The above scenario demonstrates how telemedicine can improve older adults' day-to-day lives. As Stronge et al. point out in their review, telemedicine systems have benefited older adults "by increasing peer support interactions, providing health-care access to older adults in rural communities, reducing the cost of health care, increasing exercise, reducing pain and depression, and, perhaps most important, improving functional independence" (Stronge et al., 2007, p. 1). Furthermore, family medicine physicians are also rediscovering the advantages of home care, "in light of the aging population, advances in portable medical technology, and changes in Medicare reimbursement" (Landers, 2006, p. 366). Recent studies have underscored the crucial need for the successful adoption of technology for the functional independence of older adults (Czaja et al., 2006). Again, the implementation of the previously mentioned technologies in developing countries will be dependent on significant increases in per capita income.

Legal and Ethical Issues

Ethics of Aging Research

In the United States, the institutional review board (IRB) of any research institution considers all research on older adults to involve a vulnerable group, comparable to doing research with children or pregnant women. The IRB has to review all research done with older adults, such as basic cognitive aging research involving memory differences between young and older adults (cf. Mitchell & Bruss, 2003). However, in practice, it is routine for the IRB to grant permission to use the same consent forms used for younger adults with healthy older adults. When research participants have some degree of cognitive impairment, such as Alzheimer's disease (Mitchell & Schmitt, 2006), the participant's ability to understand and sign an informed consent form can be a significant issue (High & Doole, 1995). If the research participant is too cognitively impaired, the IRB will usually require a consent form signed by the participant's spouse (or other legal guardian or caregiver), as well as an assent provided verbally by the participant (Fazio & Mitchell, 2007).

IRBs were created through legislature in 1974 in the United States via the National Research Act, which established a National Commission for the Protection of Human Subjects of Biomedical and Behavioral Research. This was based on the Declaration of Helsinki, made at the 18th World Medical Assembly in Helsinki, Finland in 1964, which was in turn based on the Nuremberg Code. The latter was an outcome of the Nuremberg War Crimes Trials in 1947, in which 23 Nazi German physicians were found guilty of "performing medical experiments upon concentration camp inmates and other living human subjects, without their consent, in the course of which the defendants committed murders, brutalities, cruelties, tortures, atrocities, and other inhuman acts." The court prescribed guidelines for permissible medical experiments, including voluntary consent, benefits outweighing risks, and the ability of subjects to terminate participation. The 1996 revision of the Helsinki declaration from the 48th General Assembly states: "Concern for the interests of the subject must always prevail over the interests of science and society."

The World Health Organization (WHO) has an international Research Ethics Review Committee and states that "all research involving human participants must be conducted in an ethical manner that respects the dignity, safety and rights of research participants" (WHO, 2006). Most of the current ethical concerns revolve around vaccines, cloning, and HIV. Although WHO singles out children, adolescents, and women as vulnerable populations, they say little about research ethics specific to older adults. At the UN-sponsored World Conference on Human Rights in Vienna, 1993, it was determined that "neither ageing as a process, nor older persons as a group, are specifically mentioned in the text of the Convention" (Loza, 2001, p. 72). Clearly, different cultural and political systems and values affect the ethics of research procedures (and related legislation) followed in specific countries. On the other hand, there is a growing interest in the establishment of universal standards for the concept of international elder law (Doron, 2005).

In *smart house* environments, big brother issues are raised, since the elderly person is being monitored 24 hours a day, 7 days a week. Rogers and Fisk (2006) asked their aware home participants how they felt about the compromise of their privacy by the technology in their home. Of the nearly 3000 replies, some of the comments they received included (Rogers & Fisk, p. 29):

- "If this [monitoring system] would keep me independent longer, I wouldn't mind as much."

- "If it's only my daughter who monitors me, it's alright."
- "If you really need it, privacy becomes secondary."

(Incidentally, note that residents in nursing homes and even assisted-living arrangements already sacrifice a great deal of privacy.)

Euthanasia

Everybody has got to die, but I have always believed an exception would be made in my case. Now what?

—William Saroyan, final statement published after his death at age 72

Euthanasia is not specifically an aging issue, but is often addressed in a death and dying unit at the end of gerontology courses and textbooks. Assisted suicide is still illegal in most of the United States (Oregon is the exception), but has been legalized in some countries. In Holland, in 1995 alone, 3600 patients died via assisted suicide or euthanasia (Stern, 1998). This trend is viewed by many health professionals and ethicists as a slippery slope (cf. Foley & Hendin, 2002). The most visible proponent and conductor of assisted suicide, Dr. Jack Kevorkian, served a prison sentence from 1999–2007 for second-degree murder in the poisoning of a 52-year-old man in Michigan. Obviously, different countries and cultures have vastly differing views on euthanasia, but that is beyond the scope of this chapter.

Influences of Politics, Economics, Culture, and Religion

Ageism

Among the myriad topics covered in this book, one issue unique to the field of aging is *ageism*. Ageism is defined as "a process of systematic stereotyping and discrimination against people because they are old, just as racism and sexism accomplish this for skin color and gender" (Butler, 2001a, p. 38). An entire *Encyclopedia of Ageism* (Palmore, Branch, & Harris, 2005) exists, with coverage ranging from *abuse* to *voice quality*. For the purposes of this chapter, we ask if ageism varies as a function of culture. Other than the United States, the encyclopedia entries only include Japan. However, at least one study found ageism still prevalent among British physicians (Young, 2006). Given that the awareness of the issue and phenomenon of ageism is relatively new in progressive countries (Butler, 1969; Palmore, 1990), it is likely to be widespread around the globe.

Elder Abuse

Elder abuse is an extreme version of ageism, involving both attitude and behavior. In the late 1970s, the issue of elder abuse and neglect began to receive more attention in the United States "due to the increasing awareness of the burgeoning number of older adults"

(Quinn, 2001, p. 324). In 1998, the US Administration on Aging published a report, the *National Elder Abuse Incidence Study*, which revealed that "at least one half million older persons in domestic settings were abused and/or neglected, or experienced self-neglect" (Quinn, 2001, p. 325). Recently, elder abuse in other cultures has also begun to receive more attention, both from researchers and government policy makers. For example, Chakraborti (2004) reports that widows, in particular, constitute a disproportionately large number of the elderly in Asia, because women in those cultures tend to marry men who are 10 to 15 years older than themselves. As a result, they "have to endure longer periods of widowhood. Their conditions are worsened by the fact that they are unable to fend for themselves." Even worse, "abandonment of elderly widows, even from educated families, is on the rise" (Chakraborti, 2004, pp. 26–27).

Culture

The experiences of older adults vary widely around the world, not only because of individual differences in biological and psychological aging, but also because the "frameworks of social beliefs and values" (Wilson, 2000, p. 17) vary dramatically across different cultures.

Research in many non-Western cultures is lacking. For example, regarding Asia:

> Although ageing research has been well-developed and well documented in Europe and other developed countries, including Japan, it has yet to take shape in most other parts of Asia. To a great extent the lack of interest in aging research in Asia owes its origin to the belief that the family support system is and will continue to be foolproof insurance against all the problems faced during old age. (Chakraborti, 2004, pp. 25–26).

Family Support for the Elderly

A long-standing American myth is that the Walton Family (a 1970s television show in which an extended family including parents, children, and grandparents live under one roof) was the norm, and that now older adults are relegated to a lonely incarceration in nursing homes. Although loneliness is an issue for many older adults—especially widows (Lopata, 2001)—only about 5% of those aged over 65 are residents of any long-term institution (Palmore, 1998).

Outside of America, "the family is an effective provider of old-age support in India and most other Asian countries." (Chakraborti, 2004, p. 26). In contrast to most countries in the Western world—where many programs have been developed specifically to support needs of older adults—"many Asian countries have barely begun to think about their elderly; and given the pace of population aging in Asia and the corresponding lack of adjustment mechanisms, a 'time bomb' or 'age quake' may not be very far" (Chakraborti, 2004, p. 27). Chakraborti (2004, p.29) goes on to say that glaciers might provide a more appropriate metaphor for rapid aging, "since a glacier moves at a slow pace but with enormous effects wherever it goes and with a long-term momentum that is unstoppable."

Developed countries, mostly in Europe and North America, have established institutions for dealing with older adults' health needs, in contrast to Asian countries, where family-based support of the elderly is the norm. Between these two extreme scenarios, Australia provides an interesting comparison, having the distinction of "a European tradition and an Asian future" (Kendig & Quine, 2006, p. 431). Ninety percent of the Australian population is concentrated in coastal urban areas. (For an interesting analysis of growing old in cities, specifically New York, London, Paris, and Tokyo, see Rodwin & Gusmano, 2006). Australia's population aging profile is similar to that of the United States, in which older adults are projected to comprise 18% of the total population by 2021. Also similar to the United States, over 90% of older adults live in private households, with the remainder living in nursing homes or boarding houses in 1998 (Kendig & Quine, 2006). Among older adults with disabilities, 77% have "some informal support from family or friends," and 53% receive some "formal support" in the form of community or private services (Kendig & Quine, 2006, p. 433). Although Australia—unlike most Asian countries—has formal community services available, "children have strong values of family obligation for frail older parents who wish to remain independent" (Kendig & Quine, 2006, p. 434). Thus, Australia continues to provide a fascinating microcosm of the phenomenon of world population aging in the twenty-first century.

Respect and Status

Modernization theory—"how individuals and societies respond and adapt to processes of demographic, political, economic, and social changes" (Achenbaum, 2001, p. 709)—has been applied to population aging. This theory predicts that "the status of elders . . . decline[s] with the degree of modernization" (Luborsky & McMullen, 1999, p. 83). Cowgill and Holmes (1972) found support for their modernization hypothesis by looking across 15 societies varying from preliterate to peasant to industrial. However, the relationship between cultural changes and the position of elderly is quite complex, as revealed by a summary of 10 key propositions listed in Table 18-2. Achenbaum (2001) summarized 50 years of modernization theory scholarship as follows: "How social scientists study connections between old age, population aging, and modernization has changed, but the theory's original raison d'être remains salient" (p. 710).

In the Jewish religion, there is great respect for older adults, regardless of the culture where the Jews are living. Instead of 65 years old, the operational definition of elder (*zaken* in Hebrew, which also means *wise*) is age 70 and older. For example, Jewish law specifies that one should stand up when any person 70 years of age and older enters a room. In practice, children in religiously observant homes (i.e., orthodox) stand up when either their parents or any other older person enters a room. In Israel, children and teenagers have been observed to leap to their feet to offer their seat on the bus to an older adult. This kind of respect is also true of many other religions and cultures, but even when this tenet is observed, does it translate into a lack of prejudice and discrimination in milieus such as the workplace, or treatment of patients? Unfortunately, respect for elders is *not* a tenet of

TABLE 18-2   Proposed Relationships Between Modernization and Aging

1. The concept of old age itself appears to be relative to the degree of modernization.

2. Longevity is directly and significantly related to the degree of modernization.

3. Modernized societies have a relatively high proportion of older people in their populations.

4. The aged are the recipients of greater respect in societies where they constitute a low proportion of the total population.

5. Societies that are in the process of modernizing tend to favor the young, while the aged are at an advantage in more stable, sedentary societies.

6. Respect for the aged tends to be greater in societies in which the extended family is prevalent, particularly if it functions as if they are part of the household unit. (The implication here is that modernization breaks down the extended family.)

7. In nonindustrial societies the family is the basic social group providing economic security for dependent aged, but in industrial societies the responsibility tends to be partially or totally that of the state.

8. The proportion of aged who retain leadership roles in modern societies is lower than in industrial ones.

9. Religious leadership is more likely to be a continuing role of the aged in preindustrial societies than in modern societies.

10. Retirement is a modern invention found only in modernized, high-productivity societies.

Sources: Luborsky and McMullen, 1999; Holmes and Holmes, 1995.

all cultures. For example, in India, it is not uncommon for older widows to be abandoned by their families (Chakraborti, 2004).

Cognitive Neuroscience and Aging

Cognitive neuroscience issues in aging and culture have begun to receive some attention (Park & Gutchess, 2006). Although the basic neurological and psychological mechanisms of perception, memory, and cognition—which by and large are affected negatively by normal aging—would not be expected to vary across cultures, some unusual phenomena (e.g., picture naming as a measure of semantic memory, cf. Mitchell, 1989) are being explored across different languages and cultures (Yoon, Feinberg, & Gutchess, 2006). Indeed, one study found a positive correlation between attitude towards aging and explicit memory performance; older Chinese had both a more positive attitude and higher memory scores compared to a group of older Americans (Levy & Langer, 1994). Even something as fundamental as hearing loss (a ubiquitous aging phenomenon) has been found to be correlated with negative attitudes about hearing held by older adults ages 70 to 96 themselves (Levy, Slade, & Gill, 2006).

Aging Phenomena in South America

In South American countries, more attention is being focused on the lives of older women (Loza, 2001), who suffer from poverty and have disproportionate illiteracy rates. In Brazil, researchers have documented dramatic differences in aging cultures as a function of socioeconomic status, meaning those who are marginalized versus the well-to-do "self-sufficient" (Leibing & Py, 2005). Leibing (2005) examined historical changes in Brazilian culture and attitudes spanning from 1967 to 2002. Her investigation revealed a shift from an emphasis on old age to a *third age* label. Leibing describes third age as a phase between adulthood and old age, in which successful aging involves the "empowerment of elderly persons by fighting against aging stereotypes and for better living conditions" (Leibing, 2005, p. 18). This phenomenon was epitomized in Fernanda Montenegro, considered by many to be Brazil's most talented actress, who was nominated for an Academy Award at age 70. Although Montenegro called herself "the old lady from Ipanema," (cf. Tom Jobim & Vinicius de Morae's song, "Garota de Ipanema") and did not try to conceal the visible effects of aging ("prominent wrinkles"), Leibing's analysis still portrays a class of people who use fame and financial power to transcend a more traditional life course (i.e., avoiding superficial signs of aging). Although positive aging stereotypes are welcome, in Brazil, it is only the rich and the famous who can afford to continue fighting and spending in the " struggle against becoming old" (Leibing, 2005, p. 22). In a country with significant poverty, the beautiful old lady is the exception, not the rule.

Case Study Examples

Ageism: Two Case Studies

Dr. Robert Butler, a physician who founded the National Institute on Aging in the United States, relates the following incident involving a centenarian friend. His 100-year-old friend had a pain in his left knee, and so went to see his internist about it. After examining the patient, the doctor concluded that it was just "old age." Dr. Butler's friend retorted, "But doc, my right knee is also 100 years old, and it doesn't hurt!" In this case, the physician's lack of knowledge (or at least inadequate diagnosis) resulted in a fairly benign outcome, although the patient's left knee did not receive treatment. However, it is difficult to imagine a 25-year-old being told that an ailment was the result of "youth."

Dr. Kevin Hendler specializes in geriatric dentistry at Emory Healthcare in Atlanta, Georgia, and related the following incident (Hendler, 2005). A 97-year-old woman presented with the need for some dental work. The patient and her family were not very enthusiastic about dental work, assuming that the older lady did not have much longer to live anyway, given her age. However, Dr. Hendler convinced her to go ahead with the dental work, and the lady went on to live to the age of 108. Imagine how different the last 11 years of her life would have been without the ability to chew food. If this dentist had succumbed to ageism, his patient would have lost many years of normal eating. At the other end of the life span, no one would suggest depriving 11 years of normal life from a growing child. Dr. Hendler says "treatment decisions by patients or family members should not be based solely on the number that represents age, but rather on health and quality of life" (personal communication, September 22, 2006). Patients who decided not to have the recommended dental work have subsequently told him that had they known they would live so long they would have done things differently. Sometimes patients tell Dr. Hendler, "I don't know how much longer I have," and he replies, "That's right, you don't know, so you should be comfortable because it may be a while" (personal communication, September 22, 2006). Sometimes patients in their 70s will say they do not want better treatment because they will not need it for very long; Dr. Hendler's reply is, "How do you know?"

This case is only one concrete example of how attitudes toward the elderly can make such an enormous difference. Unfortunately, a number of studies (271 citations in a 2006 MEDLINE search) reveal that ageism is alive and well among health professionals. Dr. John Young (2006), head of the Academic Unit of Elderly Care and Rehabilitation at St. Luke's Hospital in England, writes that institutionalized ageism in his country is endemic, based on a number of recent medical studies. For example, a recent population-based study found that patients over the age of 80 years with minor stroke and transient ischemic attacks were underreferred and undertreated (Fairhead & Rothwell, 2006). However, Dr. Young expresses hope for the future, as the "UK government has recently been embarrassed into action" (Young, 2006, p. 509). Mortality rates from heart disease and cancer declined in Britain after a policy initiative was established called the National Service Framework for Older People. Perhaps other governments around the world will follow suit in the twenty-first century.

Centenarians

Following are some vignettes of vibrant centenarians, taken from volunteers at the Georgia Centenarian Study (University of Georgia, 2006):

- At 104, Mary Sims Elliott was working on her autobiography, writing poetry, and trying to influence her church's position on social issues. Now she is 105 and her autobiography, titled *My First One Hundred Years*, was just published.

- At 105, Geneva McDaniel taught aerobics daily at her senior citizens center. Now she is 107 and recruiting residents of her retirement community to exercise with her.

- At 106, former sharecropper Jessie Champion and his 86-year-old wife, Fronnie, were weeding and harvesting their garden. Recently, Fronnie passed away and Jessie, now 107, lives and gardens with his daughter.

The researchers at the Georgia Centenarian Study generally agree that the secret of longevity is still a mystery. First, according to Director Leonard Poon, no two centenarians are the same: "For as many optimistic people, we find as many who are grumpy" (University of Georgia, 2006). Furthermore, "centenarians are far more different than they are alike," according to Dr. Peter Martin, who codirects the centenarian study (University of Georgia, 2006). "There are many paths to longevity, and each situation is very different." As for a family history of longevity, Dr. Poon says: "People aren't likely to live long just because their parents did. It seems the genetic contribution is important for some centenarians who come from a long line of long-lived people. But we have as many people who do not come from long-lived families" (University of Georgia, 2006). On the other hand, other researchers have found a select group of centenarians living in Nova Scotia (Duenwald, 2003). This province has approximately 21 centenarians per 100,000 people, compared to a rate of 18 per 100,000 people in the United States and only 3 per 100,000 people worldwide. In Nova Scotia, it appears that longevity does run in families.

Religious Lifestyle in Israel

Bnei Brak, Israel's most religious city (Rosenblum, 2001), was found to have the highest global life expectancy in 2001: 81.1 years for women, 77.4 years for men (slightly higher records were held in 2006 by Japan and Iceland). What is most interesting about this small city's longevity record is that life is long in spite of other demographics: Bnei Brak is also Israel's poorest city, confounding the normal correlation between poverty and poor health (Rosenblum, 2001). In addition, the orthodox Jewish residents are known neither for engaging in exercise nor for maintaining a low-fat diet. The most likely formula for long life in this community appears to be a highly engaged level of religious enthusiasm. Although the conclusions are not unequivocal, a majority of studies investigating the relationship between religious practice and health have found a positive correlation (Schaie, Krause, & Booth, 2004). In Israel, a very exhaustive study (N = 3900 over a 16-year period) compared 11 religious versus 11 secular *kibbutzim* (best translated as *egalitarian collectives*). It was found that the mortality rate in the religious groups was less than half at 3.9% versus the 9.1% of the secular groups (Kark et al., 1996). The authors ruled out potential confounds due to a variety of sociodemographic variables, including education, ethnic origin, and social support. The only explanation remaining was an "embracing protective effect of religious observance" (Kark et al., p. 346).

It will be interesting to see future studies of this relationship in other cultures around the world. To date, very few international or cross-national studies are available (Schaie et al., 2004). In one notable exception (Musick, Traphagan, Koenig, & Larson, 2000), researchers compared religious and spiritual practices in the United States with those in Japan, and found a very different perspective on the relationship between spirituality and health. Older religious Japanese "employ religious activity in an attempt to avoid a decline into poor health as they grow older," including visits to *pokkuridera* (sudden death temples), "at which they pray for a sudden, peaceful, death devoid of excessive suffering" (Musick et al., p. 84).

Conclusion

La vejez no es una enfermedad, es una etapa de nuestra vida.

—Betsie Hollants (cited in Loza, 2001)

Old age is not a disease and cannot be cured.

—Élie Metchnikoff, biologist

Although Metchnikoff (1912) published his insight nearly a century ago, only a few biologists and even fewer gerontologists have grasped this message (Hayflick, 2006). According to Hayflick (in press), the best strategy at our disposal for slowing the rate of aging is to promote good health. Or, as many gerontologists have said—in light of some of the medical advances that can keep a person alive longer via artificial means—our goal should not be to add years to life, but rather, to add "life to years" (i.e., improve people's health and decrease the proportion of old age spent in morbidity). James Fries has called for health policy promoting the compression of morbidity by shortening the period "between an increasing average age of the onset of disability and the age of death" (Fries, 2001, p. 234). This is certainly a worthwhile goal to pursue globally, particularly in developing countries.

Acknowledgments

Support for the preparation and writing of this chapter was provided by grants from the WellStar College of Health and Human Services and from the Foley Family Foundation. Thanks to Deborah Garfin for her unswerving logistical support and to Sandi Nelson for her invaluable bibliographic support.

References

Achenbaum, W. A. (2001). Modernization theory. In G. L. Maddox (Ed.), *The encyclopedia of aging* (3rd ed., Vol. II, pp. 708–710). New York: Springer.

Allard, M., Lèbre, V., & Robine, J.-M. (1998). *Jeanne Calment: From Van Gogh's time to ours: 122 extraordinary years* (B. Coupland, Trans.). New York: W. H. Freeman & Co.

Arking, R. (2006). *The biology of aging: Observations and principles* (3rd ed.). New York: Oxford University Press.

Browning, R. (1942). Rabbi Ben Ezra. In P. Loving (Ed.), *The selected poems of Robert Browning* (pp. 260–266). Roslyn, NY: Walter J. Black.

Butler, R. N. (1969). Ageism: Another form of bigotry. *The Gerontologist, 9,* 243–246.

Butler, R. N. (2001a). Ageism. In G. L. Maddox (Ed.), *The encyclopedia of aging* (Vol. I, pp. 38–39). New York: Springer.

Butler, R. N. (2001b). Geriatrics. In G. L. Maddox (Ed.), *The encyclopedia of aging* (3rd ed., Vol. I, pp. 435–436). New York: Springer Publishing Company.

Chakraborti, R. D. (2004). *The greying of India: Population ageing in the context of Asia.* New Delhi: Sage Publications.

Clark, E. (1995). *Growing old is not for sissies II: Portraits of senior athletes.* Rohnert Park, CA: Pomegranate Artbooks.

The Columbia world of quotations. (1996). New York: Columbia University Press. Retrieved August 2, 2007, from http://www.bartleby.com/66

Cowgill, D. O., & Holmes, L. D. (1972). *Aging and modernization.* New York: Appleton-Century-Crofts.

Czaja, S. J., Charness, N., Fisk, A. D., Hertzog, C., Nair, S. N., Rogers, W. A., et al. (2006). Factors predicting the use of technology: Findings from the Center for Research and Education on Aging and Technology Enhancement (CREATE). *Psychology and Aging, 21,* 333–352.

Doron, I. (2005). From national to international elder law. *The Journal of International Aging, Law, & Policy, 1,* 43–67.

Duenwald, M. (2003, January). Puzzle of the century. *Smithsonian,* 73–80.

Fairhead, J. F., & Rothwell, P. M. (2006). Underinvestigation and treatment of carotid disease in elderly patients with transient ischaemic attack and stroke: Comparative population based study. *Bristish Medical Journal, 333,* 525–534.

Fazio, S., & Mitchell, D. B. (2007). *Persistence of self in individuals with Alzheimer's disease: Evidence from language and visual recognition.*Unpublished manuscript, Kennesaw State University.

Foley, K., & Hendin, H. (Eds.). (2002). *The case against assisted suicide: For the right to end-of-life care.* Baltimore: Johns Hopkins University Press.

Fries, J. F. (2001). Compression of morbidity/disease postponement. In G. L. Maddox (Ed.), *The encyclopedia of aging* (3rd ed., Vol. I, pp. 234–236). New York: Springer.

Greenberg, S. (2005). *A profile of older Americans: 2005.* Retrieved August 2, 2007, from http://www.aoa.gov/PROF/Statistics/profile/2005/profiles2005.asp

Haub, C. (2006). *2006 world population data sheet.* Retrieved August 2, 2007, from http://www.prb.org

Hayflick, L. (1996). *How and why we age.* New York: Ballantine Books.

Hayflick, L. (2004). "Anti-aging" is an oxymoron. *Journal of Gerontology: Biological and Medical Sciences, 59A,* 573–578.

Hayflick, L. (2006). La dolce vita versus la vita sobria. *The Gerontologist, 46,* 413–416.

Hayflick, L. (in press). Good health is the slowest rate of aging. *Journal of Gerontology: Biological and Medical Sciences.*

He, W., Sengupta, M., Velkoff, V. A., & DeBarros, K. A. (2005). *65+ in the United States: 2005.* Washington, DC: U.S. Census Bureau.

Helping elderly stay at home. (2006, 6 November). *Howick and Pakuranga Times, New Zealand.*

Hendler, K. (2005, June). *The relationship between oral health and general health: New research in health maintenance and promotion.* Paper presented at the Consortium on Active Retirement and Aging, Kennesaw State University, Kennesaw, GA.

High, D., & Doole, M. (1995). Ethical and legal issues in conducting research involving elderly subjects. *Behavioral Sciences and the Law, 13,* 319–335.

Holmes, E. R., & Holmes, L. (1995). *Other cultures, elder years.* Thousand Oaks, CA: Sage.

Kark, J. D., Shemi, G., Friedlander, Y., Martin, O., Manor, O., & Blondheim, S. H. (1996). Does religious observance promote health? Mortality in secular vs. religious kibbutzim in Israel. *American Journal of Public Health, 86,* 341–346.

Kastenbaum, R. (2001). Gerontology. In G. L. Maddox (Ed.), *The encyclopedia of aging* (3rd ed., Vol. I, pp. 441–443). New York: Springer Publishing Company.

Kendig, H., & Quine, S. (2006). Community services for older people in Australia. In H. Yoon & J. Hendricks (Eds.), *Handbook of Asian aging* (pp. 431–451). Amityville, NY: Baywood Publishing Company.

Kinsella, K., & Phillips, D. R. (2005). Global aging: The challenge of success. *Population Bulletin, 60*(1), 3–42.

Landers, S. H. (2006). Home care: A key to the future of family medicine? *Annals of Family Medicine, 4*, 366–368.

Leibing, A. (2005). The old lady from Ipanema: Changing notions of old age in Brasil. *Journal of Aging Studies, 19*, 15–31.

Leibing, A., & Py, L. (2005). The new old—aging and gerontology in Brasil. *AGHExchange, 28*(3), 1–19.

Levy, B., & Langer, E. (1994). Aging free from negative stereotypes: Successful memory in China and among the American deaf. *Journal of Personality and Social Psychology, 66*, 989–997.

Levy, B. R., Slade, M. D., & Gill, T. M. (2006). Hearing decline predicted by elders' stereotypes. *Journal of Gerontology: Psychological Sciences, 61B*, P82–P87.

Lopata, H. Z. (2001). Loneliness. In G. L. Maddox (Ed.), *The encyclopedia of aging* (3rd ed., Vol. I, pp. 615–616). New York: Springer Publishing Company.

Loza, M. D. (2001). Ageing in transition: Situation of older women in Latin America region. In United Nations Programme on Aging (Ed.), *The world ageing situation: Exploring a society for all ages* (pp. 70–98). New York: United Nations.

Luborsky, M. R., & McMullen, C. K. (1999). Culture and aging. In J. C. Cavanaugh & S. K. Whitbourne (Eds.), *Gerontology: An interdisciplinary perspective* (pp. 65–90). New York: Oxford University Press.

Maddox, G. L. (1994). Social and behavioural research on ageing: An agenda for the United States. *Ageing and Society, 14*, 97–107.

Metchnikoff, É. (1912). *The prolongation of life: Optimistic studies* (P. C. Mitchell, Trans.). New York: G. P. Putnam's Sons and The Knickerbocker Press.

Mitchell, D. B. (1989). How many memory systems? Evidence from aging. *Journal of Experimental Psychology: Learning, Memory, and Cognition, 15*, 31–49.

Mitchell, D. B., & Bruss, P. J. (2003). Age differences in implicit memory: Conceptual, perceptual, or methodological? *Psychology and Aging, 18*, 807–822.

Mitchell, D. B., & Schmitt, F. A. (2006). Short- and long-term implicit memory in aging and Alzheimer's disease. *Aging, Neuropsychology, and Cognition, 13*, 611–635.

Morgan, R. (2006, August). The medium is still the message. *Observer, 19*, 21–24.

Mundorf, N., & Brownell, W. (2001). Communication technologies and older adults. In G. L. Maddox (Ed.), *The encyclopedia of aging* (3rd ed., Vol. I, pp. 224–226). New York: Springer Publishing Company.

Musick, M. A., Traphagan, J. W., Koenig, H. G., & Larson, D. B. (2000). Spirituality in physical health and aging. *Journal of Adult Development, 7*, 73–86.

National Research Council. (2001). *Preparing for an aging world: The case for cross-national research.* Washington, DC: National Academy Press.

Nesselroade, J. R. (2001). Individual differences. In G. L. Maddox (Ed.), *The encyclopedia of aging* (3rd ed., Vol. I, pp. 532–533). New York: Springer Publishing Company.

Palmore, E. (1990). *Ageism.* New York: Springer.

Palmore, E. (1998). *The facts on aging quiz* (2nd ed.). New York: Springer.

Palmore, E., Branch, L., & Harris, D. K. (Eds.). (2005). *Encyclopedia of ageism.* Binghamton, NY: Haworth Pastoral Press.

Park, D., & Gutchess, A. (2006). The cognitive neuroscience of aging and culture. *Current Directions in Psychological Science, 15*, 105–108.

"People in U.S. Living Longer" (2005, March 1). *Los Angeles Times*, p. 1.

Perls, T. T. (2004). The oldest old. *Scientific American Special Edition, 14*(3), 6–11.

Perls, T. T., & Silver, M. H. (1999). *Living to 100: Lessons in living to your maximum potential at any age.* New York: Basic Books.

Quinn, M. J. (2001). Elder abuse and neglect. In G. L. Maddox (Ed.), *The encyclopedia of aging* (3rd ed., Vol. I, pp. 324–327). New York: Springer Publishing Company.

Riggs, K. E. (2004). *Granny@work: Aging and new technology on the job in America.* New York: Routledge.

Rodwin, V. G., & Gusmano, M. K. (2006). *Growing older in world cities: New York, London, Paris, and Tokyo.* Nashville: Vanderbilt University Press.

Rogers, W. A., & Fisk, A. D. (2006). Aware home technology: Potential benefits for older adults. *Public Policy and Aging Report, 15*, 28–30.

Rosenblum, J. (2001, 16 February). L'chaim in Bnei Brak. *Jerusalem Post.*

Rowe, J. W., & Kahn, R. L. (1998). *Successful aging.* New York: Pantheon.

Schaie, K. W., Krause, N., & Booth, A. (Eds.). (2004). *Religious influences on health and well-being in the elderly.* New York: Springer.

Stern, Y. (1998, March). Hospice care: Can it have a Jewish heart? *The Jewish Observer, 21–25.*

Stronge, A. J., Rogers, W. A., & Fisk, A. D. (2007). Human factors considerations in implementing telemedicine systems to accommodate older adults. *Journal of Telemedicine and Telecare, 13*, 1–3.

Tae-gyu, K. (2006, November 6). Robot maids for elderly to make debut in 2013. *The Korea Times.*

United Nations. (2002). *World population ageing: 1950–2050*: United Nations publication, Sales No. E.02.XIII.3.

United Nations Programme on Aging. (2001). A society for all ages: Evolution and exploration. In United Nations Programme on Aging (Ed.), *The world ageing situation: Exploring a society for all ages* (pp. 1–12). New York: United Nations.

University of Georgia, Institute of Gerontology, College of Public Health. (2006). *Georgia centenarian study.* Retrieved August 11, 2007, from http://www.geron.uga.edu/research/centenarianstudy.php

US Census Bureau. (2006). *Nation's population to reach 300 million on Oct. 17.* Retrieved August 11, 2007, from http://www.census.gov/Press-Release/www/releases/archives/population/007616.html

"U.S. Life Expectancy up to 77.6" (2005, March 1). *The Boston Globe*, p. 1.

Vaupel, J. W., & Jeune, B. (1995). The emergence and proliferation of centenarians. In B. Jeune & J. Vaupel (Eds.), *Exceptional longevity: From prehistory to the present.* Odense, Denmark: Odense University Press.

WHO. (2006). *Research ethics review committee.* Retrieved August 11, 2007, from http://www.who.int/rpc/research_ethics/en

Wilson, G. (2000). *Understanding old age: Critical and global perspectives.* London: Sage Publications.

Yoon, C., Feinberg, F., & Gutchess, A. H. (2006). Pictorial naming specificity across ages and cultures: A latent class analysis of picture norms for younger and older Americans and Chinese. *Gerontology, 52*, 295–305.

Young, J. (2006). Ageism in services for transient ischaemic attack and stroke. *Bristish Medical Journal, 333*, 507–508.

Appendix 18-A: 20 Questions about Global Aging

1. *True or false?* In the year 2000, children under the age of 15 still outnumbered elderly people (aged 65 and over) in almost all nations of the world.

2. The world's elderly population is increasing by approximately how many people each month?

   a. 50,000   b. 300,000   c. 500,000   d. 800,000

3. Which of the world's developing regions has the highest aggregate percent elderly?

   a. Africa   b. Latin America   c. The Caribbean   d. Asia (excluding Japan)

4. China has the world's largest total population (more than 1.2 billion people). Which country has the world's largest elderly (65+) population?

   a. Japan   b. Germany   c. China   d. Nigeria

5. *True or false?* More than half of the world's elderly today live in the industrialized nations of Europe, North America, and Japan.

6. Of the world's major countries, which had the highest percentage of elderly people in the year 2000?

   a. Sweden   b. Turkey   c. Italy   d. France

7. *True or false?* Current demographic projections suggest that 35 percent of all people in the United States will be at least 65 years of age by the year 2050.

8. *True or false?* The number of the world's "oldest old" (people aged 80 and over) is growing more rapidly than that of the elderly as a whole.

9. More than one-third of the world's oldest old live in which three countries?

   a. Germany, the United States, and the United Kingdom

   b. India, China, and the United States

   c. Japan, China, and Brazil

   d. Russia, India, and Indonesia

10. Japan has the highest life expectancy at birth among the major countries of the world. How many years can the average Japanese baby born in 2000 expect to live?

    a. 70 years   b. 75 years   c. 81 years   d. 85 years

11. *True or false?* Today in some countries life expectancy at birth is less than 40 years.

12. What are the leading killers of elderly women in Europe and North America?

     a. Cancers   b. Circulatory diseases   c. Respiratory diseases   d. Accidents

13. *True or false?* Elderly women outnumber elderly men in all developing countries.

14. There are more older widows than widowers in virtually all countries because:

     a. Women live longer than men

     b. Women typically marry men older than themselves

     c. Men are more likely than women to remarry after divorce or the death of a spouse

     d. All of the above

15. In developed countries, recent declines in labor force participation rates of older (55 and over) workers are due almost entirely to changing work patterns of:

     a. Men   b. Women   c. Men and women

16. What proportion of the world's countries have a public old-age security program?

     a. All   b. Three-fourths   c. One-half   d. One-fourth

17. Approximately what percent of the private sector labor force in the United States is covered by a private pension plan (as opposed to, or in addition to, public Social Security)?

     a. 10%   b. 25%   c. 33%   d. 60%

18. In which country are elderly people least likely to live alone?

     a. The Philippines   b. Hungary   c. Canada   d. Denmark

19. *True or false?* In developing countries, older men are more likely than older women to be illiterate.

20. *True or false?* In most nations, large cities have younger populations (i.e., a lower percent elderly) than the country as a whole.

Answers

1. **True**. Although the world's population is aging, children still outnumber the elderly in all major nations except six: Bulgaria, Germany, Greece, Italy, Japan, and Spain.

2. **d.** The estimated change in the total size of the world's elderly population between July 1999 and July 2000 was more than 9.5 million people, an average of 795,000 each month.

3. **c.** The Caribbean, with 7.2% of all people aged 65 or older. Corresponding figures for other regions are: Asia (excluding Japan), 5.5%; Latin America, 5.3%; and Africa, 3.1%.

4. **c.** China also has the largest elderly population, numbering nearly 88 million in 2000.

5. **False**. Although industrialized nations have higher percentages of elderly people than do most developing countries, 59% of the world's elderly now live in the developing countries of Africa, Asia, Latin America, the Caribbean, and Oceania.

6. **c.** Italy, with 18.1% of all people aged 65 or over. Monaco, a small principality of about 32,000 people located on the Mediterranean, has more than 22% of its residents aged 65 and over.

7. **False**. Although the United States will age rapidly when the Baby Boomers (people born between 1946 and 1964) begin to reach age 65 after the year 2010, the percent of population aged 65 and over in the year 2050 is projected to be slightly above 20% (compared with about 13% today).

8. **True**. The oldest old are the fastest-growing component of many national populations. The world's growth rate for the 80+ population from 1999 to 2000 was 3.5%, while that of the world's elderly (65+) population as a whole was 2.3% (compared with 1.3% for the total [all ages] population).

9. **b.** India has roughly 6.2 million people aged 80 and over, China has 11.5 million, and the United States 9.2 million. Taken together, these people constitute nearly 38 percent of the world's oldest old.

10. **c.** 81 years, up from about 52 in 1947.

11. **True.** In some African countries (e.g., Malawi, Swaziland, Zambia, and Zimbabwe) where the HIV/AIDS epidemic is particularly devastating, average life expectancy at birth may be as much as 25 years lower than it otherwise would be in the absence of HIV/AIDS.

12. **b.** Circulatory diseases (especially heart disease and stroke) typically are the leading cause of death as reported by the World Health Organization. In Canada in 1995, for example, 44% of all deaths occurring to women at age 65 or above were attributed to circulatory disease. The percentage was virtually the same for elderly men.

13. **False.** Although there are more elderly women than elderly men in the vast majority of the world's countries, there are exceptions such as India, Iran, and Bangladesh.

14. **d.** All of the above.

15. **a.** From the late 1960s until very recently, labor force participation rates of older men in developed countries were declining virtually everywhere, whereas those for women were often holding steady or increasing. But because older men work in much greater numbers than do older women, increases in female participation were more than offset by falling male participation.

16. **b.** Of the 227 countries/areas of the world with populations of at least 5,000, 167 (74%) reported having some form of an old age/disability/survivors program circa 1999.

17. **d.** The share of the private sector U.S. labor force covered by private pension plans was about 60% in the mid-1990s. However, not all employees who are covered by such plans actually participate in them.

18. **a.** The Philippines. The percent of elderly people living alone in developing countries is usually much lower than that in developed countries; levels in the latter may exceed 40%.

19. **False.** Older women are less likely to be literate. In China in 1990, for example, only 11% of women aged 60 and over could read and write, compared with half of men aged 60 and over.

20. **We do not know.** Data for selected cities/countries are presented in Chapter 5. Some literature from developed countries suggests that the statement is false; evidence from certain developing countries suggests that it is true. Both the Census Bureau's International Programs Center and the National Institute on Aging's Behavioral and Social Research Program would be most interested in empirical input from interested parties. Understanding global aging is a dialectical process.

Source: Kinsella, K., & Velkoff, V. A. (2001). *An aging world: 2001* (No. P95/01-1): Washington: U.S. Census Bureau.

Chapter 19

Establishing Medical and Nursing Education Programs in the Country of Georgia

Judith L. Wold, H. Kenneth Walker, and Natia Partskhladze

Introduction

A functional healthcare system is a critical cornerstone of any country. The health and well-being of a country's population is vital to its economic progress. This chapter describes in detail the efforts of a group of partners in Atlanta, Georgia, in the United States, and the country of Georgia, a former republic of the Soviet Union. A vital goal of the partnership has been to elevate the profession of nursing in this country in order to improve the quality of health care and to have an impact upon other sectors. Nurses and the nursing profession form the foundation for the critical healthcare sector of any national healthcare system. Nurses are crucial caregivers and leaders in every facet of the healthcare sector including rural areas, outpatient clinics, hospitals, primary care, and public health. The nursing profession is particularly vital in developing countries that are in transition from totalitarian governments to democracy. The nursing profession in these countries, almost without exception, is at a very low professional level. Transitional countries make little use of the enormous potential that nurses have to make an impact upon every part of the healthcare sector.

This chapter presents a model that can be applied to other similar transitional nations. The partnership has been engaged extensively in other areas of the healthcare sector, with the aim of revitalizing and modernizing the sector through capacity building, organizational development, and the institutionalization of contemporary practices. All of these activities are outlined in detail.

The country of Georgia is located at the crossroads of the Western and the Eastern hemispheres. Technically located in southwest Asia, Georgia is bordered on the west by the Black Sea and Turkey, the east by Azerbaijan, the north by Russia (the longest of its land borders) and the south by Armenia. Georgia is approximately the size of the US state of South Carolina. Its capitol is the city of Tbilisi. Located on the Silk Road, a well known

Figure 19-1 Dhvari Georgian Orthodox monastery in the Causasus Mountains.

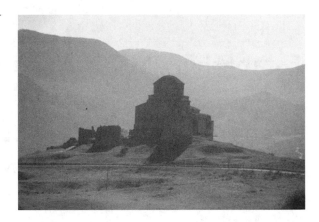

and historically significant Chinese trade route extending 7,000 miles eastward from the Mediterranean Sea to the Yellow River, Georgia has been conquered innumerable times in its long history. Rich in heritage, the people of Georgia are an intelligent, highly educated society with a literacy rate of almost 100%. Although it has been a Christian country for many centuries, a number of religious sects coexist peacefully in Georgia (see Figure 19-1).

The people of Georgia, who now number under 5 million, are warm and gracious to a fault, going above and beyond expectations to treat visitors to the country hospitably. As a former satellite country of the former Soviet Union, Georgia was quite well to do by Soviet standards, serving as the wine capital and Black Sea summer playground of the Soviet elite. With the crumbling of the Soviet Union, Georgia suffered the same rapid economic decline that all of the republics suffered. With the economic destabilization of Georgia and the concomitant problems of providing social protection, poverty among its citizens has risen sharply. The poorer segments of the population are enduring the greatest hardships because of the lack of governmental spending on social services, infrastructure, and health (Bunnell, Hoover, Day, Yetter, & Dersham, 2005). In 2004 there were still 240,000 persons internally displaced from the civil conflicts that Georgia had endured. Georgia ranks as number 100 on the human development index (HDI) among 177 ranked countries (UNDP, 2006a). The HDI is calculated from life expectancy, education, and gross domestic product indices, which are accurate human development measures of long and healthy life, knowledge, and a decent standard of living (UNDP, 2006b).

During their transition from communism to democracy, the gross domestic product of Georgia fell by 75%, and in 1994 per capita healthcare expenditures fell from $95.50 to $0.90 (Skarbinski et al., 2002). Aside from agriculture (arable land accounts for approximately 12% of the country's land), Georgia has few natural resources, making economic recovery for this country difficult. In a 2005 report, Brunnell et al. presented data suggesting that even though there is little interaction with governmental officials, Georgian communities still expect the government to take care of their needs. This is not a sur-

Figure 19-2 Open air market in Tbilisi.

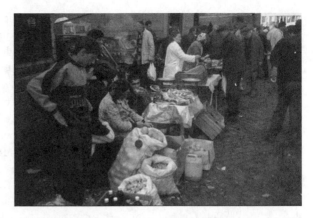

prising holdover from the former Soviet era. Infrastructure deterioration in electricity, roads, gas, and water supply, especially in the rural areas, is a serious issue. Although there is little evidence of entrepreneurial spirit, likely because of depleted savings and investment deterioration, an increasing number of people are leaving rural areas due to lack of employment opportunities (Brunnell et al., 2005). However, one positive action made by the government has been its attempt to decrease bureaucratic red tape and paperwork in order to make doing business in Georgia easier (International Finance Corporation, 2006). Figure 19-2 depicts an "open air" market in Tbilisi.

Environmental problems directly affecting health in Georgia are "air pollution . . .; heavy pollution of Mtkvari River and the Black Sea; inadequate supplies of potable water; and soil pollution from toxic chemicals" (Central Intelligence Agency [CIA], 2006, p. 2). Georgia is a mountainous country with the greater Caucasus Mountains in the north and the lesser Caucasus Mountains in the south (CIA, 2006). Many of the roads in Georgia are in an advanced state of disrepair, making travel, especially in an emergency medical situation, treacherous and slow.

Because of its location and the fact that Georgia is a Christian country, it has become a strategic ally of the United States. President Saakashvili's courting of the Western world, among other issues, has kept the Georgia–Russia relationship in turmoil. Georgia depends on Russia for much of its oil and electricity and has suffered poor or no service on numerous occasions. Additionally, Russia supports regional separatist activities in the areas of Abkhazia and South Ossetia, and most recently in Armenia (Axis, 2005), which further antagonizes the Georgian government. There are now oil pipelines from the Caspian Sea running through Georgia to the Black Sea. The construction of these pipelines has helped to bolster Georgia's economy. With the economic need of Georgia to attract business, the necessity of a modern healthcare system is of primary importance.

Following the 1991 collapse of the former Soviet Union, the American International Health Alliance (AIHA) was formed through the United Stated Agency for International Development (USAID) with the goal of advancing global health. Their work began in the newly independent states (NIS) in 1992 with a partnership model. The partnership model paired healthcare entities in the United States with hospitals and communities in the NIS in an attempt to address the problems experienced by the decimated NIS health-care systems. The US healthcare entities volunteered their expertise and committed to helping through these partnerships, with AIHA providing the support services and management systems (AIHA, 2006). The only AIHA remuneration for the partners was essentially reimbursement of travel expenses for trips to and from the partnership countries. The time and expertise of the partners was in-kind funding. This partnership model has proven extremely successful, and so AIHA has broadened its scope of influence to the central and eastern European (CEE) countries and beyond. AIHA's programmatic approach was based on the concept that all partnerships would most likely share common concerns and problems within their healthcare systems. With this concept instilled in partnership philosophy, partners collaborated in a number of areas including emergency medicine, nursing, women's health, health management, infection control, primary health care, and neonatal resuscitation among others to transform healthcare in the NIS and CEE countries (American International Health Alliance [AIHA], 2006). Partnerships in most of the NIS ran for a specified length of time (3 or 4 years) and then "graduated" from AIHA oversight and funding. Over the years this has included 105 partnerships linking volunteers in the United States with communities, institutions, and colleagues in the countries of central and eastern Europe and the former Soviet Union in successful efforts to improve health-related services and strengthen human and organizational capacity in countries with limited resources. One of the longest-standing partnerships resulting from the original AIHA partnerships in the NIS is the Atlanta–Tbilisi healthcare partnership (ATHP). Also known as the "Georgia to Georgia" project, the endeavor that started with a single partner hospital has grown in scope and influence in both Georgias. In 2002, the Atlanta–Tbilisi project evolved into the nongovernmental organizations (NGO) *Partners for International Development (PfID)* and its in-country counterpart *Partners for Health (PfH)*.

The United Nations defines an NGO as:

> A nongovernmental organization is a not-for-profit, voluntary citizens' group that is organized on a local, national, or international level to address issues in support of the public good. Task-oriented and made up of people with a common interest, NGOs perform a variety of services and humanitarian functions, bring citizens' concerns to governments, monitor policy and program implementation, and encourage participation of civil society stakeholders at the community level. They provide analysis and expertise, serve as early-warning mechanisms and help monitor and implement international agreements. Some are organized around specific issues, such as human rights, the environment, or health (UN, 2006).

Here a grant writer on the Atlanta–Tbilisi project describes its successes:

> Begun in 1992 the Atlanta–Tbilisi Healthcare Partnership (ATHP) has brought together educational and governmental institutions in Atlanta, Georgia, and in the country of Georgia for the purpose of sharing information and expertise to improve health care in Georgia. Other important relationships have been forged under the Fogarty Fellowships, the Muskie Fellowships, the World Bank health reform project, the Epidemic Intelligence Service programs of CDC, the World Health Organization (WHO) Collaborating Center in Maternal and Perinatal Health programs, USAID projects for infectious disease surveillance, and the Association of University Programs in Health Administration (Henry, A. 2002, p.1).

Georgia partners are the Government of Georgia, Ministry of Labour, Health and Social Affairs, the Caucasus School of Business, Georgian Technical University, and Tbilisi State University. The Atlanta institutions include Emory University, Georgia State University, Georgia Institute of Technology, Grady Memorial Hospital, and the Morehouse School of Medicine. Although the partnership has received public-sector funding, sizeable contributions by the US partner institutions and their volunteer health professionals have more than matched the US government's support.

The partnership has been involved in many aspects of the healthcare arena in Georgia over the span of this partnership association. Assessment has been an ongoing task with the partnership and priorities changed as some of the more pressing problems have been addressed. After addressing the Georgian healthcare system and communicable diseases, the areas of assistance that will de discussed in this chapter will include healthcare reform, access to information, nursing and nursing education, women and children, medical education, business education, healthcare management, scholarly activities, emergency care, and other activities.

The Georgian Healthcare System

From 1921 until 1991, the Georgian healthcare system was part of the greater Soviet healthcare system. In this centralized system of health care, known as the Semashko model, health care for every Soviet citizen was provided by the government from general public revenues. The Semashko model was based on a hospital inpatient medical model, which was extremely costly with little to no focus on prevention or primary care. There were a huge number of hospital beds in this system with an equally huge number of doctors and other medical personnel staffing them. Assessment of this system did not report on quality of care, but rather quantitative indicators such as number of beds, occupancy rates, or number of referrals were used as markers. Outcomes reported were usually congruent with whatever the Soviet superiors wanted achieved.

With the collapse of the Soviet Union came economic blight for all of the countries of that union. Georgia was no exception. The healthcare system in Georgia declined rapidly because of the poor financial situation in the country resulting from civil war, stagnant economy, and inflation. Although healthcare system reform has been on the table since 1995, the system is still not meeting the needs of its citizens, especially the poorer segment of the population. The following text is a partial representation of Georgian healthcare reform legislation, from the Law of Georgia on Health Care, Section 4, from December 10, 1997 (World Health Organization, 2006a).

The principles of state policy in the field of health care are the following:

1. To provide the population with universal and equal access to medical care within the framework of state-funded medical programs

2. To assure the protection of human rights and freedoms in the field of health care, as well as the recognition of the patient's dignity, honor, and autonomy

3. To recognize the independence of the physician and other medical personnel within the framework prescribed by Georgian legislation

4. To adapt the health system to the country's economic development strategy and ensure that the national health system is properly managed

5. To protect against discrimination, during the provision of medical care, toward detained or imprisoned persons, as well as persons suffering from certain disease

6. To implement and strengthen internationally recognized standards of medical ethics in the healthcare field

7. To provide the population with full information on all existing forms of medical care and the modalities of access to such care

8. To promote cooperation with international organizations working in the field of health care

9. To assign responsibility to the state for the extent and quality of the medical services determined by the compulsory health insurance program

10. To accord priority to primary health care and emergency medical care, with the participation of the public and private sectors

11. To assign responsibility to the state for the licensing and certification of medical personnel, health establishments, medical faculties, and medical training establishments

12. To ensure that the state, society, and every citizen participate in the adoption of a healthy lifestyle and also the protection of the working, home, and recreational environments

13. To assure the diversity of organizational and legal structures and forms of ownership in the field of medical service, as well as the equality of their rights

14. To apply administrative and legal sanctions against acts that are harmful to the population's health

15. To provide for state funding through an overall program and specific programs, and to assure the autonomy of the management system as well as financial and economic contractual relations in order to permit the self-management of state-funded health establishments, in accordance with the legislation

16. To provide for the state funding of biomedical and healthcare research in keeping with existing resources and to create, to this end, favorable conditions for attracting funds from the private sector

17. To ensure that professional and other nongovernmental organizations participate in the creation of a modern and efficient health system through consultations, scientific and professional discussions, the development of relevant projects, and participation in the protection of patients' rights

In principle the legislation looks laudable, but economic circumstances have prevented forward movement. In 2005 healthcare-sector expenditures were 5–5.5% of the gross domestic product (GDP); however, the government expenditures were not more than 30% of that amount. At this writing, the government does not yet have a clear roadmap with which to advance the healthcare system. The infrastructure of Georgia's healthcare system is antiquated and unable to meet the present needs of its citizenry in quality or geography (Open Society Georgia Foundation, 2006). A study conducted by the Curatio International Foundation (Gotsadze, Bennett, Ranson, & Gzirishvili, 2005), based on a 2000 Tbilisi household survey, found that the poorest households spend almost a quarter of their income on out-of-pocket healthcare expenses compared to only 15% spent by wealthier families. Additionally, 55% of this money was spent on medicines that are not covered by government programs. Over half of the people in this survey reported that they self-treat, and at least 11% don't seek treatment at all. When people do seek care, they turn to a specialist first, probably an acquaintance, which negates the country's push for less expensive primary care. Many seek emergency treatment because they wait too long to attend to their health in a less costly fashion. Because salaries of healthcare professionals are so low, out-of-pocket payments directly to healthcare personnel to receive better care (or any care at all) are commonplace (Belli, Gotsadze, & Shahriari, 2004). The current supply of healthcare professionals greatly exceeds demand. Figure 19-3 shows a typical Georgian hospital emergency room.

Health Indicators

According to the WHO (2006b), Georgia is an economy in transition. Life expectancy at birth for Georgians is 70 years for males and 77 years for females, although *healthy* life expectancy is almost 10 years less than these figures. Adult mortality rates indicate a huge disparity between males and females with male mortality standing at 161 per 1000 while female mortality was 60 per 1000. Total health expenditure per capita was $US174 in 2003. The health of nations is usually measured by its maternal and infant mortality rates. In 2004, infant mortality rate stood at 40 per 1000, (compared to 7 per 1000 in the United

Figure 19-3 Typical Georgian hospital emergency room.

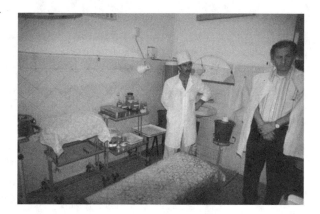

States) while the child mortality rate of children younger than 5 years was 43 per 1000 (compared to 8 per 1000 in the United States). Abortion rates are high and live births per 1000 have steadily decreased since the year 2000. John Snow International is working with women in Georgia to improve reproductive health.

The deterioration of the healthcare system in Georgia is slowly being repaired under the auspices of many international aid agencies. One major problem with vaccines was the inability to maintain refrigeration, which invalidated their effectiveness. UNICEF and other international organizations have worked with the Georgian government on maintaining the ability to refrigerate and increasing the number of World Health Organization (WHO) (2006b) reports on immunization coverage in Georgia from 1993 to 2005 for bacille Calmette-Guérin (BCG), diphtheria-pertussis-tetanus 3 (DPT3), oral polio vaccine 3 (OPV3), measles containing vaccine 1 (MCV1), and hepatitis B 3 (HepB3). Immunization coverage has risen from 30–50% to more than 80–90% for BCG, DPT, OPV, and measles but less so for hepatitis B, which was only introduced in 2001. In July of 2002, Georgia received its polio-free certification.

AIDS

The first case of HIV in Georgia was diagnosed in 1989. Through December of 2004, a total of 637 cases of HIV infection have been reported. However, WHO estimates that the true number of infections in Georgia may be closer to 3000. Seventy percent of reported cases are, or have relations with, injection drug users. The stage is set in Georgia for a devastating HIV/AIDS epidemic (Tkeshelashvili-Kessler, del Rio, Nelson, & Tsertsvadze, 2005). The main contributing factors are: a dire economic environment; an increasing incidence of drug trafficking and use of illicit drugs; a large prison population; rise in sexually transmitted infections (STIs); increased migration and internally displaced populations; rising incidence of HIV infection in neighboring countries such as the Ukraine; and a burgeoning commercial sex trade. In addition, hepatitis C is widespread and tuberculosis is epidemic which could prove to be as destructive as it is in Africa. USAID (2006) reports that in 2005 over 12,000 people at high risk for HIV were reached with prevention interventions, which, among other things, lowered the use of needle sharing from 79.2% in 2002 to 42.9% in 2005.

The partnership has supported promising young Georgians to come to Emory University for training. There have been many collaborative research projects, resulting in eight publications and presentations. Eighteen Georgians have received short- and long-term training. In-country training has been given. Of particular importance was an *Ethical Conduct of Research* course, as this helped Georgian scientists and institutions to apply to improve conduct in order to have their Institutional Review Boards registered and approved by the US Department of Health and Human Services, which is a prerequisite for applying for research funding from US government agencies. Additional US partners have included the Bloomberg School of Public Health of Johns Hopkins University, State University of New York Downstate Medical Center, the Centers for Disease Control and Prevention (CDC), and the Sparkman Center of the University of Alabama. The US partners have also collaborated with a successful Comprehensive International Research Program on AIDS (CIPRA) RO3 application and have worked closely on an U19 CIPRA application recently submitted to the National Institutes of Health.

Tuberculosis

Tuberculosis (TB) has emerged as a serious public health problem in Georgia (Weinstock et al., 2001). The annual incidence of disease is approximately 100 TB cases per 100,000 people, and the prevalence is 150 per 100,000 people (Khechinashvili, Mdivani, & Blumberg, 2004). Rates of multiresistant TB are high and exceed 10% of newly diagnosed cases. HIV coinfection appears to be low, but HCV coinfection is common, affecting nearly a quarter of all TB patients (Richards et al., 2002). The 30 TB dispensaries in Georgia are generally dilapidated with limited laboratory facilities and frequently with poorly trained personnel. The National Tuberculosis Program leadership has embraced the directly observed therapy (DOTS) short-course program and there have been limited pilot projects. DOTS implementation is greatly needed to improve TB control in Georgia and establish the infrastructure necessary for the treatment of MDR-TB patients (i.e., through DOTS-plus). Although there is resistance to DOTS from physicians trained in the Soviet era, there have been nine DOT (direct observation therapy) spots newly established in Tbilisi. These DOT spots have increased patient compliance with TB treatment therapy from 28% to 91%; the TB treatment success rate in Tbilisi reached 71% in 2005 versus 60% in 2003 (USAID, 2006).

Collaborative research activities of the partnership have focused on investigating the clinical and molecular epidemiology of tuberculosis in Georgia. Five short-term trainees have come to the United States for laboratory or epidemiologic training for the duration of several months and 15 Emory medical students have gone to Georgia to carry out collaborative research projects with the National Tuberculosis Program and AIDS Center colleagues. These projects have been supported by grants from the US Civilian Research Development Foundation and the US DHHS Biotechnology Exchange Program. The NIH Fogarty International Center has funded the Emory–Georgia TB Research Training Program, which focuses on addressing the research needs and gaps in the current expertise in Georgia. The goal of the program is to help build human resource capacity for high quality TB-related research in Georgia by providing long-, medium- and short-term training to a diverse group of researchers with outstanding potential; it will build the in-country research capacity so it can support evidence-based translation of research into policy and practice in Georgia.

Healthcare Reform

In 1994, a member of the partnership spent a year in Georgia with the specific purpose of assisting the government in legislative reform. Faculty members from the Rollins School of Public Health at Emory University worked with her and provided extensive consultation to the Georgian government during the partnership, including mentoring 10 Georgians who received their MPH at Emory. They also assisted with the strategic development of the State Health Insurance Fund. A partial result of this collaboration was the drafting and issuing of presidential Decree 400 in December 1994, which established state healthcare funding, specified licensure of medical facilities, created registration and quality control of medications and supplies, and established certification and licensure of healthcare providers.

Access to Information

During the initial years of the partnership it became quite clear that enhancing access to information for the Georgian partners would be a vital accomplishment. There was no access to medical literature, and practitioners were not in the habit of reading medical journals to update their knowledge base. The National Information Learning Center was established in 1996, with a fast Internet connection, computers, and servers. Document delivery and classes for the public in searching databases such as MEDLINE are now provided. There is dial-up access and a local area network for institutions in Tbilisi. The Uniformed Services University for the Health Sciences has contributed significantly to the project. A bulletin, *Contemporary Medicine*, has summaries of topical articles from the current Western medical press translated into Georgian alongside English. A Web page is maintained about health care in Georgia. Videoconferencing, telemedicine, and distance learning are provided. Clinical practice guidelines have been developed in association with Atlanta partners and are being implemented (Burns, Kirtava, & Walker, 2005).

Nursing

Nursing has been a key presence in the work of the partnership since its inception. Acting as advisors to Georgian nursing leaders, the partnership has made an extensive effort to improve the knowledge level and professional acceptance of the profession of nursing in the country of Georgia. The nurse participants from both sides of the partnership have put forth a great deal of effort in implementing a three-pronged approach to upgrade the nursing profession in Georgia. The plan has encompassed the enhancement of skills of practicing nurses (ongoing), strengthening the political base of nursing within the country, and the implementation of a university-based program for nursing education.

In 1993, a delegation of nurses, which included hospital nurse administrators and a university nursing educator, visited Tbilisi with the specific goals of assessing both the Georgian nursing education system and the level of nursing care and skills in the partner hospital, City Hospital #2. These objectives were accomplished, and were reported in their meetings with the Minister of Health. One of the most important features of this partnership was the regular and continuing US interaction with the highest governmental officials for the country of Georgia.

By and large, nursing education in Georgia was and is carried out by both the government and private schools, which is called "middle and higher technical medical education." Though called *nursing colleges*, no nursing education takes place in institutions of higher education; therefore, none of the graduates from these programs have the degree that would allow them to teach in a university-level baccalaureate nursing education program. Thus, nursing is taught by physicians, and nursing education is carried out in schools with little funding, few learning resources, and, when compared to nursing education in the United States, low expectations of their graduates. Students interested in pursuing a nursing career enter nursing school out of the 9th or 11th year of high school and spend 2 to 3 years in "nurses training." Students take an examination at the end of their program, which, if they pass, qualifies them to take a nursing position at a hospital or clinic. There is no countrywide licensure examination for nursing. There is little oversight of the quality of nursing education because of the many private nursing schools and also because of the economic situation in the country. There are between 50 and 70 nursing schools in Georgia. The Ministry of Education and Science of Georgia is responsible for the oversight and accreditation of schools but only conducts institutional accreditation.

An interesting twist in nursing education is that medical students (who enter medical school immediately after high school) can practice as nurses after 2 years of medical school. If these medical students decide to practice as nurses while attending medical school, they may take positions from less well-prepared technical nurses. In Georgia, there are more physicians than nurses. In 2003 there were 20,962 physicians or 409 per 100,000 people in Georgia, and there were 17,807 medical nurses or 347 per 100,000 people. Midwives numbered 1495 or 290 per 100,000, and dentists numbered1438 or 280 per 100,000. Health expenditure per capita in Georgia in 2002 was $US123 dollars as compared to $5274 per capita for the United States (WHO, 2006b). Salaries for both physicians and nurses are very low. A nurse's salary is less than $US150 per month, and a physician's pay is anywhere between $50 and $300 if salaried (personal communication, Kirtava October 10, 2006). Of course, the out-of-pocket payments by their patients can raise that salary significantly.

During the initial nursing delegation visit to Georgia, the level of hospital nursing was also assessed. Although conditions have somewhat improved, in 1993 there was a desperate shortage of medical supplies and equipment. Assessment revealed that nurses in Georgia are trained at a level somewhere between our nursing assistants and licensed practical nurses (LPNs). Nurses in Georgia make few independent decisions regarding patient care nor do they write in the medical records in the hospitals, and they are historically not allowed to carry out many procedures considered standard for American nurses. The nurse's role is seen basically as "handmaiden" to the physician. As mentioned, there is no countrywide licensure for nurses and no real mechanism or mandate for continuing nursing education. At the end of this first 1993 visit, the US and Georgian nurse partners agreed on the three-pronged approach previously mentioned as the guiding framework for their subsequent work. This approach was imparted to the Ministry of Labor, Health, and Social Affairs (MoLHSA) and to the AIHA who agreed with this approach.

For both political and educational reasons, the US partners assisted the Georgian nurses in developing a nursing association. In 1995, the Georgian Nurses Association (GNA) was instituted as a mechanism to unite nurses in the country and to deliver continuing education under its auspices. A small fee for membership was assessed and the association began in earnest. At about the same time as the inauguration of the GNA, the Georgian parliament passed a law making nursing a distinct profession and the Minister of Health appointed a chief nursing officer (CNO) for the country. At that time, the CNO was also elected as the first President of the GNA, a situation that eventually became a liability for both the GNA and the CNO. A National Learning Resource Center for nursing was set up, staffed and equipped through AIHA funding in the government's National Health Management Center in 1997. The NLRC still provides classes for nurses in the Georgian countryside (Wold, Mullis, & Wolk, 1998).

After the peaceful overthrow of the Shevardnadze government in 2003 (called the Rose Revolution), Mikhail Saakashvili was elected president of Georgia. Saakashvili's first mission was to clean up corruption in Georgia. Many people and their families were implicated in corrupt dealings. The fallout from those early proceedings resulted in a family implication of the CNO, who then lost favor with the government and was ousted. Saakashvili's new Minister of Labor, Health, and Social Affairs (MoLHSA) did not appoint another chief nurse, and although the GNA still exists on paper and has officers, there is no money in the organization's treasury and little enthusiasm for revitalizing the organization at this writing.

The second prong of the approach, which is closely tied to continuing education, was the quest to institute a university-based baccalaureate nursing education program. Because baccalaureate education of nurses in a US model requires both sciences and liberal arts, the partnership made the decision to align itself with a multipurpose institution instead of a medical university. It was felt that a medical university would continue with a heavy medical influence and limit nursing from becoming its own profession. In 1996, the partnership forged an agreement with Javakhishvili Tbilisi State University (TSU) to cooperate in instituting a Bachelor of Science nursing program. This arrangement was approved by the Minister of Health (MOH) at that time with the promise of start-up funding in the amount of 50.000 Lari (GEL) (approximately $25,000 USD). The funding never materialized as a result of both the dire financial straits of the government and eventually by the revolution that occurred.

However, two delegations of Georgian physicians have been to the United States to be trained to conduct the baccalaureate program. Knowing the realities of teaching in a university system, the partnership knew there were no technically trained Georgian nurses qualified to teach in a university. There were physicians who had worked as nurses or who had also taught in technical "colleges" of nursing. The first delegation of three physicians came to the United States for a month. These physicians sat in on university nursing courses, visited clinical rotations in hospitals, and carried extensive course material and nursing texts back to their country. Hundreds of volumes of donated nursing texts were shipped to the TSU library. Negotiations continued in an attempt to implement the baccalaureate program but government funding did not materialize.

After the partnership re-formed into Partners for International Development (PfID) and Partners for Health (PfH), implementing a university-based approach to nursing education continued to be a priority. Figure 19-4 presents the PfID-PfH Model for Nursing Education for Georgia. The partners know that worldwide, nurses at a modern professional level of education have enormous responsibility for patient care in hospitals, outpatient clinics, and rural areas. Research shows that patient outcomes suffer if nurses are not educated and prepared to meet the challenges of a modern system of health care (Scott, Sochalski, & Aiken, 1999). In the villages of Georgia, a nurse often serves as a combination of nurse clinician and public health worker. Better education for Georgian nurses can produce better patient outcomes. Well-educated nurses are pivotal in executing the primary care, health promotion, and disease prevention model of health care desired by the country of Georgia. This seems even more important as there is, as of yet, no specific curriculum and training outline for nurses in the sizable project of Georgia's primary healthcare system restructuring, supported by the World Bank (WB), Department of International Development (DFID of the United Kingdom), and European Union (EU). Partnership trainers could successfully play a role in that development as well. Nurse educators could be prepared to offer a full range of the courses needed to train highly qualified primary healthcare nurses. Trainers could also conduct health and wellness events and educate Georgian nurses on how to provide health promotion and disease prevention methods to populations in both urban and rural areas of the country. Prevention of disease in a time of scarce monetary resources is one way to reduce healthcare expenditures. Moreover, more comprehensively educated nurses will be able to provide expert care at the bedside that will be required as Georgia acquires a more technologically advanced medical care system.

A second attempt to prepare trainers to implement a BS program occurred in 2005 with funding from AIHA, the Soros Foundation, Open Society Georgia Foundation

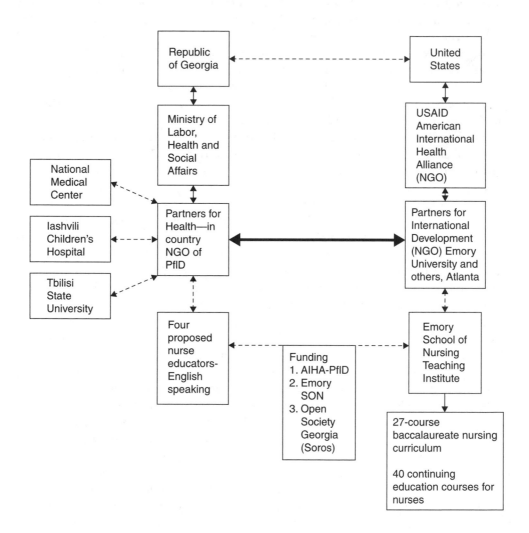

Figure 19-4   PfID-PfH Model for Nursing Education for Georgia.

(OSGF), and the Nell Hodgson Woodruff School of Nursing (NHWSN) at Emory University (OSGF, 2006). From the group of Georgian nurses actively involved in this work, four nurse trainers were selected by the partnership to participate in the proposed project. The nursing education director of the partnership had been leading the nursing education component of the partnership for the past 12 years and was very familiar with nursing, nursing education, and human resources in the country. Criteria for the selection process were the following:

- Being closely involved with the nursing profession in Georgia
- Being closely involved with the Atlanta–Tbilisi partnership
- Having graduated from medical university and so being eligible to teach in a higher-education program for nurses in Georgia
- Being familiar and in a working relationship with the current partner hospitals (National Medical Center and Central Children's Hospital)
- Being involved in development of training and other materials, workshops and other activities in these hospitals
- Fluent in both speaking and writing in the English language

Four physicians spent an entire semester in the NHWSN at Emory. Not only were they enrolled in the Nursing Teaching Institute, but they were guided in this teaching institute in developing a culturally specific 27-course baccalaureate nursing curriculum, completely translated into Georgian. Each course had an accompanying updated American text. Additionally, 40 continuing education (CE) courses were developed in the areas outlined in Table 19-1.

The development of the CE courses were of prime importance because continuing education has always been a mainstay of the partnership and is a fallback approach in the continuing efforts to undergird better nursing education. These trainers returned to Tbilisi in June of 2005 to begin an ambitious CE plan for nurses in the partner hospitals and to continue to negotiate for the university-based program.

As mentioned above, continuing education for nurses has always been a mainstay of the Atlanta–Tbilisi partnership. Figure 19-5 shows a group of Georgian nurses in one of the partnership's newly furnished hospital learning laboratories. Over the years there have been many exchange nurses coming to the United States for observation and training in nursing leadership, education, and skills. A *train the trainer* approach was the preferred method of education for the partnership. In the early years of the partnerships, AIHA was very involved in developing nurse leaders in the NIS countries and held annual nurse leadership conferences that were attended by both partners. Numerous CE seminars have been held on such topics as nursing triage, nursing assessment, infection control, intravenous therapy, pain management, pre- and postoperative care, community focused care, and other topics. Complete plans for setting up a modern nursing care system have been provided for the partner hospitals, many of them translated into Georgian. These include

TABLE 19-1   Nursing Continuing Education Programs Developed in the
Teaching Institute at Emory University, 2005

Nurses and Nursing Assessment

Fundamentals of Nursing

(Vital signs, bed making, hygiene, oral care, transferring patients, injections, transfusions, infection control)

Infection Control

Trauma and Triage Nursing Skills

Cardiovascular-LymphaticSystem, Pathology (Patho)/Pharmacology (Pharm)/Skills/Patient (Pt.) education

Respiratory System, TB, Patho/Pharm/Skills/Pt. education

Gastrointestinal System, Patho/Pharm/Skills/Pt. education

Neurological System, Patho/Pharm/Skills/Pt. education

Endocrine System, Patho/Pharm/Skills/Pt. education

Immune System, Patho/Pharm/Skills/Pt. education

Renal and Urologic System, Patho/Pharm/Skills/Pt. education

Preoperative care, Nursing Skills/Pt. education

Postoperative care, Nursing Skills/Pt. education

Musculoskeletal System, Patho/Pharm/Skills/ Pt. education

Integument, Patho/Pharm/Skills/ Pt. education

Mental Health Conditions, Nursing Skills/Pt. education

Care of Older Patients, Nursing Skills/Pt. education

Critical Care, Patho/Pharm/Skills/Pt. education

Cancer, Patho/Pharm/Skills/Pt. education

Pain Management, Patho/Pharm/Skills/Pt. education

Infectious Diseases, STDs, Patho/Pharm/Skills/Pt. education

Reproductive and Pregnancy-Related Considerations, Patho/Pharm/Skills/Pt. education

nursing structure standards (protocols, procedures, forms), infection control, hospital safety, human resources policy manual, and a health system operational policy manual among others.

By June 2005, nursing education centers, funded by AIHA through the PfID and PfH partners, were established at the Central Children's Hospital (CCH) in 2004 and the National Medical Center in 2005 on the model of the previously mentioned nursing learning resource center (NLRC). The nursing educators were hired by CCH at the con-

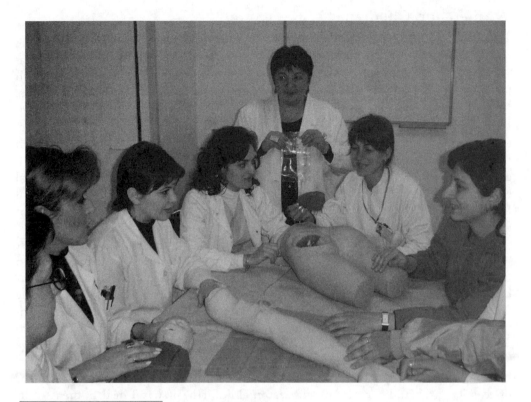

Figure 19-5 Georgian nurses in learning lab.

tinuous professional education (CPE) unit to provide continuous certificate courses and in-service nursing education to the partner hospitals and in other priority areas (primary healthcare, etc.) using the curricula developed at NHWSN. Follow-up of the CE activities with nurses who attended all sessions showed an overall knowledge retention rate of 84% and a skills usage rate of 75% among the 72 nurses sampled (Partskhladze et al., 2006).

Nursing skills have improved in a number of targeted facilities in Georgia. There are many NGOs operating in the country with programs that include the upgrading of nursing skills. As in the United States, the development of nursing as a respected profession will take time and money. Georgia needs in-country nursing champions with political influence because upgrading the profession of nursing is a both a cultural change and an economic issue. It will require an investment and a commitment on the part of the Georgian government to upgrade nursing education in a university setting. Although this partnership has sought and received approval for its plans, continuously met its objectives, and kept governmental officials informed of all outcomes, a university-based education for nursing is not yet a reality in Georgia.

Women and Children

Numerous exchanges have focused on perinatal medicine with an emphasis on public health problems. For example, an Emory medical student analyzed blood from 500 placentae and discovered an incidence of 60% hypothyroidism in newborns, a study which helped lead to corrective measures of the government and international organizations. Neonatal mortality in Georgia in the 1990s was five to seven times that in the European Union. Monitoring of the fetus during gestation by sonogram or during labor by electronic monitoring was rudimentary. Figure 19-6 shows a typical hospital newborn nursery. A group of Emory physicians, composed of an obstetrician and several neonatologists, assessed care practices in the maternity houses throughout Georgia. Educational exchanges occurred, focusing on obstetric monitoring and neonatal care. The Neonatal Resuscitation Program of the American Academy of Pediatrics had 30 participants from the regions of Georgia. This group has now trained instructors throughout the Caucasus.

The Atlanta–Kutaisi Partnership was inaugurated in 1999, establishing the first Women's Wellness Center (WWC) in Western Georgia. The Susan Komen Foundation provided $150,000 in grants for a project promoting breast health. In 2000 the center was opened in a renovated building. Carelift International participated in furnishing the facility. The WWC provides screening and preventative healthcare, contraception, nutrition, prenatal care, breast health education, reproductive counseling, pap smears, ultrasound, loop electrocautery excision procedures, and colposcopy. Over 36,000 women have been educated in personal breast examination. The partners established a community health council, a project in secondary schools on reproductive and psychiatric assessment of teenage girls, and community classes on childbirth, prenatal health, breast self-examination, and breast feeding.

Figure 19-6 Typical newborn nursery in Georgia.

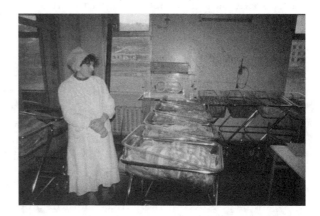

Medical Education

Since 1991, medical education in Georgia bears many similarities to the United States during the pre-Flexner era, with a plethora of private medical schools existing primarily to provide income for the teachers. There are 58 medical schools and 17,000 students in this country with under 5 million in population.

Forty students from Georgia have spent from 2 to 6 months doing clinical rotations at Emory and thirty graduates have been accepted into residency programs at Emory in specialties such as internal medicine, psychiatry, radiation oncology, and neurology. Twenty-eight Emory medical students have spent 1 to 2 months doing electives in Tbilisi. Each Emory student has had a specific project with some of these projects having an impact on public health policies in Georgia.

Business Education

In 1992 Georgia State University (GSU) of Atlanta began assisting with the establishment of business education programs in Tbilisi. This was followed by the establishment of the Caucasus School of Business (CSB) in 1998, in collaboration with the Georgian Technical University and Tbilisi State University. Funding for the project was obtained through the United States Department of State, Bureau of Educational and Cultural Affairs, in addition to USAID and with substantial cost sharing by Georgia State University. The Robinson College of Business at Georgia State University helped to develop the MBA and BBA curricula, trained Georgian faculty and administrators, and developed computer and distance-learning facilities, as well as library and audiovisual facilities. Over 90% of the Georgian faculty members have been trained in Atlanta during semester-long faculty development programs and have been awarded certificates to teach specific courses. Furthermore, each year, five Georgian students are admitted to Georgia State University for one semester, on a competitive basis. CSB has experienced dramatic growth: a faculty of 63 that teaches a student body of 800; BBA and MBA degrees are offered, and there are plans to include PhD and MHA degrees.

Healthcare Management

Hospital management is a new and developing field in the country of Georgia. Under the Soviet-designed Semashko model, healthcare planning, financing, and management decisions were centralized. Chief doctors served as administrators. These doctors were clinicians by training, had no management education, and were only held responsible for volume indicators. Poor performance resulted in the application of administrative measures or removal. Since the Georgian independence, hospital executives have struggled with multiple restructuring efforts to decentralize decision-making, reduce costs, and improve efficiency. However, the old management structures are poorly prepared to manage resources and financial obligations.

Georgian partners with significant American hospital leadership experience have provided the new administrators intensive instruction in budgeting, reimbursement, wage administration, performance monitoring and improvement, staffing, quality improvement programming, and service consolidation. The learning curve is significant and the talent pool shallow. The partnership is now awarding a Certificate in Health Services Management to enhance middle-management capabilities and is in process of designing an academic-based masters of health administration to broaden the base of individuals qualified to lead a financially sound and outcome-based health system.

Scholarly Activities and Biomedical Research

The training environment established by the partnership has enabled 14 Emory medical students, one internal medicine resident from Cornell, and one infectious diseases fellow from Emory to work on collaborative research projects about HIV, TB, and Hepatitis B/C in Georgia; funding has been from multiple grants and Emory University.

The partnership has collaborated with other US institutions as well. A medical anthropologist from the graduate faculty of political and social science at the New School investigated cultural aspects of tuberculosis control and DOTS implementation in contemporary Georgia (Koch, 2004). Koch's dissertation, called *Governing Tuberculosis: Competing Cultures of Disease and Medicine in Post-socialist Georgia*, focuses on the impacts of the Soviet medical infrastructure collapse on disease incidence, local institutions, and the role of international donors in healthcare reform. There are immediate implications for health and service delivery practices as a result of the experiences of professionals working in the TB sector and changing forms and standards of expertise. As patients bypass clinical services and self-medicate in readily available pharmacies and outdoor markets, the risk of the spread of drug-resistant tuberculosis escalates. The anthropological perspective highlights the cultural meanings and unintended consequences of well-intended policies and technical interventions. A Stanford medical student explored the effects of post-Soviet healthcare reforms and economic deterioration on access to care and healthcare financing among ill patients in 248 households in Tbilisi (Skarbinski et al., 2002).

The partnership supported and participated in a visit by leading Georgian physician scientists to the Fogarty International Center of the NIH and the National Institute of Allergy and Infectious Diseases. The NIH has sent senior scientists on fact-finding visits to Georgia, and has conducted workshops on grantsmanship.

Emergency Medical Care and Other Initiatives

Emergency medicine was practiced in the West while on-site resuscitation was unknown in the former Soviet Union. The partnership opened an Emergency Medical Services (EMS) training center in October 1995, for the purpose of training individuals in prehospital care. By 1998, 60 courses had been given to the public, including students, guards, mountain guides, and pipeline company workers; a total of 1492 people were trained. A

Figure 19-7 A Georgian child's view of an ambulance.

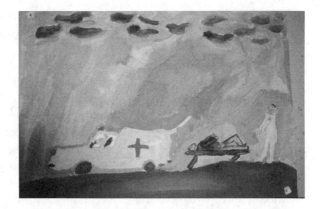

Web page was produced, three manuals published in Georgian and a learning resource for emergency medicine established.

A productive relationship has evolved between pediatric emergency medicine faculty in Atlanta and a newly opened modern emergency room in Central Children's Hospital, the premier pediatric hospital in Georgia. The goal is to transition medical staff who are trained in pediatrics and critical care medicine into the role of emergency medicine practitioners. New concepts were introduced, including the role of an emergency medicine physician, nursing triage, patient tracking, and flow through an emergency department. A Western-style pediatric emergency facility was opened in 2005 at the Iashvili Pediatric Hospital in Tbilisi with the assistance of this partnership. Figure 19-7 shows a Georgian child's drawing of an ambulance. The new ER is serving as a model for the country, indeed the whole Caucasus, and has been instrumental in providing modern health care to hundreds of pediatric patients throughout Georgia. A number of other initiatives have been carried out, including assessment of the radiological services of the country and training in echocardiography and cardiac catheterization (Casarella, 1993).

Discussion

The partnership began when the American International Healthcare Alliance (AIHA) came to Atlanta in the spring of 1992 and invited the leaders of Emory University School of Medicine, Morehouse School of Medicine, and Grady Hospital to participate in a partnership with the country of Georgia. AIHA was formed in 1992 by a consortium of major healthcare provider associations and professional medical education organizations in response to an initiative made by the US Agency for International Development (USAID) to develop healthcare partnerships between the United States and the former Soviet Union. AIHA guided the Georgia–Georgia partnership with wisdom and advice. In addition to providing direct funding and administrative support for the partnership, AIHA also provided substantial region-wide resources in support of many of the partnership's initiatives including emergency medical services, nursing, women's health care, infection control, evidence-based practice and informatics, and health management and administration.

The funds spent during the 12 years are estimated at approximately 12 million dollars: 4 million from USAID, in-kind contributions from the Atlanta partners of 7 million, and funds from other sources at 1 million. The Atlanta–Tbilisi Partnership has been formalized with the establishment of a nongovernmental organization, the Partners for International Development. The partnership is becoming more productive with time. A richly collaborative relationship has formed an effective unit of individuals and institutions from both countries. The results span over a surprisingly wide range of societal sectors. The Caucasus School of Business has educated many young Georgians in the methodology of a market-oriented economy, and they are having a pervasive effect upon business in Georgia. The school is forming the basis of education in healthcare administration. Georgian and US medical students have benefited from cross-cultural medical and educational experiences. Over 30 Georgian medical school graduates are now fully trained and certified in specialties in the United States; 3 are on the faculty of Emory University. Their attempts in going back to practice in Georgia have not been successful due to the present lack of technology. They are experimenting with how to best help Georgia without returning there. One has enlisted her US colleagues and is planning to establish a modern radiation oncology center in Georgia, which only has a few old cobalt units. Another graduate is working to establish modern cardiology in Georgia through equipment donation and training. The Women's Wellness Center has introduced new concepts in the care of women and children. Collaborative research on AIDS and TB has produced new information that can be applied not only to Georgia but also to other transitioning countries, and has resulted in the establishment of a burgeoning modern research environment. Young Georgian scientists have been trained in current scientific rigor and methods, including ethics in science, making them eligible to compete for grants on the international scene. Ingrained societal behaviors and perceptions are transforming: the professional status of nurses is improving; medical students and professionals continuously update their knowledge by reading current journals; and new concepts are taking root, such as measuring patient satisfaction, evidence-based medicine, and the use of clinical practice guidelines.

Current activities include the development of a nursing school, a division of healthcare management in the Caucasus School of Business, and a pediatric radiation oncology center. The planning for a public health school is beginning. Plans for the next several years include reforming the current curriculum of medical schools, more training for emergency health practitioners, postgraduate residency training, and continuing medical education for practitioners.

The changing nature and role of societal institutions shapes and is shaped by political, economic, and cultural changes already underway within the healthcare sector as well as more generally. Academic collaborations represented by this partnership provide a vehicle for institution building and a model for future international development. Information technology remains crucial to providing access to electronic databases in the fields of health and business and in order to connect sites in countries such as Georgia with each other and with the West.

These results highlight the unique resources that academic institutions can bring to foreign aid and development. The universities of the West are replete with a vast amount of information that can be used by countries such as Georgia. Western scholars can collaborate with the scholars of developing countries to produce new information that can be used by all countries.

References

American International Health Alliance. (2006). *AIHA web page*. Retrieved October 6, 2006, from http://www.aiha.com/index.jsp

Axis Information and Analysis. (2005) *Moscow sacrifices Armenia to destroy Georgia*. Retrieved November 8, 2006, from http://www.axisglobe.com/ article.asp?article=449

Belli, P., Gotsadze, G., & Shahriari, H. (2004). Out-of-pocket and informal payments in health sector: Evidence from Georgia. *Health Policy 70*(1), 109–123.

Bunnell, R., Hoover, B., Day, M., Yetter, S., & Dersham, L. (2005). *Georgia employment and infrastructure initiative: Socioeconomic inventory assessment*. Retrieved October 6, 2006, from http://georgia.usaid.gov/programs/pdf/3_1.pdf

Burns, C., Kirtava, Z., & Walker, K. (2005). The role of information access in sustainable healthcare in Georgia: The Atlanta–Tbilisi Health Partnership model. *Information Services & Use, 25*, 125–135.

Casarella W. (1993). Radiology in Tbilisi: The legacy of 70 years of soviet government. *American Journal of Radiology, 161*, 23–25.

Central Intelligence Agency. (2006). *World factbook*. Retrieved November 8, 2006, from https://www.cia.gov/cia/publications/factbook/geos/gg.html

Gotsadze, G., Bennett, S., Ranson, K., & Gzirishvili, D. (2005). Health care seeking behaviour and out-of-pocket payments in Tbilisi, Georgia: Household survey findings. *Health Policy and Planning, 20*(4), 232–242.

Henry, A. (2002). *Proposal for capacity building to support health care reform in Georgia with emphasis on nursing, distance education, healthcare management and public health*. Unpublished grant document. Atlanta, GA: Partners for International Development.

International Finance Corporation. (2006). *Doing business: Georgia is this year's top reformer*. Retrieved October 6, 2006, from http://www.doingbusiness.org/documents/Press_Releases_07/ DB07CISpressrelease.pdf

Khechinashvili, G., Mdivani, N., & Blumberg, H. M. (2004). Lessons learned from implementation of DOTS (Directly Observed Therapy, short course) tuberculosis control strategy in the Republic of Georgia. *42nd Annual Meeting of Infectious Diseases Society of America*. Boston: Infectious Diseases Society of America.

Koch, E. (2004). Governing tuberculosis: Competing cultures of disease and medicine in post-socialist Georgia. Unpublished Ph.D. dissertation, Graduate Faculty of Political and Social Science, The New School. New York, NY.

Open Society Georgia Foundation. (2006). *Public health program: HealthCare system in Georgia*. Unpublished document.

Partskhladze, N., Gogashvili, M., Jashi, M., & Mindadze, S. (2006). AIHA monitoring and evaluation—FY 2006 indicator: Percentage of targeted healthcare providers applying training *(Nurses)*. Unpublished report for the AIHA.

Richards, D. C., Mikiashvili, T., Parris, J. J., Shubladze, N., Tertsvadze, T., Khechinashvili, G., et al. (2002). Risk of hepatitis C virus (HCV) and HIV co-infection among tuberculosis (TB) patients in the Republic of Georgia. *2002 Southern Regional Meetings of the American Federation for Medical Research*. New Orleans.

Scott, J. G., Sochalski, J., & Aiken, L. (1999). Review of magnet hospital research: Findings and implications for professional nursing practice. *Journal of Nursing Administration, 29*(1), 9–19.

Skarbinski, J., Walker, H. K., Kobaladze, A., Kirtava, Z., Baker, L. C., & Raffin, T. A. (2002). Ten years of transition: The burden of out-of-pocket payments for health care in Tbilisi, Republic of Georgia. *Journal of the American Medical Association, 287*(8), 1043–1049.

Tkeshelashvili-Kessler, A., del Rio, C., Nelson, K., & Tsertsvadze, T. (2005). The emerging HIV/AIDS epidemic in Georgia. *International Journal of STD & AIDS, 16*, 61–67.

United Nations. (2006). *NGO definition*. Retrieved September 27, 2006, from http://www.un.org/dpi/ngosection/brochure.htm

United Nations Development Program. (2006a). *UNDP Human development reports: Refugees and armaments*. Retrieved October 6, 2006, from http://hdr.undp.org/statistics/data/indicators.cfm?x=217&y=3&z=1

United Nations Development Program. (2006b) *Technical note 1: Calculating the human development indices*. Retrieved November 9, 2006, from http://hdr.undp.org/docs/statistics/indices/technote_1.pdf

United States Agency for International Development. (2006). *Georgia health and social development: Successes*. Retrieved November 10, 2006, from http://georgia.usaid.gov/programs/health_and_social_development.html

Weinstock, D. M., Hahn, O., Wittkamp, M., Sepkowitz, K. A., Khechinashvili, G., & Blumberg, H. M. (2001). Risk for tuberculosis infection among internally displaced persons in the Republic of Georgia. *International Journal of Tubercular Lung Disease, 5,*164–169.

Wold, J., Mullis, R., & Wolk, J. (1998). Establishing health and human service professional education in the former Soviet Union: The Georgia to Georgia Project. *Journal of Allied Health, 27*(1), 25–29.

World Health Organization. (2006a). Georgia. Law of Georgia on health care, December 10, 1997. (Sakartvelos k'anoni, 31 December 1997, No. 47–48, 126–145, Text No. 1139-Is). *WHO International Digest of Health Legislation*. Retrieved October 6, 2006, from http://www3.who.int-/idhl-rils/frame.cfm?language=english

World Health Organization. (2006b). *Georgia*. Retrieved November 8, 2006, from http://www.who.int/countries/geo/en

Chapter 20

A Unique Perspective
on Health Care in Panama

Larry Purnell

Overview

To understand the Republic of Panama, one must be knowledgeable about the people and their heritages, the unique topography and biocultural ecology of the country, the history of the Panama Canal, and the relationship of Panama with the United States. The republic is a mixture of cosmopolitanism and traditionalism, wealth and poverty, advanced allopathic medicine and traditional medicine, migration and immigration, and biodiversity and multiculturalism, which includes traditional indigenous Indian populations. Moreover, the involvement of the Delaware–Panama Partners of the Americas, a grassroots nongovernmental organization, has had a major impact on Panama.

The Republic of Panama, meaning "plenty of fish," is located on the narrowest and lowest part of the s-shaped Isthmus of Panama that links North America and South America. Panama is slightly smaller than South Carolina, approximately 77,082 sq km (29,761 sq mi). The country's two coastlines are the Caribbean on the north and the Pacific on the south. To the east is Colombia and to the west Costa Rica. The highest point in the country, Volcán Barú near the Costa Rican border, rises to almost 3500 m (11,483 ft). The lowest elevation is in the middle of the country where the Panama Canal crosses. The population of 3.2 million as of 2004 has a growth rate of 1.26%. The Capital, Panama City, contains one third of the population. The unit of currency is the balboa, which is equal to the US dollar. Balboas are available only in coins; otherwise Panama uses the US dollar. Spanish is the official language, although the US influence in the Canal Zone reinforces the use of English as a second language. November 3 is celebrated as the official date of independence in Colombia, which was won from Spain in 1821.

Panama is divided into nine provinces and three provincial-level *comarcas*, which are similar to reserves: Embera, Kuna Yala, and Ngobe-Bugle. The nine provinces are Bocas del Tora, Chiriqui, Cocle, Colon, Darien, Herrera, Los Santos, Panama, and Veraguas. Each province is somewhat unique in its history, culture, and lifestyle. The provincial borders have not changed since they were determined at independence from Colombia in 1903. Over 350 San Blas Islands, near Colombia, are strung out for more than 160 km along the sheltered Caribbean coastline. Other principal islands are those of the Archipiélago de las Perlas in the middle of the Gulf of Panama, the penal colony on the Isla de Coiba in the Gulf of Chiriquí, and the decorative island of Taboga, a tourist attraction that can be seen from Panama City. In all, some 1000 islands are off the Pacific coast of Panama.

Panama has a tropical climate. Temperatures are uniformly high, as is the relative humidity, with little seasonal variation. Diurnal ranges are low; on a typical day during the dry season in the capital city, the early morning minimum may be 24°C (75°F) and the afternoon maximum 29°C (84°F). The temperature seldom exceeds 32°C (90°F) for more than a short time. Temperatures are markedly cooler in the mountain ranges in western Panama where frosts occur. Panama's tropical environment supports an abundance of plants. Forests dominate, interrupted in places by grasslands, scrub, and crops. Although nearly 40% of Panama is still wooded, deforestation is a continuing threat to the rain-drenched woodlands.

Almost 500 rivers traverse Panama, with many originating as highland streams. The Río Chagres is one of the longest rivers, a part of which was dammed to create Gatun Lake, which forms a major part of the transit route between the locks near each end of the Panama Canal.

Transportation

There are three separate, unconnected railroad systems totaling 238 km (148 mi), including one main line between Panama City and Colón plus two in the west, originating in David and Almirante and continuing across the Costa Rican border. Over 9535 km (5925 mi) of roadside twine through Panama. The Pan-American highway, running from Costa Rica through Panama ends in Darien. Existing roads do not connect from Darien into Colombia. Sixty percent of the roadways are unpaved and not passable during parts of the rainy season. Of 105 airports, only 44 are paved. One international airport, Tocumen, is near Panama City. The transisthmian pipeline completed in 1982 runs from Puerto Armuelles to Chiriquí Grande and brings crude oil from Ecuador.

People of Panama

Because the isthmus holds a central position as a transit zone, Panama has long enjoyed a measure of ethnic diversity. This diversity, combined with a variety of regions and environments, has given rise to a number of distinct subcultures. Most Panamanians view their society as composed of three principal groups: the Spanish-speaking Roman Catholic mestizo majority, the English-speaking Protestant Antillean blacks, and tribal Indians. The precise racial and ethnic divisions are 66% mestizo (mixed Amerindian and white), 14% West Indian (Amerindian and mixed), 14% white Spanish, and 6% Amerindian. Included in these groups are Chinese, Middle Eastern, Swiss, Yugoslavian, and North American immigrants; all have contributed to the multiculturalism of

Panama. Only 6.4% of the population is over the age of 65 years and 9.8% is under the age of 14 years. Panama has a young median population of 26.18 years.

A few retired US citizens, mostly former Canal Zone employees, reside in Chiriquí. Small groups of Hispanic blacks, *playeros*, and Hispanic Indians, *cholos*, live along the Atlantic coast lowlands and in Darién. Their settlements date from the colonial era and are concentrated along waterways. They rely on farming and raising livestock that have adapted to the tropical forest environment.

The Guaymí, related to the Nahatlan and Mayan Nations of Mexico and Central America, are concentrated in Bocas del Toro, Chiriquí, and Veraguas. In the 1980s, the government began developing a copper mine, a highway, a pipeline, and a hydroelectric plant on Guaymi land in the province of Chiriquí. The Guaymi have attempted to protect their land and publicize their misgivings about the projects because the government has had a lack of interest in their plight about the impact on their lands and about the effect of dam construction on fishing and water supplies. The matter has not been fully resolved.

Ethical Issue. An *ethical principle of distributive justice* is that basic goods should be distributed so that the least advantaged members of society are benefited. Distributive justice also means that the rights of one group are balanced against another. What is your opinion about the Panamanian government developing copper mines, traversing roads, and building pipelines through Guayamí Indian territory?

The Cuna, also referred to as the Kuna, are concentrated mainly along the Caribbean coast, east of Colón on the San Blas islands, which are small coral islands, each only a few feet above sea level. The largest of these islands, Aligandí, is only 32 acres (13 hectares). Daily 20-minute flights from Panama City carry passengers back and forth from the mainland and Aligandí. Only native Kuna are allowed on the island overnight and only with prior permission from their independent government. Kuna homes are made with cane walls and guava-thatched roofs. Bathroom facilities are a short walk to the end of piers where outdoor toilets have the Atlantic Ocean as their automatic flushing system. Fresh water is piped from the mainland. In addition, a small number of Kuna are scattered in the remote mountains of western Panama and the interior of Darién.

The Bribri, part of the Talamanca tribe of Costa Rica, have substantial contact with outsiders. Many are employed on banana plantations. The Bókatá live in eastern Bocas del Toro and have little exposure to outsiders. Since the early 1980s, a small dirt road serves the area, which is only passable in dry weather. The Chocó (or Embera) occupy the southeastern portion of Darién along the border with Colombia. Most are bilingual in Spanish and Chocó.

All tribes are under the jurisdiction of both the provincial and national governments. The indigenous policy section of the Ministry of Government and Justice bears primary responsibility for coordinating programs that affect Indians, serving as a liaison between the tribes and the national government. The 1972 constitution required the government to establish reserves, *comarcas,* for indigenous tribes, but the extent to which this mandate had been implemented varies. Most settlements of any size have a primary school; a few also have secondary schools.

Urban society includes virtually all members of the elite. Centered mainly in Panama City, this group is composed of old families of Spanish descent and newer families of immigrants. All elite families are wealthy; the immigrant families are linked with commerce and are part of Panama's twentieth-century development as a transit zone. Older families think of themselves as aristocracy from birth. Newer families have less prestige and social status. Until the dominance of General Torrijos, whose power base was the National Guard, an oligarchy of older elite families virtually controlled the country's politics under the auspices of the Liberal Party. Politics is considered the quintessential career for a young man of elite background. The old, aristocratic families have long provided the republic's presidents, cabinet ministers, and many members of the legislature. Older elite families are closely interrelated and in the past were careful to avoid racially mixed unions.

Antillean blacks have little success in attaining elite status, even when wealthy; however, Spanish-speaking Roman Catholic blacks are able to gain acceptance. An increasing degree of admixture with mestizo and more recent immigrant elements is occurring. Many such families enter the elite and intermarry with members of the older families. Commercial success has become a substitute for an illustrious family background. The popular saying "Money whitens everyone" describes this phenomenon.

The middle socioeconomic class is predominantly mestizo, but it includes children and grandchildren of black Antilleans, the descendants of Chinese laborers on the railroad, Jews, and more recent immigrants from Europe and the Middle East. Like the elite, the middle class is largely urban, although many small cities and towns of the interior have their own middle-class families. The middle class encompasses small businessmen, professionals, managerial and technical personnel, and government administrators. Middle-class parents make great sacrifices to send their children to the best schools possible. Young men are encouraged to acquire a profession, and young women are steered toward office jobs in government or business. In contrast with the elite, the middle class views teaching as a respected occupation for a young woman.

The lower socioeconomic class constitutes the bulk of the country's urban population. As a group, they are stratified by employment and race, and they comprise artisans, vendors, manual laborers, and servants. Ethnically, the lower socioeconomic class has three principal components: mestizo migrants from the countryside; children and grandchildren of Antillean blacks; and Hispanicized blacks who are descendants of former slaves. The split between Antillean blacks and the rest of the populace is particularly marked. Although there is some social mixing and intermarriage, religious and cultural differences isolate the Antilleans. They are gradually becoming more Hispanicized, but the first generation usually remains oriented toward its Caribbean origins. The second and third generations are under North American influence through exposure to US citizens in the former Canal Zone, where most Antilleans are employed. Because the majority of rural migrants to the metropolitan region are women, women outnumber men in many larger urban areas. Many come in search of work as domestics. Young, single mothers constitute a significant proportion of the urban population.

History, Politics, and Government

Perhaps as early as 8000 BC, people used the Isthmus of Panama to continue their southward migration and settle in South America. Whether they used land routes or sea routes or a combination of these to make their journeys is not known, but long before the arrival of Europeans, the Indians of North and South America had established ocean routes for trade and cultural commerce along the Pacific coast. The Caribbean coast may also have had some maritime commerce among the Indians.

In 1502, Columbus landed in Panama on his fourth voyage. In 1510, Vasco de Balboa crossed the isthmus and was the first European to see the Pacific Ocean. Pizarro used the isthmus for his subjugation of the Incas, whose empire collapsed in 1532. As a result of Pizarro's actions, Charles V, ordered the first survey for a proposed canal in 1534. Although no construction was undertaken, a cobblestone mule trail, called Las Cruses, was built to support the conquest of South America's Pacific coast and to carry tons of gold being shipped to Spain from Peru. Parts of that trail are still visible today. Subsequently, the indigenous population of Panama was greatly reduced and Spanish control over the area was established.

In 1821, the Spanish colonies revolted against Spain and thus Panama became a province of New Granada, which included Colombia, Ecuador, and Venezuela, under the leadership of Simon Bolivar, the Latin American revolutionary who hoped to unite South America into a single confederated state. Regional rivalries doomed the unified state, and by 1830, only Colombia and Panama remained united despite some efforts to create a separate state for Panama. In 1882, the French began work on the Panama Canal along the route of the 1855 Panama railroad; however, financial troubles, yellow fever, malaria, tuberculosis, cholera, diphtheria, smallpox, and bubonic plague among the workers ended the project. In 1885, the Republic of Colombia was formed with Panama as a Colombian province. Only in 1903, after Colombia's first civil war had killed nearly 100,000 people, did Panama gain independence with US support.

When Panama declared independence from Colombia, Panama and the United States entered into a treaty by which the United States undertook the construction of an interoceanic ship canal across the isthmus. The following year (1904), the United States purchased the rights and the equipment from the French. Despite the problems of tropical disease, the unusual geology of the isthmus, the enormous size of the locks and volume of excavation required, and the need to reestablish communities, plans were made to build the canal. Before any work could begin, the United States appointed an American physician, William Gorgas, to examine the area. Gorgas and his medical team eradicated yellow fever and brought malaria under control, making it possible to build the canal.

During the building of the canal, Gatun Lake was formed by constructing a dam across the Chagras River, creating an artificial lake to fuel the locks. This dam created the largest artificial lake in the world at the time and required relocating certain indigenous groups. The locks were manufactured in the United States and transported to the site in sections.

Ethical Issue.   The *ethical principle respecting autonomy* means that individuals are free to decide how they live their lives as long as their decisions do not negatively impact the lives of others. This principle is balanced with distributive justice. What are your thoughts and concerns about forced relocation of people to create a dam that has international implications?

The 1904 constitution gave the United States the right to intervene in any part of Panama and to reestablish public peace and constitutional order. This confirmed Panama's status as a de facto protectorate of the United States. This provision gave the United States the right to add additional territory to the Canal Zone whenever it believed this was necessary for defensive purposes. These grants of power to the United States were to cause increasing discontent in Panama, particularly in the 1950s and 1960s.

The 51-mile canal, completed in 1914, was operated exclusively by the United States until 1979, at which time a 1977 treaty established the Panama Canal Commission to allow the Panamanians to take increased responsibility for its operations of the canal. On December 31, 1999, the entire operations of the canal were transferred to the government of the Republic of Panama. The Panama Canal Authority (PCA), an autonomous body, has operated the Panama Canal since that time. The canal is to remain a neutral zone, and the United States is legally entitled to intervene to maintain its neutrality.

A Hong Kong-based entity operates the ports at both entrances to the canal, which is a concern to some in the United States. Because many of today's ships are larger than the original construction of the canal was designed to handle, the PCA is widening it to allow larger container vessels to pass through. At the Pacific entrance of the canal, the Bridge of the Americas spans 5,425 feet across Panama Bay (Panama, 2005).

An interesting structure in the Panama Canal Zone is Fort Sherman, a 23,100-acre world heritage site on Panama's Atlantic side. Over half of Fort Sherman's land area is tropical forest with a full range of jungle terrain and vegetation: tall grass lands, mountains, swamps, blue and brown water, and single and double canopy jungle. The United States maintained its jungle operations training center there until 2000. In addition, extensive coral reefs exist along the Caribbean coast near Fort Sherman. Today the interest is in preserving Fort Sherman's biodiversity.

The Panamanian form of government, similar to the United States, is divided into three branches: the executive, the legislative, and the judiciary. The executive branch has one president and two vice presidents, all elected by popular vote for 5-year terms. The legislative branch is the Unicameral National Assembly; the members are also elected by popular vote and serve 5-year terms. In the judiciary branch, the Supreme Court of Justice has nine appointed judges who serve 10-year terms.

Personalism, giving one's political loyalties to an individual rather than to a party, has influenced the political scene of Panama since its independence. Whereas government officials giving special privileges and positions to a family member is not unique to Panama, a high rate of nepotism occurs in Panama. From 1968 until his death in 1981, General Omar Torrijos dominated politics. In 1984, Nicolas Barletta, a puppet of Manuel Noriega, became the first elected president in 16 years. One year later, Vice President Eric Devalle, another supporter of Noriega who was head of the Panamanian National Guard, replaced him. In 1988, Noriega was indicted in the United States for drug trafficking. When Devalle tried to fire Noriega in 1989, the National Assembly named Noriega the leader and declared the United States and Panama to be in a state of war. The United States seized Panama City trying to capture Noriega, who surrendered 1 month later. Noriega was taken to Miami where he was eventually convicted and remains in US custody.

Ethical Issue.   Balancing the rights of one individual against another is the *ethical principle of justice*. What concerns do you have with appointing and promoting family members over others who may be more qualified for a position?

After Noriega's capture, Ernesto Balladares was installed as president. During his tenure, Panama's military, including the National Guard, was abolished and the Panamanian Public Forces were created. A constitutional amendment prohibits the creation of a standing military force. Four years later in 1994, Omar Trojillo was elected president. The first female president, Mireya Moscoso, the widow of former president Arias from the 1960s, was elected in 1999. Martin Torjillos, son of the former dictator, is the current president. Politics seem to be somewhat stable at the time of this writing.

Economics

With a per capita income of $6,900 (up from $2,509 in 1999), 37% of Panamanians still live in poverty, and 18.5% live in extreme poverty. Poverty rates are higher in rural areas than in urban areas. The 2004 unemployment rate of 12.6% is significantly lower than it was in the early 1990s. Over 40% of women are employed, up significantly from the early 1980s. The average wage for women is 87% of that for men.

Panama's main crops are bananas, sugarcane, rice, corn, coffee, beans, tobacco, melons, and flowers. Livestock, forestry, and fishing are major commercial enterprises. Natural resources include copper, mahogany forests, shrimp, and hydropower. Only 6.2% of the land is arable. Major industries include construction, petroleum refining, brewing, manufacturing cement and other construction materials, and sugar milling. The country has an oversupply of nonskilled workers. International banking is also big business with an offshore financial center.

An extensive shoreline is responsible for Panama being a major transshipment point and primary laundering center for narcotic and money-laundering activities, especially in the Colon free trade zone. Most of the country's exports go to the United States, Costa

Rica, Germany, Belgium, and Italy. About one third of Panama's imports come from the United States, another third from other industrial countries, and one third from Latin America.

In addition to the substantial income generated by the Panama Canal, ecotourism is another major source of income. A land full of history, art, and culture, Panama's privileged geographical position shelters a rich and abundant natural flora and fauna, resulting in one of the most important natural areas of the word. More than 50% of the world's floral species can be found in Panama, consisting of vascular plant flowers, moss, lichens, algae, and fungi. The national flower, *Peristeria elata*, an orchid, is one of over 1200 floral species in Panama.

Panama is also a destination for bird-watchers with 940 species of birds, which is more than the United States and Canada combined. Of these 940 species, 127 are migratory and 23 are endemic. The national bird of Panama, the harpy eagle, is considered the most powerful bird of prey in the world. Panama also claims 214 species of reptiles, 143 species of amphibians, 225 species of mammals, and 1,500 species of butterflies. The maritime wealth is also fascinating, considering the word *panama* means land of fish, and includes 207 species of fish, algae, cetaceans, and coral reefs. Overall, Panama has 15 national parks.

Technology

The long-standing concern of reliable telephone communication seems to now be solved. Until the early 2000s, Panama had only one telephone company, Cable and Wireless Panama, and it took Panamanians in some areas up to 6 months to get telephone services. The impetus for improved services and competition started with the introduction of Radio Shack, where one could purchase a telephone and get immediate telephone service. As of January 2003, the government has awarded numerous new concessions for fixed-line telephone services. Additional mobile services will be added in 2008.

In October 2000, the Global Academy Institute for Integrative Medicine convened a conference called "Health Today: Realities, Obstacles and Perspectives" to offer the medical community and other constituencies of the healthcare sector of Panama and the surrounding region a variety of health and medical perspectives from across the Americas. Cosponsors were the Foreign Ministry of Panama, the Health Ministry of Panama, Global Academy Genome Institute, Pan-American Health Organization, and the United Nations Development Program.

The health conference coincided with the meeting of health ministers of Latin America, Spain, and Portugal. The health ministers' meeting took place as part of the annual meeting of the Ibero–American Summit of Governments. The presentations and dialogues focused on the following themes: (a) integrative medicine and its relevance in terms of the traditional healing systems of the Americas and its potential for low-cost medical services; and (b) genetic technology and its impact on the future of health care. This conference demonstrates the importance Panamanians see for technology in their future.

In June 2003, Panama hosted "Info Com 2003," a trade event aimed at promoting e-business and information technology in Panama and the Latin American region. "Info Com 2003" is an initiative of the committee of technology of the American Chamber of Commerce and Industries of Panama. The main purpose of this event was to stimulate executives to find the most effective and efficient ways to administer resources, take advantage of new opportunities, and increase the use of the best technological options. "Info Com 2003" promoted the concept of the *new* Panama Canal . . . a roadway of cutting-edge information technology and telecommunications.

The objectives of "Info Com 2003" were to (a) offer a global vision of the technological solutions related to information systems, company management, client relations, logistics, telecommunications, Internet access, electronic commerce, and network infrastructure; (b) present new business opportunities that arise from technology; and (c) educate on the latest developments in information technology and telecommunications and their applications at the enterprise level.

Several hundred participants from the scientific and medical communities, academia, policy makers, civil society representatives, the media, and the general public attended this conference. The conference was not only an educational event, but also an opportunity for members to exchange their views. The conference was broadcast by Panamanian television to increase access to a broader public, a key strategy used by the Global Academy wherever possible.

The engineering and maintenance units in the Ministry of Public Health encourage health facilities to use common methods for procuring, installing, and maintaining biomedical equipment. They have also attempted to draft technical specifications for the procurement of biomedical equipment. Preventive maintenance continues to be problematic. The social security hospitals and clinics appear to have adequate and better equipment than the hospitals and clinics operated by the Ministry of Public Health. The few smaller, private hospitals appear to have adequate emergency equipment.

Education

Overview of Education

Public education began in Panama soon after independence from Colombia was gained in 1903. The system presented an extremely paternalistic view of education as evidenced in a 1913 meeting of the First Panamanian Educational Assembly that stated, "The cultural heritage given to the child should be determined by the social position he will or should occupy. For this reason, education should be different in accordance with the social class to which the student should be related" (Library of Congress, 2004a).

This elitist focus changed under US influence. Since that statement was made, education has been recognized as a mark of status; thus, almost people of elite status receive a university education. Most attend private schools either at home or abroad, and many study a profession, with law and medicine being the most favored. Having a profession is viewed not as a means of livelihood, but as a status symbol and as an adjunct to a political career.

By the 1920s, successive Panamanian governments gave high priority to developing a system of universal primary education. Adult literacy, which was only 30% in 1923, rose to 50% in less than a decade. By the early 1950s, adult literacy increased to more than 70%, to 87% in 1980, and is currently over 90%. Men and women are equally represented among the literate with more women then men attending college. The most notable disparity in education is between urban and rural Panamanians. School attendance is compulsory for children from ages 6 to 15 years, or until the completion of primary school. However, several insolated areas of Panama still do not have a secondary school.

Ethical Issue. The *principle of justice* requires meaningful equality among individuals for those positions in society that bring greater economic and social rewards. What are your thoughts about the government not providing facilities for secondary education in some rural areas of Panama?

Two types of secondary school programs follow a 6-year primary cycle: an academic-oriented program and a vocational-type program. The academic program, which represents nearly three quarters of all secondary-school enrollment, involves two 3-year cycles. The lower cycle has a standard curriculum that includes Spanish, social studies, religion, art, and music. The upper cycle consists of two academic courses of study: arts and sciences, leading up to entrance to the university, or a less rigorous course of study, representing the end of a student's formal education.

In addition to academic programs, vocational secondary-school programs offer professional or technical courses aimed specifically at giving students the technical skills for employment following graduation. Roughly one quarter of all secondary students pursue this type of course. Like the more academic-oriented secondary school programs, the vocational-type programs are divided into two cycles. Students can choose their studies from a variety of specializations, including agriculture, art, commerce, and industrial trades.

The oldest, largest, and most highly regarded institution of higher education, the University of Panama, has produced many public figures and thus is known as the "nest of eagles". Drawing most of its student body from upwardly mobile rather than long-established elements of the elite, students are well known for their political activism. Nearly three quarters of all university students attended the University of Panama. The university has regional centers and extensions.

The University of Santa Maria la Antigua, a private Roman Catholic institution established in 1965, has an enrollment of 5,000 to 6,000 students. A third university, the Technical University founded in 1981, accounts for approximately 7,000 students. A fourth university, the Autonomous University of Chiriqui, is rapidly expanding after separating from the University of Panama in 2000. Over 5,000 students attend this university. In addition, some small, private universities with English as the language of instruction are located in Panama City.

Education for the Health Professions

Panama has one public medical school, which is located at the University of Panama, as well as two private ones. The university also has a master's program in health promotion geared to multidisciplinary needs and is located in the School of Public Health. Paramedic programs are at the baccalaureate level. Nurse midwives work in many rural areas and inner-city clinics. The government finances higher education in public universities, but housing and books are not included. The cost of textbooks is high, so often students share in the cost of a book, then cut it up and make copies for their cohort students to share.

Only baccalaureate nursing programs exist in Panama; there is one at the University of Panama and one at the Autonomous University of Chiriquí in David. Baccalaureate nursing programs have 144 hour credits per semester, which is equivalent to many master's degree programs in the United States. In the senior year, students experience providing health care to a community, sometimes in extremely remote areas where the student may travel 2 to 3 days on horseback to get to the destination, and then be the only healthcare provider in the area. Their living arrangements may be in an elementary schoolhouse without heat or air-conditioning. All students complete a senior research thesis.

Panama has a master's degree program in nursing administration in which this author consults and teaches. Many nursing faculty have their master's and doctorates from American universities. Others have master's degrees in nursing from Colombia, Costa Rica, and Mexico. The role of advanced-practice nurses is being developed. Two private universities are starting nursing programs; their success in recruiting students is unknown.

Communication

The official language of Panama is Spanish. However, many of the population are bilingual in Spanish and English. Some speak a third language such as Chinese, Japanese, Portuguese, or Italian. Most of the indigenous populations are bilingual in their native languages and Spanish.

Contextual speech patterns among Panamanians can include a high-pitched, loud voice and a rate that seems extremely fast to the untrained ear. The language uses apocopation, which accounts for this rapid speech pattern. An apocopation occurs when one word ends with a vowel, and the next word begins with a vowel. This creates a tendency to drop the vowel ending of the first word and results in an abbreviated rapid-sounding form. For example, the Spanish phrase for "how are you?," "*¿Cómo está usted?,*" may become "*¿Comestusted?*" The last word, *usted,* is frequently dropped. Some may find this fast speech difficult to understand. However, if one asks the individual to enunciate slowly, the effect of the apocopation or truncation is less pronounced. For the first 3 days of each trip to Panama, this author has a mantra, *Habla mas despacio, por favor,* or "speak more slowly, please," until becoming accustomed to the rapid speech patterns.

Using Spanish to communicate with Panamanian clients is important. However, the healthcare provider who assumes a total understanding of Panamanian Spanish may negatively impact their interactions. Attempt speaking Spanish, but do not be overly confident; the idiomatic expressions are numerous and change from country to country.

Respect (*respeto*) is extremely important, especially when meeting a Panamanian for the first time. Always greet the person formally, unless told to do otherwise. Greeting the person with Señorita (Miss), Señora (Mrs.), Señor (Mister), Doña (Madam), Don (Sir), and Doctor or Doctora, sets the stage for formal communication. *Familism*, the value of family, is also an important concept. For health teaching to be effective, the provider must engage the entire family.

Approaching the Panamanian client with *personalism,* being friendly, and directing questions to the family spokesperson (usually the male) may help to facilitate more open communication. However, one must remember that the spokesperson is not necessarily the decision maker. The woman may make the decision, but the culturally prescribed role is for the man to transmit the message. *Personalism* emphasizes people and family orientation and is essential for building confidence, promoting health, and establishing a cultural connection. On repeat visits, polite conversation includes briefly asking about family members. The concept of *personalism* may be difficult for some healthcare professionals because many are socialized to form rigid boundaries between the caregiver and the client and family.

Cultural Communication Patterns

While some topics such as income, salary, and investments are taboo, Panamanians generally like to express their inner beliefs, feelings, and emotions once they get to know and trust a person. Meaningful conversations are important, often becoming loud and seemingly disorganized. To the outsider, the situation may seem stressful or hostile, but this intense emotion means that the participants in the conversation are having a good time and enjoying each other's company.

Panamanians place great value on closeness and togetherness, including when they are in an inpatient facility. They frequently touch and embrace others and like to see relatives and significant others. Touch between a man and a woman, between two men, and between two women, is acceptable. To demonstrate respect, compassion, and understanding, healthcare providers should greet the Panamanian client with a handshake. On establishing rapport, providers may further demonstrate approval and respect through backslapping, smiling, and affirmative nods of the head.

Many Panamanians consider sustained eye contact when speaking directly to an older person as rude. Direct eye contact with teachers, physicians, nurses, and superiors may be interpreted as insolence. Avoiding sustained and direct eye contact with superiors is a sign of respect. This practice may or may not be seen in the younger generation, but it is imperative that healthcare providers take cues from the client and family. Many among the indigenous Indian populations do not maintain eye contact with persons older than themselves or people in hierarchical positions.

Out of respect for the healthcare provider, many Panamanians may avoid disagreeing, expressing doubts, or asking questions. Certainly, any negative feelings about the healthcare encounter would not be expressed. However, encouraging patients to ask questions, even if it is through an interpreter, is considered polite behavior.

Temporal Relationships

Many Panamanians, especially those from lower socioeconomic groups, are focused on the present, out of choice and necessity. Many individuals do not consider it important or do not have the income to plan ahead financially. The trend is to live in the "more important" here and now, because *mañana* (tomorrow) cannot be predicted. With this emphasis on living in the present, preventive health care and immunizations may not be a priority. *Mañana* may or may not really mean tomorrow, but rather it often means "not today" or "later."

Some Panamanians perceive time as relative rather than categorically imperative. Deadlines and commitments are flexible, not firm. Punctuality is generally relaxed, especially in social situations. This concept of time is innate in the Spanish language. For example, semantically, one cannot be late for an appointment; one can only arrive late.

Because of their more relaxed concept of time, Panamanians may arrive late for appointments, although the current trend is toward greater punctuality. Healthcare facilities that use an appointment system for clients may need to make special provisions to see clients whenever they arrive. Healthcare providers must listen carefully for subtle cues when discussing appointments. Disagreeing with healthcare providers who set the appointment may be viewed as rude or impolite. Therefore, some Panamanians will not tell you directly that they cannot make the appointment. In the context of the discussion, they may say something like, "My husband goes to work at 8:00 a.m. and the children are off to school, then I have to do the dishes . . ." The healthcare professional should ask: Is 8:30 a.m. on Thursday okay for you? The person might say "yes," but the healthcare professional must still intently listen to the conversation and then possibly negotiate a new time for the appointment. Many consider it rude to openly disagree in social situations. Because it might be seen as rude to directly say no, the Panamanian may say "yes." However, "yes" may mean "I hear you, but I am not going to follow your instructions," "I hear you, and I do not agree," "I will think about it," "I am not sure what you mean, but I do not want to embarrass myself or you to explain it more," or may mean "I understand you, agree with you, and will follow your instructions and advice."

Format for Names

Names in most Spanish-speaking populations seem complex to those unfamiliar with the culture. A typical name is La Señorita Olga Gaborra y Rodriguez. Gaborra is the name of her father, and Rodriguez is her mother's surname. When she marries a man with the surname name of Guiterrez, she becomes La Señora (denotes a married woman) Olga de

Guiterrez y Gaborra y Rodriguez. The word *de* is used to express possession, and the father's name, which is considered more important than the mother's name, comes first. However, this full name is rarely used except on formal documents and for recording the name in the family Bible. Out of respect, most Panamanians are more formal when addressing nonfamily members. Thus, the best way to address Olga is not by her first name, but rather as Señora de Guiterrez. Titles such as *Don* and *Doña* for older respected members of the community and family are also common.

Healthcare providers must understand the role of the elderly when providing care to people of Panamanian culture. To develop confidence and *personalismo,* an element of formality must exist between healthcare providers and elderly people. Becoming overly familiar by using physical touch or using first names may not be appreciated early in a relationship. As the healthcare professional develops confidence in the relationship, becoming familiar may be less of a concern. However, using the first name of an elder client might never be appropriate.

Spirituality and Religion

The religious affiliations of Panamanians are 85% Roman Catholic, 5% Protestant, and 5% other, which includes Islamic and Jewish. The constitution prescribes that there shall be no prejudice with respect to religious freedom, and the practice of all forms of worship is authorized. However, the constitution recognizes that the Roman Catholic faith is the country's predominant religion and contains a provision that it be taught in the public schools. However, such instruction or other religious activity is not compulsory. The constitution does not specifically provide for the separation of church and state, but it implies the independent functioning of each.

Members of the clergy may not hold civil or military public office, excepting the posts that may be concerned with social welfare or public instruction. The constitution stipulates that senior officials of the church hierarchy in Panama must be native-born citizens. The church has a long tradition of noninvolvement in national politics. A weak organization and a heavy dependence on foreign clergy (only 40% of the nation's priests are native-born Panamanians) inhibit the development of strong hierarchical positions on political issues.

Ethical Issue.   *Respecting autonomy* is an ethical principle, which allows groups to make decisions about their lives and organization as long as they do not have a negative effect on the decisions of other groups. Do you think that requiring church officials in hierarchal position to be native-born Panamanians violates this principle?

Church concern over social issues increased notably in the 1960s and 1970s with conflicts between the hierarchy and the Torrijos government. In the late 1980s, Archbishop Marcos Gregorio McGrath, a naturalized Panamanian citizen and a leader among the Latin American bishops, headed the church hierarchy. McGrath and the other bishops strongly supported Panama's claims to sovereignty over the Canal Zone and urged ratification of the Panama Canal treaties.

The devout Panamanians regard church attendance and the observance of religious duties as regular features of everyday life, and even the most casual or nominal Roman Catholics adjust their daily lives to the prevailing norms of the religious calendar. Although some sacraments are observed more scrupulously than others, baptism is almost universal; in fact, baptism is generally considered the most significant religious rite. Throughout the country, birth and death are marked by religious rites observed by all but a very few.

Virtually every town has its own Roman Catholic church, but many do not have a priest in residence. Many rural inhabitants receive only an occasional visit from a busy priest who travels among a number of isolated villages. In rural areas, families often have to travel some distance to the nearest parish center. This trip is important and people willingly undertake it in order to practice religious rites.

The Antillean black community is largely Protestant. Indians follow their own indigenous belief systems, although both Protestant and Catholic missionaries are active among the various tribes. However, Roman Catholicism permeates the social environment culturally as well as religiously. Religious attitudes, customs, and beliefs differ between urban and rural areas, although many members of the urban working class and recent migrants from rural regions usually retain their folk beliefs.

Panamanians, regardless of their religious affiliation, take their religion seriously. Purnell's study (1999) reported that 81% of participants prayed for good health; however, the most important thing in their lives was family, followed by religion. If healthcare delivery is to be effective for Panamanians, care and health teaching must be delivered in the family context.

Research and Demonstration Projects

The National Geographic research station near Panama City as well as the American Institute of Biological Sciences conduct research on marine studies, fungal infections in frogs, and other environmental concerns. A cagelike steel gondola on top of a crane gives researchers a bird's eye view of the jungle canopy where research studies are conducted. A number of archeological and anthropological studies are also being conducted.

For many years, the Institute of Nutrition of Central America and Panama at the University of Panama has had an ongoing research project on breast-feeding among diverse populations in Panama. A popular finding is a belief that maternal milk plays a definite role in the etiology of diarrheal diseases. One of the explanatory models of diarrheal disease in children is the hot–cold theory of illness and disease causation; if the mother is too hot or too cold at the time of breast-feeding, the child will get diarrhea. Examples of this were explained to this author while teaching and taking nursing and dietetic students to Panama: (a) if ironing (a hot activity), wait a while before breast-feeding; (b) if the mother has been in the hot sun, she should cool off before breast-feeding, (c) if exposed to cold wind, the mother should wait until warm before breast-feeding, and (d) she should not immediately breast-feed if she has consumed cold liquids or been exposed to the open door of a cold refrigerator.

The City of Knowledge, created in 1995 and governed by a private, nonprofit organization, is an international complex for education, research, and innovation located at the former Fort Clayton military base in the Panama Canal Zone. The City of Knowledge offers facilities and support for establishing programs in education, research, and technological development and helps develop and strengthen the relationship between the academic, scientific, and business worlds with an international orientation. Opportunities are made available in association with the Panamanian International Center for Sustainable Development, the United Nations Program for Development, and the Inter-American Biodiversity Information Network. Current researchers in this complex come from the National Environment Authority, University of Delaware, Purdue University, and Iowa State University, to name a few.

The academic component of the City of Knowledge offers programs through a variety of methodologies, including traditional classroom education and distance education. The business component, Panama's International Technopark, offers services dedicated to fostering interaction and technology transfers. They also focus on the added value between national and foreign businesses that apply high technology to develop innovative products or services that are international in their projection. The International Organizations Component is linked closely with sustainable human development in Latin America and Panama.

The City of Knowledge has only been fully functional for about 4 years. Research in a number of areas such as health and biodiversity are underway, but its future is still not fully established.

Partners of the Americas: Delaware–Panama Partners of the Americas

Partners of the Americas has had a significant, sustained, and positive influence on peoples lives in Panama and in the state of Delaware through Delaware–Panama Partners of the Americas. In 1963, President John F. Kennedy launched the Alliance for Progress, a program of government-to-government economic cooperation across the Western Hemisphere. At the same time, he called for a parallel people-to-people initiative, one that would allow private citizens to work together for the good of the Americas. These initiatives were established as part of the US Agency for International Development.

Soon after its founding, Alliance for Progress shifted to the private sector and changed its name to Partners of the Americas. In the following years, the organization expanded into the Caribbean and ultimately formed 120 volunteer chapters involved in 60 partnerships, of which Delaware–Panama Partners is one. This partnership developed because both Delaware and Panama are international banking centers, each has only one major university, both have a canal (Delaware Canal and the Panama Canal), and each have shared interests in farmer-to-farmer programs. Beekeeping for the production of honey and research on bee venom for allergies are also shared interests. Delaware–Panama Partners has had numerous projects and some noteworthy research. Health and health research programs became an interest when this author received the first grant for these initiatives in 1990.

Partners of the Americas believes, as stated in the mission, that working together across borders builds understanding and improves the lives of people in the Western Hemisphere. Partners of the Americas was built and continues to thrive upon enduring relationships across borders at the grassroots level. Working together, the staff and volunteers throughout the Americas bring expertise in the areas of civil society and governance, exchanges and fellowships, gender and equality, youth and children, and agriculture and environment.

Although Partners is not a research-oriented organization, it has produced many noteworthy research projects. On the research side, faculty from the University of Delaware and the University of Panama have completed the following research studies and projects:

1. Young women's attitudes and involvement towards future needs of the elderly for caregiving

2. Panamanian health beliefs and the meaning of respect afforded them by healthcare providers

3. Folic acid project financed by the March of Dimes to increase the awareness of the importance of folic acid in the diet of women of childbearing age in Panama and in Delaware and the development of bilingual materials because of the increased risk of Hispanic populations for spina bifida and other neural tube defects that are related to folic acid deficiency

4. Culturally appropriate material for tobacco use prevention geared to a variety of age groups as well as to aid teachers, physicians, and other health personnel with new approaches

5. Environmental impact and clean up of the Panama Canal Zone because of the effect that contamination has had on the environment and health of the people living in the Canal Zone

6. Graduate student and faculty exchanges were made in pediatric oncology, disabilities studies, and disaster management. The US Center for Disaster Management is located at the University of Delaware.

7. A family-life project to develop reproductive health education materials suitable for use in Panama and the Latin American community in Delaware

8. Culturally relevant health information for emergency preparedness

9. Higher education linkages to develop ongoing programs in higher education that are self sustaining

10. Promotion of knowledge of women's rights to build awareness of the revised code of family law as it affects women's rights

11. A service-learning program to promote and train participants in school and community leadership

Ethical Issue. The ethical *principle of nonmaleficence* means that we as individuals, groups, or organizations should not engage in activities that run the risk of harming others. The US military used the Panama Canal Zone as a dumping ground for biohazardous waste. What responsibility do you think the United States should have in cleaning up the Canal Zone, even though it is now under the control of the Panamanian government? Do you think the *ethical principle of beneficence,* in which one's actions should actively promote the health and well-being of others, has been violated?

Healthcare Practices

Overview of the Healthcare System

The Panamanian constitution guarantees the right to medical and health care throughout the nation's territories. The public health sector is comprised of the Ministry of Health, which covers 60% of the population, the Social Security Fund, which covers 40% of the population, and the Institute for National Water Supply and Sewerage Systems. The current government's health objectives are to offer universal access to comprehensive health programs, to improve the quality of the services, and to reduce gaps through a decentralized model of care that emphasizes primary health care. In the last 15 years, the number of private health insurance packages available has become widely increased.

The Department of Environmental Health is charged with administering rural health programs and maintaining a safe water supply for communities of fewer than 500 inhabitants, communities that make up roughly one third of the total population. The National Water and Sewage Institute and the Ministry of Public Works share responsibility for urban water supplies. Public health, especially for rural Panamanians, is a high priority. Under the slogan "Health for All by the Year 2000," the government has embarked on an ambitious program to improve the delivery of health services and sanitation in rural areas. The program is aimed at changing the emphasis from curative, hospital-based medical care to community-based preventive medicine.

The Ministry of Health bears primary responsibility for public health programs. At the district and regional levels, medical directors are responsible for maintaining healthcare services at healthcare centers and hospitals and monitoring outreach programs for the communities surrounding these facilities. The Social Security Institute maintains a medical fund for its members and operates a number of healthcare facilities, which members can use for free and nonmembers for a nominal fee. The Social Security Institute and the Ministry of Health have attempted, with limited success, to coordinate what in essence are two separate public healthcare systems in an effort to eliminate redundancy. The World Bank has provided financial assistance to help with this endeavor.

Panama's social security system covers most permanent employees. Principal disbursements are for retirement and health care. Permanent employees pay taxes to the Social Security Institute, and the self-employed contribute on the basis of their income as reported on income tax returns. Agricultural workers are generally exempted.

Substantial improvements in a wide variety of areas have come to fruition. Village health committees communicate the needs of villagers to healthcare officials. The program enjoyed its most notable successes in the early 1970s with the construction of water delivery systems and latrines in a number of previously underserved rural areas. Village health committees also organize community health education courses, immunization campaigns, and medical team visits to isolated villages. These federations lend money to villages for the construction of sanitation facilities, to assist them in contacting the Ministry of Health personnel for specific projects, and to help with financing medical visits to the villages.

Village health committees are most successful in regions where land and income are relatively equitably distributed. The regional medical director is pivotal and assigns a high priority to preventive health care. However, many committees are inoperative. In general, rural healthcare funding has been adversely affected by government cutbacks. Facilities tend to be heavily used and poorly maintained. Marked disparities in health care between urban and rural regions continue.

Ethical Issue. What ethical principles have been violated with poor distribution of healthcare services in Panama? How is this different from the United States and other more- or less-developed countries?

Healthcare Workforce

Panama has more physicians than nurses with 12.6 physicians and 11.3 nurses for every 10,000 people. The ratio per 10,000 for dentists is 2.9; for radiologists, 1.4; and for laboratory technicians, 3.2. The number of nurses is inadequate to meet Panama's needs, and the supply is unevenly distributed. Nurses who are willing to practice in remote areas receive up to a 50% increase in pay. The country is also short on laboratory technicians. All health professionals in the public sector are protected by union contracts, which set the pay scales. Nurses' salaries are good compared to other professionals. Physicians start at a monthly base salary of $1025.00 and nurses at $750.00, although differentials are given for merit and for specialization (PAHO, 2001).

Ethical Issue. Higher education is free in Panama. The health sector distribution and statistics are not what one expects for a developing country. What do you suggest to address the *ethical principles of justice, beneficence, autonomy,* and *nonmaleficence?*

The birthrate of 29.1 per 1000 in rural areas and 23.1 in urban areas has been gradually decreasing over the past 3 decades. Infant mortality below 1 year is 16.8 per 1000 and 26.2 per 1000 for age under 5 years. Most deaths from infant mortality are caused by congenital abnormalities, pneumonia, intestinal infections, and protein-calorie malnutrition. The leading causes of death in children ages 1 to 5 years are accidental injuries, multiple forms of violence, intestinal disorders, and pneumonia. Death for ages 6 to 10 years parrot the deaths for ages 1 to 5 years, but in a different order. In the 10 to 14 age group, the death rate is 37.6 per 100,000 and for ages 15 to 19, the death rate is 88.1 per 100,000 with a vast difference between the sexes: 108 in males and 53 in females.

Rural Panama has disproportionately high infant and maternal mortality rates. Rural babies are roughly 20% more likely to die than their urban counterparts; childbearing is five times more likely to be fatal in rural Panama than in cities. The infant mortality rate of Panama Province is one third that of Bocas del Toro and one fourth that of Darién.

Ethical Issue.   What ethical principles are involved with health disparities in Panama? Can you make suggestions for addressing these disproportionate health disparities? How are these disparities different from or similar to wealthier nations?

The overall fertility rate of 2.6 per woman varies significantly from urban to rural areas. In their research, Warren et al. (1987) and Purnell (1999) report that nonuse of family planning services might be due in part to indigenous Indians' strong cultural values of family. Female sterilization remains a prevalent method of birth control, followed by oral contraceptives (Warren et al., 1987). The crude death rate is 4.4% with a maternal mortality rate of 6.4%. The life expectancy for women is 77.93 years and 72.68 years for men.

Service Facilities and Quality of Services

Panama has 22 hospitals, some of which are privately owned. The province of Panama has 12 hospitals, many of which are specialty-specific, such as psychiatry, maternal-child, pediatrics, or medical and surgical. Chiriqui Province has 3 hospitals. The provinces of Herrera, Veraguas, Los Santos, Chorrera, Colon, and the San Blas Islands each has 1 hospital. The provinces of Bocas del Toro, Cocle, and Darien do not have any hospitals but do have clinics. Medical facilities, including nearly all laboratory and special-care facilities, are concentrated in the capital city. Roughly 87% of the hospital beds are in publicly owned and operated by institutions, mostly located in Panama City.

Medical facilities and personnel are concentrated beyond what might reasonably be expected, even given the capital city's share of total population. Panama City has roughly two and a half times the national average of hospital beds and doctors per capita and nearly three times the number of nurses per capita. The effect of this distribution is seen in continued regional disparities in health indicators.

Ethical Issue.   What ethical principles are involved with the maldistribution of healthcare facilities in Panama?

The overall perceptions of Panamanians on healthcare delivery is that (a) private care is best but too costly, (b) the social security facilities are better than those administered by the Ministry of Health, (c) the care is trusted and sophisticated despite long delays in accessing trusted providers, and (d) the rural, indigenous population voice basic needs without regard to quality (Moises, 2003). Because most hospitals have waiting lists for surgery, an effort is underway to extend operating room hours, increase budgets for purchasing drugs and medical and surgical supplies, and procure services from the private sector. Sandiford and Salvetto (2002) reported that inequalities in health care in rural areas of Panama result from low utilizations rates, which are related to the travel time to get to a facility and the perceived low quality when care was accessed.

Ethical Issue.   The *ethical principle of distributive justice* has been violated in the distribution of health services in Panama. What can individuals, groups, and the government do to help correct the poor distribution of health services?

To this author's knowledge, only one hospital has a quality-improvement program, which was started by one of his students from the graduate nursing program at the University of Panama. Other students and faculty of the nursing school from the University of Panama were prime movers to help enact the current seatbelt law in Panama.

Most hospitals have active infection-control programs. Specialty women's hospitals have active milk banks. In public hospitals that cater to the indigenous rural populations, facilities are available where one family member can stay in the hospital with the patient, while the rest of the family can camp out on hospital property.

Illness, Disease, and Injury Profile

The illness, disease, and injury profile of Panama is changing from one of infectious diseases to one similar to the more developed nations. However, some infectious diseases that were almost eliminated in the past are reemerging, and newer ones are arising. The leading causes of death are (a) malignant neoplasms; (b) accidents, self-inflicted injuries, assaults, and other acts of violence; (c) cerebrovascular diseases; (d) ischemic heart disease; (e) chronic diseases of the lower respiratory tract; and (f) diabetes mellitus. The rate for communicable diseases has decreased significantly over the last 15 years. However, tuberculosis is on the rise and diseases caused by the human immunodeficiency virus represent 1 of 10 leading causes of death with a rate of 15.2 per 100,000; rates are higher in men (23.3) than in women (7.0).

The leading causes of morbidity treated at public health facilities are influenza, diarrhea and gastroenteritis, rhinopharyngitis, the common cold, and malnutrition. Health workers, nurses in urban areas, and either nurses or community health promoters in rural areas are trained to provide follow-through on mental health programs, control of vector-borne diseases, tuberculosis, and cervical cancer. The leading discharge diagnoses in public health hospitals are problems related to childbirth and the puerperium, diseases of the respiratory tract, multiple trauma, infectious parasitic diseases, and problems with the newborn and the perinatal process.

Although the country supposedly has an adequate blood supply, places in remote areas such as the San Blas Islands do not have storage facilities. When someone on these islands needs a transfusion, the donor and recipient lie side by side on tables while the transfusion occurs. Testing for HIV does not exist. All but one resident in the San Blas Islands have type B+ blood. HIV in the rest of the country is on the rise with 44% transmitted through heterosexual activity, 40% through homosexual or bisexual activity, 10% through intravenous drug use, 1% through blood transfusions, and 5% perinatally (total number with HIV $\approx$ 16,000).

The largest of the San Blas Islands, Aligandi, has its own hospital with 8 beds. However, when missionary groups perform surgery, the hospital may expand to 100 beds with patients being housed on the verandas and every available room, including the guesthouse and physician's private quarters.

A wide variety of medicines are available over the counter in Panama, as are herbal and traditional remedies. Family members may go to the pharmacy and purchase drugs, such as injectable diazepam, and then take them to the hospital and administer it to a relative or friend.

Drug abuse is considered a priority health problem for younger groups and constitutes the leading cause of violence and crime in the country. Alcohol is the drug of choice for the population as a whole. Men are more likely to abuse illicit drugs and women are more likely to abuse less powerful tranquilizers. Cocaine is on the rise, mainly in the young-adult population.

Infectious Diseases

The Gorgas Memorial Institute of Tropical and Preventive Medicine, founded in 1921, was named after William C. Gorgas, a US Surgeon General known throughout the world as the conqueror of malaria and yellow fever. His pioneer efforts in halting an epidemic of yellow fever enabled the United States to complete the Panama Canal. The institute, which was moved in 2002 to the University of Alabama, had a mission to create a health education program to train researchers in tropical health, disease, and medicine and to establish a research institute focusing on tropical and preventative medicine in Panama. After decades of health care and research projects, the hospital is now a specialty oncology hospital financed by the Japanese.

Because of Gorgas hospital, much research on infectious disease has been completed in Panama. Despite the progress made in eliminating many tropical and infectious diseases, there has been a reemergence of cholera, classical dengue and dengue hemorrhagic fever, malaria, tuberculosis, and Venezuelan equine encephalitis.

Research on a number of health concerns and the environment is continuing, much of it by universities from the United States and Great Britain. One project contains drug-related studies on infectious diseases (Kursar, Capson, Corley, Corley, Gupta, Harrison, et al., 1999), and the other involves the detection of depression by nurses in primary care (Moreno, Saravanan, Kohn, & Miranda, 2003).

Hantavirus pulmonary syndrome (HPS), transmitted by rodents, made its debut in Panama in 1999. HPS is an infectious disease typically characterized by fever, myalgia, and headache and followed by dyspnea, noncardiogenic pulmonary edema, hypotension, and shock. Common laboratory findings include elevated hematocrit, leukocytosis with the presence of immunoblasts, and thrombocytopenia. The case-fatality rate can be as high as 52%. Hantaviruses are most often transmitted to humans through the inhalation of infectious rodent feces, urine, or saliva. However, strain-specific virus transmission may occur from person-to-person contact.

HPS was first recognized in 1993 in the Four Corners region of the United States. Since then, 363 cases of HPS have been confirmed in the United States. Before 2000, no human hantavirus infections had been reported in Central America. An outbreak of hantavirus pulmonary syndrome occurred in the province of Los Santos, Panama, in late 1999 and early 2000. Eleven cases were identified; three of which were fatal. The outbreak was investigated by the Panamanian Ministry of Health, Gorgas Memorial Institute for Health Studies, the US Centers for Disease Control and Prevention (Atlanta, GA), and the Pan–American Health Organization, and was conducted in collaboration with local medical and public health officials. To monitor the spread of disease, an outbreak communications center was established at the Ministry of Health in Panama City and staffed by physicians, public health officials, and health educators. Operations of this center included (a) passive surveillance for suspected cases of HPS, (b) a public hotline that addressed symptoms and signs of HPS as well as methods of prevention, and (c) nationwide distribution of HPS educational materials. Panama appears to be able to initiate epidemiological surveillance quickly and competently.

Arthropod-borne Diseases

Arthropod-borne diseases common in Panama are malaria, Chagas disease, dengue fever, leishmaniasis, filariasis, and yellow fever. A brief description of these diseases follows:

- Malaria, an infectious disease characterized by cycles of chills, fever, and sweating, is caused by a protozoan of the genus *Plasmodium* in red blood cells, which is transmitted to humans by the bite of an infected female anopheles mosquito. The period between the mosquito bite and the onset of malarial illness is usually 1 to 3 weeks. Prevention and treatment are frequently the same: chloroquine phosphate and primaquine are the most common but other drugs are also used such as artemether, artesunate, quinidine, doxycycline, mefloquine, and sulfa preparations.

- Chagas disease, also called trypanosomiasis, is caused by the parasite *Trypanosoma cruzi* and is transmitted by reduviid bugs, kissing bugs, primarily found in cracks and holes in substandard housing. Infection is spread to humans when an infected bug deposits feces on a person's skin, usually while the person is sleeping. The person accidentally rubs the feces into the bite wound, in an open cut, the eyes, or mouth. An infected mother can pass infection to her baby during pregnancy, at delivery, or while breast-feeding. Chagas disease is characterized by fever and enlargement of spleen and lymph nodes. Acute symptoms only occur in about 1% of the time; most people do not seek medical treatment.

- Dengue fever, a tropical disease transmitted by *Aedes aegypti* mosquitoes, is characterized by high fever, rash, headache, and severe muscle and joint pain. The disease usually occurs in 5-year cycles and strikes people with low levels of immunity. The mosquito flourishes in rainy seasons and can breed year round in water-filled flowerpots, plastic bags, and cans. The incubation period ranges from 3 to 15 days. Only supportive therapy is available in the form of treating or preventing dehydration.

- Leishmaniasis, caused by a flagellate protozoan, is transmitted to humans by bloodsucking sand flies. The parasites can live in animals or in humans and affect white blood cells. The more serious type affects internal organs causing fever, anemia, splenomegaly, and discoloration of the skin. Untreated, it can become fatal. Treatment is with amphotericin B, drugs containing antimony, or the newest drug available, miltefosine, which had a 95% effectiveness in clinical trials in 2003.

- Yellow fever, a tropical disease caused by a bite from the female *Aedes aegypti* and haemagogus mosquitoes, is characterized by high fever, jaundice, and gastrointestinal hemorrhaging. In severe cases, prostration and renal failure may occur. Because there is no specific treatment, vaccination is important. Symptoms appear suddenly after an incubation period of 3 to 5 days.

- Filariasis, also called lymphatic filiariasis or elephantiasis, is caused by thread-like parasitic round worms (nematodes) and their larvae and is transmitted by mosquitoes. Acute episodes of local inflammation involving skin, lymph nodes and lymphatic vessels often accompany the chronic lymphedema or elephantiasis. Some of these symptoms are caused by the body's immune response to the parasite, but most are the result of bacterial infection of skin where normal defenses have been partially lost due to underlying lymphatic damage. In endemic communities, some 10 to 50% of men suffer from genital damage, especially hydrocele, and elephantiasis of the penis and scrotum. Elephantiasis of the entire leg, the entire arm, the vulva, or the breast swelling up to several times normal size can affect up to 10% of men and women. The worst symptoms of the chronic disease generally appear in adults and in men more often than in women. Treatment is with albendazole and diethylcarbamazine.

These are recommendations to help prevent arthropod-borne diseases:

- Wear a long-sleeved shirt and long pants while outside to prevent illnesses carried by insects.

- Use insect repellent containing DEET (diethylmethyltoluamide) in 30–35% strength for adults and 6–10% for children.

- Use a bed net impregnated with the insecticide permethrin.

- Properly dispose of household trash.

- Do not leave water-filled flowerpots with standing water.

- Eliminate other sources of standing water.

Food- and Waterborne Illnesses

Common waterborne and food-borne diseases are amoebiasis, brucellosis, cholera, hepatitis A, and typhoid fever. Other diseases include rabies and hepatitis B. Myiasis, a condition caused by a botfly, is endemic in Central America. A brief description of these illnesses follows:

- Amoebiasis, an infection caused by pathogenic amebas, especially *Entamoeba histolytica*, is usually contracted by ingesting water or food contaminated by amoebic cysts. Symptoms include diarrhea, abdominal pain or discomfort, and fever. Symptoms take from a few days to a few weeks to develop and manifest themselves in about 2 to 4 weeks. This is synonymous to the following: It may take 5 years for cardiovascular diseases to develop but symptoms do not become manifested until many years later. Most infected people are asymptomatic, but this disease has the potential to make the sufferer dangerously ill, especially if there is immunocompromise.

- Brucellosis, a bacterial disease caused by *Brucella*, is transmitted by contact with infected animals or through contaminated milk or milk products. The disease is also called undulant fever because of the rising and falling of fevers, sweats, malaise, weakness, anorexia, headache, and muscle and back pain.

- Cholera, an infectious disease caused by the bacteria *Vibrio cholerae*, is characterized by profuse watery diarrhea, vomiting, muscle cramps, and severe dehydration. The disease can be mild with little to no symptoms.

- Hepatitis A, also called infectious hepatitis, is an infection of the liver caused by an RNA virus and is transmitted by ingesting infected food and water or through contact with infected feces. Symptoms range from flulike symptoms to more severe symptoms such as nausea, poor appetite, abdominal pain, fatigue, jaundice, and dark urine. Recovery can be complete in a few weeks to months. Very few cases progress to death. Treatment is symptomatic with rest and fluids.

- Typhoid fever, a highly infectious disease caused by *Salmonella typhi,* is transmitted by contaminated food or water and is characterized by fever, headache, coughing, intestinal hemorrhaging, and rose-colored spots on the skin. Treatment includes antibiotics such as ampicillin, chloramphenicol, trimethoprim-sulfamethoxazole, or ciprofloxacin.

- Myiasis, the condition caused by botfly, is endemic in Central America and is caused by parasitic dipterous fly larvae feeding on the host's necrotic or living tissue. Botflies lay their larvae in open wounds. The larvae stage appears as maggots, which then live off the tissue. Treatment is removing larvae through pressure or the maggots with forceps and then cleaning and disinfecting the wound.

These are some recommendations to prevent food- and waterborne illnesses:

- Vaccinations for hepatitis A or immune globulin (IG)
- Hepatitis B or immune globulin vaccination
- Rabies vaccination, if you might be exposed to wild or domestic animals through your work or recreation
- Typhoid vaccination is particularly important because of the presence of *S. typhi* strains resistant to multiple antibiotics in this region.
- A booster for tetanus and diphtheria—f not vaccinated within the last 10 years
- Yellow fever vaccination

Also helpful is this overall general advice for staying healthy:

- Wash your hands often with soap and water.
- Drink only boiled water or water and carbonated (bubbly) drinks in cans.
- Avoid tap water, fountain drinks, and ice cubes.
- Eat only thoroughly cooked food or fruits and vegetables you have peeled yourself.
- Do not eat fruit purchased from street vendors.
- Boil it, cook it, peel it, or forget it.

Other Health Concerns

Other illnesses commonly found in Panama include contact dermatitis caused by pesticides and fungicides among banana plantation workers, especially in the western provinces where Chiquita Banana and United Fruit Banana are major employers (Penagos, 2002). Efforts to teach workers how to protect themselves are being made, along with translating written materials into indigenous languages for those for whom Spanish and English are a second language.

In addition, drowning as a result of strong currents and undertows are common throughout Panama. One should always check with local authorities before attempting to swim in coastal areas. The problem is not the surf but the unusual undertows from the surf.

A survey conducted in rural Chiriqui estimated a heavy prevalence of dental caries with a large need for treatment. A convenience sample of 2597 subjects showed a mean decayed, missing, and filled teeth index of 4.08 for 12-year-olds, 6.40 for 15-year-olds, 13.20 for the 35 to 44 age group, and 18.88 for the 65 to 74 age group ($P < .001$). No statistically significant differences by gender were found. These findings rank rural Panama with Mexico and Haiti when compared to the results of other Central American community studies. The percentage of caries-free 12-year-olds was 6.8%. Of the total sample, 74.7% of individuals required one or multiple surface restorations and 47.9% required at least one extraction. Restorative need was greatest in the 15-year-olds. The severity of dental caries in this sample was moderately severe, and the treatment need was extraordinarily high (Asroth, Berg, McDowell, Hamman, & Mann, 1998).

Traditional Practitioners and Herbal Medicine

Traditional Practitioners

Panamanians from all socioeconomic levels rely on traditional care providers. Healers include *curanderos(as), sobadores(as), espiritistas, brujos(as), masajistas,* and *(y)jerberos(as)*. Traditional practitioners, who are usually well known by the family, are often consulted before and during biomedical treatment. Although usually no contradictions or contraindications to traditional remedies arise, healthcare providers must always consider the client's use of these practitioners to prevent conflicting treatment regimens.

Curanderos receive their talents from God or serve an apprenticeship with an established practitioner. *Curanderos* have great respect from the community, accept no monetary payment (but may accept gifts), are usually a member of the extended family, and treat many traditional illnesses. *Curanderos* do not usually treat illnesses caused by witchcraft. Currently, *curanderos* prescribe drugs, a practice the physicians are trying to stop. However, because *curanderos* can only prescribe over-the-counter medicines, this practice is likely to continue. One can purchase a wide variety of antibiotics and other medicines without a prescription.

The *yerberos* (also spelled *jerberos*) are folk healers with specialized training in growing herbs, teas, and roots and who prescribe these remedies for the prevention and cure of illnesses. A *yerbero* may suggest that the person go to a *botanica* (herb shop) for specific herbs. In addition, these traditional practitioners frequently prescribe the use of laxatives. *Sobadores* subscribe to treatment methods similar to those of a western chiropractor. The *sobador* treats illnesses that primarily affect the joints and musculoskeletal system by using massage and manipulation.

Brujos (witches) treat illnesses and conditions caused by witchcraft. Specific rituals are performed to eliminate the evils from the body.

Espiritistas, spiritualists, work with clients in terms of their spiritual connections, including religious connections. They do not usually prescribe medications but might prescribe herbal remedies and religious icons.

Herbal Medicine

Multiple studies have been completed on Mexican and Mexican-American herbal remedies. However, the only research study found in the literature on herbal medicine of Panamanians was conducted by Purnell (1999). In this study, 61% of Panamanians regularly used herbs and herbal teas to maintain their health. Moreover, 74% used herbs and teas when they were ill. People grow herbs in their yards. In the home in which this author stays when in Panama, the middle-class family grows a number of herbs. If they have an overabundance of herbs, they are sold to the local pharmacist who dries and prepares them for sale to the general public. For some of the preparations, leaves are use; for others, the roots are used. See Table 20-1 for a list of teas and their uses.

Case Study

McDowell Memorial Medical Center and a state university have joined forces to sponsor sending 10 nursing students and 10 nursing staff to Panama for a 2-week cross-cultural learning experience. Students and staff come from maternal–child, pediatric, medical–surgical, community, and psychiatric nursing. All students and staff identify with the dominant American culture. Only one student and two staff nurses have traveled outside the United States. Their travel experiences were in Rio de Janeiro, Brazil; Ontario, Canada; and London, England. Three of them have limited experience with the Spanish language from high school. The remainder only knows a few expressions in Spanish.

Brenda Polek, a nurse manager from the Medical Center, and Alan Hardy, a faculty member from the university, will accompany the group. Both feel they have a "fair" understanding of the Spanish language. The main reason for students to participate in this experience is for an elective course on international nursing. Multidisciplinary staff nurses are participating in the trip to specifically learn about the Panamanian culture because the medical center has increasing numbers of Panamanians on maternal–child, pediatric, and medical–surgical inpatient units and outpatient departments. All students and staff will be housed with Panamanian families throughout their travels.

All students in this cultural immersion experience will be able to attend classes in the nursing programs while in Panama. When in the clinical areas, staff and students will be accompanied with staff nurses in outpatient clinics and on inpatient units. Not all students and staff will get the same clinical rotations. They will be in formal learning experiences 4 days each week and have 3 days each week for traveling and sightseeing. Journaling, where students and staff record their observations and experiences, will be a large part of this program.

TABLE 20-1   Herbal Teas and Conditions for Use

Herbal Tea	Conditions for Use
Aguacate (avocado)	Hypertension, aphrodisiac
Ajo (garlic)	Bronchitis, respiratory conditions, hypertension, anti-inflammatory, infections, lower cholesterol
Canella con aniz (cinnamon)	Toothache, flu, coughs, pain, ulcers
Cebola (onion)	Bronchitis, respiratory conditions, flu
Cipres (cypress)	Whooping cough
Eucalyptus	Colds, coughs, allergies
Ginseng	Aphrodisiac, anemia, heart problems, diabetes, depression, hypertension, ulcers
Guanabano	Diarrhea, vomiting
Guava	Colds, diarrhea
Limon (lemon)	Colds, flu, calms nerves, sleep, headache, stomachache
Llanten (plantain)	Liver problems, stomachache
Malazana (tuberlike yam)	Colic
Manzanilla (chamomile)	Nerves, calms children, antispasmodic, diaphoretic, ulcers, aids digestion
Marano (mangrove)	Inflammation, edema
Mastranto	Colds, headache, stomachache, nerves, stress in children
Naranjo (orange)	Colds, flu, stomachache
Tilo (lime)	Colic, quiets nerves, flu, stomachache, ulcers
Toronjo (grapefruit)	Stomachache
Valleriana	Sleep, sedation, hypertension
Sabila (aloe)	Colds, gives strength, headache
Salvia (sage)	Worms, diabetes, ulcers, stomachache, headache, gives strength, strengthens nerves, stops sweating

Brenda Polek and Alan Hardy, in conjunction with faculty and staff in Panama, will arrange housing and clinical experiences; some of them will be with indigenous Indian groups. The students and staff nurses will plan any other details before they leave for Panama.

   1. How do you feel about staying with a family in Panama when you do not speak the Spanish language well?

2. How might you prepare to improve your Spanish language skills before you depart from home?

3. What are the passport and visa requirements for traveling to Panama? These requirements will change depending on your country of origin.

4. What vaccinations or medications will you take before you leave home? Where will you go to find out what is currently recommended for traveling to Panama?

5. What kind of clothing and uniforms will you need to take with you?

6. What do you need to know about verbal communication practices of Panamanians in order to not violate social taboos?

7. What do you need to know about nonverbal communication practices of Panamanians in order to not violate social taboos?

8. How might you go about visiting a traditional healer while in Panama?

9. A few Panamanians, especially the younger generation, are anti-American because of US influence in the Canal Zone, the environmental concerns left by the military in the Canal Zone, and the Noriega experience. How might you handle negative comments from Panamanian students about Americans?

10. As part of your immersion experience, you are required to attend a religious service while in Panama. Which type of service would you want to attend?

11. Make a list of experiences and sightseeing trips you might like to do while in Panama. Where would you obtain this information before you leave for Panama?

12. If you have the opportunity to accompany your host family on a trip without your cohort group, would you take them up on this opportunity?

13. What do you need to know about arthropod-borne diseases and food- and waterborne illnesses you may encounter on your trip?

14. Make a list of at least 10 strategies to maintain your health, your personal safety, and the safety of your group while traveling in Panama.

15. You are expected to take "a small gift" reflecting your home country for your host family. What gift will you take?

16. What would be at least one souvenir that you would want to bring home with you?

Critical Thinking Questions

1. Identify strategies for integrating allopathic healthcare providers and practices with traditional healthcare practices and providers.

2. How might churches and religious leaders assist healthcare providers in educating communities for health promotion and wellness, as well as illness, disease, and injury prevention?

3. What are some key elements that nurses should include in delivering educational programs to vulnerable populations with low literacy and with Spanish as a second language?

4. Identify infectious diseases and food- and waterborne diseases. What prevention strategies might you use?

5. What are some positive and negative influences that the United States has had on the health of Panamanians?

Bibliography and References

Astroth, J., Berg, R., Berkey, D., McDowell, J., Hamman, R., & Mann, L. (1998). Dental caries prevalence and treatment in Chiriqui Province, Panama. *International Dentistry Journal, 18*(3), 203–209.

Business Panama. (2005). *Panama at a glance.* Retrieved January 18, 2006 from http://www.business-panama.com/about_panama/glance.php

CIA. (2004). *Panama government.* Retrieved January 18, 2006, from http://www.cia.gov/cia/publications/factbook/geos/pm.html

CIA. (2005). *CIA world factbook online: Panama.* Retrieved January 2, 2006, from http://www.cia.gov/cia/publications/factbook/geos/pm.html

City of Panama. (2005). *Information technology in Panama.* Retrieved January 6, 2006, from http://www.e-panama.gob.pa/foro/forum_program.htm

El Ciudad del Saber. (2006). *The city of knowledge.* Retrieved January 25, 2006, from http://www.cdspanama.org

Finding Aid to the Gorgas Memorial Institute of Tropical and Preventive Medicine Records, 1899–1992. Retrieved December 27, 2005, from https://www.nlm.nih.gov/hmd/manuscripts/ead/gorgas212.html

Frysinger, G. R. (2003). *Panama City, Panama.* Retrieved January 5, 2006, from http://www.galenfrysinger.com/panama_city.htm

Global Academy. (2001). *Health today–Realities, obstacles, and perspectives.* Retrieved December 25, 2005, from http://theglobalacademy.org/conf_panama.asp

GlobalSecurity.Org. (2004). *Engineer jungle warfare course.* Retrieved August 3, 2005, from http://www.globalsecurity.org/military/facility/fort-sherman.htm

Hollenberg, N. K., Rivera, A., Meinking, T., Martinez, G., McCullough, M., Passan, D., et al. (1999). Age, renal perfusion and function in island-dwelling indigenous Kuna Amerinds of Panama. *Nephron, 82*(2), 131–138.

Hurtado, E. (1989). Breastfeeding in the etiology of diarrhea. *Archives of Latin American Nutrition, 39*(3), 278–291.

Kursar, T. A., Capson, T. L., Coley, P. D., Coley, D. G., Gupta, M. B., Harrison, L. A., et al. (1999). Ecologically guided bioprospecting in Panama. *Pharmaceutical Biology, 37*(Suppl. 1), 114–126.

Library of Congress. (2004a). *Panama country studies.* Retrieved January 2, 2006, from http://countrystudies.us/panama

Library of Congress. (2004b). *Panama: The constitution.* Retrieved January 18, 2006, from http://countrystudies.us/panama/51.htm

Library of Congress. (2004c). *Panama: Education.* Retrieved December 25, 2005, from http://countrystudies.us/panama/39.htm

Library of Congress. (2004d). *Panama religion.* Retrieved January 18, 2006, from http://countrystudies.us/panama/38.htm

Moises, L. (2003). Perceptions of health care quality in Central America. *International Journal for Quality in Health Care, 15*, 67–71.

Moreno, P., Saravanan, Y., Kohn, R., & Miranda, C. T. (2003). Evaluation of the PAHO/WHO training program on the detection and treatment of depression for primary care nurses in Panama. *Acta Psychiatrica Scandinavica, 108*(1), 61.

Outbreak of hantavirus pulmonary syndrome, Los Santos, Panama, 1999–2000. (2000, March). *Mortality and Morbidity Weekly Review, 17*(49), 205–207.

PAHO. (2004). *Profile of the health services system of Panama.* Washington, DC: PAHO.

PAHO. (2005). *Information on health: Panama.* Retrieved January 2, 2006, from http://www.paho.org/English/D/P39.pdf

Panama.(2005). *Pictures of Panama.* Retrieved February 11, 2006, from http://www.info-panama.com/panama-gallery/index.php?lang=english

Panama Canal: A tight squeeze. (2005, July 23). *The Economist*, p. 36.

Panama Canal Authority. (2006). *Welcome to the Panama Canal.* Retrieved January 18, 2006, from http://www.pancanal.com/eng

Partners of the Americas web site. (2005). Retrieved December 27, 2005, from http://www.partners.net/index.htm

Penagos, H. G. (2002). Contact dermatitis caused by pesticides among banana plantation workers in Panama. *International Journal of Occupational and Environmental Health, 8*(1), 14–18.

Purnell, L. (1999). Panamanian health beliefs and the meaning of respect afforded them by health-care providers. *Journal of Transcultural Nursing, 14*(4), 331–340.

Sandiford, P., & Salvetto, M. (2002). Health inequities in Panama. *Gaceta Sanitaria, 16*(1), 70–81.

Warren, C. W., Monteith, R. S., Johnson, J. T., Santiso, E., Guerra, F., & Oberle, M. W. (1987). Use of maternal-child health services and contraception in Guatemala and Panama. *Journal of Biosocial Sciences, 19*(2), 229–243.

Wikipedia. (2005). *Hospitals in Panama.* Retrieved February 11, 2006 from http://en.wikipedia.org.wiki/List_of_hospitals_in_Panama.

World Bank. (2004). *Panama at a glance.* Retrieved December 27, 2005 from http://devdata.worldbank.org/AAG/pan_aag.pdf

Chapter 21

Health and Environmental Design: The Relationship Between Health and Place in a Philippine Urban Setting

Mary Anne Alabanza Akers

Timothy A. Akers

Introduction

When you enter a place, whether it be inside a building, plaza park, or forest, do you notice its effect on you as a human being? Does the space make you tense, or does it have a calming effect on your nerves? Is there mystery and discovery that holds your interest to stay there? Does the place meet your needs? Does it give you aesthetic pleasure?

These are questions that design professionals throughout the world (e.g., urban planners, landscape architects, architects, and interior designers) address in their work in order to build better places. Beyond the basic functions that a place provides, these professionals also consider its aesthetics and impact on people's well-being. However, their assignments can neither be completed nor can they be sustainable if they work in a vacuum. Collaborating with health professionals and social scientists (e.g., psychologists, sociologists, and anthropologists) is an essential ingredient to creating healthy places for people. The US Centers for Disease Control and Prevention (CDC) defines healthy places as

> Those designed and built to improve the quality of life for all people who live, work, worship, learn, and play within their borders—where every person is free to make choices amid a variety of healthy, available, accessible, and affordable options. (Centers for Disease Control and Prevention, n.d.)

Parallel to this definition is the World Health Organization's (WHO) concept of a healthy city, which is, "one that improves its environments and expands its resources so that people can support each other in achieving their highest potential" (Takehito, 2003).

Using the CDC and WHO definitions as a starting point, this chapter introduces the reader to an emerging field of environmental design and health. This area of study often overlaps with medical geography, a subdiscipline of geography that examines the spatial implications of human disease and health, as well as environmental health, which emphasize the direct and indirect pathological effects of chemical and biological factors in the environment. However, the environmental design and health field differs from medical geography and environmental health to the extent that it encompasses the study of everyday aesthetics and how they influence people's health. Furthermore, environmental design implies the creation, construction, and organization of physical and natural places to enhance and promote quality living. While the medical geographer tracks the incidence of lead poisoning among preschool-aged children on a map, for example, the environmental health scientist conducts scientific research to find the origins of the contaminant. On the other hand, the environmental designer conducts a site inventory of the children's home, immediate neighborhood, and district. Using the information gathered, a plan is formulated to redesign the environment. If the contaminant is found in the playground soil, and remediation has been accomplished, the environmental designer restructures the place to support a full range of child development (e.g., coordination with other children, manipulative play, discovery, and expression). The designer may suggest an adventure playground without the conventional monochromatic glare of concrete as ground or boring playscapes that do not encourage creative play. Instead, the designer may intentionally place natural features in the site including pebbles and sand, so children can creatively explore their properties, or safe deciduous trees or shrubs for children to understand their annual cycles. Thumbing and arranging fallen leaves entices children into imaginative play, in addition to strengthening their fine motor skills.

Dr. Jacques M. May, a physician–geographer, highlights the different perspectives offered by medical geographers, environmental health scientists, and health design professionals in this quote:

> Disease, any disease—and let me remind you that by disease I mean maladjustment to the environment—can never occur without the combination of three orders of factors converging in time and space; that is, there must be a stimuli from the environment, there must be responses from an agent, and there must be the conglomeration of thoughts and traits that we call culture (May, 1961).

By culture, Dr. May refers to the specific geographic features of a site (e.g., rainfall, soil types, temperature), as well as physical elements of human settlements that either "encourage or inhibit a relation between agent and host" (Koch, 2005, 216). Environmental designers examine these site characteristics that make up Dr. May's concept of culture.

By illustrating divergent ways that geographers, health environmentalists, and designers work, we can now focus on the main thesis of this chapter—the relationship between environmental design and health, or, in other words, the influence of everyday aesthetics on people's well-being. To address the topic, we present a case study of street vendors in Baguio City, Philippines. These informal microentrepreneurs who set up their tiny ventures along public sidewalks, corners, and parking spaces have been the target of our multiyear, longitudinal study since 1999. In this chapter, we ask the following questions:

- What past research supports the connection between health and place, and how does environmental design address the issues?

- How do urban landscapes in developing countries, such as the Philippines, impact people's quality of life?

- What role do the design professions have in building healthy places for street vendors?

Health and Place

Hipprocrates is a pivotal figure in linking health and place. In his treatise, *On Airs, Waters, and Places*, he exhorts physicians and medical students to investigate health and disease in the context of a community's location and local climate (Hippocrates, 400 BCE). Temperature, wind direction, qualities of the waters, elevation, position of the stars, and other physical phenomena, if observed regularly, can explain and even predict physical conditions and incidence of diseases. For example, he attributes the differences between European groups and Asian people to seasonal changes, topography, and other place elements. Among European tribes, Hippocrates further observed that contrasts in stature, shape, and courage are caused by diverse geographical elements.

Early Environmental Design Health Interventions

In the 1850s, Dr. John Snow, a notable physician who studied the link between health and place, argued that environmental elements augmented the transmission of cholera in London. Contrary to the popular medical belief that cholera spread through noxious air generated by urban waste in poor districts, he advanced the notion that cholera was transmitted through personal contact and contaminated water. Using mortality and water-source data, he created a map to support his case and, through basic calculations, found a strong correlation between cholera severity and an interface of the city's water sources and sewage flow (Koch, 2005). This discovery became the impetus for urban infrastructure design.

Interestingly, American urban planning is rooted in similar health circumstances. At about the same period, a surge of urban migration to major cities, such as New York City, induced large concentrations of people in certain districts, which facilitated the transmission of diseases such as cholera, malaria, and typhoid fever. Sewer systems were dysfunctional because they served as drainage channels for storm waters and not organic wastes (Peterson, 1983). However, there were no disposal areas for excrement, so it ended up in these sewers. Weak and irregular water flow prevented the wastes from being carried out, and the sewers eventually became cesspools. The import of a "water carriage" system from Europe, from which our present-day toilet system was derived, proved to be the key to addressing urban health (Levy, 2000). However, the design of the piping network throughout the city was instrumental to its success in America. Large-scale planning, which considered topography, population density, and existing street layout, was essential in making the "water carriage" system function.

Landscape architecture evolved to incorporate the need to address health and sanitation concerns as well. Frederick L. Olmsted, the father of American landscape architecture, believed in the significant role that nature plays in people's well-being. Known for his work in creating Central Park in New York City, Olmsted promoted this project as the "lungs of the city." Because of health epidemics caused by the substandard conditions of congested tenement housing in New York City, a park was to serve as a therapeutic and relaxing place for residents.

Current Environmental Design Approaches to Health

Children's Places

Playgrounds

The World Health Organization (WHO) accounts 25–33% of the global burden of disease to environmental risk factors, and of this percent range, 40% involve children less than 5 years of age (Wargo, 2004). Children are more vulnerable to environmental disease than adults because toxicants can impede the growth and development of their body organs and systems. Because of their smaller body masses, it is more difficult for them to detoxify and excrete toxins, which can stay in their systems much longer. In addition, children are more heavily exposed to environmental toxins that settle on the ground because they play outside and have more hand-to-mouth contact than adults. A study of preschoolers in Makati, metropolitan Manila, Philippines, show that playground soils are a source of lead exposure to preschool children (Sharma & Reutergardh, 2000). An interesting feature about this study is that all of the examined sites were neighborhood playgrounds in high-income subdivisions. Several Australian studies also give evidence to the link between lead exposure and children's play areas (New South Wales Department of Environment and Conservation, 2003). Contaminated play areas were found near major transportation routes and old industrial sites.

This health concern can be addressed at various levels. City planners can designate land away from high-volume traffic streets for parks and playgrounds. In fact, the Australian studies show that the distance from highly traveled thoroughfares correlates with the degree of lead contamination. However, in cases where moving these parks is not feasible, another environmental design approach can be applied. On-site planning and design strategies grounded in environmental principles can help "clean up" a play area. Inasmuch as capping the soil by pouring concrete is an option, this method does not improve play areas because it increases injury risk. A more environmentally sound strategy is phytoremediation technologies, meaning processes involving plants that absorb contaminant hard metals, such as lead. Environmental engineers work closely with city planners and landscape architects to ensure proper phasing of park improvement. It is essential that specific areas be designated for phytoremediation and should be off limits to any human activity. Although it may take a while for this method to be effective, it is gentler to the environment and can produce safe and visually pleasing parks with abundant natural features.

Schools

Many urban schools in the developing world are located at undesirable sites (e.g. along highways, major transportation arteries, and depots), which expose children to vehicle exhaust throughout the day. An estimated 50 million annual cases of chronic cough and wheezing among children younger than 14 years old can be attributed to outdoor air pollution (Wargo, 2004). Identifying "safe and clean" areas for schools is a land-use planning tool for mitigating health problems associated with outdoor air pollution. However, only a few developing communities have the option to select their school sites. A site-based plan, which involves installing trees and other types of vegetation, may positively affect air quality. A mixture of air pollutants and high temperatures produces a harmful ozone layer, but the presence of trees can cool urban sites and also, to a certain extent, alleviate deteriorated air. Trees can also absorb certain pollutants and serve as interceptors of toxic airborne particles (Nowak, 1998). Ecological schoolyard design, which integrates sustainable practices with educational settings, can have positive health effects.[1]

Homes

In low-income countries, acute lower respiratory infections are the leading causes of mortality in children between 5 and 14 years old (Wargo, 2004). Respiratory problems are location-based because high levels of air pollution are usually found in homes. The burning of solid fuels (e.g., dung, wood, coal, and agricultural scraps) in cramped residential quarters contributes significantly to indoor pollution. Typically, the less advantaged suffer from this condition. A report about the global burden of disease indicates that in India, China, and Africa, approximately 70% of households continue to depend on solid fuels for cooking and heating (WHO, 2002a). Rampant usage of this fuel type warrants intervention, especially because about 800,000 of the deaths of very young children are due to pneumonia caused by indoor air pollution (WHO, 2002a). As much as common interventions often introduce other energy technologies (e.g., gas stoves, electricity, and solar energy) and improve stove efficiency, an environmental design response to this health problem is to modify the microenvironment at the pollution source. Architecturally, the home can be redesigned to rectify air circulation by incorporating

---

[1]Ecological schoolyards have physical features such as school gardens with indigenous plants, forested areas, water forms, and energy models (e.g., wind turbines).

simple features such as chimneys, smoke hoods to extract indoor smoke, reducing the eave spaces, and adding or enlarging windows in the cooking area. Furthermore, repositioning or rearranging the kitchen and living areas to take full advantage of wind direction is another aesthetic solution in mitigating indoor pollution.

Places for the Elderly

The elderly is another group susceptible to health problems triggered by environmental factors. Among some of the most common elderly health problems are falls and injuries. A European Union report states that 30% of elderly people fall at least once a year, and 70% of accidental deaths among this group are attributed to falls (EU Project, 2006). Inappropriately designed indoor environments for the elderly contribute to this health concern. Residential features that affect risk for falls include vinyl bathroom floors, a lack of handrails on staircases, poor lighting, furniture arrangement, and clutter. Architects and interior designers have a role in modifying home environments to make them safer places. For example, architects can design elderly homes with special attributes such as stair railings, minimal presence of stairs, lower cupboards and shelves, and slip-resistant flooring. The American Disability Act (ADA) provides standards for these types of residential quarters. For example, an 11-inch tread for a stair is wide enough to prevent falls. Other ADA requirements such as room dimensions, toilet spaces, and door widths ensure safe mobility for elderly use.

Research has revealed that older adults are more susceptible to falls and injuries in outdoor environments than inside their living spaces (Li et al., 2006). Their study in northern California is consistent with other studies throughout the world (e.g., Canada, England, Norway, Israel, and Japan), which identify outdoor environmental qualities as prime factors contributing to this health hazard. In this study, sidewalks, curbs, and streets were the most common places in which the elderly fell. Physical characteristics such as uneven surfaces, cracks, obstacles, high curb height, and slippery pavements precipitated falls. Simple management practices such as evening cleaning of these walking surfaces will improve their environments. Nevertheless, landscape architects and traffic engineers can also reduce risks of falling by creating innovative solutions for street design. For example, installing different color pavement material at the edge of a sidewalk can mark the curb from the walkway, considering that many elderly experience visual impairments. Furthermore, design decisions to mitigate glare outdoors, especially in walking areas may include designing paths along existing vegetation.

Outdoor spaces for the elderly are an essential ingredient for their health. Research has shown that the elderly require well-designed spaces, such as patios, courtyards, gardens, and nearby parks, for good health and well-being. A study of elderly Japanese gives evidence to the link between green spaces and longevity (Takano, Nakamura, & Watanabe, 2002). It demonstrated that access to green spaces such as parks and tree-lined streets encouraged outdoor activity among senior citizens, which lengthened their lives. Aside from providing green spaces, environmental designers also examine elements, such as microclimate, in designing quality spaces. Since the elderly are susceptible to extreme temperature changes, designers consider drafts, wind currents, and sun movements in planning an outdoor space (Marcus & Francis, 1998). Courtyards that are exposed to the winter winds and hot summer sun are unhealthy and will certainly not be used. The placement of these outdoor spaces is carefully chosen by designers so that senior citizens can enjoy the winter sun in a controlled setting and cool summer breezes under shaded areas.

The Environment and Health

For people to be healthy, one must examine the places in which they live, work, socialize, recreate, and even run errands. These places should not only be free of disease-producing matter but, more fundamentally, should enhance people's well-being while being environmentally friendly. Conserving our natural resources and mitigating the harmful effects of our self-built environments have a strong bearing on addressing the state of our health. An evolving concept of *ecosystem health* recognizes that people's level of health is proportional to the healthy functionality of their ecosystems (McCally, 2002). Promoted by biologists, ecologists, and health professionals, this concept examines the impact of human patterns on large-scale ecological changes. These changes, in turn, cause many of our human health problems. Scientific evidence has shown that the earth's temperatures have been increasing, due largely to human behavior and lifestyles. This climate change has been deemed the cause of 2.4% of worldwide diarrhea and 6% of malaria in middle-income countries (WHO, 2002b). Hot temperatures also induce cardiovascular problems among vulnerable groups because their bodies have to work harder to keep cool. Diseases such as the West Nile, cholera, and Lyme disease are spreading in North America and Europe because the changing climates help the carriers to thrive (e.g., ticks, mosquitoes, and mice). It is estimated by WHO that warmer weather contributes to more than 150,000 deaths and 5 million illnesses each year (Eilperin, 2005).

Loss of vegetation is another environmental factor found to have a connection with disease. A study observed that clustered forest and herbaceous cover (e.g., pastures, row crops, and grass) mitigated the incidence of Lyme disease in suburban areas (Jackson, 2005). The conventional American suburban landscape with green spaces interspersed among residential subdivisions was associated with increased incidence of Lyme disease. In other words, patchy forested areas in low-density suburban regions encourage contact between people and animals that are familiar with humans, such as the white-tailed deer and white-footed mouse. Therefore, it is suggested that environmental designers conserve larger forested areas and innovatively cluster housing in more suitable residential land, referred to as conservation subdivisions (Arendt, 1996).

The relationship between deforestation and human health is manifested in several studies. In the Peruvian Amazon, a team of researchers found that malaria-inducing mosquitoes bite people 200 times more in cleared areas than in forests (Cascio, 2006). Similar findings were found in Africa (Patz & Olson, 2006). The Nipah virus in Southeast Asia is thought to have come from the transmission of the vector from bats, to pigs, and then to humans (Chua, Chua, & Wang, 2002). The degradation of the bats' natural habitat forced them to migrate to orchards near farms, where they transferred the pathogen to pigs, eventually impacting human health. Likewise, vegetation loss is linked to new and emerging and reemerging diseases as people forage closer to deep forests. Micro-organisms look for new hosts (i.e., humans) when the survival of their primary host (i.e., animals) is threatened by the loss of their habitat. Diseases such as Ebola, SARS, dengue, and malaria are the results of these drastic land-use changes. With the nature of global commerce and a pronounced increase in international travel, these pathogens are readily transmitted across world regions. An Ethiopian sneezing, for example, could lead to a Californian catching the cold (Armelagos & Harper, 2005).

Many of these world health problems are larger than what environmental designers, in general, are able to tackle. Though environmental planners address issues at larger regional scales, extensive social and behavioral change must occur throughout the world. We must not be overwhelmed, however, with the severity of the task, or we will be stymied into doing nothing. As designers shape communities and influence land-use patterns, they can make a significant difference in the quality of our environments, and thereby improve our health. To illustrate the relationship between health and design, a case study undertaken by the authors of this chapter of a Philippine upland urban center is described. The longitudinal study, initiated in 1999, focused on establishing a link between the physical environment and health of a vulnerable population—pauperized street vendors.

Urbanization in Asia

More than half of the world's population resides in Asia. The United Nations Population Division claims that of the estimated 6.5 billion people in the world, 3.9 reside in Asia alone (United Nations, 2004). Specifically, China and India account for about 37% of the world's population. A significant trend in population dynamics is the unprecedented rate of urbanization among world regions. Projections for the year 2030 indicate that 60% of the people in the world will be living in urban environments. Asia is forecasted to be the region where a significant portion of urban residents will dwell (United Nations, 2005). Rapid urbanization produces health concerns in many developing countries. Urban infra-structure and services cannot catch up with the massive demands placed on them. Sewer systems, transportation networks, housing, medical care, and educational services are not adequate to meet the needs of an expanding population. As a result, residential and work environments are so substandard that people's health is threatened.

The Philippines has one of the fastest urbanization rates in the world. From 1960 to 1995, the annual growth rate of urban areas was 5.14% (World Bank Group, 2002). It is estimated that 60% of the Philippine population will live in urban areas. As observed, rapid urbanization exists in periurban areas outside of metropolitan Manila, and sec-ondary cities, such as Baguio City. The following section describes the development of

Baguio City based on a health need, and further describes how its current urbanizing trends impact the health of its residents, particularly street vendors working in the central business district.

Baguio City: A City Founded on Health and Healing

A prime example of the relationship between health and place is Baguio City, Philippines. Baguio City, because of its high elevation, became a colonial hill station in the early 1900s. Hill stations were prevalent in Southeast Asia as settlements for sick colonial soldiers (Reed, 1999). Through memoirs and chronicles of military physicians, soldiers' health was documented to have improved significantly when they recuperated in the highlands of India, Burma, Thailand, Vietnam, Cambodia, and the Philippines. Debilitating tropical diseases and extreme heat in the lowlands made it unbearable for European colonialists to survive, so they retreated to mountainous, convalescent places. As these village centers evolved, not only were soldiers assigned here, but civil servants, missionaries, plantation owners, merchants, and other westerners visited these cool and refreshing hill stations to heal, rejuvenate, and strengthen their physical, emotional, and spiritual health (Reed, 1999).

In 1898, when Spain sold the Philippines to the United States, American occupation began in the islands. Similar to the European experience, the brutal heat in the lowlands, exposure to diseases (e.g., malaria, cholera, typhoid, and dysentery), and absence of the four seasons put a severe strain on the American colonialists. They looked for an upland place to develop, and in 1900, identified Baguio's current location as the most ideal spot for the country's summer capital and health resort. Major infrastructure such as roads and public buildings were built, and in 1909, the settlement was established as a chartered city.

The construction of a principal military recreational base (Camp John Hay), the rise of a gold-mining industry, and formation of educational institutions contributed to the development of Baguio as a major city in northern Philippines. Today, it is a thriving regional center with about 250,000 people and an annual growth rate of 1.95% (Baguio City, 2006). Projections show that in 2010, the city will reach a population of 300,000. Migration from other provinces has increased the number of residents significantly.

Baguio City's economy is based on a service sector, primarily its colleges and universities. This contributes to a significantly young population in which 65.5% of residents are younger than 30 years old. Other services include retail, commercial, and medical services. In addition, an important job generator is the export-processing district outside the city core.

A Case Study of Health and Place: Street Vendors in Downtown Baguio

In spite of Baguio City's economic opportunities, the number of jobs is not adequate for its increasing population. As in the case of many cities in the developing world, a shortage of formal employment encourages the rise of the informal sector. The *informal sector* is often defined as economic activities that lack the formalistic or regulatory structures expected of traditional businesses, such as standardized systems for taxation and licensure (Akers & Akers, 2005). Measuring the extent of the informal sector is a difficult task because of its elusive nature. In fact, the International Labour Organization reports that the informal sector in the developing world ranges from 10% to 90% (International Labor Organization, 2002). However, high percentages are found in east and west Africa, south and Southeast Asia, and parts of Latin America. Lower percentages of informal participation rates are found in eastern Europe.

Obtaining precise statistics is difficult because of this sector's ambiguity and lack of standard surveillance measures across various national governments and international agencies. For example, the Philippine Department of Labor reveals that the informal sector is made up of approximately 13.4 million Filipinos, or about 46% of the labor force (Indon, 2002). The ILO, on the other hand, reports that 19 million Filipinos, or 70% of the Philippine workforce is engaged in unregulated livelihood activities (Asanza, 2003a). Nevertheless, the informal sector is a thriving group that will not go away.

Informal activities are roughly divided into two subsectors; the home-based businesses, and outdoor microenterprises located on streets, corners, and alley spaces. As mentioned, street vending is often a response to a decline in the formal economy. For example, a sharp rise in street vendors was observed during the Asian crisis of 1998 (Bhowmik, 2005). It seems that this sector provides a safety net for the masses, especially those highly dependent on the ebbs and flows of the formal economy. Although cities often implement punitive laws that curtail these microenterprises, they provide benefits to most urban dwellers. Aside from supplying affordable goods and services to pedestrians, they are convenient because they are scattered throughout the city, and they serve as "observers" for street safety. A world-renowned urbanist proclaims that the more "eyes" there are on the street, the safer the place is (Jacobs, 1961).

The Study

Research on street vendors is minimal and often inaccessible (Bhowmik, 2005). The few published works available have focused mainly on labor dynamics, political and economic nature, and social networks of street vending. To date, except for studies published by this chapter's authors, no study has involved an interdisciplinary approach to understanding street vendors and their environments. Since 1999, data were collected in several phases (see Table 21-1). Various professionals were involved as members of the research team in the different study phases (e.g., city planner, health researcher, public relations expert, environmental health specialist, medical physician, and nurse). This chapter will focus mainly on the 2003, 2004, and 2006 research phases because the data collected link health and environmental design more closely than the previous phases.

Street Vendors and Their Physical Environments

To examine the connection between health and environmental design, it was necessary to target street vendors who had fixed physical locations. The ambulatory vendors, those

TABLE 21-1   Interdisciplinary Project on Street Vendors: Project Phases

Year	Research Focus	Research Methodology	Disciplines Represented
1999	Social networks, microeconomic nature of street enterprises, and environmental assessment	Survey of 219 vendors, physical inventory of vendor sites	City planning, urban affairs, and urban health
2000	Relationships between street vendors and adjacent formal businesses	Visual documentation and informal interviews	City planning, public relations
2003	Health and environmental assessment	Survey of 187 vendors, physical inventory of vendor sites	City planning, urban affairs, urban health, and nursing
2004	Air quality	Air quality monitoring on 30 vendors sites and one central fixed site	City planning, urban affairs, urban health, and environmental health
2006	Health screening	Medical testing for 15 vendors (e.g., physicals, blood tests, oximeter readings at vendor sites), in-depth health survey for 10 vendors	City planning, urban affairs, urban health, medicine, nursing

who sell from place to place, were excluded from our samples because it was difficult to control for transient physical environments. As a result of this target sampling, most of the informal traders were women (80%) with an average age of 40 years old. Studies from other countries reveal that male vendors tend to be ambulant because they are physically able to carry their goods around with them. In terms of educational status, some vendors had finished elementary school (30%), while others were high school graduates (40%) or individuals with some college education (26%). Nine respondents had no schooling at all.

Street vendors in Baguio City have been involved in these economic activities for an average of 11 years. They work long hours—10 hours a day, Monday to Sunday—and earn only about US$20 a week (Akers, Sowell, & Akers, 2004). Similar to vendors in other Asian countries, most of them work in challenging environments such as very steep sidewalks, overcrowded spaces, polluted air, and locations that do not protect them from the elements (Akers & Akers, 2005). Baguio City's central business district (CBD), which is situated in a valley, is the hub for economic, political, medical, educational, social, and cultural activities. Its streets and public spaces are often congested with pedestrians and vehicles that run on diesel fuel. In spite of urban stressors such as noise, dust, traffic, crowding, and so on, the CBD thrives on the energy created by street activities continuing 24 hours a day.

The major question we put forward is: How do the physical environments in the CBD impact street vendor health? Considering that vendors work long hours and are constantly exposed to various climactic elements and stressors, to what extent do these factors affect their health and well-being? To answer these questions, we first divided the CBD into 35 sites, which represented specific places where vendors congregated. For several years, we monitored, measured, and observed these sites. In 2003, a health survey was conducted among 187 vendors in various places around downtown Baguio. Questions about their health conditions and use of medical services were asked. In addition, a physical evaluation of their workplaces was conducted. The next year, we measured air quality in the same sites. After statistical tests were applied, we concluded that relationships between place and health do exist. The following section summarizes the study results.

The Link Between Place and Street Vendor Health

Magsaysay Avenue Site

Of the 31 sites examined, the most problematic, in terms of vendors experiencing ailments, is Magsaysay Avenue, a highly congested place at the bottom of the valley. It is one of the main arteries that lead to the CBD's core. This particular site is just across from the main city market, where most goods are dropped off to be distributed throughout the city. The street vendors there complain about colds, asthma, high blood pressure, and arthritis. Environmental factors may contribute to these health conditions. For example, compared to other streets in the CBD, the sidewalk width in this site is narrower. With major universities within the area and the site's proximity to the marketplace, the Magsaysay Avenue site experiences the highest pedestrian volume in downtown (40 persons per minute). Such jam-packed conditions can lead to the transmission of airborne diseases such as colds and influenza Figure 21-1 shows the high-density pedestrian flow in Magsaysay Avenue. Influenza is the third leading cause of morbidity in the Cordillera Autonomous Region, in which Baguio City is located (Philippine Department of Health, 2002). The exchange of money and products between vendors and pedestrians also increases the transmission of viruses and bacteria.

Figure 21-1 Pedestrian congestion on Magsaysay Avenue.

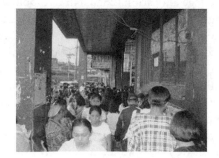

Another characteristic of the Magsaysay Avenue site is its microclimate. Although the buildings' overhangs, which span almost the entire sidewalk width, protect some vendors from the monsoon rains, they also create a tunnel effect. With concrete walls and sidewalks, as well as its west-facing orientation, this workplace can be very cold. Due to Baguio City's elevation of 5,000 feet above sea level, its temperatures during the cold months of December to February can go as low as 50°F (10°C). During these months, street vendors brace the extreme cold when they set up shop as early as 5 a.m. The cold and damp tunnel effect caused by the physical features of the area threatens the immune systems of vendors, which may make them vulnerable to colds, cough, and other ailments (Figure 21-2). The cold environment in the Magsaysay Avenue is hostile to street vendors who complain about arthritic problems as well.

Furthermore, air quality monitoring revealed that the Magsaysay Avenue site is one of the most polluted places in the CBD, especially during the afternoon rush hour. High traffic volume, idling vehicles that run on diesel fuel, and disrupted circulation flow as public vehicles drop off their passengers in undesignated spots, are responsible for the poor air quality in this street. Vendors suffer from asthma, intense headaches, and high blood pressure.

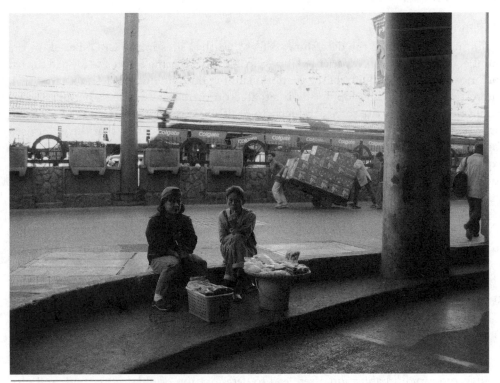

Figure 21-2 Cold and dark physical environments along Magsaysay Avenue.

Assumption Street Site

On the average, vendors got sick twice in 2003, the year the health survey was conducted. However, vendors located at Assumption Street claimed they were sick seven times that year. Among some of the health problems they experienced were colds, tightness in the chest, trouble breathing, and intense headaches. The air quality is very poor during the morning rush hour compared to other sites. An explanation to this is the fact that vendors are located along a steep one-way street leading to several elementary schools. Heavy morning traffic consists of diesel fuel vehicles idling on an incline. Such a substandard environment may be causing some of vendors' health problems.

The physical characteristics of the Assumption Street site may also contribute to the vendors' health conditions. For example, compared to the average curb height throughout sidewalks in the CBD, the site's sidewalk is very low. During the monsoon season (June through September), Baguio City gets an exorbitant amount of rainfall, which constantly rushes down the slopes of Assumption Street. Because of the sidewalk's low height, it is not unusual for rainwater to sweep into the vendors' locations. Furthermore, unlike the Magsaysay Avenue site that has an overhang extending the sidewalk's width, the Assumption site only has about half of the sidewalk covered. Vendors do not have adequate shelter from the rains.

Healthy Sites

Preliminary analysis of the data shows a few "healthy" sites in the CBD. Based on the number of times vendors experienced illness in 2003, the Kayang Street site topped the list for "most healthy," with 60% of the vendors claiming they did not get sick at all that year. Interestingly, this highly sloping site is situated on the central market's periphery. One would not expect the site to be conducive to healthiness, since the wet market is located right on this street. Sanitary conditions are questionable considering that the water used for cleaning the meat and fish products is drained next to individual vendor stalls. One explanation may be that "used water" never reach the vendor sites because they are surrounded with drainage holes. Another possible cause is that Kayang Street is not a through street but a location for public passenger vehicle parking, which explains its relatively low traffic volume.

The Harrison Street sites are other "healthy" sites based on their air quality. Compared to other sites with similar levels of traffic, these sites have some of the best air quality conditions. A major explanation for such good air quality is that the two sites on Harrison Street are adjacent to the main park in Baguio City. Burnham Park has about an acre green that stretches beside Harrison Street. With trees and good wind circulation, the negative impact of vehicle exhaust is lessened. See Figure 21-3 for a view of Harrison Street.

These descriptive examples give evidence to the link between environmental features and health conditions of street vendors in Baguio City. Even as environmental designers conceptualize urban spaces and do their best to create quality places, the processes of change and rapid urbanization often lead to deterioration of physical settings, and ulti-

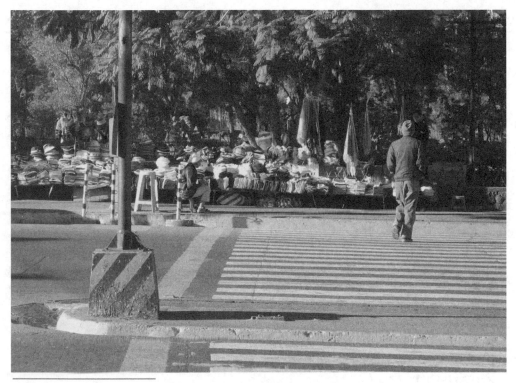

Figure 21-3   Harrison Street, adjacent to Burnham Park.

mately, poor health of its users. Unless the same space-makers monitor and evaluate their development projects, these places will continue to degrade. Therefore, it is essential that environmental designers propose continuous improvements to the urban places they build.

An Environmental Design Proposal to Address Health in Baguio City's Central Business District

One of the major problems of Baguio City's downtown is vehicular and pedestrian congestion. Although the conventional traffic engineering solution is to build highway bypasses around the urban core, a more sustainable approach is proposed here. To preserve the character of the city's center, highways should not be built inside in the CBD. These monstrous structures will increase the dark and cold tunnel effect in the urban spaces underneath. Cold, moist air and lack of sunlight will negatively affect, not only vendors' environments, but pedestrians, businesses, and other downtown users.

A transportation plan that decentralizes traffic volume should be conceptualized. A framework that encourages satellite service centers around the city will decrease the number of vehicles entering the urban core. Banks, professional offices, medical offices, etc., can relocate to disperse services around the city.

An important part of the environmental design plan is to "pedestrianize" several streets in the CBD. This move will decongest the sidewalks and encourage the use of urban spaces for more community-oriented activities (e.g., social, leisure, cultural, and arts) and active living, while increasing their economic vitality. Vibrant street life, which encourages walking, is a proven ingredient for successful, healthy, urban downtowns. Several Asian cities in India and Indonesia have closed major streets to accommodate pedestrians (Institute for Transportation and Development Policy, 2003). Evaluations of these planning strategies have yielded positive results. Businesses have increased their sales, air quality improves, users are more encouraged to stay in these places, crime decreases, and urban spaces are enlivened.

Lastly, to improve the health of street vendors and urban residents living, working, or visiting the CBD, a greening movement should be embarked upon. Restoring existing parks to better health as well as planting vegetation around the CBD are some of the ways to blend the natural environment with the physical structures typical of highly urbanized areas. Planting vegetation will improve the air quality and decrease the effects of the urban heat during the hot, summer months.

Conclusion

This chapter provides a case study that describes the relationship between the physical environment and health. As evident in our study of street vendors in Baguio City, Philippines, the characteristics of their workplaces are correlated with health problems. Working long hours in cold and damp places, flooded sites, crowded conditions, sloping streets, and highly polluted areas impacts the health of street vendors tremendously. Environmental designers, while having a significant role in mitigating these physical environments, have to collaborate with health professionals to ensure effective solutions.

References

Akers, M. A. A., Sowell, R., & Akers, T. (2004). A conceptual model for planning and designing healthy landscapes in the Third World: A study of street vendors in the Philippines. *Landscape Review, 9*(1).

Akers, M. A. A., & Akers, T. 2005. Urbanization, land use and health in Baguio City, Philippines. In G. Guest (Ed.), *Globalization, health, and the environment: An integrated perspective*. Lanham, MD: Altamira Press.

Asanza, A. L. (2003a). Extension of social protection in the Philippines. Manila: International Labour Organization. Retrieved April 25, 2003, from http://www.ilo.org/public/English/region/asro/manila/2003/mar/espp.htm

Asanza, A. L. (2003b, January–July). Health micro-insurance for the excluded: Women in the informal economy. *International Labour Organization Manila Newsletter, 2*(1). Retrieved October 15, 2006, from http://www.ilo.org/public/english/region/asro/manila/downloads/vol2i1.pdf

Arendt, R. G. (1996). *Conservation design for subdivisions: A practical guide to open space networks.* Washington DC: Island Press.

Armelagos, G. J., & Harper, K. (2005). Disease globalization in the third epidemiological transition. In G. Guest (Ed.), *Globalization, health, and the environment: An integrated perspective.* Lanham, MD: Altamira Press.

Baguio City Official Website. (2006). Retrieved October 1, 2006, from http://www.baguio.gov.ph/index.php?option=content&task=view&id=106

Bhowmik, S. K. (2005). Street vendors in asia: A review. *Economic and Political Weekly,* May 28–June 4.

Cascio, J. (2006, January 16). Deforestation and malaria. *World Changing.* Retrieved September 1, 2006, from http://www.worldchanging.com/archives/003997.html

Centers for Disease Control and Prevention (CDC). (n.d.). *Designing and building healthy places.* Retrieved August 11, 2007, from http://www.cdc.gov/healthyplaces

Chua, K. B., Chua, B. H., & Wang, C. W. (2002). Anthropogenic deforestation, El Nino and the emergence of Nipah virus in Malaysia. *Malaysian Journal of Pathology, 24*(1), 15–21. Retrieved September 1, 2006, from http://www.ncbi.nlm.nih.gov/entrez/query.fcgi?db=pubmed&cmd=Retrieve&dopt=AbstractPlus&list_uids=16329551&itool=iconabstr&query_hl=2&itool=pubmed_docsum

Eilperin, J. (2005, November 17). Climate shift tied to 150,000 fatalities. *The Washington Post.* Retrieved 1, 2006, from http://www.washingtonpost.com/wp-dyn/content/article/2005/11/16/AR2005111602197.html

EU project develops method to detect falls among the elderly. (2006, May 20) *Healthcare Mergers, Acquisitions & Ventures Weekly,* p. 72.

Hippocrates. (400 BCE). *On airs, waters, and places.* (F. Adams, Trans.). Retrieved August 11, 2007, from http://classics.mit.edu/Hippocrates/airwatpl.1.1.html

Indon, R. M. (2002). The Philippine urban informal sector. *Philippine Studies, 50*(1st qtr.).

Institute for Transportation and Development Policy. (2003). Pedestrianizing Asian cities. *Sustainable Transport,* 22–25. Retrieved November 10, 2006, from http://www.itdp.org/ST/ST15/ST15.pdf

International Labour Organization. (2002). *ILO compendium of official statistics on employment in the informal sector* (STAT Working Paper No. 1-2002). Retrieved October 1, 2006, from http://www-ilo-mirror.cornell.edu/public/english/bureau/stat/download/comp2a.pdf

Jackson, L. E. (2005). *The relationship of land-cover pattern to Lyme disease.* (Doctoral Dissertation, University of North Carolina, Chapel Hill).

Jacobs, J. (1961). *The death and life of great American cities.* New York: Vintage Books.

Koch, T. (2005). *Cartographies of disease: Maps, mapping, and medicine.* Redlands, California: ESRI Press.

Levy, J. M. (2000). *Contemporary urban planning* (5th ed.). Upper Saddle River, New Jersey: Prentice Hall.

Li, W., Keegan, T. H. M., Sternfeld, B., Sidney, S., Quesenberry, C. P., Jr., & Kelsey, J. L. (2006). Outdoor falls among middle-aged and older adults: A neglected public health problem. *American Journal of Public Health, 96*(7), 1192–1200.

Marcus, C. C., & Francis, C. (1998). *People places: Design guidelines for urban open space.* New York: John Wiley & Sons, Inc.

May, J. M. (1961). *Studies in disease ecology.* New York: Hafner Publishing. In T. Koch (Ed.), *Cartographies of disease: maps, mapping, and medicine.* Redlands: California: ESRI Press.

McCally, M. (Ed.). (2002). Environment, health, and risk. *Life support: The environment and human health* (pp. 1–14). Cambridge, Massachusetts: MIT Press.

New South Wales Department of Environment and Conservation. (2003). *Pathways of exposure to lead.* Retrieved October 3, 2006, from http://www.environment.nsw.gov.au/leadsafe/leadinf8.htm#soil

Nowak, D. J., McHale, P. J., Ibarra, M., Crane, D., Stevens, J. C., & Luley, C. J. (1998). Modeling the effects of urban vegetation on air pollution. In S. Gryning & N. Chaumerliac (Eds.), *Air pollution modeling and its application XII* (pp. 399–407). New York: Plenum Press. Retrieved August 11, 2007, from http://www.fs.fed.us/ne/syracuse/Pubs/Downloads/02_DN_etal_Compensatory.pdf

Patz, J., & Olson, S. (2006, April 11). Malaria risk and temperature: Influences from global climate change and local land use practices. *PNAS.* Retrieved September 1, 2006, from http://www.sage.wisc.edu/pubs/articles/M-Z/Patz/Patz+OlsonPNAS2006.pdf

Peterson, J. A. (1983). The impact of sanitary reform upon American urban planning. In D. A. Krueckberg (Ed.), *Introduction to planning history in the United States.* New Brunswick, NJ: Rutgers University Center for Urban Policy Research.

Philippine Department of Health. (2002). *Morbidity: Ten leading causes.* Retrieved September 20, 2006, from http://www.doh.gov.ph/data_stat/html/fhsis/morbidity_region.pdf

Reed, R. R. (1999). *City of pines: The origins of Baguio as a colonial hill station and regional capital* (2nd. ed.). Baguio City, Philippines: A-Seven Publishing.

Sharma, K., & Reutergardh, L. B. (2000). Exposure of preschoolers to lead in the Makati area of metro Manila, the Philippines. *Environmental Research Section A, 83,* 322–332.

Takano, T., Nakamura, K., & Watanabe, M. (2002). Urban residential environments and senior citizens' longevity in megacity areas: The importance of walkable green spaces. *Journal of Epidemiology and Community Health, 56,* 913–918.

Takehito, T. (Ed.). (2003). *Healthy cities and urban policy research.* London: Spon Press, Taylor and Francis Group.

United Nations. (2004). *World population prospects: The 2004 revision analytical report,* (Vol. 3). Washington DC: United Nations Department of Economic and Social Affairs, Population Division. Retrieved September 2, 2006, from http://www.un.org/esa/population/publications/WPP2004/WPP2004_Vol3_Final/Chapter1.pdf

United Nations. (2005). *World population prospects: 2005 revision, executive summary.* Washington DC: United Nations Department of Economic and Social Affairs, Population Division. Retrieved 2, 2006, from http://www.un.org/esa/population/publications/WUP2005/2005WUPHighlights_Exec_Sum.pdf

Wargo, J. (2004). *The physical school environment: An essential element of a health-promoting school.* Geneva, Switzerland: World Health Organization, Department of the Protection of the Human Environment.

World Health Organization. (2002a). *Regional burden of disease due to indoor air pollution.* Retrieved October 3, 2006, from http://www.who.int/indoorair/health_impacts/burden_regional/en/index.html

World Health Organization. (2002b). *World health report 2002: Reducing risks, promoting health life.* Geneva, Switzerland: WHO. Retrieved September 25, 2006, from http://www.who.int/globalchange/climate/summary/en/index.html

Chapter 22

Building Cultural Competence: A Nursing Practicum in Oaxaca, Mexico

David Bennett

Carol Holtz

The United States is experiencing the largest sustained immigration wave in its history with an estimated 44.3 million documented and undocumented immigrants arriving each year, the majority from Latin America. People of Latin American or Hispanic descent now compose 15% of the United States population. The US Census Bureau reports that Hispanics have surpassed African-Americans to become the largest minority group in the United States. By 2050 the number of Latino and persons of Hispanic descent could increase to 102.6 million or 24% of the US population. In late 2003, the state of Georgia reported having experienced one of the highest rates of recent Mexican immigrants of all of the United States. The Latino population in metropolitan Atlanta, Georgia, increased by 400% over the last decade. Traditionally the US healthcare system, both public and private, was designed to accommodate patients who were mainly Caucasian (European-American) or black (African-American). The immigration of Spanish-speaking healthcare consumers has challenged providers to structure a system with personnel who are culturally competent and have at least a functional understanding of the Spanish language (US Census Bureau, 2007).

With the goals of increasing the cultural competence and language skills of nursing students at Kennesaw State University (KSU) in 1995–1996, the faculty planned and implemented an intense 2-week nursing practicum in the capital city of the state of Oaxaca, Mexico (*wa-ha-ka*).

This program reflects both the mission of KSU and the WellStar School of Nursing to increase intercultural contacts, cultural competence, and global understanding for both faculty and students. The development and implementation of this experience and the outcomes experienced by participants will be described.

Need for Cultural Competence

Nursing as a profession has focused on the improvement of care delivery for clients of varying ethnicities, nationalities, and socioeconomic levels. Clients from cultures other than that of the nurse often do not fully benefit from nursing care due to miscommunication, misunderstanding, and potential conflicts of values, beliefs, norms, and mutually stereotypical attitudes. Comprehensive knowledge of the culture of the client is imperative in order to adequately assess, plan, implement, and evaluate nursing care (Leininger, 1978; Purnell & Paulanka, 2003; Spector, 2004). Cultural competence is an ongoing process of developing cultural awareness, knowledge, skill, and the opportunity for cultural encounters (Camphina-Bacote, 1994). Hall, Stevens and Meleis (1994) propose that the future of nursing depends on the ability to meet the needs of an increasingly diverse population. Self-awareness of personal prejudices, attitudes, and stereotypical perceptions is essential before one can learn about people of other cultures. Leininger (1978) proposed that it is not the client's responsibility to be understood, but the nurse's responsibility to understand and meet the clients' needs.

Impact of Study Abroad and Immersion Experiences on Cultural Competence

Although cultural competence can be achieved by working with clients of other cultures in the nurse's home country, many studies have shown that a deeper understanding of culture and language competence can be achieved by study-abroad programs that immerse students in the culture and language of the country. Lutterman-Aguilar and Gingerich (2002) reported that we are now living in a period of tremendous growth in study-abroad programs with an estimated 2 million American students studying abroad in 2000. These authors proposed that growth in study abroad has increased the sense of interconnectedness and globalization in unprecedented terms in the past 30 years. With the unprecedented wave of migration to US cities from countries around the world, the understanding achieved by study abroad is essential to absorption of immigrants and maintaining a functioning society. These programs not only provide exposure of students to different cultures, but they also give the student opportunities to experience the unique feeling of being a member of a minority in a different culture, in which the student communicates both verbally and nonverbally in a different language.

Language Acquisition and Increased Fluency

As demographics change, differing languages present a special challenge to care providers. Isabelli-Garcia (2000) documented improvement in Spanish fluency and communication skills of students who participated in a semester-long study abroad experience in Argentina. Isabelli-Garcia defined fluency in terms of the number of words used in a response, the number of pauses in the students' communication, and the number of times the students struggled when communicating in the language. The researcher found improvements in the levels of fluency of all students after a semester-long immersion experience. The KSU faculty believe that the requirement for preimmersion exposure to the language, the around-the-clock immersion for the 2-week period in Oaxaca, and the frequent use of Spanish language in clinical settings in Georgia all combine to improve student fluency and decrease the fear of communicating in another language, not to mention the overall outcomes of improving patient care and the building of trust.

Experiential Learning

Dewey (1997) proposed that experiences in study-abroad programs are not innately educational simply because they are conducted in another country. Dewey maintains that not all experiences have equal merit and that unless planned with purpose and supported by reflection, critical analysis, and synthesis, some experiences may actually result in negative learning instead of the desired outcomes. As Geary (1995) described, meaning is not inherently associated with experiences, rather, knowledge is socially constructed as students observe, reflect, and interpret the meanings of the experience to their own lives. Kolb (1984) observed that reflection and analysis are essential components of experiential education. The faculty members planning the KSU immersion experience determined that immersion alone was insufficient to achieve the desired outcomes of the experience. Time for discussion and reflection during the experience and reflection, synthesis, and analysis in the post-immersion period had to be intentionally planned into the course activities in order to foster the conversion of experience into knowledge. Faculty members must be able to promote reflection and group learning through group facilitation and individual journaling.

Affective learning occurs more efficiently when emotional connections are made with the content being studied. To promote connectedness, the faculty planned experiences to connect the student with people so the content of the course can come alive (Wallace, 1993). Wallace (1993) also proposed that having functioned successfully in a different environment can increase self-confidence, increase the awareness of personal strengths and weaknesses, and promote the knowledge of how to approach other human beings. KSU faculty members intentionally decided that living with Mexican families and having interactions with care givers from the Mexican culture would improve the affective and experiential learning of the students.

Problem-Based Learning

Dewey (1997) also found that experiential learning must relate to real-life problems. Student recognition of problems in their areas of interest can arouse curiosity and increase seeking of information and the analysis of the problem. The focus of problem-based learning is not just problem solving, but the critical analysis of a problem and reflection on the multitude of potential solutions. Therefore KSU faculty members decided to develop learning strategies that required students to identify a problem, research literature related to the problem, and perform critical analysis of the situation.

Achieving Praxis

Another consideration of the faculty member planning the nursing study-abroad program was the transfer of transcultural nursing theory and preexperience preparation in language, history, and culture into meaningful learning, both during and after the immersion experience. Rolfe (1996) defined *praxis* as an alternative to the traditional scientific paradigm that proposes that the purpose of nursing theory is to inform and direct practice. In the praxis paradigm, the relationship between formal theory and practice is much more complex and involves informal theory development achieved by the process of reflection and reliance on personal experience learned from paradigm patient cases. Personal knowledge drawn from paradigm cases in the nurse's individual repertoire is used to construct informal theory that influences actual practice. The process of reflection influences the development of this personal knowledge. Reflection-in-action involves a cyclical process of hypothesis testing and on-the-spot experimenting. Reflection-on-actions informs personal practice through a process of examining situations that have occurred with an eye toward improving practice in similar situations in the future. The processes of journaling and faculty mentoring are important to promote reflection as a means of understanding and achieving cultural competence. As a result, journaling, postexperience discussions, in-hospital faculty guidance, and postexperience reflection and problem solving were included in learning activities to encourage praxis.

Development of the Study-Abroad Practicum

The Setting

The state of Oaxaca is one of the most ethnically diverse states in Mexico, with a population of over four million inhabitants of a variety of indigenous ethnic groups, speaking primarily Spanish but also an estimated 30 other indigenous dialects. Oaxaca is one of the poorest states in Mexico; however, it is very rich in cultural diversity and history. Economic factors have resulted in the immigration (both legal and illegal) of young people from Oaxaca to the United States for work. These workers often come to the metropolitan Atlanta region to seek employment and live in large communities with other recent Latino immigrants. They seek health care in local hospitals, from private physicians, and from nurse-managed clinics.

The city of Oaxaca (currently now the capital of the state of Oaxaca) was founded in 1529 by Hernan Cortes and is an urban center of 400,000 inhabitants. The tapestry of languages, cultures, archaeological sites and colonial architecture makes the city ideal for a cultural immersion experience. The state of Oaxaca relies on tourism and agricultural production to support the population (Ewing, 1996).

Oaxaca is also an excellent setting for studying the healthcare system of Mexico and the healthcare practices of the population. Students often hold the assumption that health care is available to all, but find in Oaxaca that poor and rural populations are increasingly unable to compete for scarce health resources. In Oaxaca the maternal mortality rate is twice that of the national Mexican average. Health problems include the inability to access fresh, clean water; childhood malnutrition; and exposure to communicable diseases, which all contribute to common causes of morbidity and mortality. Mexico ranks second in Latin America in incidence of HIV/AIDS and 11th in the world. Air pollution is a major problem throughout the country resulting in chronic bronchitis, emphysema, asthma, lung cancer, and eye infections. Cholera and other gastrointestinal disorders resulting from poor sanitation and unclean water are particularly devastating to infants and children (Barry, 1992). Many employed workers carry private health insurance, but the majority of people receive their health care from the government's Pronasol program. Lustig (1992) states that the IMSS (Mexican Institute of Social Security), one of the national health insurance programs, has been strained by the inflationary economy. Infant and preschool mortality and morbidity have increased due to avitaminosis and other nutritional deficiencies (Lustig, 1992).

Several universities, schools of nursing, and medicine and language schools make Oaxaca a city with a large population of students. Although KSU students are reminded to maintain measures to protect personal security, Oaxaca remains a comparatively safe city for students. The healthcare infrastructure is welcoming to students and provides a rich diversity of primary, secondary, and tertiary care experiences with very diverse populations. KSU faculty members decided that these characteristics made Oaxaca an ideal site for a clinically based nursing study-abroad course.

Initial Connections

The initial process in developing the practice began by visiting the area to determine the feasibility of establishing a study-abroad nursing elective course. Contact with healthcare leaders in the city produced a dialogue on such topics as the expectations of the healthcare system, the objectives of the experience, how students would pay for the trip, and whether the students expected to be paid for their work. Other discussions included the facilities and experiences available and potential benefits to the healthcare system.

The KSU student nurses would primarily work in the central, public, acute-care hospital for indigent patients with Mexican nurse preceptors and a nearby pediatric hospital outside the city of Oaxaca. These facilities serve patients coming from distant, isolated regions of Oaxaca and also indigent city dwellers. The hospitals also serve as training facilities for local medical schools and nursing schools. Students would also participate in primary care experiences in the satellite health department clinics. In these settings, students could also make home visits with nurses and social workers and provide health education to children in local schools. The use of the mentor teams (KSU student nurses and local Oaxacan nurses) addressed a major concern of the faculty member and the healthcare leaders regarding the potential for errors when working in a healthcare system based in another culture and language. Students would work under the direct supervision of the

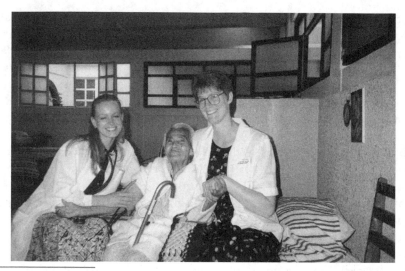

Figure 22-1 Kennesaw State University students working with elderly patients in Oaxaca, Mexico.

mentor nurse and would not administer medications or perform procedures except under the guidance and approval of the Oaxacan nurse.

Student housing was another challenge. The expectation was that in order to experience cultural immersion, the student should live with a local family that spoke only Spanish in the household. Only one student would be placed in each household to encourage interaction, integration into the family, and avoid the use of English between students while in the home. Arrangements for housing were facilitated through an existing link with a local housing coordinator who recruited and screened host families. The mothers of the host families usually take the lead in the care of the students and are paid for the room and board through the housing coordinator. To learn more about the Mexican family and culture, to improve Spanish conversational skills, and to understand what students were experiencing, the nursing faculty member elected to participate in the in-home experience and was assigned her own Oaxacan family.

Choosing appropriate field trips to archaeological sites and surrounding pueblos was necessary to increase student understanding of the socioeconomic conditions, history, and conflicts that formed the area culture. After visiting numerous sites, the faculty determined that the pre-Columbian archaeological sites of Monte Alban and Mitla were representative of the dominant indigenous cultures of the region, the Zapotec and Mixtec peoples. Inhabitants of the pueblos surrounding the capital city produce handmade items for sale in the city and for the export market. Profits supplement agricultural income and improve the standard of living in the pueblo dramatically. These experiences were planned for students as weekend excursions to augment other aspects of the practicum.

Spanish language classes to support the student's ability to interact in the hospitals and clinics are an essential component of the immersion experience. Noncredit classes were arranged at one of the many Spanish language schools in Oaxaca. Due to the diverse backgrounds and levels of Spanish proficiency, small groups of 3–4 students per local Spanish faculty member were planned. Nursing faculty members participated with a private tutor to increase their proficiency as well.

The travel arrangements, for a group of English-speaking study-abroad students going to a Spanish-speaking country, require additional coordination. To stay within a reasonable budget, an experienced travel agent and fairly definite numbers of participants are needed months in advance. Insurance for treatment and emergency evacuation in the case of accidents or illness was also obtained through sources already in use by other study-abroad programs. Other budget considerations for the program included local housing and meals, Spanish lessons, weekend cultural excursions, donations of medical supplies, a reception for the host families, and course tuition for a 3-semester credit course at KSU.

Academic Decisions in Course Development

The next step was to address the academic aspects designed to achieve course objectives. Strategically planned activities to encourage experiential learning, language-skill improvement, reflection, and problem-based learning were included. The course and learning strategies have evolved over the years; therefore, this discussion will focus on current course learning strategies and their details. The faculty divided the course planning into the three distinct stages of preimmersion, immersion, and postimmersion experiences aimed at increasing cultural competence with the general Latino population. Although the authors understand that the Latino culture is not a homogenous grouping of similar peoples, they believe that the knowledge gained from experiences in the Mexican culture is transferable to other Latino populations.

Preimmersion
The majority of the students participating in the program have never traveled abroad to another country. Orientation attendance is expected, and concerned parents and spouses are invited. All imaginable topics are covered in a discussion led by the nursing faculty members and reinforced in a comprehensive information guide. A series of articles regarding health issues among Latin Americans and the community in Oaxaca are placed on library reserve for course members. Students who are not bilingual are expected to complete a course provided on the KSU campus entitled Spanish for Health Professionals.

Learning Strategies for the Immersion and Postimmersion Phases
The grading criteria for the course include student participation in all course activities unless ill. This participative portion of the course is graded on a pass-fail basis. To promote reflection during the experience, each student is expected to keep a daily journal of his or her experiences in Oaxaca. Topics include their feelings, thoughts, and beliefs about

the Oaxacan community prior to the 2-week visit and comparisons to the realities encountered. Journals included individual daily experiences with healthcare delivery and nursing practice; observations on living with a family of a different culture; interactions with people within the community; and descriptions of sights, smells, sounds, and tastes encountered. As a learning strategy, students are encouraged to reflect on their feelings of being in a country with a different language and on both their positive and negative experiences in the culture. Students summarize this journal into a more formal, narrative paper accounting for 25% of the course grade. To allow additional reflection on the experience, analysis, and synthesis, the paper is submitted at the end of the summer semester, 8 weeks after the return from Oaxaca.

Additionally, to promote further reflection, analysis, synthesis, and problem-based learning, each student completes a formal research paper to be submitted at the end of the 8 weeks following the return from Oaxaca. Examples of topics chosen for this paper in the past include an in-depth exploration of a major health issue as identified by members of the Oaxacan community; an exploration of either the political, economic, or environmental influences of the health status of the Oaxacan community; and the application of transcultural nursing theory to give culturally congruent care to clients in the Oaxacan community or to Latino clients in Atlanta, Georgia. They are encouraged to submit their papers, and many present at a variety of professional meetings. The grade on this project represents the remaining 75% of the course grade.

Implementation of the Nursing Practicum in Oaxaca

Recruitment of Students

During the developmental phase of the study abroad program, the immediate challenge was the recruitment of at least 10 students for the program in the beginning of the new academic year. Photos of Oaxaca, the families, housing, the clinics, and the cultural sites were circulated among interested students, and students were invited to ask questions about the new course. The course was approved by all curriculum committees, and the initial class quickly filled with 13 students.

Orientation sessions were carefully planned and a detailed handout developed to give to students and interested family members. Topics included personal safety needs; documents, money, and packing needs; special health needs; housing; transportation; working in the clinics or hospitals; Spanish tutoring sessions; clinical conferences; cultural excursions; shopping; and perhaps most valuable of all, information about cultural sensitivity and appropriate dress and behavior. Oaxacan culture is more formal in dress and behavior than the US culture, and students needed this information and more to avoid cultural misunderstandings. Sessions lasted for about 2 hours and students, parents, and spouses were encouraged to ask questions. Many were very concerned about health and safety needs while others wanted to know more about the public health clinics and hospitals, the topics for the research paper, and the housing arrangements. Potential scholarship resources were also addressed.

Students and Faculty

During the past 11 years more than 100 students have taken this course. The average group size is about 13 students. Although the majority of the students are from KSU, others have participated from different nursing programs within Georgia, as well from nursing programs in other states. Other participants include recent KSU nursing graduates and nurses in the community who audit the course and receive no academic credit. Several premed, medical students, and human services students have also participated in the course with alterations in the clinical practice portions and daily activities based on levels of expertise and interests.

Medical Supplies and Equipment Donations

Faculty members planning the program noted that at times medical supplies and equipment were not available in clinics or on acute care units. To thank the Oaxacan host physicians and nurses and augment patient care, the faculty decided to include donations of healthcare materials as a part of the program activities. The collection of supplies and equipment to donate to the Oaxacan healthcare system was achieved by solicitation of donations and funded by a portion of student course tuitions. All supplies are packed in small boxes and students check them with their luggage.

Student Housing

Each student is placed with a family who provides a private bedroom and three meals a day. The families greet the students at the airport to take them to their Oaxacan homes. This transition can be stressful because suddenly the students are alone with their new families, expected to communicate in Spanish, and exposed to the crowded streets of Oaxaca City. Families are carefully screened by the Oaxaca housing coordinator and treat students like members of their own family, showing much concern about their whereabouts and offering affection and attention. Students often participate in host family activities such as attending church services, family outings, and family get-togethers. Families are warm and welcoming, but the first few days in this new environment can be stressful and students find that they tire easily.

The experiences of living with an Oaxacan family are a vivid contrast to the everyday life experiences for the students at home. Most students are in their late twenties to mid-thirties and are parents. They pay their own tuition, living expenses, often hold a part-time job, balance a busy schedule, and are full-time parents and spouses. In contrast, while living with a family in Oaxaca, they become dependent "child-adults." The families provide them their own bedroom in their houses, prepare their meals using local foods, care for them, and protect them. This experience can be disconcerting but comfortable to the more independent student. Students enjoy gathering for lunch and the afternoon nap—a family ritual "siesta" that is very much part of the whole local culture of Oaxaca. Family members often return home for lunch, and all shops, businesses, and schools in the city close from 1:30 p.m. for up to 2 hours. Students often make comparisons to this tradition and the hectic lifestyle they experience in the United States.

Spanish Lessons

Although some students are proficient in Spanish, most have taken at least a medical Spanish course as a minimum background, and others have had additional courses or previous use of Spanish in clinical settings with patients. While in Oaxaca, students receive a 1-hour, daily conversational Spanish tutoring session with a Spanish professor from the University of Oaxaca's *Centro de Idiomas* language school. The student-faculty ratio is usually four students to one professor.

Few of the inhabitants in Oaxaca speak English, so students find it necessary to speak Spanish for all daily activities to the family members in the homes where they live; to the nurses, doctors, and patients in the clinics; and to others in the community such as the taxi drivers, waiters and waitresses in the restaurants, shop owners, and street vendors. Most students speak Spanish all day long, every day, and become more relaxed and fluent. As one can imagine, misunderstandings and *faux pas* occur, but the Oaxacan population is used to tourists and non-Spanish speakers and is usually very forgiving of mistakes.

The Oaxacan Healthcare System

Students find the Oaxacan healthcare system and workers to be welcoming and enthusiastic in providing them with interesting clinical experiences. Students with a better com-

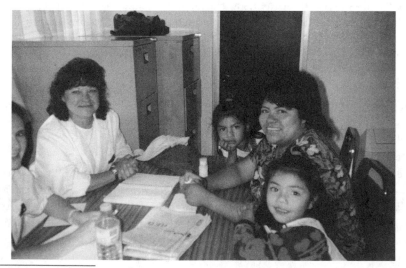

Figure 22-2 Kennesaw State University students teaching patients in a health clinic in Oaxaca, Mexico.

mand of the Spanish language and assertive personalities tend to have more rewarding experiences. Students bond with Oaxacan nurses, nursing students, physicians, and medical students. The exchange of cultural information and language lessons in English and Spanish make the bonds even stronger. Students are placed throughout the hospital with nurse mentors on each clinical unit, and faculty members circulate throughout the hospital, translating if necessary and facilitating the experience. Pairing the student with Mexican nurses eliminates much of the potential for errors in patient care. Students are involved with the Oaxacan nurses in the preparation of medications, the performance of procedures, and the activities of daily living of the patients. Students are required to spend 1 week at the central city hospital and another week at a local village pediatric specialty hospital. The majority of patients at both of these hospitals are indigent.

Student Outcomes

The outcomes students have achieved in this study-abroad practicum have been diverse, rewarding, and have affected practice patterns on return to the United States. Students have gained knowledge in a variety of healthcare issues affecting Latino immigrants, improved their Spanish language skills, developed an appreciation of the similarities and differences of cultures, and improved in their abilities to provide culturally competent care.

A review of the topics chosen by students for their analysis and synthesis papers reveals the wide range of learning that has occurred. Some examples of paper or project topics include the following:

- The Incidence of Neural Tube Defects Among Hispanics and Its Implication for Nursing Care
- Some Major Health Issues in the Oaxacan Community
- The Provision of Health Care in Mexico
- A Comparison of the Mexican and US Healthcare Systems
- Embracing Transcultural Nursing Theory Experientially
- The Problem of Dehydration of Patients in Mexico
- How the Government and Economy Affect the Quality and Availability of Healthcare in Mexico
- The Practice of Transcultural Nursing Theory in Community Care for the Oaxacan Client
- Giger and Davidhizar's Transcultural Nursing Theory Applied to Mexican Culture

Several students have presented to their *Sigma Theta Tau* (nursing honor society) chapters or the Transcultural Nursing Society. Other students presented their experiences in other nursing classes, while a few have had their papers published in refereed nursing journals. Some students have been invited to present their work at statewide study-abroad meetings sponsored by the Georgia Board of Regents.

Student Course Evaluations

Perhaps most revealing of the impact of the course on student participants are course evaluations. When asked, "What did you learn from your nursing practice in this setting?" the following responses are representative of the majority of evaluations. One student responded, "It gave me a better appreciation for the culture, the importance of family unity, and increased my language skills." Another stated, "I was impressed with what the nurses and doctors accomplished with so little supplies and materials. They were resourceful and careful. My experience in Oaxaca was very helpful to me with my nursing practice at home in Atlanta. I am better able to relate and care for my Hispanic patients." One student who is currently a labor and delivery nurse at a large urban hospital in Atlanta wrote, "This course was definitely a peak life experience for me. I have felt very drawn to Hispanic people since I have worked at my hospital. This experience, being immersed in the culture, working with nurses, mothers, and children in Mexico, living with a Hispanic family, was an opportunity to see inside a world that is rarely opened to outsiders or tourists. I am very grateful to have had this course." Another student made the following comment, "I believe that I'm more knowledgeable about the Mexican culture, especially related to health care, as well as the language and medical care. With this knowledge I have been better equipped to plan and administer care that is individualized for the Mexican population I come in contact with every day in my practice here in Georgia. I consider this course to be the best I ever had. I learned so much besides nursing: I learned about politics, economics, the Spanish language, music and art, archeology, history, etc."

Lessons Learned

Many lessons were learned from setting up this nursing elective program in Oaxaca, Mexico. First, it is imperative to have university support. The university must see the need for the program and be willing to invest time and money for faculty to go to the area and meet with local health officials, set up a housing program, review the clinical sites, and learn about the local culture, customs, and special cultural sites to visit. All faculty must be able to speak at least a functional level of Spanish and have a basic appreciation of what it is like to live, work, and study in a developing country with different customs, food, language, health issues, and cultural behaviors. Health insurance for local care for faculty and students is necessary as well as insurance for possible evacuation to the United States. Checking with the Mexican embassy or consulate is necessary beforehand when bringing in valuable supplies through customs into Mexico. Transportation, transferring planes, immigration, and customs issues with a group of students, some of whom may never have traveled before, are among the many issues that must be considered. Preparation for phys-

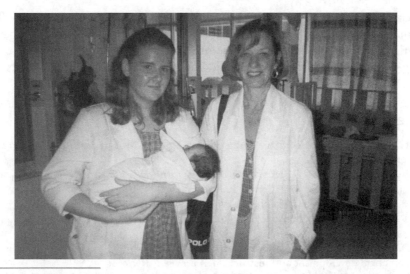

Figure 22-3 Dr. Carol Holtz with a student nurse from Kennesaw State University, caring for a pediatric patient in a municipal hospital in Oaxaca, Mexico.

ical safety; potential loss of passport, money, and plane tickets; and illness must be planned for well ahead of the trip with students. Even with the best of intentions of both Americans and Mexicans, problems will occur in language and cultural interpretation, and each experience is a lesson learned. Finally, the willingness of the Mexican healthcare administrators to tolerate placement of students with varying levels of Spanish proficiency in their hospitals and clinics is a humbling and eye-opening experience. Extensive orientation to the hospital, careful pairing of students with compatible nurses and, in some cases, placing a student with limited Spanish skills with a student with a higher level of proficiency increases the potential for successful placements. The nurses, physicians, medical students, and nursing students of Oaxaca are overwhelmingly welcoming, willing to teach, and eager to communicate. One has to ask if under similar circumstances would the American healthcare system be as welcoming?

Conclusion

The process of developing and implementing the Oaxacan study-abroad nursing program has been a challenge, especially since a new health secretary for the state is appointed every 3 years. Each year things have been slightly different, and new challenges have been encountered under varying healthcare administrators in Oaxaca.

The nursing practicum in Oaxaca is a valuable and rich learning adventure for faculty as well as students. Much preparation is necessary in order for this to be a safe and beneficial learning experience. Every aspect must be thoroughly planned, and all partici-pants must reasonably expect the unplanned and unknown to still occur. In general, the student's cultural competence has been enhanced after the experience of attending the nursing practicum in Oaxaca, Mexico, and both students and faculty are better prepared to work with Latino and Hispanic clients in their own local community.

References

Barry, T. (1992). Mexico: A country guide. Albuquerque, NM: The Inter-Hemisphere Resource Center.

Camphina-Bacote, J. (1994). *The process of cultural competence in health care: A culturally competent model of car* (2nd ed.). Wyoming, OH: Perfect Printing Press.

Dewey, J. (1997). *Experience and education.* New York: Simon and Schuster.

Ewing, R. (1996). *Six faces of Mexico: History, people, geography, government, economy, literature and art.* Tucson, AZ: The Arizona Board of Regents.

Geary, D. C. (1995). Reflections of evolution and culture in children's cognition: Implications for mathematical development and instruction. *American Psychologist, 50,* 24–37.

Hall, J. M., Stevens, P. E., & Meleis, A. I. (1994). Marginalization: A guiding concept for valuing diver-sity in nursing knowledge development. *Advances in Nursing Science, 16*(4), 32–41.

Isabelli-Garcia, C. L. (2000). Development of oral communication skills abroad. *Journal of Studies in International Education, 4*(1), 149–169.

Kolb, D. A. (1984). *Experiential learning as the source of learning and development.* Englewood Cliffs, NJ: Prentice Hall.

Leininger, M. (1978). *Transcultural nursing: Concepts, theories, and practices.* New York: John Wiley & Sons.

Lustig, L. (1992). *Mexico: The making of an economy.* Washington, DC: Brookings Institution.

Lutterman-Aguilar, A. & Gingerich, O. (2002). Experiential pedagogy for study abroad: Educating for global citizenship. *Frontiers: The Interdisciplinary Journal of Study Abroad.* Retrieved January 27, 2007, from http://frontiersjournal.com/issues/vol8/vl8_07_luttermanaguilargingerich.pdf

Purnell, L. D. & Paulanka, B. J. (Eds.). (2003). *Transcultural health care: A cultural competent approach.* Philadelphia: F.A. Davis.

Rolfe, G. (1996). *Closing the theory-practice gap: A new paradigm for nursing.* Oxford, UK: Butterworth Heinemann.

Spector, R. (2004). *Cultural diversity in health and illness.* (6th ed.). Norwalk, CT: Appleton & Lange.

US Census Bureau. (2007). *Hispanic population of the United States.* Retrieved August 11, 2007, from http://www.census.gov/population/www/socdemo/hispanic.html

Wallace, J. A. (1993) Educational values of experiential education. In T. Gochenout (Ed.), *Beyond experience: An experiential approach to cross-cultural Education* (2nd ed.). Yarmouth, ME: Intercultural Press.

Index